NURSING CARE PLANS

*Nursing Diagnosis
and Intervention*

NURSING CARE PLANS

Nursing Diagnosis and Intervention

Meg Gulanick, PhD, RN
Assistant Professor
Niehoff School of Nursing
Loyola University of Chicago
Loyola University Medical Center
Chicago, Illinois

Audrey Klopp, PhD, RN, ET
Director, Medical-Surgical Nursing
Clinical Specialist
Michael Reese Hospital and Medical Center
Chicago, Illinois

Susan Galanes, MS, RN, CCRN
Clinical Nurse Specialist
Suburban Lung Associates
Elk Grove Village, Illinois

Deidra Gradishar, BS, RN
Obstetric Outreach Educator
University of Chicago Perinatal Network
Chicago, Illinois

Michele Knoll Puzas, MHPE, RN,C
Pediatric Nurse Clinician
Michael Reese Hospital and Medical Center
Chicago, Illinois

Third Edition

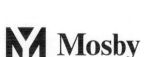 Mosby

St. Louis Baltimore Boston Chicago London Madrid Philadelphia Sydney Toronto

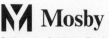 **Mosby**

Dedicated to Publishing Excellence

Publisher: Alison Miller
Editor: Timothy M. Griswold
Developmental Editor: Kathy Sartori
Project Manager: Mark Spann
Designer: David Zielinski

Printed in the United States of America
Composition by The Clarinda Company
Printing/binding by Von Hoffmann Press

Mosby—Year Book, Inc.
11830 Westline Industrial Drive
St. Louis, Missouri 63146

0-8016-7745-9

94 95 96 97 98 CL / VH 9 8 7 6 5 4 3 2 1

Contributors

Sherry Adams, RN, ADN

Cynthia Antonio, RN, BSN

Linda Arsenault, RN, MSN, CNRN

Lou Ann Ary, RN, BSN

Kathryn S. Bronstein, RN, PhD, CS

Catherine Brown, RN, MSN

Ursula Brozek, RN, MSN

Marian D. Cachero-Salavrakos, RN, BSN

Mary Leslie Caldwell, RN

Jan Colip, RN, MSN, CCRN

Eileen Collins, MSN, RN, PhD Candidate

Carol Clark, RN

Sue A. Connaughton RN, MSN, Psy.D Candidate

Adrian Cooney, RN, BSN

Margaret A Cunningham, RN, MS

Maria Dacanay, RN

Martha Dickerson, RN, MS, CCRN

Susan Eby, MS, PT

Linda Ehrlish, RN, MSN

Sandra Eungard, RN, MS

Ann Filipski, RN, MSN, CS, Psy.D Candidate

Sharon Fulcus, RN, BSN

Victoria Frazier-Jones, RN, BSN

Susan Galanes, RN, MS, CCRN

Barbara Gallagher, RN, BSN

Susan Geoghegan, RN, BSN

Margaret Gleason, RN, BSN

Cynthia Gordon, RN, BSN

Deidra Gradishar, RNC, BS

Kathleen Grady, RN, PhD

Meg Gulanick, RN, PhD

Frankie Harper, RN

Lorraine M. Heaney, RN

Jean M. Hughes, RN

Florencia Isidro-Sanchez, RN, BSN

Kathleen Jaffrey, RN

Vivian Jones, RN

Linda Kamenjarin, RN, BSN, CCRN

Maureen Kangleon, RN

Carol Keeler, RN, MSN

Audrey Klopp, RN. PhD, ET

Susan R. Laub, RN, MEd, CS

Deborah Lazzara, RN, MS, CCRN

Evelyn Lyons, RN, BSN

Donna MacDonald, RN, BS, CCRN

Marilyn Magafas, RNC, BSN, MBA

Beth Manglal-Lan, RN, BSN

Sheri Martucci, RN, MSN

Mary T. McCarthy, RN, MSN, CS

Doris M. McNear, RN, MSN

Encarnacion Mendoza, RN, BSN

Anita D. Morris, RN

Carol Nawrocki, RN, BSN

Charlotte Niznik, RN, MSN, CDE

Margaret Norton, RN, MSN

Mary O'Leary, RN, BSN

Rachel Ongsansoy, RN, BSN

Anne Paglinawan, RN, BSN

Lumie I. Perez, RN, BSN, CCRN

Gina Marie Petruzzelli, RN, BSN

Susan Pische, RN, BSN, MBA

Judith Popovich, RN, PhD

Michele Knoll Puzas, RN,C MHPE

Eileen Raebig, RN,C

Charlotte Razvi, RN, MSN, PhD

Dorothy Rhodes, RN

Linda Rosen-Walsh, RN, BSN

Rosaline L. Roxas, RN

Carol Ruback, RN, MSN, CCRN

Nancy Ruppman, RN, BSN, CURN

Marilyn Samson-Hinton, RN, BSN

Caroline Sarmiento, RN, BSN

Christa M. Schroeder, RN, MSN

Nedra Skale, RN, MS, CNA

Gail Smith-Jaros, RN, MSN

Nancy Staples, RN, BSN

Preface

Entering the 1990s, the nursing profession faced a tremendous challenge to provide quality patient care admist intensive cost containment efforts. Today, with health care reform on the horizon, and an ever-increasing emphasis on continous quality improvement, the new challenge demands that nurses be creative and efficient in planning for their patients' needs. In addition, nurses will be called upon as never before to assume more and more responsibility for providing America's health care. The comprehensive care plan guides in this book can serve as reference standards from which nurses can individualize patient care and improve not only the efficiency but also the quality of care.

Michael Reese Hospital and Medical Center's Department of Nursing has been a leader in the development of such care plan guides since publication of its *Comprehensive Nursing Care Plan Guidebook* in 1984. That initial book contained 75 guides, and attracted the attention of the C.V. Mosby Co. which subsequently published the first and second editions of *Nursing Care Plans: Nursing Diagnosis and Intervention*. These nationally acclaimed books were larger compilations of care plans for the clinical problems and treatments most widely encountered at major teaching hospitals. The editors of those earlier editions now proudly present an even more comprehensive edition, which includes additional "state-of-the-art" care plan guides, while recognizing the trend toward increased acuity in the inpatient setting.

The inclusion of both nursing diagnoses and medical problems continues to be an important feature of this book. Chapter One, the core of the book, specifically addresses 52 NANDA-approved nursing diagnoses, including some newly-recognized diagnoses such as high risk for aspiration, health seeking behaviors, caregiver role strain, and high risk for infection. This chapter allows a "pure" approach to nursing diagnosis and ensures that any patient care issue can be addressed. Wherever appropriate, Agency For Health Care Policy & Research recommendations have been incorporated into these care plans (pain, incontinence, skin integrity). The subsequent chapters are organized by body system or clinical specialty and include the latest trends in nursing and medical practice. Each body system/clinical specialty includes updated or completely new guides reflective of current trends and practices. Examples are automatic implantable defibrillator, lung cancer, radical neck surgery, breast cancer, laparoscopic abdominal surgery, peripheral stem cell transplant, ovarian cancer, and surgical closure of pressure sores.

This third edition also contains an expanded Neurology chapter, consolidated Gastrointestinal chapter, and Hematology plans reflective of higher acuity problems such as aplastic anemia, hemophilia, and sickle cell pain crisis.

To assist the reader in planning truly comprehensive care, one care plan may include references to several other related care plan guides. In addition, the table of contents is newly organized, to ease location of the needed care plans.

The most requested and useful update in this edition is the expansion of rationales given for most interventions and for many assessments. These explanations serve as helpful teaching aids, and may eliminate the need for an additional reference book. The intervention section includes "Ongoing" as well as initial nursing assessment. In addition, Ongoing Assessment and Therapeutic Interventions are highlighted with symbols defining their collaborative or independent nature. This important feature increases the reader's awareness of collaborative management and clearly defines when it is used. "Potential Problems" have been reworked to conform to NANDA's "high risk for" terminology, and risk factors for high-risk problems are included. This format change will assist all nurses, but especially those involved in preventative health education/management. Expanded definitions for both nursing and medical diagnoses are included and both related factors and defining characteristics are listed under each diagnosis.

A concerted effort was made to maintain a strict separation of the components of the nursing process. Ongoing assessments and defining characteristics are clearly separated from therapeutic interventions and expected outcomes, which have been written to be more measurable. Likewise, defining characteristics are separated from related factors.

The changes made to this book's format and content aid both the student and practitioner in deriving the appropriate nursing diagnoses and formulating a complete plan of care collaboratively and independently.

Nursing Care Plans reflects the evolution of nursing practice and nursing diagnosis. The care plan guides simultaneously incorporate both independent and collaborative nursing interventions according to priority need, depicting nursing practice in the "real world." Nurses of all levels of expertise will find this book helpful. Its content serves as a self-contained teaching guide and source of support for the novice nurse, while serving as a review or organizational tool for the experienced nurse.

Reflecting the clinical expertise of hundreds of nurses, this clinical reference is truly a one-of-a-kind book developed *by* nurses, *for* nurses.

ACKNOWLEDGMENTS

This book could not have been written without the support and contributions of many people. A special thanks goes to the talented nurse authors who shared their clinical expertise with us. We also wish to acknowledge our Nurse Specialist colleagues who provided the necessary encouragement and assistance to see this project to fruition. And finally, we are forever grateful to Emma Glover and Rosalie Clay for their quality work in preparing the manuscript materials for this book.

Meg Gulanick   Susan Galanes   Michele Knoll Puzas
Audrey Klopp   Deidre Gradishar

Contents

How to Individualize
Nursing Care Plans

Nursing is defined as the diagnosis and treatment of human responses to actual or potential health problems. Gordon defines a nursing diagnosis as "an actual or potential health problem which a nurse, by education and experience, is capable and licensed to treat." Inherent in these definitions is the nurse's ability to identify actual or potential problems, and to identify methods of assisting the patient to a resolution of those problems.

Nurses care for large numbers of patients, many or all of whom have complex care needs. Some nursing activities are independent interventions, such as teaching and comfort measures. The nursing process (assessment, diagnosis, planning, implementation, and evaluation) is the organizing framework for these activities. Other activities represent interdependent activities, in which nurses carry out the physician's plan of care and address the patient's response to those interventions. Medication administration is an example of an interdependent activity. Both independent and interdependent activities take place in a complex health care environment, where nurses function as coordinators, arranging the various aspects of health care delivery in a way which best meets patients' needs. Tremendous amounts of information for large numbers of patients must be available to the nurse in a concise, well-organized format.

While nursing diagnosis is clearly an exciting development for nursing, nurses at the bedside are often acutely reminded that the state-of-the-nursing-diagnosis-art is still very much a state of becoming. Most research related to nursing diagnosis has addressed only the label, etiologic factors, and defining characteristics; the interventional strategies have begun to be formally organized, but are largely unresearched. This situation leaves the bedside nurse with a label (or diagnosis), possible related factors, and defining characteristics, but without the plan of care related to the diagnoses which pertain to the patient's needs. The nursing care plan guides in this book have recognized both the independent and interdependent role of the nurse, have clustered groups of nursing diagnoses in such a manner as to facilitate the nurse's coordinative role in today's complex health care environment, and provide structure and substance for the complex set of behaviors known as the nursing process. Most importantly, these nursing care plan guides assist the nurse in planning comprehensive, individualized care.

COMPONENTS OF THE CARE PLAN

Each care plan guide throughout this book includes the following information: actual nursing diagnoses, related factors and defining characteristics, or diagnoses for which the patient is at risk, with risk factors. All nursing care plan guides include assessments, interventions, and measurable expected outcomes.

NURSING DIAGNOSIS

The nursing diagnosis is the summary judgment which the professional nurse makes about the data gathered during the nursing assessment. Almost all nursing diagnoses used throughout this book have been approved by NANDA (North American Nursing Diagnosis Association, an organization charged with the responsibility of classifying and developing nursing diagnoses) and are expressed in NANDA's nomenclature. This standardization assists nurses in developing a common language to improve professional communication. However, some original diagnostic labels have been incorporated into the care plan guides formulated for medical diagnoses at the discretion of the clinical nurse. Definitions of the NANDA diagnoses are included with each care plan guide in Chapter One. Some definitions were developed by NANDA; others were created by the clinical nurse authors based on review of the literature and their clinical expertise.

RELATED FACTORS/RISK FACTORS

Before developing a treatment plan for a nursing diagnosis, an evaluation must be made of those factors thought to be related to or the probable cause of the problem. Such factors may be physical, psychological, environmental, social, or spiritual. Each diagnosis in this book lists several contributing or risk factors which may be related to the diagnosis. These factors serve to direct the selection of subsequent nursing interventions.

DEFINING CHARACTERISTICS

Each actual nursing diagnosis in this book lists observable signs and symptoms that are usually present when the health problem exists; these descriptive signs are known as the defining characteristics for that diagnosis. Some characteristics are quite specific, must be present before a diagnosis can be made, and are considered critical data. Other characteristics are less precise, appear in several diagnoses, and are considered supportive data. The defining characteristics are gathered during the nursing assessment. A valid diagnosis must be based on actual assessment, not assumptions, regarding defining characteristics. Accuracy of a diagnosis can be verified by comparing the assessed defining characteristics with those listed for the standard care plan.

The defining characteristics in this book are a representative, though not an exhaustive listing of the common characteristics associated with a nursing problem. Many of the identified characteristics were modified from NANDA's listing for each diagnosis.

EXPECTED OUTCOME

Expected outcomes are concise statements that should identify a specific, observable, realistic and measurable goal. All expected outcomes in this edition have been written in present tense (e.g. the patient demonstrates) with observable, measurable language (e.g., the patient demonstrates dressing change using aseptic technique).

Expected outcomes must be evaluated within a specific time frame to assist in determining whether the plan of care needs revision or resolution. Because of the individuality and complexities of patient care, no standard time frames were identified in these guides. The readers will have to make this adaptation based on professional judgment.

NURSING INTERVENTIONS

Nursing interventions are those actions or prescriptions that assist in meeting the defined goal or outcome. They include two components of the nursing process: assessments and planned interventions. The *ongoing assessments* listed for each diagnosis are related to the defining characteristics or risk factors. Because the presence of a specific cluster of characteristics represents an actual problem, ongoing assessments are needed both to validate actual presence of the problem and to measure or document progress in treating or alleviating the problem. *Therapeutic interventions* are those measures required to accomplish the desired outcome. Since these are orders, they begin with a verb and clearly direct the nurses' actions and each is denoted with a symbol indicating whether the nurse performs the function collaboratively or independently. The ongoing assessments also have this feature. They include actual nursing therapies, documentation of actions and results, and consultation and communication with other health professionals.

Most interventions reflect treatments that nurses can perform independently. However, the editors did include collaborative (interdependent) practice measures commonly observed in practice (e.g. monitoring diagnostic and laboratory tests, administering medications and oxygen, providing care according to critical care protocols). Many of these therapeutic interventions reflect changing national trends in nurses' professional responsibilities, and, in some practice areas, nurses already perform them independently. This is nursing practice in the "real world". There were also times when it was more difficult to clearly designate an intervention as independent vs. collaborative (e.g., "anticipating/preparing for procedures or surgery, referring patients to pastoral care, notifying physicians of abnormalities). Decisions were made depending on the intent of the intervention, the severity of the situation, and the setting in which it was occuring.

Not every suggested intervention is appropriate for all patients throughout their hospitalization or illness. A broad range of nursing actions are presented here to provide the practitioner with options when adapting the care plan to specific patient needs. As a patient's condition changes, some of the interventions for a specific nursing diagnosis will assume higher priority than others. For example, during the acute phase of "Ineffective Breathing Pattern", immediate physical therapies supercede follow-up care concerns.

The nursing intervention section also includes patient education. These actions are presented in several different formats throughout the book. In the generic nursing diagnosis section in Chapter One, patient education interventions are listed in a separate section. In the chapters which contain medical diagnoses and procedures, some teaching interventions are included in many of the subcategories of nursing diagnoses found in that standard care plan; most have been significantly expanded.

RATIONALES

Rationales are incorporated into most nursing interventions to explain the purpose for or necessity of particular nursing actions; these rationales serve as learning tools for both the novice and experienced practitioner. Inclusion of such rationale may eliminate the need for an additional reference book.

GENERAL VS. SPECIFIC CARE PLAN GUIDES

Chapter One includes general, comprehensive care plan guides for the NANDA-approved nursing diagnoses most commonly used in clinical practice. These guides provide a framework for designing an individual patient's care plan. Patients may present with one or several nursing diagnoses; careful initial nursing assessment is required for selection of the most appropriate diagnoses. The nursing interventions for these general care plan guides are comprehensive, reflecting several approaches to treating the health problem. Not all interventions may be appropriate for a specific patient. An extensive listing of possible related or risk factors is provided to direct selection of appropriate nursing activities.

Although these general guides allow almost any patient care issue to be addressed, our nurse authors identified the need to develop additional guides for those medical problems and treatments most commonly encountered in their daily practices. While recognizing that all patients are individuals with unique health needs, most patients do share common concerns and problems. These specific care plans focus on similarity among patients, and their use can therefore optimize efficient delivery of nursing care. These guides include clustering of the common nursing diagnoses most frequently assessed with each medical problem.

In these guides, nursing diagnoses are presented according to priority needs. For example, airway problems or pre-op teaching needs tend to be first. Actual problems are presented before "high-risk for" problems; discharge teaching and planning concerns are usually addressed last. Since the nursing diagnosis is now related to a more specific etiology, the nursing interventions are more specific and concise. For example, interventions for decreased cardiac output related to pacemaker failure include many interventions not found in the general decreased cardiac output care plan guide in Chapter One. Many care plans also contain procedural interventions (e.g., complex cardiac care plans) to assist the novice nurse in providing optimal care. When appropriate, references to other pertinent care plans are made within a specific care plan to assist the nurse in providing truly comprehensive care.

USE OF THE CARE PLAN GUIDES

These care plans were written to be used both as guides for nursing practice and as tools to assist nurses and institutions in meeting J.C.A.H.O., state and local requirements. While expectations that individualized plans of care be developed and used for each patient exist, other responsibilities and time constraints often limit care planning efforts.

There are a variety of ways in which *Nursing Care Plans* can be utilized both individually by nurses and collectively by institutions; uses include clinical practice, teaching/education, quality improvement, and research. On the clinical units, standardized care plans can be used to write a plan of care for a particular patient, or they can serve as a guide to the care of a patient population in general. Nurses can use the care plan guides as quick references, especially when caring for new or infrequently encountered types of patients. Using these care plans increases efficiency by allowing nurses to spend their scarce time individualizing and adapting care plans rather than creating new ones. High-lighting applicable information, lining out inappropriate information, or writing in parameters and dates particular to one patient are quick methods of individualization.

The care plan guides in this book are educational tools; each guide encapsulates the plan of care in a logical, rational manner. Establishing the information contained in the care plan guides as standards on a particular unit or for a specific population of patients allows for assessment of staff learning needs, and may be used with students, new staff members, and other health care team members as instructional guides to patient care. The guides can also be used to evaluate individual nursing practice or to address deficiencies noted in nursing care following quality assurance activities.

These care plan guides are also unique quality improvement tools. Quality improvement activities are based on locally, regionally, and nationally accepted standards of care and practice; this collection of care plan guides reflects the expertise of hundreds of practicing staff nurses as well as nationally recognized advanced practice nurses who served as resources in the development of these guides. Individual guides can be used to identify and define standards, so that nurses involved in quality improvement activities, as well as nurse managers, can identify problem areas in specific aspects of care. Documentation issues, often the focus of quality assurance activities, may be addressed using the care plan guides as the basis for evaluating care given. The importance of such monitoring activities is increasing as third party payers and certifying/surveying agencies require increasing amounts of evidence of the plan of care, as well as care provided.

The care plan guides also provide a framework for research. The development, refinement, and validation of nursing diagnoses, efficacy of therapeutic interventions, validity of expected outcomes, acuity systems' reliability, and issues of nurse-generated revenue and direct reimbursement for nursing care rendered are applicable topics for research activities.

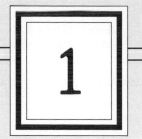

Nursing Diagnosis Care Plans

Activity intolerance

A state in which a person has insufficient physical or psychological energy to endure or perform desired physical activities.

RELATED FACTORS / DEFINING CHARACTERISTICS	EXPECTED OUTCOMES AND NURSING INTERVENTIONS / *RATIONALE* (■ = INDEPENDENT; ▲ = COLLABORATIVE)

RELATED FACTORS

Generalized weakness
Deconditioned state
Sedentary life-style
Insufficient sleep or rest periods
Lack of motivation/depression
Prolonged bedrest
Imposed activity restriction
Imbalance between O_2 supply and demand
Pain

DEFINING CHARACTERISTICS

Verbal report of fatigue or weakness
Inability to begin/perform activity
Abnormal heart rate or BP response to activity
Exertional discomfort or dyspnea

EXPECTED OUTCOMES

Patient maintains activity level within capabilities, as evidenced by normal heart rate, blood pressure during activity, and absence of shortness of breath, weakness, and fatigue.
Patient verbalizes and utilizes energy conservation techniques.

ONGOING ASSESSMENT

- Determine patient's perception of causes of fatigue/activity intolerance. *May be temporary or permanent, physical or psychological. Assessment guides treatment.*
- Assess patient's level of mobility. *Aids in defining what patient is capable of, which is necessary prior to setting realistic goals.*
- Assess nutritional status. *Adequate energy reserves are required for activity.*
- Assess potential for physical injury with activity.
- Assess need for ambulation aids: bracing, ADL equipment modification.
- Assess patient's cardiopulmonary status before activity:
  Heart rate, orthostatic BP changes.
  Need for O_2 with increased activity.
  How Valsalva maneuver affects heart rate when patient moves in bed. *Valsalva maneuver, which requires breath holding and bearing down, can cause bradycardia and related reduced cardiac output.*
- Monitor patient's sleep pattern and amount of sleep achieved over past few days.
- Observe and document response to activity. *Close monitoring serves as a guide for optimal progression of activity.*
  Report:
  Rapid pulse (>20 beats over resting rate or 120 BPM).
  Palpitations.
  Significant increase in systolic BP (>20 mm Hg).
  Significant decrease in systolic BP (drop of ≥20 mm Hg).
  Dyspnea, labored breathing, wheezing.
  Weakness, fatigue.
  Lightheadedness, dizziness, pallor, diaphoresis.
- Assess emotional response to change in physical status.

THERAPEUTIC INTERVENTIONS

- Encourage adequate rest periods, especially *before* ambulation, diagnostic procedures, and meals *to reduce cardiac workload.*
- Refrain from performing nonessential procedures *to promote rest.*
- Anticipate patient's needs (e.g., keep telephone, tissues within reach).
- Assist with ADL as indicated *to reduce energy expenditure* but avoid doing for patient what he/she can do for himself/herself; *increases patient's self-esteem.*
- Provide bedside commode as indicated *to reduce energy expenditure. Note: bedpans require more energy than commode.*
- Encourage physical activity consistent with patient's energy resources.
- Plan activities for times when patient has the most energy.
- Encourage verbalization of feelings regarding limitations. *Acknowledgement that living with activity intolerance is both physically and emotionally difficult aids coping.*
- Progress activity gradually *to prevent overexerting the heart and to promote attainment of short-range goals:*
  Active ROM exercises in bed progressing to sitting/standing.
  Dangling 10-15 min t.i.d.
  Deep breathing exercises t.i.d.
  Sitting up in chair 30 min t.i.d.
  Walking in room 1-2 min t.i.d.
  Walking in hall 25 ft, then slowly progressing, saving energy for return trip.
- Encourage active ROM exercises t.i.d. *to maintain muscle strength and joint range of motion;* if further reconditioning needed, confer with rehabilitation medicine personnel.
- Provide emotional support while increasing activity. Promote a positive attitude regarding abilities.
- Encourage patient to choose activities that gradually build endurance.
- Improvise in adapting ADL equipment/environment.

RELATED FACTORS / DEFINING CHARACTERISTICS	EXPECTED OUTCOMES AND NURSING INTERVENTIONS / *RATIONALE* (■ = INDEPENDENT; ▲ = COLLABORATIVE)

PATIENT EDUCATION

- Teach patient/significant others to recognize signs of physical overactivity. *Promotes awareness of when to reduce activity.*
- Involve patient/significant others in goal setting and care planning. *Setting small attainable goals can increase self-confidence and self-esteem.*
- Encourage significant others to bring ambulation aid: walker or cane.
- Teach the importance of continued activity once at home *to maintain strength/ROM/ endurance gain.*
- Assist in assigning priority to activities *to accommodate energy levels.*
- Teach energy conservation techniques. *They reduce oxygen consumption, allowing more prolonged activity.* Some examples include:
    Sitting to do tasks. *Standing requires more work.*
    Changing positions frequently. *Distributes work to different muscles to avoid fatigue.*
    Pushing rather than pulling.
    Sliding rather than lifting.
    Working at an even pace. *Allows enough time so not all work is done in a short period of time.*
    Storing frequently used items within easy reach *to avoid bending and reaching.*
    Resting for at least 1 hour after meals before a new activity *because energy is needed to digest food.*
    Using wheeled carts for laundry, shopping, and cleaning needs.
    Organizing a work-rest-work schedule.
- Teach appropriate use of environmental aids (e.g., bed rails, elevation of head of bed while patient gets out of bed, chair in bathroom, hall rails) *to conserve energy and prevent injury from fall.*
- Teach ROM and strengthening exercises.
- Encourage patient to verbalize concerns about discharge and home environment.

By: Meg Gulanick, RN, PhD
John Lorocco, PT
Susan Eby, PT, MS

Airway clearance, ineffective

A state in which an individual is unable to clear secretions or obstructions from the respiratory tract to maintain airway patency.

RELATED FACTORS / DEFINING CHARACTERISTICS	EXPECTED OUTCOMES AND NURSING INTERVENTIONS / *RATIONALE* (■ = INDEPENDENT; ▲ = COLLABORATIVE)

RELATED FACTORS

Decreased energy and fatigue
Tracheobronchial: infection, obstruction (including foreign body aspiration), secretions
Perceptual/cognitive impairment
Trauma

DEFINING CHARACTERISTICS

Abnormal breath sounds (crackles, rhonchi, wheezes)
Changes in respiratory rate or depth
Cough
Cyanosis
Dyspnea
Fever

EXPECTED OUTCOMES

Patient's secretions are mobilized and airway is maintained free of secretions as evidenced by: clear breath sounds, eupnea, normal skin color, ability to effectively cough up secretions following treatments and deep breaths.

ONGOING ASSESSMENT

- Auscultate lungs for presence of breath sounds as needed. *Routine assessment of breath sounds allows for early detection and correction of abnormalities.*
- Assess respirations; note quality, rate, pattern, depth, flaring of nostrils, dyspnea on exertion, evidence of splinting, use of accessory muscles, position for breathing.
- Assess changes in orientation and behavior pattern.
- Assess changes in vital signs and temperature.
- Assess patient's knowledge of disease process.
- Assess effectiveness and productivity of cough.
- Note presence of sputum; assess quality, color, and consistency.
- ▲ Monitor arterial blood gases (ABGs); note changes.

Continued.

Nursing Diagnosis Care Plans

RELATED FACTORS / DEFINING CHARACTERISTICS	EXPECTED OUTCOMES AND NURSING INTERVENTIONS / *RATIONALE* (■ = INDEPENDENT; ▲ = COLLABORATIVE)

THERAPEUTIC INTERVENTIONS

- Position patient with proper body alignment for optimal breathing pattern (if tolerated, head of bed at >45 degrees). *This promotes better lung expansion and improved air exchange.*
- Routinely check the patient's position *so he/she does not slide down in bed, causing the abdomen to compress the diaphragm, which would cause respiratory embarrassment.*
- Assist with incentive spirometry as appropriate.
- If abnormal breath sounds are present, assist patient with coughing.
    Administer pain relief medications before the attempt.
    Splint any incisional/injured area.
    Instruct patient how to cough effectively.
    Utilize cough techniques as appropriate (e.g., quad, huff).
    Coach the patient through the process.
- ▲ If cough is ineffective, use oropharyngeal or tracheal suction as needed:
    Explain procedure to patient.
    Utilize soft rubber catheters *to prevent trauma to mucous membranes.*
    Use curved-tip catheters and head positioning (if not contraindicated) *to facilitate secretion removal from a specific side (right vs. left lung).*
    Use universal precautions: gloves, goggles, and mask as appropriate.
    Instruct the patient to take several deep breaths before and after each nasotracheal suctioning and use supplemental O_2 as appropriate *to prevent suctioning-related hypoxia.*
    Stop suctioning and provide supplemental O_2 (assisted breaths by ambu bag as needed) if the patient experiences bradycardia, an increase in ventricular ectopy, and/or desaturation.
- ▲ Provide humidity (when appropriate) via bedside humidifier (positioned near patient) and humidified O_2 therapy *to prevent drying of secretions.*
- Encourage oral intake/fluids within the limits of cardiac reserve *to maintain hydration.*
- Instruct and/or change patient's position (e.g., ambulate, turn every 2 hr). *This will help to facilitate secretion movement and drainage.*
- ▲ Administer medications (antibiotics, bronchodilators, diuretics) as ordered, noting effectiveness and side effects.
- Assist with oral hygiene every 4 hr or as needed *to decrease oral flora.*
- Maintain adequate airway. Anticipate the need for an artificial airway (intubation) if secretions cannot be cleared.
- ▲ With respiratory therapy department, coordinate optimal time for postural drainage and percussion, i.e., at least 1 hr after eating *to prevent aspiration.*
- Pace activities *to prevent fatigue.* Maintain planned rest periods.
- Instruct patient to avoid restrictive clothing *that could prevent adequate respiratory excursion.*

PATIENT EDUCATION

- Demonstrate and teach coughing, deep breathing, and splinting techniques *so patient will understand the rationale and appropriate techniques to keep the airway clear of secretions.*
- Instruct patient on indications for, frequency, and side effects of medications.
- Instruct patient how to use prescribed inhalers, as appropriate.
- Teach patient about environmental factors that can precipitate respiratory problems.
- Explain effects of smoking, including second-hand smoke.
- Refer patient and/or significant others to stop-smoking group, as appropriate.
- Instruct patient on warning signs of pending/recurring pulmonary problems.
- Consult with pulmonary clinical nurse specialist, as appropriate.

By: Sue Galanes, RN, MS, CCRN

Anxiety

A vague uneasy feeling that usually stems from an impending or anticipated circumstance or event. It can be focused on an activity, object, or situation or unfocused and more generalized. It is believed to be primarily internally motivated, and its source may be nonspecific or unknown to the person experiencing it. The feeling may be experienced as diffuse and is generally categorized into four levels: mild, moderate, severe, and panic.

RELATED FACTORS / DEFINING CHARACTERISTICS	EXPECTED OUTCOMES AND NURSING INTERVENTIONS / *RATIONALE* (■ = INDEPENDENT; ▲ = COLLABORATIVE)

RELATED FACTORS

Threat or perceived threat to physical and emotional integrity

Change in health status and associated changes in role function

Intrusive diagnostic and surgical tests and procedures

Changes in environment and routines

Threat or perceived threat to self-concept

Threat to (or change in) socio-economic status

Situational and maturational crises

Intrapersonal conflicts caused by unmet needs and/or emotional fixation at an earlier level of development

Interpersonal conflicts

DEFINING CHARACTERISTICS

Physiological:

Increase in blood pressure, pulse, respirations

Dizziness, light-headedness

Perspiration

Frequent urination

Flushing

Dyspnea

Palpitations

Dry mouth

Headaches

Nausea and/or diarrhea

Restlessness

Pacing

Voice quavering

Pupil dilation

Insomnia, nightmares

Trembling

Feelings of helplessness and discomfort

Physiological/Behavioral

↑ Tension

Worry

Vague uneasy feeling

Scared

Jittery

Feeling helpless

Distress

Apprehension

↑ Wariness

Fearfulness

EXPECTED OUTCOMES

Patient recognizes anxiety signs at a low-intensity level.

Patient demonstrates a positive coping method.

Patient describes a reduction in the level of anxiety experienced.

ONGOING ASSESSMENT

- Assess patient's level of anxiety. *Mild anxiety enhances patient's awareness and ability to identify and solve problems. Moderate anxiety limits awareness of environmental stimuli. Problem solving can occur but may be more difficult, and patient may need help. Severe anxiety decreases patient's ability to integrate information and solve problems. Panic is severe anxiety. Patient is unable to follow directions. Hyperactivity, agitation, and immobilization may be observed.*
- Assess patient's coping mechanisms in handling anxiety. *This can be done by interviewing patient and significant others. This assessment helps determine the effectiveness of coping strategies currently used by patient.*
- Document behavioral and verbal expressions of anxiety. *Symptoms often provide information regarding the degree of anxiety. Physiological symptoms and/or complaints intensify as the level of anxiety increases.*

THERAPEUTIC INTERVENTIONS

- Acknowledge awareness of patient's anxiety. *Acknowledgment of patient's feelings validates the feelings and communicates acceptance of those feelings.*
- Reassure patient that he/she is safe. Stay with patient if this appears necessary. *The presence of a trusted person assures patient of his/her security and safety during a period of anxiety.*
- Maintain a calm and tolerant manner while interacting with patient. *Staff's anxiety may be easily perceived by patient. The patient's feeling of stability increases in a calm and nonthreatening atmosphere.*
- Establish a working relationship with patient through continuity of care. *An ongoing relationship establishes a basis for communicating anxious feelings.*
- Orient patient to the environment as needed. *Orientation and awareness of the surroundings promotes comfort and a decrease in anxiety.*
- Use simple language and brief statements when instructing patient about diagnostic and surgical tests. *When experiencing moderate to severe anxiety, patients are unable to comprehend anything more than simple, clear, and brief instructions.*
- Reduce sensory stimuli by maintaining a quiet environment; keep "threatening" equipment out of sight. *anxiety may escalate with excessive conversation, noise, and equipment around patient.*
- Encourage patient to notify staff when anxious feelings occur. *Staff availability reinforces a feeling of security for patient.*
- Encourage patient to talk about anxious feelings and examine the anxiety-provoking situation. Assist patient in assessing the situation realistically and recognizing factors leading to the anxious feelings. Avoid false reassurances.
- As patient's anxiety subsides, encourage to explore specific events preceding both the onset and reduction of the anxious feelings. *Recognition and exploration of factors leading to or reducing anxious feelings are important steps in developing alternative responses. Patient may be unaware of the relationship between emotional concerns and anxiety.*
- Assist in developing anxiety-reducing skills (relaxation, deep breathing, positive visualization, reassuring self-statements, etc). *Utilizing anxiety-reduction strategies enhances patient's sense of personal mastery and confidence.*
- Assist patient in developing problem-solving abilities. *Learning to identify a problem and evaluate alternatives to resolve it help patient to cope.* Emphasize the logical strategies patient can use when experiencing anxious feelings.
- ▲ Administer antianxiety medications as appropriate.

Continued.

Anxiety—cont'd

RELATED FACTORS / DEFINING CHARACTERISTICS	EXPECTED OUTCOMES AND NURSING INTERVENTIONS / *RATIONALE* (■ = INDEPENDENT; ▲ = COLLABORATIVE)
DEFINING CHARACTERISTICS— cont'd *Physiological/Behavioral* Feeling of inadequacy Crying Poor eye contact *Cognitive* Difficulty concentrating Confusion ↓ ability to problem-solve Forgetfulness	**PATIENT EDUCATION** • Assist patient in recognizing symptoms of increasing anxiety; explore alternatives to use to prevent the anxiety from immobilizing her/him. *The ability to recognize anxiety symptoms at lower-intensity levels enables patient to intervene more quickly to manage his/her anxiety. Patient will be able to use problem-solving abilities more effectively when the level of anxiety is low.* • Remind patient that anxiety at a mild level can encourage growth and development and is important in mobilizing changes. • Instruct patient in the proper use of medications and educate him/her to recognize adverse reactions. *Medication may be used if patient's anxiety continues to escalate and the anxiety becomes disabling.*

By: Ursula Brozek, RN, MSN
   Meg Gulanick, RN, PhD

Aspiration, high risk for

The state in which an individual is at risk for entry of gastric secretions, oropharyngeal secretions, or exogenous food or fluids into tracheobronchial passages as a result of dysfunction or absence of normal protective mechanisms.

RISK FACTORS	EXPECTED OUTCOMES AND NURSING INTERVENTIONS / *RATIONALE* (■ = INDEPENDENT; ▲ = COLLABORATIVE)

RISK FACTORS
Reduced level of consciousness.
Depressed cough and gag reflexes.
Presence of tracheotomy or endotracheal tube.
Presence of gastrointestinal tubes.
Tube feedings/medication administration.
Decreased gastrointestinal motility.
Impaired swallowing.
Facial/oral/neck surgery or trauma.
Situations hindering elevation of upper body.
	EXPECTED OUTCOMES
	Patient maintains patent airway.
	Patient's risk of aspiration is decreased as a result of ongoing assessment and early intervention.
	
	ONGOING ASSESSMENT
	• Monitor level of consciousness. *A decreased level of consciousness is a prime risk factor for aspiration.*
	• Assess cough and gag reflex. *A depressed cough or gag reflex increases the risk of aspiration.*
	• Monitor swallowing ability:
	  Assess for cough or throat clearing after a swallow.
	  Assess for residual food in mouth after eating.
	  Assess for regurgitation of food or fluid through nares.
	  Monitor for choking during eating or drinking.
	• Auscultate bowel sounds every shift *to evaluate bowel motility. Decreased gastrointestinal motility increases the risk of aspiration because food/fluids accumulate in the stomach.*
	• Assess for presence of nausea/vomiting.
	• Assess pulmonary status for clinical evidence of aspiration. Auscultate breath sounds for development of crackles and/or rhonchi. *Aspiration of small amounts can occur without coughing or sudden onset of respiratory distress, especially in patients with a decreased levels of consciousness.*
	▲ In patients with endotracheal or tracheostomy tubes, monitor the effectiveness of the cuff. Collaborate with the respiratory therapist, as needed, to determine cuff pressure. *An ineffective cuff can increase the risk of aspiration.*

THERAPEUTIC INTERVENTIONS

- Keep suction setup available and use as needed *to maintain a patent clear airway.*
- Notify the physician immediately of noted decrease in cough and/or gag reflexes, or difficulty in swallowing. *Early intervention protects the patient's airway and prevents aspiration.*
- Position patients who have a decreased level of consciousness on their side, *so that the airway is protected. Proper positioning can decrease the risk of aspiration.*
- Supervise/assist patient with oral intake *to detect abnormalities early.*
- Offer foods with consistency that patient can swallow. *Semisolid foods like pudding and hot cereal are most easily swallowed. Liquids and thin foods like creamed soups are most difficult for patients with dysphagia.*
- Encourage patient to chew thoroughly and eat slowly during meals. Instruct patient not to talk while eating.
- Place whole or crushed pills in soft foods, (e.g., custard); (first ask the pharmacist which pills should not be crushed; as appropriate, request medication in elixir form.)
- ▲ Utilize speech pathology consultation as appropriate. *A speech pathologist can be consulted to perform a dysphagia assessment that will help to determine the need for video fluoroscopy or barium cookie swallow.*
- Elevate head of bed, and keep patient upright for 30 to 45 minutes after feeding. *The upright position facilitates the gravitational flow of food/fluid through the alimentary tract. If the head of bed cannot be elevated (because of patient's condition), use a right side-lying position after feedings to facilitate passage of stomach contents into the duodenum.*
- In patients with NG or gastrostomy tubes:
  Check placement prior to feeding. *A displaced tube may erroneously deliver tube feeding into the airway.*
  Check residuals prior to feeding. Hold feedings if residuals are high and notify the physician. *High amounts of residual can cause distention of the stomach and lead to reflux emesis.*
  Place dye (e.g. methylene blue) in NG feedings. *Detection of the color in pulmonary secretions would indicate aspiration.*

PATIENT EDUCATION

- Explain to patient/significant other the need for proper positioning *to decrease the risk of aspiration.*
- Instruct patient/significant other on proper feeding techniques.
- Instruct patient/significant other on upper-airway suctioning techniques *to prevent accumulation of secretions in the oral cavity.*
- Instruct patient/significant other on signs and symptoms of aspiration. *Aids in appropriately assessing high-risk situations and determining when to call for further evaluation.*
- Instruct significant other on what to do in the event of an emergency.

By: Sue Galanes, RN, MS

Body image disturbance

A disturbance or alteration in the attitude a person has about the actual or perceived structure or function of all or part of the body. This attitude is dynamic and altered through interaction with other persons and situations and is influenced by age and developmental level.

RELATED FACTORS / DEFINING CHARACTERISTICS	EXPECTED OUTCOMES AND NURSING INTERVENTIONS / *RATIONALE* (■ = INDEPENDENT; ▲ = COLLABORATIVE)
RELATED FACTORS Situational changes (e.g., pregnancy, temporary presence of a visible drain/tube, dressing, attached equipment)	**EXPECTED OUTCOMES** Patient demonstrates enhanced body image and self-esteem as evidenced by ability to look at, touch, talk about, and care for actual or perceived altered body part/function.

Continued.

Body image disturbance—cont'd

RELATED FACTORS / DEFINING CHARACTERISTICS	EXPECTED OUTCOMES AND NURSING INTERVENTIONS / *RATIONALE* (■ = INDEPENDENT; ▲ = COLLABORATIVE)

RELATED FACTORS— cont'd

Permanent alterations in structure and/or function (e.g., mutilating surgery, removal of body part [internal or external])

Malodorous lesions, change in voice quality

DEFINING CHARACTERISTICS

Verbal identification of feeling about altered structure/function of a body part

Verbal preoccupation with changed body part or function

Naming changed body part or function

Refusal to discuss/acknowledge change

Focusing behavior on changed body part and/or function

Actual change in structure/function

Refusal to look at, touch, or care for altered body part

Change in social behavior (withdrawal, isolation, flamboyance)

Compensatory use of concealing clothing, other devices

ONGOING ASSESSMENT

- Assess perception of change in structure/function of body part (also proposed change). *Extent of response is more related to the value or importance patient places on the part or function than the actual value or importance.*
- Assess perceived impact of change on ADL, social behavior, personal relationships, occupational activities.
- Note patient's behavior regarding actual or perceived changed body part/function.
- Note frequency of self-critical remarks.

THERAPEUTIC INTERVENTIONS

- Acknowledge normalcy of emotional response to actual or perceived change in body structure/function. *Stages of grief over loss of a body part or function is normal, and typically involves a period of denial.*
- Help patient identify actual changes. *Patients may perceive changes that are not present/real.*
- Encourage verbalization of positive or negative feelings about actual or perceived change.
- Assist patient in incorporating actual changes into ADL, social life, interpersonal relationships, occupational activities. *Opportunities for positive feedback may hasten adaptation.*
- Demonstrate positive caring in routine activities. *Professional caregivers represent a microcasm of society, and their actions/behaviors will be scrutinized as the patient plans to return home, to work, etc.*

PATIENT EDUCATION

- Teach patient adaptive behavior to compensate for actual changed body structure/function, such as: use of adaptive equipment, clothing that conceals altered body part or enhances remaining part/function, use of deodorants, etc.
- Help patient identify ways of coping that have been useful in the past.
- Encourage patient to seek out/attend support groups made up of individuals with similar alterations. *Laypersons in similar situations offer a different type of support, which is perceived as helpful. Examples: United Ostomy Association, Why Me?, I Can Cope, Mended Hearts.*

By: Audrey Klopp, RN, PhD, ET

Body temperature, altered, high risk

A state in which an individual is at risk for failure to maintain a normal body temperature.

RISK FACTORS	EXPECTED OUTCOMES AND NURSING INTERVENTIONS / *RATIONALE* (■ = INDEPENDENT; ▲ = COLLABORATIVE)

RISK FACTORS

Extremes of weight or age

Dehydration

Illness

Trauma

Drugs

Environment: exposure to *hot/cold*

Inappropriate clothing

Vigorous activity or inactivity

EXPECTED OUTCOMES

Patient maintains body temperature within a normal range.

ONGOING ASSESSMENT

- Assess for presence of risk factors.
- Assess for precipitating event.
- Use a continuous temperature measuring device, preferably a tympanic or rectal probe. *Provides temperatures close to core. Continuous monitoring assists with diagnosis and management in labile cases.*
- Measure temperature at frequent intervals. Use the same instrument and method at each interval. If method is changed (e.g., axillary versus rectal), document route. *A change of this type usually causes a variance in the temperature obtained.*
- Monitor other physical indicators:

  Heart and respiratory rate   Fluid balance

  Blood pressure   Electrolytes

  Skin condition   Mental status

▲ Assist with diagnostic exams. *Specific diagnosis is necessary for illness and trauma risks to be treated.*

Continued.

RISK FACTORS	EXPECTED OUTCOMES AND NURSING INTERVENTIONS / *RATIONALE* (■ = INDEPENDENT; ▲ = COLLABORATIVE)

THERAPEUTIC INTERVENTIONS

▲ Provide preventive measures as necessary.
  Control environment.
  Provide appropriate clothing/covering.
  Provide adequate fluid and dietary intake.
  Administer medications as ordered.
■ Notify physician of changes in physical status, especially temperature.
■ If altered body temperature becomes a problem, refer to appropriate care plan:
  Hypothermia, p. 38
  Hyperthermia, p. 37

PATIENT EDUCATION

■ Explain risk factors and rationale for temperature measurement.
■ Explain prevention of risk factors and consequences of development of temperature alterations.
■ Provide community resources, consultants as needed.

By: Michele Knoll Puzas, RN,C, MHPE

Bowel incontinence

The state in which an individual experiences involuntary passage of stool. Bowel incontinence may occur as a result of traumatic injury to rectal, anal, or nervous tissue; damage to these tissues because of infection or radiation; neurologic diseases/problems (stroke, multiple sclerosis, diabetes mellitus); dementia; changes in the musculature of bowel elimination because of age, fecal impaction, diarrhea, or inability to reach the toilet in a timely manner.

RELATED FACTORS / DEFINING CHARACTERISTICS	EXPECTED OUTCOMES AND NURSING INTERVENTIONS / *RATIONALE* (■ = INDEPENDENT; ▲ = COLLABORATIVE)

RELATED FACTORS

Neuromuscular problems:
  Stroke, multiple sclerosis, diabetes, dementia, nerve trauma
Musculoskeletal problems:
  Pelvic floor relaxation, nerve trauma, damage to sphincters
Radiation
Infection
Postoperative injuries
Fecal impaction
Medications
Immobility
Lack of accessible toileting facilities

DEFINING CHARACTERISTICS

Involuntary passage of stool

EXPECTED OUTCOMES

Patient is continent of stool.

ONGOING ASSESSMENT

■ Assess patient's normal bowel elimination pattern. *There is a wide range of "normal" for bowel elimination; some patients have two bowel movements per day, while others may have a bowel movement as infrequently as every third or fourth day. If there is current pathology that may affect bowel elimination, determine pre-morbid bowel elimination pattern.*
■ Determine cause of incontinence (i.e., review related factors).
■ Perform manual check for fecal impaction. *When patient has a fecal impaction (hard, dry stool that cannot be expelled normally), liquid stool may leak past the impaction.*
■ Assess whether current medications/treatments may be contributing to bowel incontinence. *Hyperosmolar tube feedings, bowel preparation agents, some chemotherapeutic agents, and certain antibiotic agents may cause explosive diarrhea that the patient cannot control.*
■ Assist in preparing patient for diagnostic measures to determine cause(s) of bowel incontinence. *Tests include flexible sigmoidoscopy, barium enema, colonoscopy, and anal manometry (study to determine function of rectal spincters).*
■ Assess degree to which patient's daily activities are altered by bowel incontinence. *Patients may restrict their own activity or become isolated from work, family, and friends because they fear odor and embarrassment.*
■ Assess use of diapers, sanitary napkins, incontinence briefs, fecal collection devices, and underpads.
■ Assess perineal skin integrity. *Stool can cause chemical irritation to the skin, which may be exacerbated by the use of diapers, incontinence briefs, and underpads.*
■ Assess patient's ability to go to the bathroom independently.
■ Assess patient's environment for availability of accessible toilet facility.
■ Assess fluid and fiber intake. *Both are related to normal bowel evacuation.*

Continued.

■ **Bowel incontinence—cont'd**

RELATED FACTORS / DEFINING CHARACTERISTICS	EXPECTED OUTCOMES AND NURSING INTERVENTIONS / *RATIONALE* (■ = INDEPENDENT; ▲ = COLLABORATIVE)

THERAPEUTIC INTERVENTIONS

- Ensure fluid intake of at least 3000 cc per day, unless contraindicated. *Moist stool moves through the bowel more easily than hard, dry stool.*
▲ Provide high-fiber diet under the direction of a dietician, unless contraindicated. *Fiber aids in bowel elimination because it is insoluble and absorbs fluid as the stool passes through the bowel; this creates bulk. Bulky stool stimulates peristalsis and expulsion of stool from the bowel.*
- Manually remove fecal impaction, if present.
- Encourage mobility/exercise if tolerated. *This enhances gravity, stimulates peristalsis, and aids in bowel evacuation.*
- Provide a bedside commode and assistive devices (cane, walker) or assistance in reaching the commode/toilet.
▲ Institute a bowel program. *Facilitating regular bowel evacuation will prevent the bowel from emptying sporadically (i.e., decrease incontinence):*
    Encourage bowel elimination at the same time every day *(shortly after breakfast is a good time because the gastrocolic reflex is stimulated by food/fluid intake).*
    Following breakfast (or a warm drink), administer a suppository and perform digital stimulation every 10-15 minutes until evacuation occurs.
    Place patient in an upright position for defecation. *Flexion of the thighs (e.g., sitting upright with feet flat on floor) facilitates muscular movement that aids in defecation.*
- Treat any perianal irritation with a moisture barrier ointment.
- Discourage the use of pads, diapers, or collection devices as soon as possible.
- Use a fecal incontinence device selectively over pads, diapers, and rectal tubes. *These devices (pouches that adhere to skin around the rectum) allow for collection and disposal of stool without exposing the perianal skin to stool; odor and embarrassment are controlled because the stool is contained.*

PATIENT EDUCATION

- Teach patient the causes of bowel incontinence.
- Teach patient the importance of fluid and fiber in maintaining soft, bulky stool.
- Teach patient the importance of establishing a regular time for bowel evacuation.
- Teach caregiver use of fecal incontinence device.
- Teach patient to manage perianal irritation prophylactically using moisture barrier ointment.
- Teach patient the importance of a regular exercise program.

By: Audrey Klopp, RN, PhD, ET

Breathing pattern, ineffective

A state in which an individual's respiratory pattern (cycles of inhalation and exhalation) does not enable adequate ventilation.

RELATED FACTORS / DEFINING CHARACTERISTICS	EXPECTED OUTCOMES AND NURSING INTERVENTIONS / *RATIONALE* (■ = INDEPENDENT; ▲ = COLLABORATIVE)

RELATED FACTORS

Inflammatory process:
  Viral or bacterial
Hypoxia
Neuromuscular impairment
Pain
Musculoskeletal impairment
Tracheobronchial obstruction
Perception or cognitive impairment
Anxiety
Decreased energy and fatigue
Decreased lung expansion

EXPECTED OUTCOMES

Patient's breathing pattern is maintained as evidenced by: eupnea, normal skin color, and regular respiratory rate/pattern.

ONGOING ASSESSMENT

- Assess respiratory rate and depth by listening to breath sounds at least every shift. *Respiratory rate and rhythm changes are early warning signs of impending respiratory difficulties.*
- Assess for dyspnea and quantify (i.e., note how many words per breath patient can say); relate dyspnea to precipitating factors.
- Monitor breathing patterns: bradypnea, tachypnea, hyperventilation, Kussmaul respirations, Cheyne-Stokes, apneustic, Biot's, and ataxic patterns.
- Note muscles used for breathing (i.e., sternocleidomastoid, abdominal, diaphragmatic).
- Monitor for diaphragmatic muscle fatigue (paradoxical motion).

RELATED FACTORS / DEFINING CHARACTERISTICS	EXPECTED OUTCOMES AND NURSING INTERVENTIONS / *RATIONALE* (■ = INDEPENDENT; ▲ = COLLABORATIVE)

DEFINING CHARACTERISTICS

Dyspnea
Tachypnea
Fremitus
Cyanosis
Cough
Nasal flaring
Respiratory depth changes
Altered chest excursion
Use of accessory muscles
Pursed-lip breathing/prolonged expiratory phase
Increased anteroposterior chest diameter

ONGOING ASSESSMENT

- Note retractions, flaring of nostrils.
- Assess position patient assumes for normal/easy breathing.
- ▲ Monitor ABGs; note differences.
- Monitor for changes in orientation, increased restlessness, anxiety, air hunger.
- Assess skin color, temperature, capillary refill; note central versus peripheral cyanosis.
- Monitor vital capacity in patients with neuromuscular weakness.
- Assess presence of sputum for quantity, color, consistency.
- Note changes in activity tolerance.

THERAPEUTIC INTERVENTIONS

- Position patient with proper body alignment for optimal breathing pattern. *If not contraindicated, a sitting position allows for good lung excursion and chest expansion.*
- Ensure that O_2 delivery system is applied to the patient *so that the appropriate amount of oxygen is continuously delivered and the patient does not desaturate.*
- Encourage sustained deep breaths by:
    Demonstration (emphasizing slow inhalation, holding end inspiration for a few seconds, and passive exhalation).
    Use of incentive spirometer (place close for convenient patient use).
    Asking patient to yawn, *to promote deep inspiration.*
- Maintain a clear airway by encouraging patient to clear own secretions with effective coughing. If secretions cannot be cleared, suction as needed to clear secretions.
- Use universal precautions: gloves, goggles, and mask, as appropriate.
- Pace and schedule activities providing adequate rest periods *to prevent dyspnea resulting from fatigue.*
- Provide reassurance and allay anxiety by staying with patient during acute episodes of respiratory distress. *Air hunger can produce an extremely anxious state.*
- Provide relaxation training as appropriate (biofeedback, imagery, progressive muscle relaxation).
- Encourage diaphragmatic breathing for patient with chronic disease.
- ▲ Use pain management as appropriate.
- Anticipate the need for intubation and mechanical ventilation if patient is unable to maintain adequate gas exchange with the present breathing pattern.

PATIENT EDUCATION

- Explain all procedures prior to performing, *to decrease patient's anxiety.*
- Explain effects of wearing restrictive clothing *so that respiratory excursion is not compromised.*
- Explain use of O_2 therapy.
- Explain environmental factors that may worsen patient's pulmonary condition (e.g., pollen, second-hand smoke), and discuss possible precipitating factors (e.g., allergens and emotional stress).
- Explain symptoms of a "cold" and impending problems. *A respiratory infection would increase the work of breathing.*
- Teach patient/significant others appropriate breathing, coughing, and splinting techniques *to facilitate adequate clearance of secretions.*
- Teach patient how to count own respirations and relate respiratory rate to activity tolerance. *Patient will then know when to limit activities in terms of his/her own limitations.*
- Teach patient when to inhale and exhale while doing strenuous activities. *Appropriate breathing techniques during exercise are important in maintaining adequate gas exchange.*
- Prepare patient/significant other for at-home care:
    Teach signs of respiratory compromise.
    Refer significant other to participate in basic life support class for CPR, as appropriate.
- ▲ Refer to Social Services or social worker for further counseling and/or support groups related to patient's condition.
    Instruct about the oxygen therapy to be used at home.
    Instruct about medications: indications, dosage, frequency, and potential side effects.
    Review the use of at-home monitoring capabilities, as appropriate, and refer to resources for rental equipment.

By: Sue Galanes, RN, MS, CCRN

Cardiac output, decreased

A state in which the left and/or right ventricle is unable to maintain a cardiac output sufficient to meet the needs of the body. Common causes of reduced cardiac output include myocardial infarction, hypertension, valvular heart disease, congenital heart disease, cardiomyopathy, arrhythmias, drug effects, fluid overload, decreased fluid volume, and electrolyte imbalance.

RELATED FACTORS / DEFINING CHARACTERISTICS	EXPECTED OUTCOMES AND NURSING INTERVENTIONS / *RATIONALE* (■ = INDEPENDENT; ▲ = COLLABORATIVE)

RELATED FACTORS

Increased/decreased ventricular filling (preload)
Alteration in afterload
Impaired contractility
Alteration in heart rate/rhythm/conduction
Decreased oxygenation
Cardiac muscle disease

DEFINING CHARACTERISTICS

Variations in hemodynamic parameters (BP, heart rate, CVP, pulmonary artery pressures, SVO$_2$, cardiac output, neck veins)
Arrhythmias, ECG changes
Rales, tachypnea, dyspnea, orthopnea, cough, abnormal ABGs, frothy sputum
Weight gain, edema, decreased urine output
Anxiety, restlessness
Syncope, dizziness
Weakness, fatigue
Abnormal heart sounds
Decreased peripheral pulses, cold clammy skin
Confusion, change in mental status
Angina
EF <40%
Pulsus alternans

EXPECTED OUTCOMES

Patient maintains: BP within normal limits; warm, dry skin; regular cardiac rhythm; clear breath sounds; and strong bilateral, equal peripheral pulses.

ONGOING ASSESSMENT

- Assess physical status closely, document changes, report significant changes in parameters.
  Arterial BP, orthostatic changes, pulsus paradoxus.
  Apical/radial pulses; peripheral pulses (strength, equality).
  Heart rate.
  Respirations, breath sounds.
  Heart sounds, murmurs, rubs.
  Jugular venous distention.
  Skin color, temperature, moisture.
  Fluid balance, presence of peripheral edema.
  I & O, weight (same scale and amount of clothing).
  Chest pain/pressure.
- ▲ Monitor diagnostic/laboratory studies (e.g., ECG changes, ABGs, Hgb, CRIT, chest x-ray).
- ▪ Assess for changes in mental status.
- ▲ If hemodynamic monitoring is in place:
  Monitor BP, central venous/RAP, PAP (systolic, diastolic, and mean), pulmonary capillary/artery wedge pressure.
  Monitor SVO$_2$ continuously *(change in oxygen saturation of mixed venous blood is one of the earliest indicators of reduced cardiac output).*
  Perform cardiac output determination.
- ▪ Monitor continuous ECG as appropriate.
- ▪ Monitor ECG for rate, rhythm, ectopy, and change in PR, QRS, and QT intervals. *Tachycardia, bradycardia, and ectopic beats can compromise cardiac output.*
- ▪ Assess response to increased activity. *Physical activity increases the demands placed on the heart. Close monitoring of patient's response serves as a guide for optimal progression of activity.*
- ▪ Assess contributing factors *so appropriate plan of care can be initiated.* (Also see Fluid volume deficit, p. 25; Myocardial infarction, p. 132; Cardiogenic shock, p. 159; Cardiac dysrhythmias, p. 114; Chest trauma, p. 188; etc.).

THERAPEUTIC INTERVENTIONS

- ▲ Administer medication as prescribed, noting response and watching for side effects and toxicity. Clarify with physician parameters for withholding medications. (Common medications include digitalis therapy, diuretics, vasodilator therapy, and inotropic agents.)
- ▲ Maintain optimal fluid balance:
  Administer fluid challenge as prescribed, closely monitoring effects.
  Maintain hemodynamic parameters at prescribed levels.
  Restrict fluid and Na as prescribed.
- ▲ Maintain adequate ventilation/perfusion:
  Place patient in semi- to high-Fowler's position *to reduce preload and ventricular filling*; place in supine position *to increase venous return, promote diuresis.*
  Administer humidified O$_2$ as ordered.
- ▲ Maintain physical and emotional rest:
  Restrict activity *to reduce O$_2$ demands.*
  Provide quiet, relaxed environment. *Emotional stress increases cardiac demands.*
  Organize nursing and medical care *to allow rest periods.*
  Monitor progressive activity within limits of cardiac function.
  Administer stool softeners p.r.n.
  Monitor sleep patterns; administer sedative p.r.n.

RELATED FACTORS / DEFINING CHARACTERISTICS	EXPECTED OUTCOMES AND NURSING INTERVENTIONS / *RATIONALE* (■ = INDEPENDENT; ▲ = COLLABORATIVE)

THERAPEUTIC INTERVENTIONS

- If arrhythmia occurs, determine patient response, document, and report if significant or symptomatic. *Both tachyarrhythmias and bradyarrhythmias can reduce cardiac output and myocardial tissue perfusion.*
- Have antiarrhythmic drugs readily available.
- ▲ Treat arrhythmias according to medical orders or protocol and evaluate response. See treatment under Myocardial infarction: acute phase, p. 132.
- ▲ If invasive adjunct therapies are indicated (e.g., intra-aortic balloon pump, pacemaker), maintain within prescribed protocol.

PATIENT EDUCATION

- Explain symptoms and interventions for decreased cardiac output related to etiology.
- Explain drug regimen, purpose, dose, and side effects.
- Explain progressive activity schedule and signs of overexertion.
- Explain diet restrictions (fluid, sodium).

By: Meg Gulanick, RN, PhD

Caregiver role strain   *A caregiver's felt difficulty in performing the caregiver role.*

RELATED FACTORS / DEFINING CHARACTERISTICS	EXPECTED OUTCOMES AND NURSING INTERVENTIONS / *RATIONALE* (■ = INDEPENDENT; ▲ = COLLABORATIVE)

RELATED FACTORS

Care recipient requires assistance of caregiver in management of: bowel incontinence, bladder incontinence, self-care deficits, impaired mobility, alteration in thought process, sleep pattern disturbance, and potential for violence.

Caregiver has health problems.

Caregiver has knowledge deficit regarding management of care.

Caregiver's personal and social life is disrupted by demands of caregiving.

Caregiver has multiple competing roles.

Caregiver's time and freedom is restricted because of caregiving.

Past history of poor relationship between caregiver and care recipient.

Caregiver feels care is not appreciated.

Social isolation of family/caregiver.

Caregiver has no respite from caregiving demands.

Caregiver unaware of available community resources.

Caregiver reluctant to use community resources.

Community resources not available.

Community resources not affordable.

EXPECTED OUTCOMES

Caregiver demonstrates competence and confidence in performing the caregiver role by meeting care recipient's physical and psychosocial needs.

Caregiver expresses satisfaction with caregiver role.

Caregiver verbalizes positive feelings about care recipient and their relationship.

Caregiver reports that formal and informal support systems are adequate and helpful.

Caregiver uses strengths and resources to withstand stress of caregiving.

Caregiver demonstrates flexibility in dealing with problem behavior of care recipient.

Family system drawn closer by caregiving experience.

ONGOING ASSESSMENT

- Establish relationship with caregiver and care recipient to facilitate assessment and intervention.
- Assess caregiver-care recipient relationship.
- Assess family communication pattern. *Open communication in the family creates a positive environment whereas concealing feelings creates problems for caregiver and care recipient.*
- Assess family resources and support systems. *Family and social support is related positively to coping effectiveness.*
- Assess caregiver's appraisal of caregiving situation, level of understanding, and willingness to assume caregiver role. *Individual responses to potentially stressful situations are mediated by an appraisal of the personal meaning of the situation.*
- Assess for neglect and abuse of care recipient and take necessary steps to prevent injury to care recipient and strain on caregiver.
- Assess caregiver health.

Continued.

RELATED FACTORS / DEFINING CHARACTERISTICS	EXPECTED OUTCOMES AND NURSING INTERVENTIONS / *RATIONALE* (■ = INDEPENDENT; ▲ = COLLABORATIVE)

DEFINING CHARACTERISTICS

Caregiver expresses difficulty in performing patient care.
Caregiver verbalizes anger with responsibility of patient care.
Caregiver worried that own health will suffer because of caregiving.
Caregiver states that formal and informal support systems are inadequate.
Caregiver regrets that caregiving responsibility does not allow time for other activities.
Caregiver expresses problems in coping with patient's behavior.
Caregiver expresses negative feeling about patient or relationship.
Caregiver neglects patient care.
Caregiver abuses patient.

THERAPEUTIC INTERVENTIONS

- Encourage caregiver to identify available family/friends who can assist with caregiving.
- Suggest that caregiver use available community resources such as Respite, Home Health Care, Adult Day Care, etc.
- Encourage caregiver to set aside time for self.
- Acknowledge to caregiver the role he/she is carrying out and its value.
- Encourage care recipient to thank caregiver for care given. *Feeling appreciated decreases feeling of strain.*
- Provide time for caregiver to discuss problems, concerns, and feelings. Ask caregiver how he/she is managing.
- Inquire about caregiver's health. Offer to check blood pressure and to perform other health checks.
- ▲ Refer for family counseling if family amenable.
- Encourage involvement of other family members to relieve pressure on primary care giver. *Caring for a family member can be mutually rewarding and satisfying family experience.*
- ▲ Refer to social worker for referral for community resources and/or financial aid, if needed.
- Encourage family to become involved in community effort, political process, and policy making to effect legislation that supports caregivers, (i.e., family leave policy, availability of affordable community resources).

PATIENT EDUCATION

- Provide information on disease process and management strategies. *Accurate information increases understanding of care recipient's condition and behavior.*
- Instruct caregiver in management of care recipient's nursing diagnoses. Demonstrate necessary caregiving skills and allow sufficient time for learning before return demonstration. *Increased knowledge and skill will increase caregiver's confidence and decrease strain.*

By: Kathleen M. Perry, RN, MS, CS

Communication, impaired verbal

The state in which an individual's ability to use or understand language in human interaction is decreased or absent.

RELATED FACTORS / DEFINING CHARACTERISTICS	EXPECTED OUTCOMES AND NURSING INTERVENTIONS / *RATIONALE* (■ = INDEPENDENT; ▲ = COLLABORATIVE)

RELATED FACTORS

Impaired cerebral tissue perfusion secondary to stroke, head injury, or brain tumor
Tracheostomy
Intubation
Structural problem (e.g., cleft palate, postlaryngectomy)
Wired jaws
Cultural difference (i.e., speaks different language)
Dyspnea
Fatigue

DEFINING CHARACTERISTICS

Inability to recognize or understand words
Difficulty articulating words
Inability to recall familiar words, phrases, or names of known persons, objects, and places
Unable to speak dominant language

EXPECTED OUTCOMES

Patient able to use or understand language, *or an acceptable alternative form of communication, as evidenced by effective use of language to communicate needs, etc.*

ONGOING ASSESSMENT

- Assess the following:
  Ability to speak spontaneously.
  Ability to understand spoken word.
  Ability to understand written words, pictures, gestures.
- Assess conditions/situations that may hinder ability to use or understand language, such as:
  Alternate airway (e.g., tracheostomy, oral/nasal intubation). *When air does not pass over vocal cords, sounds are not produced.*
  Oro-facial-maxillary problems (e.g., wired jaws). *Words are articulated by coordinated movement of mouth and tongue.*
- Determine primary language spoken.
- Assess for presence of expressive aphasia *(inability to convey information verbally).*
- Assess for presence of/history of dyspnea.
- Assess energy level. *Fatigue and/or shortness of breath can make speaking difficult or impossible.*
- Assess knowledge of sign language, as appropriate.

THERAPEUTIC INTERVENTIONS

- Place call light within reach. *Reduces anxiety.*
- Anticipate needs to *decrease feelings of helplessness.* Pay attention to nonverbal cues.
- Encourage patient to speak; praise attempts and achievements.
- Listen attentively when patient attempts to communicate.
- Never talk in front of patient as though he/she comprehends nothing. *This will increase frustration and sense of helplessness.*
- Keep distractions such as television, radio at a minimum when talking to patient to *keep patient focused and assist nurse's ability to listen.*
- Do not speak loudly unless patient is hearing-impaired.
- Maintain eye contact with patient when speaking. Stand close, within patient's line of vision, generally midline. *Patient may have defect in field of vision. Nurse's eye contact and position provide support and encouragement; facilitate use of body language/lip reading.*
- Give ample time to respond. *It is difficult for patient to respond under pressure; allow time to organize responses.*
- Praise patient's accomplishments. Acknowledge his/her frustrations.
- If vocabulary is limited to yes and no answers, try to phrase questions so that patient can use these responses.
- Use short sentences. Ask only one question at a time. *Allows patient to stay focused on one thought.*
- Speak slowly and distinctly, repeating key words. *Prevents confusion.* Supplement with gestures, if necessary. *Provides as many sensory channels as possible.*
- Give concrete directions that the patient is physically capable of doing (e.g., "Point to "; "Open your mouth"; "Turn your head").
- Avoid finishing sentences for patient. Say word slowly and distinctly if help is requested. Be calm and accepting during attempts; do not say you understand if you do not, *for this may increase frustration and decrease trust.*
- When patient has difficulty with verbal expressions, give practice in repeating words after you. Begin with simple words, then progress (e.g., "Yes"; "No"; "This is a cup").
- When patient cannot identify objects by name, give practice in receiving word images (e.g., point to an object and clearly enunciate its name; "cup," "pen").
- Correct errors. *Not correcting errors reinforces undesirable performance, and will make correction more difficult later on.*
- Provide list of words patient can say; add new words to it.
- Provide patient with word-and-phrase cards, writing pad and pencil, or picture board. *Especially helpful for intubated/tracheal patients or those whose jaws are wired.*
- Carry on one-way conversation with totally aphasic patient.
- ▲ Consult speech therapist for additional help. See that patient is well rested before each session with speech therapist. *Fatigue may have an adverse effect on learning ability.*
- ▲ Consider use of electronic speech generator in postlarygectomy patients.

PATIENT EDUCATION

- Inform patient/significant others of the type of aphasia patient has and how it affects speech, language skills, and understanding.
- Offer significant others the opportunity to ask questions about patient's communication problem.
- Encourage significant others to talk to patient even though patient may not respond. *Decreases patient's sense of isolation, and may assist in recovery from aphasia.*
- Encourage patient to socialize with family and friends. *Explain that communication should be encouraged despite impairment.*
- Explain that brain injury decreases attention span.
- ▲ Provide patient with an appointment with a speech therapist, if not already done.
- Inform patient/significant others to seek information about aphasia from the American Speech-Language-Hearing Association, 10810 Rockwell Pike, Rockville, Maryland 20852.

By: Maria Dacanay, RN

Constipation/impaction

A change in normal bowel habits characterized by a decrease in the frequency and/or passage of hard, dry stool, a decrease in stool volume, or the oozing of liquid stool past a collection of hard, dry stool. Constipation may be "imagined" when the patient expects a daily bowel movement and does not have one. Constipation may be severe enough to cause rupture of the bowel but is more typically remedied by increased fluid and fiber.

RELATED FACTORS / DEFINING CHARACTERISTICS	EXPECTED OUTCOMES AND NURSING INTERVENTIONS / *RATIONALE* (■ = INDEPENDENT; ▲ = COLLABORATIVE)

RELATED FACTORS

Inadequate fluid intake
Low-fiber diet
Immobility
Fear of pain
Medication use
Lack of privacy
Pain
Laxative abuse
Pregnancy
Tumor or other obstructing mass
Neurogenic disorders

DEFINING CHARACTERISTICS

Straining at stools
Passage of liquid fecal seepage
Frequent but nonproductive desire to defecate
Anorexia
Abdominal distention
Nausea and vomiting
Dull headache, restlessness, and depression
Verbalized pain/fear of pain

EXPECTED OUTCOMES

Patient passes soft, formed stool at a frequency perceived as "normal" by the patient.
Patient/significant other verbalizes measures that will prevent recurrence of constipation.

ONGOING ASSESSMENT

- Assess usual pattern of elimination; compare to present pattern. Include size, frequency, color, and quality.
- Evaluate laxative use, type, and frequency.
- Evaluate reliance on enemas for elimination. *Abuse/overuse of cathartics and enemas can result in dependence on them for evacuation, because the colon becomes distended and does not respond normally to the presence of stool.*
- Evaluate usual dietary habits, eating habits, eating schedule, and liquid intake; compare with hospital regimen. *Change in mealtime, type of food, disruption of usual schedule, and anxiety related to hospitalization can lead to constipation.*
- Assess food preferences.
- Assess activity level. *Prolonged bed rest and lack of exercise contribute to constipation.*
- Auscultate for bowel sounds every shift. *Bowel sounds are caused by peristaltic movement of the small intestine, and are not normally altered in constipation, which is a colonic phenomenon.*
- Evaluate current medication usage, *which may contribute to constipation. Drugs that can cause constipation include: narcotics, antacids with calcium or aluminum base, antidepressants, anticholinergics, antihypertensives, and iron and calcium supplements.*
- Assess privacy for elimination (i.e., enforced use of bedpan).
- Evaluate fear of pain.
- Assess degree to which patient's procrastination contributes to constipation. *Ignoring the defecation urge eventually leads to chronic constipation, because the rectum no longer senses the presence of stool. The longer the stool remains in the rectum, the drier and harder (and more difficult to pass) it becomes.*
- Assess for hemorrhoids, *which may cause pain, and hesitancy to defecate.*
- Assess for history of neurogenic diseases, such as multiple sclerosis, Parkinson's disease. *Neurogenic disorders may alter the colon's ability to perform peristalsis.*

THERAPEUTIC INTERVENTIONS

- Encourage and provide daily fluid intake of 2000-3000 ml/day, if not contraindicated medically.
- Encourage increased fiber in diet (e.g., raw fruits, fresh vegetables [if appropriate]). *Fiber passes through the intestine essentially unchanged. When it reaches the colon, it forms a gel, which adds bulk to the stool, and makes defecation easier.*
- ▲ Consult dietitian if appropriate.
- Encourage patient to eat prunes, prune juice, cold cereal, bean products, etc. (if appropriate). *These are "natural" cathartics.*
- Orient patient to location of bathroom.
- Increase patient's physical activity by planning ambulation periods if possible. *Ambulation and/or abdominal exercises strengthen abdominal muscles that facilitate defecation.*
- Provide a regular time for elimination (e.g., after breakfast or at patient's usual time). *Many persons defecate following first meal or coffee, as a result of the gastro-colic reflex.*
- Offer a warm bedpan to bedridden patient. Assist patient to assume a high Fowler's position with knees flexed. *This position best utilizes gravity and allows for effective Valsalva maneuver.* Curtain off the area; allow patient time to relax.
- Initiate occupational/physical therapy consultation as needed.
- Assist with passive/active ROM exercises.
- Instruct in isometric abdominal and gluteal exercises *to strengthen muscles needed for evacuation* unless contraindicated.

RELATED FACTORS / DEFINING CHARACTERISTICS	EXPECTED OUTCOMES AND NURSING INTERVENTIONS / *RATIONALE* (■ = INDEPENDENT; ▲ = COLLABORATIVE)

THERAPEUTIC INTERVENTIONS

- ▲ Utilize pharmacologic agents as appropriate:
  - Metamucil: *increases fluid, gaseous, and solid bulk of intestinal contents.*
  - Stool softeners (e.g., Colace).
  - Chemical irritants (e.g., castor oil, cascara, Milk of Magnesia). *These irritate the bowel mucosa and cause rapid propulsion of contents of small intestines.*
  - Suppositories: *aid in softening stools and stimulate rectal mucosa; best results occur when given 30 min before usual defecation time or after breakfast.*
  - Oil retention enema *to soften stool.*
- · Digitally remove fecal impaction.
- ▲ Minimize rectal discomfort:
  - Warm sitz bath.
  - Hemorrhoidal preparations.

PATIENT EDUCATION

- · Explain to patient/significant others the importance of:
  - Balanced diet that contains adequate fiber, fresh fruits, vegetables, grains. *20 grams/ day is recommended.*
  - Adequate fluid intake (8 glasses/day).
  - Regular meals.
  - Regular time for evacuation and adequate time for defecation.
  - Regular exercise.
  - Privacy for defecation.
  - Administration of rectal suppositories, enemas, or laxatives when necessary.
- · Teach patients/significant others to read product labels to determine fiber content per serving.
- · Encourage patient to increase fiber intake gradually; *a precipitous increase can result in gaseous distention, bloating, and abdominal discomfort.*

By: Marian D. Cachero-Salavrakos, RN, BSN
Audrey Klopp, RN, PhD, ET

Coping, impaired family

Insufficient or compromised support by a primary supportive person (family member or close friend) of a hospitalized patient.

RELATED FACTORS / DEFINING CHARACTERISTICS	EXPECTED OUTCOMES AND NURSING INTERVENTIONS / *RATIONALE* (■ = INDEPENDENT; ▲ = COLLABORATIVE)

RELATED FACTORS

Unfamiliar environment
Separation of family members
Loss of dominant figure in family structure
Knowledge deficit regarding illness prognosis
Inaccurate/incomplete/ conflicting information
Overwhelming situation
Inadequate coping method
Prolonged disease that exhausts supportive capacity of caregivers

DEFINING CHARACTERISTICS

Expressed concern inappropriate to need
Verbalization of problem
Disregard for patient's needs
Inappropriate behavior

EXPECTED OUTCOMES

Family members identify effect patient's hospitalization has on the family unit.
Family members identify resources available for help with coping.

ONGOING ASSESSMENT

- · Assess family's knowledge and understanding of the need for hospitalization and treatment plan.
- · Assess level of family's anxiety.
- · Assess normal coping patterns in family, including strengths, problems, and resources. *Successful adjustment is influenced by previous coping success. Families with a history of unsuccessful coping may need additional resources.*
- · Assess support systems available to family.
- · Assess role of hospitalized patient in family structure.

THERAPEUTIC INTERVENTIONS

- · Approach patient in calm, reassuring manner *to reduce stress.*
- · Encourage questions or expressions of concern. *Coping difficulties vary depending on developmental level, extent of social contacts outside the family, and former experience with hospitalization.*
- · Provide honest, appropriate answers to family members' questions. *Appropriate information can relieve stress.*

Continued.

Coping, impaired family—cont'd

RELATED FACTORS / DEFINING CHARACTERISTICS	EXPECTED OUTCOMES AND NURSING INTERVENTIONS / *RATIONALE* (■ = INDEPENDENT; ▲ = COLLABORATIVE)

DEFINING CHARACTERISTICS— cont'd

Limited interaction with patient
Intolerance
Agitation/depression
Abandonment

THERAPEUTIC INTERVENTIONS

- Discuss ways families can continue to be involved in daily care. Address questions or concerns they have about their involvement in the patient's care.
- Relay pertinent questions to physician. *Physician may be able to provide additional information, reassurance, or confrontation.*
- Schedule care conferences *to address impact of family coping.*
- Maintain flexibility in visiting schedule. *Facilitating family/significant other visiting may reduce separation anxiety and increase sense of security.*
- Offer assistance in notifying clergy, other family members, etc., of patient's status. *Can promote a sense of connectedness with significant others.*
- ▲ Refer family to social service, pastoral care, etc. Request social work or psychological consults as indicated.

PATIENT/FAMILY EDUCATION

- Orient to:
    Surroundings (cafeteria, parking, telephone, etc).
    Patient's room (call light, TV, etc.).
    Equipment.
    Health professionals.
- Discuss patient's condition and needed care with the patient and the family. *Distorted ideas, if not clarified, may be more frightening than realistic preparation.*
- Provide information on the stress response *to help families understand what they are experiencing.*
- Provide information about the resources available to assist families under stress (e.g., social services, hot lines, self-help groups, educational opportunities).

By: Nedra Skale, RN, MS, CNA, Meg Gulanick, RN, PhD

Coping, impaired individual

Impaired ability to meet life's demands and role expectations because of maladaptive behaviors or lack of knowledge, support, or problem-solving skills.

RELATED FACTORS / DEFINING CHARACTERISTICS	EXPECTED OUTCOMES AND NURSING INTERVENTIONS / *RATIONALE* (■ = INDEPENDENT; ▲ = COLLABORATIVE)

RELATED FACTORS

Change in or loss of body part
Diagnosis of serious illness
Recent change in health status
Unsatisfactory support system
Inadequate psychological resources (poor self-esteem; lack of motivation)
Personal vulnerability
Inadequate coping method
Situational crises
Maturational crises

DEFINING CHARACTERISTICS

Verbalization of inability to cope
Inability to make decisions
Inability to ask for help
Destructive behavior toward self
Inappropriate use of defense mechanisms

EXPECTED OUTCOMES

Patient identifies own maladaptive coping behaviors.
Patient identifies available resources/support systems.
Patient describes/initiates alternative coping strategies.
Patient describes positive results from new behaviors.

ONGOING ASSESSMENT

- Assess for presence of defining characteristics.
- Assess specific stressors. *Accurate appraisal can facilitate development of appropriate coping strategies.*
- Assess available/useful past and present coping mechanisms. *Successful adjustment is influenced by previous coping success. Patients with history of maladaptive coping may need additional resources.*
- Evaluate resources/support systems available to patient while in hospital and at discharge.
- Assess level of understanding and readiness to learn needed life-style changes.
- Assess decision-making/problem-solving ability.

THERAPEUTIC INTERVENTIONS

- Establish a working relationship with patient through continuity of care. *An ongoing relationship establishes trust.*
- Provide opportunities to express concerns, fears, feelings, expectations.

RELATED FACTORS / DEFINING CHARACTERISTICS	EXPECTED OUTCOMES AND NURSING INTERVENTIONS / *RATIONALE* (■ = INDEPENDENT; ▲ = COLLABORATIVE)

DEFINING CHARACTERISTICS— cont'd

Physical symptoms such as:
  Overeating; lack of appetite
  Overuse of tranquilizers
  Excessive smoking/drinking
  Chronic fatigue
  Headaches
  Irritable bowel
Chronic depression
Emotional tension
High illness rate
Insomnia
General irritability

THERAPEUTIC INTERVENTIONS

- Convey feelings of acceptance and understanding. Avoid false reassurances.
- Encourage patient to identify own strengths and abilities.
- Assist patient to evaluate situation and own accomplishments accurately.
- Explore attitudes and feelings about required life-style changes.
- Encourage patient to seek information that will increase coping skills. *Patients who are not coping well may need more guidance initially.*
- Encourage patient to set realistic goals *to help gain control over situation.*
- Assist patient to problem solve in a constructive manner.
- Discourage decision making when under severe stress.
- Provide information that patient wants and needs. Do not provide more than patient can handle. *Patients who are coping ineffectively have reduced ability to assimilate information.*
- ▲ Meet with medical team to discuss treatment plan *to facilitate consistent care.*
- Reduce stimuli in environment that could be misinterpreted as threatening.
- Provide outlets that foster feelings of personal achievement and self-esteem.
- Point out signs of positive progress or change. *Patients who are coping ineffectively may not be able to assess progress.*
- Encourage patient to communicate feelings with significant others. *Unexpressed feelings can increase stress.*
- Point out maladaptive behaviors *so patient can focus on more appropriate strategies.*
- ▲ Involve social services, psychiatric liaison, pastoral care for additional and ongoing support resources.
- Assist in development of alternative support system. Encourage participation in self-help groups as available. *Relationships with persons with common interests and goals can be beneficial.*
- ▲ Administer tranquilizer, sedative as needed *to facilitate ability to cope.*
- Assist to grieve and work through the losses of chronic illness/change in body function if appropriate.

PATIENT EDUCATION

- Instruct in need for adequate rest and balanced diet *to facilitate coping strengths. Inadequate diet and fatigue can themselves be stressors.*
- Teach use of relaxation, exercise, and diversional activities as methods to cope with stress.

By: Meg Gulanick, RN, PhD

Diarrhea

A change in normal bowel habits characterized by frequent passage of loose, fluid, or unformed stools. Diarrhea may result from infectious processes, primary bowel diseases (such as Crohn's disease), drug therapies (e.g., antibiotics), increased osmotic loads (e.g., tube feedings), or increased intestinal motility, such as irritable bowel disease.

RELATED FACTORS / DEFINING CHARACTERISTICS	EXPECTED OUTCOMES AND NURSING INTERVENTIONS / *RATIONALE* (■ = INDEPENDENT; ▲ = COLLABORATIVE)

RELATED FACTORS

Stress
Anxiety
Medication use
Bowel disorders:
  Inflammation
  Malabsorption

EXPECTED OUTCOMES

Patient passes soft, formed stool no more than 3×/daily.

ONGOING ASSESSMENT

- Assess for abdominal pain, cramping, frequency, urgency, loose/liquid stools, and hyperactive bowel sensations.

Continued.

Diarrhea—cont'd

RELATED FACTORS / DEFINING CHARACTERISTICS	EXPECTED OUTCOMES AND NURSING INTERVENTIONS / *RATIONALE* (■ = INDEPENDENT; ▲ = COLLABORATIVE)

RELATED FACTORS—cont'd

Enteric infections
Disagreeable dietary intake
Tube feedings
Radiation
Chemotherapy
Bowel resection
Short bowel syndrome

DEFINING CHARACTERISTICS

Abdominal pain
Cramping
Frequency of stools
Loose/liquid stools
Urgency
Hyperactive bowel sounds/
sensations

ONGOING ASSESSMENT

- Inquire regarding:
  Drugs patient is or has been taking. *Laxatives and antibiotics may cause diarrhea.*
  Idiosyncratic food intolerances. *Spicy, fatty, or high carbohydrate foods may cause diarrhea*
  Method of food preparation. *Fried food or food contaminated during preparation may cause diarrhea.*
  Osmolality of tube feedings. *Hyperosmolar food or fluid will draw excess fluid into the gut and may stimulate peristalsis.*
  Change in eating schedule
  Level of activity
  Adequacy or privacy for elimination
  Current stressors. *Some individuals respond to stress with hyperactivity of the GI tract.*
- Check for history of:
  Previous GI surgery. *Following bowel resection, a period (1-3 weeks) of diarrhea is normal.*
  GI diseases.
  Abdominal radiation.
- Assess impact of therapeutic or diagnostic regimes on diarrhea. *Preparation for radiograph or surgery, and radiation or chemotherapy predisposes to diarrhea by altering mucosal surface and transit time through bowel.*
- Assess hydration status:
  I & O. *Diarrhea can lead to profound dehydration and electrolyte imbalance.*
  Skin turgor.
  Moisture of mucous membrane.
- Assess condition of perianal skin. *Diarrheal stools may be highly corrosive, due to increased enzyme content.*

THERAPEUTIC INTERVENTIONS

- ▲ Give antidiarrheal drugs as ordered. *Most antidiarrheal drugs suppress GI motility, thus allowing for more fluid absorption.*
- Provide dietary alterations as allowed:
  Bulk (cereal, grains, Metamucil).
  "Natural" antidiarrheals (e.g., pretzels, matzos, cheese).
  Avoidance of stimulants (e.g., caffeine, carbonated beverages).
- Check for fecal impaction by digital examination. *Liquid stool (apparent diarrhea) may seep past a fecal impaction.*
- Minimize emotional impact of illness, hospitalization, and soiling accidents by providing: privacy and opportunity for verbalization.
- Compensate for malabsorption (i.e., provide fluids, consider nutritional support).
- Evaluate appropriateness of physician's radiograph protocols for bowel preparation on basis of age, weight, condition, disease, and other therapies. *Elderly, frail, or those patients already depleted may require less bowel preparation or additional IV fluid therapy during preparation.*
- Assist with/administer perianal care after each BM.
- See Skin integrity, impaired, p. 59.

PATIENT EDUCATION

- Teach patient those etiologic factors that can be controlled:
  Avoid spicy, fatty foods.
  Broil, bake, or boil foods; avoid frying.
  Avoid foods that are disagreeable.
  Report diarrhea that occurs with prescription drugs.
- Teach patient measures that control diarrhea:
  Take antidiarrheal medications as ordered.
  Use "natural" antidiarrheals *(these may differ person to person).*
- Teach patient importance of fluid replacement during episodes.
- Teach patient importance of good perianal hygiene after each BM, *both to control perianal skin excoriation as well as to minimize risk of spread of infectious diarrhea.*

By: Audrey Klopp, RN, PhD, ET

Diversional activity deficit

The state in which an individual experiences a decreased stimulation from or interest or engagement in recreational or leisure activities.

RELATED FACTORS / DEFINING CHARACTERISTICS	EXPECTED OUTCOMES AND NURSING INTERVENTIONS / *RATIONALE* (■ = INDEPENDENT; ▲ = COLLABORATIVE)

RELATED FACTORS

Prolonged hospitalization
Environmental lack of diversional activity
Usual hobbies cannot be undertaken in hospital
Lack of usual level of socialization
Physical inability to perform tasks: isolation, traction, oxygen therapy, and IV therapy

DEFINING CHARACTERISTICS

Verbal expression of boredom
Preoccupation with illness
Frequent use of call light in absence of physical need
Excessive complaints
Withdrawal
Depression

EXPECTED OUTCOMES

Patient's attention is diverted to interests other than illness and hospitalization.

ONGOING ASSESSMENT

- Explore the importance of activity. *Theories of human occupation stress that the benefit(s) of activities are related to the importance assigned.*
- Inquire about patient's interest and hobbies prior to hospitalization (e.g., art, reading, writing, sports).
- Assess attention span.
- Assess for physical limitations.
- Observe and document response to activities.

THERAPEUTIC INTERVENTIONS

- Provide frequent patient contact. Be certain that patient is aware of your presence.
- Set up a schedule with the patient *so he/she will know when to expect contact/activities.*
- Provide and assist with specific physical, cognitive, social, and/or spiritual activities that can be accomplished in current situation.
- ▲ Collaborate with physical, occupational, and/or recreational therapy to plan and implement an acceptable, achievable activity program.
- Suggest new interests (crafts, puzzles, etc.).
- Encourage family/friends to visit and bring diversional materials.
- ▲ Obtain consultants as needed: dietary, social work, psychiatric liaison, volunteers, etc.
- Provide dietary changes if possible. *Most hospital menus rotate weekly or biweekly and soon become repetitive for the long-term patient.*
- Use distraction to focus attention away from current situation.
- Spend time with patient without providing physical care. *Engaging the patient in conversation without focusing on illness will divert the patient's attention and help pass the time.*

PATIENT EDUCATION

- Instruct concerning necessity for continued hospitalization.
- Obtain instructional materials for new hobbies/interests.
- Encourage continuation of education while hospitalized. *May be formal or informal through books.*
- Teach patient/family the benefits of diversional activity (e.g., relaxation, distraction).

By: Sherry Adams, RN, ADN

Dysfunctional ventilatory weaning response (DVWR)

A state in which a patient cannot adjust to lowered levels of mechanical ventilator support, which interrupts and prolongs the weaning process.

RELATED FACTORS / DEFINING CHARACTERISTICS	EXPECTED OUTCOMES AND NURSING INTERVENTIONS / *RATIONALE* (■ = INDEPENDENT; ▲ = COLLABORATIVE)

RELATED FACTORS

Ineffective airway clearance
Sleep pattern disturbance
Inadequate nutrition
Uncontrolled pain or discomfort

EXPECTED OUTCOMES

Patient experiences a functional ventilatory weaning response as evidenced by:
BP, HR, and RR in normal range.
Expressed feelings of comfort.
Responsive/cooperative to coaching.
ABGs within baseline range.
Effective breathing pattern.

Continued.

RELATED FACTORS / DEFINING CHARACTERISTICS	EXPECTED OUTCOMES AND NURSING INTERVENTIONS / *RATIONALE* (■ = INDEPENDENT; ▲ = COLLABORATIVE)

DEFINING CHARACTERISTICS

Mild DVWR
  Restlessness
  Slight increased respiratory rate
  Expressed feelings of increased need for O_2, breathing discomfort, fatigue, and warmth

Moderate DVWR
  Slight increase in BP (<20 mm Hg)
  Slight increase in HR (<20 beats/min)
  Increase in respiratory rate (<5 breaths/min)
  Apprehension
  Diaphoresis
  Pale, slight cyanosis
  "Wide-eyed" look
  Inability to cooperate/respond to coaching
  Decreased air entry on auscultation

Severe DVWR
  Agitation
  Increase in BP (>20 mm Hg)
  Increase in HR (>20 beats/min)
  Increase in respiratory rate (>5 breaths/min)
  Deterioration in ABGs

ONGOING ASSESSMENT

- Assess for increasing restlessness, apprehension, and agitation.
- Monitor vital signs closely during weaning process, watching for increases in BP, HR, and respiratory rate. *These are signs of weaning failure.*
- Assess breath sounds.
▲ Monitor ABGs closely. If available, monitor O_2 saturation by pulse oximetry. *Pulse oximetry is useful in detecting O_2 saturation changes early.*
- Assess skin color and warmth.
- Assess patient's ability to cooperate and to respond to coaching.
- Monitor for signs of respiratory muscle fatigue (abrupt rise in $PaCO_2$, rapid shallow ventilation, paradoxical abdominal wall motion) while weaning is in progress.

THERAPEUTIC INTERVENTIONS

▲ Notify physician and anticipate altering ventilator support dependent on the degree of DVWR.
  Mild DVWR: May be able to remain at the same ventilator setting, but further weaning should be delayed.
  Moderate DVWR: Would require return to higher ventilator setting for a time.
  Severe DVWR: Would require a return to baseline ventilator support for a long rest period.
▲ Maintain the prescribed oxygen level *so that the patient does not desaturate.*
- Individualize the patient's weaning program *to provide adequate rest periods for the patient. This may include alternating periods of "training" (weaning) and resting. Slowing the tempo of the weaning plan may be necessary for a patient potentially difficult to wean or one who has failed weaning.*
- Suction airway as needed *to maintain patency.*
▲ Maintain patient's feedings *to ensure sufficient nutrients to enable weaning.* Collaborate with dietician to ensure that 50% of the diet's non-protein caloric source is fat rather than carbohydrate.
▲ Administer pain medications as appropriate *to relieve uncontrolled pain or discomfort.* However, avoid pharmacologic sedation during weaning trials.
- Assist patient with turning and repositioning during the weaning process *to decrease energy expenditure.*
- Coach the patient through ineffective breathing patterns and episodes of anxiety, assisting him/her to focus on breathing pattern.
- Give continuous feedback to patient *to help keep patient working towards weaning.*
- Establish patient trust:
  Use a calm approach.
  Demonstrate confidence in the patient's abilities.
  Explain things prior to doing them.
  Collaborate with the patient in planning his/her care.
  Provide individual attention. *Patient trust and confidence in the nurse helps to motivate the patient in the weaning process.*
- Determine significant other's effect on the patient during the weaning process. Establish and control visiting times as appropriate. *The significant other may be a positive factor and a great support during the weaning process and then should be allowed to remain at the bedside for extended periods. However, some significant others may have a negative effect, causing the patient to become restless and fight the ventilator.*
- Provide an appropriate environment for weaning: personalized space and a quiet room.
- Assist in normalizing the patient and weaning process *to improve self-esteem:* e.g., grooming; pajamas, items from home, conversation about personal activities, humor, television, music, and reading.

PATIENT EDUCATION

- Discuss with the patient the importance of actively engaging in the work of weaning.
- Discuss with the patient and significant other the importance of setting achievable goals and explain the probable weaning process, including the potential for setbacks. *Minimizing setbacks may help to motivate the patient to try again.*

By: Sue Galanes, RN, MS, CCRN

Family processes, altered

INEFFECTIVE FAMILY COPING

A situation or event that causes a change in family members' roles or expectations. The inability of one or more members to adjust or perform, resulting in family dysfunction and prevention of the growth and development of the family and members.

RELATED FACTORS / DEFINING CHARACTERISTICS	EXPECTED OUTCOMES AND NURSING INTERVENTIONS / *RATIONALE* (■ = INDEPENDENT; ▲ = COLLABORATIVE)

RELATED FACTORS

Illness of family member
Change in socioeconomic status
Births and deaths
Conflict between family members

DEFINING CHARACTERISTICS

Inability to meet physical needs of family members
Inability to function in larger society; no job, no community activity
Inability to meet emotional needs of family members (grief, anxiety, conflict)
Inability to accept or receive needed help
Ineffective family decision-making process
Rigidity in roles, behavior, and beliefs

EXPECTED OUTCOMES

Family develops improved methods of communication.
Family identifies resources available for problem-solving.
Family expresses understanding of mutual problems.

ONGOING ASSESSMENT

- Assess for precipitating events (divorce, illness, life transition, crisis). *Depending on the stressor a variety of strategies may be required to facilitate coping.*
- Assess members' perceptions of problem.
- Evaluate strengths, coping skills, and current support systems. *To utilize previously successful techniques.*
- Identify problems with the family.

THERAPEUTIC INTERVENTIONS

- Provide opportunities to express concerns, fears, expectations, or questions *to promote communication and support.*
- Explore feelings. Identify loneliness, anger, worry, and fear *because the feelings of one family member influence others in the family system.*
- Phrase problems as "family" problems, *so they are owned and dealt with by the family.*
- Encourage members to empathize with other family members *to increase understanding of other's feelings and to foster mutual respect and support.*
- Assist family in setting realistic goals *to help gain control over the situation.*
- Assist family in breaking down problems into manageable parts. Assist with problem-solving process, with delineated responsibilities and follow-through.
- Encourage family members to seek information and resources that will increase coping skills. *Families who are not coping well may need more guidance initially.*
- ▲ Refer family to social service or counseling consultations as indicated. *Professional intervention or assistance may be required.*

PATIENT/FAMILY EDUCATION

- Provide information regarding stressful situation, as appropriate.
- Identify community resources that may be helpful in dealing with particular situations, i.e., hotlines, self-help groups, educational opportunities, social service agencies, and counseling centers. *Groups that come together for mutual support/information exchange can be beneficial in helping family reach goals.*

By: Mary O'Leary, RN, BSN
    Meg Gulanick, RN, PhD

Fear

A strong and unpleasant emotion caused by the awareness or anticipation of pain or danger. This emotion is primarily externally motivated, and its source is specific. The person, place, or thing precipitating this feeling can be identified by the individual experiencing the fear.

RELATED FACTORS / DEFINING CHARACTERISTICS	EXPECTED OUTCOMES AND NURSING INTERVENTIONS / *RATIONALE* (■ = INDEPENDENT; ▲ = COLLABORATIVE)

RELATED FACTORS

Anticipation of pain
Anticipation or perceived threat of danger

EXPECTED OUTCOMES

Patient identifies source of fear.
Patient implements a positive coping mechanism.
Patient verbalizes reduction/absence of fear.

Continued.

Nursing Diagnosis Care Plans

RELATED FACTORS / DEFINING CHARACTERISTICS	EXPECTED OUTCOMES AND NURSING INTERVENTIONS / *RATIONALE* (■ = INDEPENDENT; ▲ = COLLABORATIVE)

RELATED FACTORS— cont'd

Unfamiliar environment
Environmental stimuli
Separation from support system
Treatments and invasive procedures
Threat of death
Language barrier
Knowledge deficit
Sensory impairment
Specific phobias

DEFINING CHARACTERISTICS

Identifies object of fear
Increased respirations, heart rate, and respiratory rate
Denial
Tension
Frightened
Jittery
Apprehensive
Impulsive
Scared
Alertness
Wide-eyed

ONGOING ASSESSMENT

- Determine what the patient is fearful of by careful/thoughtful questioning. *The external source of fear can be identified and current responses can be assessed.*
- Assess the degree of fear and the measures patient uses to cope with that fear (this can be done by interviewing the patient and significant others). *Helps determine the effectiveness of coping strategies used by the patient.*
- Document behavioral and verbal expressions of fear. *Symptoms will provide information regarding the degree of fear. Physiologic symptoms and/or complaints will intensify as the level of fear increases. Note that fear differs from anxiety in that it is a response to a recognized and usually external threat. Manifestations of fear are similar to those of anxiety.*

THERAPEUTIC INTERVENTIONS

- Acknowledge your awareness of the patient's fear. *This will validate the feelings the patient is having and communicate an acceptance of those feelings.*
- Stay with patient to promote safety, especially during frightening procedures or treatments. *The presence of a trusted person assures the patient of security and safety during a period of fear.*
- Maintain a calm and tolerant manner while interacting with patient. *Patient's feeling of stability increases in a calm and nonthreatening atmosphere.*
- Establish a working relationship through continuity of care. *An ongoing relationship establishes trust and a basis for communicating fearful feelings.*
- Orient to the environment as needed. *This promotes comfort and a decrease in fear.*
- Use simple language and brief statements when instructing patient regarding diagnostic and surgical procedures. Explain what physical/sensory sensations will be experienced. *When experiencing excessive fear or dread, patient may be unable to comprehend more than simple, clear, and brief instructions.*
- Reduce sensory stimulation by maintaining a quiet environment. Remove unnecessary threatening equipment. *Fear may escalate with excessive conversation, noise, and equipment around the patient. Though staff are comfortable around "high-tech"/medical equipment, patients are not.*
- Assist patient in identifying strategies used to deal with fears in the past which were helpful or comforting. *This helps patient focus on fear as a real and natural part of life that has been and can continue to be dealt with successfully.*
- As patient's fear subsides, encourage him/her to explore specific events preceding the onset of the fear. *Recognition and explanation of factors leading to fear are significant in developing alternative responses.*
- Encourage rest periods *to improve ability to cope.*
- Suggest bringing in comforting objects from home (music, pillow, blanket, pictures).

PATIENT EDUCATION

- Reinforce the idea that fear is a normal and appropriate response to situations when pain, danger, or loss of control is anticipated or experienced.
- Instruct patient in the performance of self-calming measures that may reduce fear or make it more manageable:
    Breathing modifications *to reduce the physiologic response to fear (i.e., increased BP, pulse, respiration)*
    Exercises in relaxation, meditation, or guided imagery.
    Exercises in the use of affirmations and calming self-talk *to enhance the patient's sense of confidence and reassurance.*

By: Ursula Brozek, RN, MSN
　　Meg Gulanick, RN, PhD

Fluid volume deficit

A state of vascular, cellular, or intracellular dehydration.

RELATED FACTORS / DEFINING CHARACTERISTICS	EXPECTED OUTCOMES AND NURSING INTERVENTIONS / *RATIONALE* (■ – INDEPENDENT; ▲ = COLLABORATIVE)

RELATED FACTORS

Inadequate fluid intake
Active fluid loss (diuresis, abnormal drainage/bleeding, diarrhea)
Electrolyte/acid-base imbalances
Increased metabolic rate (fever, infection)
Fluid shifts (edema/effusions)

DEFINING CHARACTERISTICS

Decreased urine output
Concentrated urine
Dilute urine
Output greater than intake
Sudden weight loss
Decreased venous filling
Hemoconcentration
Increased serum sodium
Hypotension
Thirst
Increased pulse rate
Decreased skin turgor
Dry mucous membranes
Weakness
Sunken fontanels
Possible weight gain
Edema
Changes in mental status

EXPECTED OUTCOMES

Patient experiences adequate fluid volume and electrolyte balance as evidenced by urine output >30 ml/hr, normotensive BP, HR <100/min, consistency of weight, and normal skin turgor.

ONGOING ASSESSMENT

- Assess turgor and mucous membranes for signs of dehydration.
- Assess color and amount of urine. Report urine output <30 ml/hr for 2 consecutive hours. *Concentrated urine denotes fluid deficit.*
- Weigh daily with same scale, preferably at the same time of day, *to evaluate true fluid status, and to monitor trends.*
- Monitor temperature. *Febrile states decrease body fluids through perspiration and increased respiration.*
- Monitor active fluid loss from wound drainage, tubes, diarrhea, bleeding, and vomiting; maintain accurate I & O.
- Evaluate specific etiology for fluid deficit *to guide intervention* (fever, diarrhea, fatigue at meals, GI bleeding). Refer to Diarrhea, p. 19; Nutrition, altered: less than body requirements, p. 44; Gastrointestinal bleeding, p. 311; Diabetes, p. 490.
- Determine patient's fluid preferences: type, temperature (hot/cold).
- ▲ Monitor serum electrolytes/urine osmolality and report abnormal values.
- Document baseline mental status and record during each nursing shift. *Dehydration can alter mental status.*
- Monitor and document vital signs.
- Observe for signs of orthostatic hypotension (drop of greater than 15 mm when changing from supine to sitting position). *This indicates reduced circulating fluids.*
- Evaluate whether patient has any related heart problem prior to initiating parenteral therapy. *Cardiac patients often have precarious fluid balance and are prone to develop pulmonary edema.*
- During treatment, monitor closely for signs of circulatory overload (headache, flushed skin, tachycardia, venous distention, elevated CVP, shortness of breath, increased BP, tachypnea, cough).
- ▲ Monitor hemodynamic status including CVP, MAP, PAP, and PCWP if available.

THERAPEUTIC INTERVENTIONS

- ▲ Encourage patient to drink prescribed fluid amounts. If oral fluids are tolerated, provide oral fluids patient prefers. Place at bedside within easy reach. Provide fresh water and a straw. Be creative in selecting fluid sources (Jell-O, popsicles, Gatorade).
- Assist patient if unable to feed self and encourage significant other to assist with feedings as appropriate.
- Plan daily activities *so patient is not too tired at mealtimes.*
- Provide oral hygiene *to promote interest in drinking.*
- ▲ Obtain and maintain a large-bore IV.
- ▲ Administer parenteral fluids as ordered. Anticipate the need for an IV fluid challenge with immediate infusion of fluids for patients with abnormal vital signs.
- ▲ Administer blood products as prescribed.
- ▲ Assist the physician with insertion of a central venous line and arterial line as indicated *for more effective fluid administration and monitoring.*
- ▲ Maintain IV flow rate. *Infants and elderly patients are especially susceptible to fluid overload.* Should signs of fluid overload occur, stop infusion and sit patient up or dangle *to decrease venous return and optimize breathing.*
- ▲ Institute measures to control excessive electrolyte loss (e.g., resting the GI tract, administering antipyretics as ordered).
- ▲ Once ongoing fluid losses have stopped, begin to advance the diet in volume and composition.

Continued.

Fluid volume deficit—cont'd

RELATED FACTORS / DEFINING CHARACTERISTICS	EXPECTED OUTCOMES AND NURSING INTERVENTIONS / *RATIONALE* (■ = INDEPENDENT; ▲ = COLLABORATIVE)
	PATIENT EDUCATION · Describe/teach causes of fluid losses or decreased fluid intake. · Explain/reinforce rationale and intended effect of treatment program. · Explain importance of maintaining proper nutrition and hydration. · Teach interventions to prevent future episodes of inadequate intake. · Identify symptoms to be reported. · Teach safe use and potential side effects of medications. · Inform patient/significant other of importance of maintaining prescribed fluid intake and special diet considerations involved.

By: Sue Galanes, RN, MS, CCRN

Fluid volume excess   *State of increased fluid retention and edema.*

RELATED FACTORS / DEFINING CHARACTERISTICS	EXPECTED OUTCOMES AND NURSING INTERVENTIONS / *RATIONALE* (■ = INDEPENDENT; ▲ = COLLABORATIVE)

RELATED FACTORS

Excessive fluid intake
Excessive sodium intake
Renal insufficiency or failure
Steroid therapy
Low protein intake/ malnutrition
Decreased cardiac output; chronic or acute heart disease
Head injury
Liver disease
Severe stress
Hormonal disturbances

DEFINING CHARACTERISTICS

Weight gain
Edema
Bounding pulses
Shortness of breath; orthopnea
Pulmonary congestion on x-ray film
Abnormal breath sounds: crackles (rales)
Change in respiratory pattern
Third heart sound
Intake greater than output
Decreased hemoglobin/ hematocrit
Increased blood pressure
Increased CVP
Increased pulmonary artery pressures
Jugular vein distension
Change in mental status (lethargy or confusion)
Oliguria
Specific gravity changes
Azotemia
Change in electrolytes
Restlessness and anxiety

EXPECTED OUTCOMES

Patient maintains adequate fluid volume and electrolyte balance as evidenced by: vital signs within normal limits, clear breath sounds, pulmonary congestion absent on x-ray, and resolution of edema.

ONGOING ASSESSMENT

· Obtain patient history *to ascertain the probable cause of the fluid disturbance, which can help to guide interventions.*
· Assess weight daily and consistently, with same scale, and preferably at the same time of day *to facilitate accurate measurement and to follow trends.*
· Monitor for a significant (>2 lb) weight change in one day.
· Evaluate weight in relation to nutritional status. *In some heart failure patients, weight may be a poor indicator of fluid volume status. Poor nutrition and decreased appetite over time result in a decrease in weight, which may be accompanied by fluid retention even though the net weight remains unchanged.*
· Monitor and document vital signs.
· Monitor hemodynamic status including CVP, MAP, PAP, and PCWP, if available.
· Monitor for distended neck veins, a third heart sound, and bounding peripheral pulses, *all of which are signs of fluid overload.*
· Assess for crackles in lungs, changes in respiratory pattern, shortness of breath, and orthopnea *for early recognition of pulmonary congestion.*
· Assess for presence of generalized or pitting edema by palpating over tibia, ankles, feet, and sacrum. *Pitting edema is manifested by a depression that remains after one's finger is pressed over an edematous area and then removed. Grade edema 1+ indicates edema that is barely perceptible, to grade 4+, which indicates severe edema. Measurement of an extremity with a measuring tape is another method of following edema.*
▲ *Monitor chest x-ray reports.*
· *Monitor I & O closely.*
▲ *Monitor serum electrolytes, urine osmolality, and urine specific gravity.*
· *Assess the need for an in-dwelling urinary catheter. Treatment will focus upon diuresis of excess fluid.*
· During therapy, monitor for signs of hypovolemia *to prevent complications associated with therapy.*

THERAPEUTIC INTERVENTIONS

▲ Institute fluid restrictions as appropriate:
    Discontinue or decrease PO intake.
    Discontinue or decrease IV infusion.
    Decrease oral and IV salt intake.
▲ Collaborate with the pharmacist to maximally concentrate IVs and medications *in order to decrease unnecessary fluids.*
· Apply heparin lock on IV line *to maintain patency but to decrease fluid delivered to patient in a 24-hour period.*

RELATED FACTORS / DEFINING CHARACTERISTICS	EXPECTED OUTCOMES AND NURSING INTERVENTIONS / *RATIONALE* (■ = INDEPENDENT; ▲ = COLLABORATIVE)

THERAPEUTIC INTERVENTIONS

- Administer IV fluids via infusion pump, if possible, *to ensure accurate delivery of IV fluids.*
- ▲ Administer diuretics as ordered *to promote a fluid diuresis.*
- ▲ Administer IV inotropic agents as ordered. *Patients with heart disease may develop a decrease in contractility that could be assisted by an inotropic agent.*
- Elevate edematous extremities *to increase venous return and, in turn, decrease edema.*
- Reduce constriction of vessels (use appropriate garments, avoid crossing of legs or ankles) *to prevent venous pooling.*
- ▲ Apply antiembolic stockings or bandages as ordered *to help promote venous return and to minimize fluid accumulation in the extremities.*
- Provide adequate activity/position changes as able *to prevent fluid accumulation in dependent areas.* Assist with repositioning q2h if patient is not mobile.

PATIENT EDUCATION

- Teach causes of fluid volume excess and/or excess intake to patient/significant other.
- Provide information as needed regarding the individual's medical diagnosis (e.g., CHF, renal failure).
- Explain/reinforce rationale and intended effect of treatment program.
- Identify signs and symptoms of fluid volume excess.
- Explain importance of maintaining proper nutrition and hydration, and diet modifications.
- Identify symptoms to be reported.

By: Sue Galanes, RN, MS

Gas exchange, impaired

A state in which the individual experiences an imbalance between oxygen uptake and carbon dioxide elimination at the alveolar-capillary membrane gas exchange area.

RELATED FACTORS / DEFINING CHARACTERISTICS	EXPECTED OUTCOMES AND NURSING INTERVENTIONS / *RATIONALE* (■ = INDEPENDENT; ▲ = COLLABORATIVE)

RELATED FACTORS

Altered O_2 supply
Alveolar-capillary membrane changes
Altered blood flow
Altered oxygen-carrying capacity of blood

DEFINING CHARACTERISTICS

Confusion
Somnolence
Restlessness
Irritability
Inability to move secretions
Hypercapnia
Hypoxia

EXPECTED OUTCOMES

Patient maintains optimal gas exchange as evidenced by normal ABGs and alert responsive mentation or no further reduction in mental status.

ONGOING ASSESSMENT

- Assess respirations: note quality, rate, pattern, depth, flaring of nostrils, dyspnea on exertion, evidence of splinting, use of accessory muscles, position assumed for easy breathing.
- Auscultate breath sounds every shift, noting areas of decreased ventilation and the presence of adventitious sounds.
- Monitor vital signs, noting any changes. *With initial hypoxia and hypercapnia, BP, heart rate, and respiratory rate all rise. As the hypoxia and/or hypercapnia becomes more severe, BP may drop, heart rate tends to continue to be rapid with arrhythmias, and respiratory failure may ensue, with the patient unable to maintain the rapid respiratory rate.*
- Assess for changes in orientation and behavior.
- Assess patient's ability to cough effectively to clear secretions. Note quantity, color, and consistency of sputum.
- ▲ Monitor arterial blood gases (ABGs) and note changes.
- Assess for presence of central cyanosis.
- ▲ Monitor chest x-ray reports.
- Monitor effects of position changes on oxygenation (SaO_2, ABGs, SvO_2, and end tidal CO_2).

THERAPEUTIC INTERVENTIONS

- ▲ Maintain the prescribed oxygen delivery system at appropriate levels *so that the patient does not desaturate. Note: If the patient is allowed to eat, O_2 still must be given to the patient, but perhaps in a different manner, e.g., changing from mask to a nasal cannula. Eating is an activity and more O_2 will be consumed than when the patient is at rest. Immediately after the meal, the original oxygen delivery system should be returned.*

Continued.

Gas exchange, impaired—cont'd

RELATED FACTORS / DEFINING CHARACTERISTICS	EXPECTED OUTCOMES AND NURSING INTERVENTIONS / *RATIONALE* (■ = INDEPENDENT; ▲ = COLLABORATIVE)
	THERAPEUTIC INTERVENTIONS ▲ Utilize pulse oximetry, as available, *to continuously monitor O_2 saturation and pulse rate.* Keep alarms on at all times. *Pulse oximetry has been found to be a useful tool in the clinical setting to detect changes in oxygenation.* ■ Position with proper body alignment for optimal respiratory excursion (if tolerated, head of bed at >45 degrees). *This promotes lung expansion and improves air exchange.* ■ Routinely check the patient's position so he/she does not slide down in bed, *causing the abdomen to compress the diaphragm, which would cause respiratory embarrassment.* ■ Position patient to facilitate ventilation/perfusion matching (good side down). ■ Pace activities and schedule rest periods *to prevent fatigue. Even simple activities (such as bathing) during bed rest can cause fatigue and increase oxygen consumption.* ■ Change patient's position every 2 hours. *This will facilitate secretion movement and drainage.* ■ Suction as needed *to clear secretions.* ■ Provide reassurance and allay anxiety: Have an agreed-upon method for the patient to call for assistance (e.g., call light, bell). Stay with the patient during episodes of respiratory distress. ■ Anticipate need for intubation and mechanical ventilation if patient is unable to maintain adequate gas exchange. **PATIENT EDUCATION** ■ Explain the need to restrict and pace activities *to decrease oxygen consumption during the acute episode.* ■ Explain the type of oxygen therapy being utilized and why its maintenance is important. ■ Teach the patient appropriate deep breathing and coughing techniques *to facilitate adequate air exchange and secretion clearance.*

By: Sue Galanes, RN, MS, CCRN

Grieving, anticipatory

A state in which an individual grieves before an actual loss. It may apply to individuals who suffer a perinatal loss or loss of a body part or to patients who have received a terminal diagnosis for themselves or a loved one. Intense mental anguish or a sense of deep remorse may be experienced by patients and their families as they face long-term illness or disability. This care plan discusses measures the nurse can use to help patient and family members begin the process of grieving.

RELATED FACTORS / DEFINING CHARACTERISTICS	EXPECTED OUTCOMES AND NURSING INTERVENTIONS / *RATIONALE* (■ = INDEPENDENT; ▲ = COLLABORATIVE)

RELATED FACTORS
Perceived potential loss of significant other
Perceived potential loss of physiopsychosocial well-being
Perceived potential loss of personal possession
Situational crisis
Maturational crisis
Family crisis
 	
DEFINING CHARACTERISTICS
Client shows distress at prospect of loss
	EXPECTED OUTCOMES
	Patient verbalizes feelings and establishes and maintains functional support systems.
	
	ONGOING ASSESSMENT
	■ Identify behaviors suggestive of the grieving process (see defining characteristics).
	■ Assess stage of grieving being experienced by client or significant others:
	    denial, anger, bargaining, depression, and acceptance. *Although grief is anticipatory, stages similar to actual grief may be seen, and, like grief, the patient may move from stage to stage and back again, before acceptance occurs.*
	■ Assess the influence of the following factors on coping:
	    past problem-solving abilities, socioeconomic background, educational preparation, cultural beliefs, and spiritual beliefs. *Individuals with successful coping skills may reach and maintain the stage of acceptance more easily.*
	■ Assess whether the client and significant others differ in their stage of grieving.
	■ Identify support systems available: family, peer support, primary physician, consulting physician, nursing staff, clergy, therapist/counselor, and professional/lay support group. *If the patient's main support is the object of perceived loss, the patient's need for help in identifying support is accentuated.*

RELATED FACTORS / DEFINING CHARACTERISTICS	EXPECTED OUTCOMES AND NURSING INTERVENTIONS / *RATIONALE* (■ = INDEPENDENT; ▲ = COLLABORATIVE)

DEFINING CHARACTERISTICS— cont'd

Denial of potential loss
Sorrow
Crying
Guilt
Anger/hostility
Bargaining
Depression
Acceptance
Changes in eating habits
Alteration in activity level
Altered libido
Altered communication patterns
Fear
Hopelessness
Distortion of reality

ONGOING ASSESSMENT

- Identify potential for pathologic grieving response (see Grieving, dysfunctional, p. 30). *Anticipatory grief is helpful in preparing an individual to do actual grief work. Those who do not grieve in anticipation may be at higher risk for dysfunctional grief.*
- Evaluate need for referral to social security representatives, legal consultants, or support groups.
- Observe nonverbal communication. *Body language may communicate a great deal of information.*

THERAPEUTIC INTERVENTIONS

- Establish rapport with patient and significant others. Listen and encourage patient/significant others to verbalize feelings. *This opens lines of communication and facilitates successful resolution of grief.*
- Recognize stages of grief; apply nursing measures aimed at that specific stage. *Shock and disbelief are initial responses to loss. Reality is overwhelming; denial, panic, and anxiety may be seen.*
- Provide safe environment for expression of grief.
- Minimize environmental stresses/stimuli.
- Remain with patient throughout procedures.
- Accept need to deny loss as part of normal grief process. *Realization occurs weeks to months after loss. Reality continues to be overwhelming; sadness, anger, guilt, hostility may be seen.*
- Anticipate increased affective behavior.
- Recognize need to maintain hope for future.
- Provide realistic information about health status without false reassurances or taking away hope. *Defensive retreat occurs weeks to months after loss. Patient attempts to maintain what has been lost; denial, wishful thinking, unwillingness to participate in self-care, and indifference may be seen.*
- Recognize that regression may be an adaptive mechanism.
- Support, positively reinforce efforts to perform self-care.
- Offer encouragement: point out strengths and progress to date.
- Discuss possible need for outside support systems (i.e., peer support, groups, clergy). *Acknowledgment occurs months to year after loss. Patient slowly realizes impact of loss; depression, anxiety, bitterness may be seen.*
- Help patient list importance of rehabilitation needs.
- Encourage patient's/significant others' active involvement with rehabilitation team.
- Continue to reinforce strengths, progress. *Adaptation occurs during first year, or later, after the loss. Patient continues to reorganize resources, abilities, and self-image.*
- Recognize patient's need to review (relive) illness experience.
- Facilitate reorganization by reviewing progress.
- Discuss possible involvement with peers/organizations (e.g., stroke club, arthritis foundation) that work with patient's medical condition.
- Recognize that each patient is unique and will progress at own pace. *Time frames vary widely. Cultural, religious, ethnic, individual differences impact on manner of grieving.*
Throughout the stages:
- Provide as much privacy as possible.
- Allow use of denial and other defense mechanisms.
- Avoid reinforcing denial.
- Avoid judgmental and defensive responses to criticisms of health care providers.
- Do not encourage use of pharmacologic interventions.
- Do not force patient to make decisions.
- Provide patient with ongoing information, diagnosis, prognosis, progress, and plan of care.
- Encourage significant others to assist with patient's physical care.
- Facilitate flexible visiting hours and include younger children and extended family when appropriate.
- Help patient and significant others to share mutual fears, concerns, plans, and hopes for each other.
- Help significant others to understand that patient's verbalizations of anger should not be perceived as personal attacks.
- Encourage significant others to maintain their own self-care needs for rest, sleep, nutrition, leisure activities, and time away from patient.

Continued.

Grieving, anticipatory—cont'd

RELATED FACTORS / DEFINING CHARACTERISTICS	EXPECTED OUTCOMES AND NURSING INTERVENTIONS / *RATIONALE* (■ = INDEPENDENT; ▲ = COLLABORATIVE)
	THERAPEUTIC INTERVENTIONS • Facilitate discussion with patient and significant other on "final arrangements," (e.g., burial, autopsy, organ donation, funeral). • Provide information about support groups. *Participation in group activities with others who have experienced similar circumstances may help couple successfully work through grief process.* If the grief is the result of an imminent death: • Promote discussion on what to expect when death occurs. • Encourage significant others and client/patient to share their wishes about which family members should be present at time of death. • Help significant others to accept that not being present at time of death does not indicate lack of love or caring. • Utilize a visual method to identify the patient's critical status, i.e., color-coded door marker. *This will inform all hospital personnel of the patient's status in an effort to ensure that staff do not act or respond inappropriately to crisis situation.* • Initiate process that provides additional support and resources. ▲ Refer to other resources: counseling, pastoral support, group therapy, etc. *Patient/ significant other may need additional help to deal with individual concerns.* • Provide anticipatory guidance and follow-up as condition continues. **PATIENT EDUCATION** • Involve significant others in discussions. *This helps to reinforce understanding of all individuals involved.* • Orient patient/family to hospital procedures (cafeteria, local restaurants, rest facilities/ lounges, etc.).

By: Mary Leslie Caldwell, RN, Charlotte Razvi, RN, MSN, PhD

Grieving, dysfunctional

FAILURE TO GRIEVE

A state in which an individual is unable or unwilling to acknowledge or mourn an actual or perceived loss. This subsequently may impair further growth, development, or functioning.

RELATED FACTORS / DEFINING CHARACTERISTICS	EXPECTED OUTCOMES AND NURSING INTERVENTIONS / *RATIONALE* (■ = INDEPENDENT; ▲ = COLLABORATIVE)

RELATED FACTORS
Ambivalence toward lost object
Inability to participate in socially sanctioned mourning process and rituals
Concurrent overwhelming stress
Absence of support
 	
DEFINING CHARACTERISTICS
Mild to moderate decrease in mood
Constricted affect
Avoidance of affectively charged topics
Somatic complaints
Regression
Guilt or rumination
Withdrawal from others and/or normal activities
Marked change or deviation from usual behavior pattern
"Acting out" behavior
Patient/significant others report failure to grieve
	EXPECTED OUTCOMES
	Patient begins process of grieving, as evidenced by participation in activities, ability to discuss loss, and absence of somatic complaints.
	
	ONGOING ASSESSMENT
	• Identify actual/potential loss(es).
	• Explore nature of individual's past attitudes/relationship with lost object or person. *Ambivalence toward the lost object or person may contribute to dysfunctional grief.*
	• Assess past coping style and mechanisms used in stressful situations.
	• Assess current affective state:
	   Observe for presence/absence of emotional distress.
	   Observe quality/quantity of communication (verbal and nonverbal).
	• Assess degree of relatedness to others.
	• Determine degree of insight in present situation.
	• Identify disturbing topics of conversation or experiences.
	• Estimate degree of stress currently experienced.
	
	THERAPEUTIC INTERVENTIONS
	• Communicate comfort in patient's discussion of loss and grief.
	• Offer feedback regarding patient's expressed feelings.
	• Encourage/facilitate expressions of acceptance or offers of emotional support by significant others to patient.
	• Recognize variation and need for individual adjustment to loss and change.
	• Recognize the need for the use of defense mechanisms. Do not personalize negative expressions or affect or unduly challenge some use of denial.

RELATED FACTORS / DEFINING CHARACTERISTICS	EXPECTED OUTCOMES AND NURSING INTERVENTIONS / *RATIONALE* (▪ = INDEPENDENT; ▲ = COLLABORATIVE)

THERAPEUTIC INTERVENTIONS

- ▪ Reassure patient and significant others that some negative thoughts and feelings are normal. *Concern about how others may view one's full range of feelings may lead to further impediments in grieving process and increase a sense of isolation and loss.*
- ▪ Support the use of adaptive coping mechanisms.
- ▪ Discuss the actual loss with patient:
  Support a realistic assessment of the event/situation.
  Explore with the patient individual strengths and available resources.
  Explore reasons for avoidance of feeling or acknowledging loss.
  Review common changes in behavior associated with normal grieving (e.g., change in appetite and sleep patterns) with patient and significant others. Explain that although intensity and frequency decrease with time, the mourning period may continue longer.
  Discuss normal coping behaviors in grief recovery (e.g., need for contact with others).
- ▪ Encourage sharing of common problems with others.
- ▲ Initiate referrals to others as appropriate.

PATIENT EDUCATION

- ▪ Explain that emotional response to loss is appropriate and commonly experienced:
  Describe the "normal" stages of grief and mourning (denial, anger, bargaining, depression, acceptance).
  Offer hope that emotional pain will decrease with time. *Many view the overt expression of feelings as a "weakness" or fear that they may lose control if they begin to acknowledge the depth of their emotions.*

By: Ann Filipski, RN, MSN, CS, PsyD candidate

Health maintenance, altered

Altered health maintenance reflects a change in an individual's ability to perform the functions necessary to maintain health or wellness. That individual may already manifest symptoms of existing/impending physical ailment or display behaviors that are strongly or certainly linked to disease. The nurse's role is to identify factors that contribute to an individual's ability to maintain healthy behavior and implement measures that will result in improved health maintenance activities.

RELATED FACTORS / DEFINING CHARACTERISTICS	EXPECTED OUTCOMES AND NURSING INTERVENTIONS / *RATIONALE* (▪ = INDEPENDENT; ▲ = COLLABORATIVE)

RELATED FACTORS

Presence of mental retardation, illness, organic brain syndrome
Presence of physical disabilities/challenges
Presence of adverse personal habits:
  Smoking
  Poor diet selection
  Morbid obesity
  Alcohol abuse
  Drug abuse
  Poor hygiene
  Lack of exercise
Evidence of impaired perception
Low income
Lack of knowledge
Poor housing conditions

EXPECTED OUTCOMES

Patient describes positive health maintenance behaviors, such as keeping scheduled appointments, participating in smoking and substance abuse programs, making diet and exercise changes, improving home environment, and following treatment regime.
Patient identifies available resources.
Patient uses available resources.

ONGOING ASSESSMENT

- ▪ Assess for physical defining characteristics. *Changing ability/interest in performing the normal activities of daily living may be an indicator that committment to health and well-being is waning.*
- ▪ Assess patient's knowledge of health maintenance behaviors. *A knowledge deficit is not always the cause of poor health habits, but it needs to be ruled out.*
- ▪ Assess health history over past 5 years. *This may give some perspective on whether poor health habits are recent or chronic in nature.*
- ▪ Assess to what degree environmental, social, interfamilial disruptions/changes have correlated with poor health behaviors.
- ▪ Determine patient's specific questions related to health maintenance.
- ▪ Determine patient's motives for failing to report symptoms reflecting changes in health status. *Patient may not want to "bother" the provider, or may minimize the importance of the symptoms.*

Continued.

Health maintenance, altered—cont'd

RELATED FACTORS / DEFINING CHARACTERISTICS	EXPECTED OUTCOMES AND NURSING INTERVENTIONS / *RATIONALE* (■ = INDEPENDENT; ▲ = COLLABORATIVE)

RELATED FACTORS—cont'd

Inability to communicate needs adequately (e.g., deafness, speech impediment)

Dramatic change in health status

Lack of support systems

Denial of need to change current habits

DEFINING CHARACTERISTICS

Demonstrated lack of knowledge

Failure to keep appointments

Expressed interest in improving behaviors

Failure to recognize/respond to important symptoms reflective of changing health state

Inability to follow instructions/programs for health maintenance

Physical characteristics may include:
  Body/mouth odor
  Unusual skin color, pallor
  Poor hygiene
  Clothing soiled
  Frequent infections (e.g., upper respiratory infection [URI], urinary tract infection [UTI])
  Frequent toothaches
  Obesity/anorexia
  Anemia
  Chronic fatigue
  Apathetic attitude
  Substance abuse

ONGOING ASSESSMENT

- Discuss noncompliance with instructions/programs with patient *to determine rationale for failure.*
- Assess patient's educational preparation and ability to integrate and relate information.
- Assess history of other adverse personal habits, including: smoking, obesity, lack of exercise, and alcohol/substance abuse.
- Determine whether the patient's manual dexterity or lack of mobility is a factor in patient's altered capacity for health maintenance. *Patients may need assistive devices for ambulation or to complete tasks of daily living.*
- Determine to what degree patient's cultural beliefs and personality contribute to altered health habits. *Health teaching may need to be modified to be consistent with cultural or religious beliefs.*
- Determine whether the required health maintenance facilities/equipment (e.g., access ramps, motor vehicle modifications, shower bar/chair, etc.) are available to patient.
- Assess whether economic problems present a barrier to maintaining health behaviors. *Patients may be too proud to ask for assistance or be unaware of the benefits of Medicare or insurance coverage.*
- Assess hearing, orientation to time, place, and person *to determine the patient's perceptual abilities.*
- ▲ Obtain home assessment from visiting nurse *to determine accessibility and quality of living conditions. A trained health provider may be able to identify and solve problems in critical areas.*
- Assess patient's experience of stress/disruptors as they relate to health habits. *If stressors can be relieved, patients may again be able to resume their self-care activities.*

THERAPEUTIC INTERVENTIONS

- Follow up clinic visits with telephone/home visits *to develop ongoing relationship with patient and to vocalize support for client.*
- Provide patient with a means of contacting health care providers who will be available for questions/problem solution.
- Compliment patient on positive accomplishments *to reinforce behaviors.*
- Involve family and friends in health planning conferences.
- ▲ Ensure that other agencies (Department of Children and Family Services [DCFS], Social Services, Visiting Nurse Association [VNA], Meals on Wheels, etc.) are following through with plans.
- Provide assistive devices (i.e., walker, cane, wheelchair) as necessary.

PATIENT EDUCATION

- Provide patient with rationale for importance of behaviors such as:
  Balanced diet low in cholesterol *to prevent vascular disease.*
  Smoking cessation: *smoking has been directly linked to cancer and heart disease.*
  Cessation of alcohol and drug abuse. *In addition to physical addictions, the physical consequences of substance abuse mitigate against it.*
  Regular exercise/rest *to promote weight loss and increase agility and stamina.*
  Proper hygiene *to decrease risk of infection and promote maintenance and integrity of skin and teeth.*
  Regular physical and dental checkups *to identify and treat problems early.*
  Reporting of unusual symptoms to a health professional *to initiate early treatment.*
  Proper nutrition.
  Regular inoculations.

By: Deidra Gradishar, RNC, BS

Health-seeking behavior

A state in which an individual in stable health is actively seeking ways to alter personal health habits and/or the environment in order to move toward a higher level of health. These can range from stress management, weight loss, proper diet, and exercise to smoking cessation. This care plan will give a general overview of health-seeking behavior and then focus on one specific type— smoking cessation.

RELATED FACTORS / DEFINING CHARACTERISTICS	EXPECTED OUTCOMES AND NURSING INTERVENTIONS / *RATIONALE* (■ = INDEPENDENT; ▲ = COLLABORATIVE)

RELATED FACTORS

New condition, altered health status

Lack of awareness about environmental hazards affecting personal health

Absence of interpersonal support

Limited availability of health care resources

Unfamiliarity with community wellness resources

Lack of knowledge about health promotion behaviors

DEFINING CHARACTERISTICS

Perceives optimum health as a primary life purpose

Expresses desire to seek higher level of wellness

Expresses concern about current health status

Demonstrated or observed lack of knowledge of health promotion behaviors

Actively seeks resources to expand wellness knowledge

Expresses sense of self-confidence and personal efficacy toward health promotion

Verbalizes perceived control of health

Anticipates internal and external threats to health status and desires to take preventive action

EXPECTED OUTCOMES

Patient identifies necessary environmental changes to promote a healthier lifestyle.

Patient engages in desired behaviors to promote a healthier lifestyle.

I. GENERAL:

ONGOING ASSESSMENT

- Determine cultural influences on health teaching. *Educational materials must be adapted to cultural beliefs and attitudes.*
- Question patient regarding previous experiences and health teaching. *Adults bring many life experiences to learning sessions.*
- Assess patient's individual perceptions of health problems. *According to the Health Belief Model, the patient's perceived susceptibility to and perceived seriousness and threat of disease affect health seeking behaviors.*
- Identify priority of learning need within the overall plan of care. *Patients learn material most important to them.*
- Identify any misconceptions regarding material to be taught.
- Assess patient's confidence in his/her ability to perform desired behavior. *According to the self-efficacy theory, positive conviction that one can successfully execute a behavior is correlated with performance and successful outcome.*
- Identify patient's specific strengths and competencies. *Every patient brings unique strengths to the health planning task, (i.e., motivation, knowledge, social support).*
- Identify health goals and areas for improvement. *Systematically reviewing areas for potential change can assist patients in making informed choices.*
- Identify possible barriers to change, (i.e., lack of motivation, interpersonal support, skills, knowledge, or resources). *If the patient is aware of possible barriers and has formulated plans for dealing with them should they arise, successful behavioral change is more likely to occur.*

THERAPEUTIC INTERVENTIONS

- Encourage participation of family/significant others in proposed changes. *This may enhance overall adaptation to change.*
- Assist patient in developing a self-contract. *Enhances patient's control over behavior, creating a sense of independence, competence, and autonomy.*
- Assist in developing a time frame for implementation. *Changes need to be made over a period of time to allow new behaviors to be learned well, integrated into one's lifestyle, and stabilized.*
- Allow periodic evaluation and revisions of health plan as necessary. *This provides a systematic approach for movement of patient toward higher levels of health and promotes adherence to plan.*
- Inform patient of appropriate resources in the community: use referrals and agencies that enhance the learning of specific behaviors.
- Implement the use of modeling to assist patients. *Observing the behavior of others who have successfully achieved similar goals will help exemplify the exact behaviors that should be developed to reach the goal.*
- Provide a comprehensive approach to health promotion by giving attention to environmental, social, and cultural constraints. *In The Health Promotion Model, focusing only on behavior change is doomed to failure without simultaneous efforts to alter the environment and collective behavior.*
- Use a variety of teaching methods. *Learning is enhanced when various approaches reinforce the material that is being taught.*

Continued.

■ **Health-seeking behavior—cont'd**

RELATED FACTORS / DEFINING CHARACTERISTICS	EXPECTED OUTCOMES AND NURSING INTERVENTIONS / *RATIONALE* (■ = INDEPENDENT; ▲ = COLLABORATIVE)
	II. SPECIFIC PATIENT BEHAVIORS FOR SMOKING CESSATION

■ **II. SPECIFIC PATIENT BEHAVIORS FOR SMOKING CESSATION**

- Implement a plan to quit. For example, list reasons why patient wants to quit; decide positively to quit and avoid negative thoughts; set a target day to quit; and involve others who smoke in quitting.
- Choose an approach to quitting: (1) *cold turkey*—abrupt cessation from one's addictive level of smoking; (2) *tapering*—one smokes fewer cigarettes each day until down to 0; (3) *postponing*—one postpones the time to start smoking by a predetermined number of hours each day eventually leading to 0 cigarettes. *Different approaches appeal to different individuals.*
- Avoid temptation/situations associated with the pleasurable aspects of smoking. Suggest: (1) instead of smoking after meals, brush teeth or go for a walk; (2) instead of smoking while driving, take public transportation; (3) avoid having a cocktail before dinner if it is associated with smoking; (4) limit social activities or situations to those where smoking is prohibited; (5) if in a social situation where others smoke, try to associate with the nonsmokers present; (6) develop a clean, fresh, nonsmoking environment at work.
- Find new activities to make smoking difficult, impossible or unnecessary: (e.g., swimming, jogging, tennis, handball, raquetball, aerobics, biking).
- Maintain clean taste in mouth by brushing teeth frequently and using mouthwash.
- Do things that require the use of the hands: (e.g., crossword puzzles, needlework, gardening, writing letters).
- Keep oral substitutes handy: carrots, pickles, sunflower seeds, sugarless gum, celery, apples, etc. *Oral gratification helps reduce the urge to smoke. Low-calorie foods should be chosen because exsmokers burn fewer calories, and 25% may experience a weight gain when they stop smoking.*
- Learn relaxation techniques to reduce urge: make self limp, visualize a soothing, pleasing situation. *Breathing exercises help release tension and overcome the urge to smoke.*
- Seek social support. *Commitment to remain a nonsmoker can be made easier by talking with friends and family.*
- Mark progress and reward self for not smoking. Each week, month, etc., plan a special celebration and periodically write down reasons one is glad for quitting and post them.
- Instruct patient that relapses can occur. If they do, recognize the problem, review reasons for quitting, anticipate triggers, and learn how to avoid them.
- Pursue various coping skills to alleviate further problems and re-sign a contract to remain an exsmoker. *It is difficult to remain a nonsmoker. A slip means that a small setback has occurred; it doesn't mean that one will start smoking again. Despite strong resolve to quit, patients often find themselves in situations that may encourage relapse. Being prepared to recognize these and offering other options or sources of assistance enhances the patient's ability to cope and minimize relapses.*

By: Sheri Martucci, RN, MS

Home maintenance/management, impaired

Individuals within a home establish a normative pattern of operation. A vast number of factors can negatively impact upon that operational baseline. When this happens, an individual or an entire family may experience a disruption that is significant enough to impair the management of the environment. Health or safety may be threatened. There may be a threat to relationships or to physical well-being within the home.

RELATED FACTORS / DEFINING CHARACTERISTICS	EXPECTED OUTCOMES AND NURSING INTERVENTIONS / *RATIONALE* (■ = INDEPENDENT; ▲ = COLLABORATIVE)
RELATED FACTORS	**EXPECTED OUTCOMES**
Poor planning and organization	Patient maintains a safe home environment, as evidenced by clean environment, clean clothing, proper waste disposal, and use of necessary assist devices.
Low income	Patient identifies available resources.
Inadequate/absent support systems	Patient utilizes available resources.

| RELATED FACTORS / DEFINING CHARACTERISTICS | EXPECTED OUTCOMES AND NURSING INTERVENTIONS / *RATIONALE* (■ = INDEPENDENT; ▲ = COLLABORATIVE) |

RELATED FACTORS—cont'd

Lack of knowledge
Illness or injury of the client or a family member
Death of a significant other
Prolonged recuperation following illness
Substance abuse
Cognitive, perceptual, or emotional disturbance

DEFINING CHARACTERISTICS

Patient or family expresses difficulty or lack of knowledge in maintaining home environment
Poor personal habits including:
  Soiled clothing
  Frequent illness
  Weight loss
  Body odor
  Substance abuse
  Depressed affect
Poor fiscal management
Vulnerable individuals (i.e., infants, children, elderly, infirm) in the home are neglected
Home visits reveal unsafe home environment or lack of basic hygiene measures, (i.e., presence of vermin in home, accumulation of waste, home in poor repair, improper temperature regulation)

ONGOING ASSESSMENT

- Assess whether lack of money is a cause for not maintaining the home environment. *Grants/special monies can sometimes be found to modify the home to suit the need of the physically challenged patient. Other supports and services are available to reduce financial stress.*
- Assess history of substance abuse and determine its impact upon ability to maintain home. *Financial support of a substance abuse problem can siphon money from every available resource.*
- Perform a home assessment. Evaluate for accessibility and physical barriers. Assess bathing facilities, temperature regulation, whether windows close and doors lock, presence of screens, trash disposal. *These are basic necessities for a safe environment.*
- Evaluate each member of family to determine whether basic physical and emotional needs are being met. *A distinction must be made between optimal living conditions and a safe home environment.*
- Assess patient's knowledge of the rationale for personal and environmental hygiene and safety. *Realize, however, that knowledge deficit is unlikely to be responsible for poor home maintenance in all cases.*
- Assess patient's physical ability to perform home maintenance. *For example, patients may not do laundry because they are unable to carry large boxes of detergent from the store, or may be unable to carry rubbish to the collection site because sidewalks are icy, etc.*
- Assess whether patient has all assistive devices necessary to perform home maintenance. *If unavailable, other options may need to be explored such as a homemaker, family assistance, etc.*
- Assess impact of death of relative who may have been a significant provider of care. *Aspects of home maintenance may have been performed by the decreased and a new plan to meet these needs may need to be developed.*
- Assess patient's emotional/intellectual preparedness to maintain a home. *Some patients who are mentally challenged are quite capable of living alone if provided with the appropriate supports, while the patient with Alzheimer's disease may be unable to care for self.*
- ▲ Enlist assessments by social worker or community resources that may help family/individual. *Patients may be unaware of the services to which they are entitled.*

THERAPEUTIC INTERVENTIONS

- Begin discharge planning immediately after admission *to ensure that discharge is organized to meet individual needs of family.*
- Integrate family and patient into the discharge planning process. *This will ensure patient-centered objectives and promote compliance.*
- Plan a home visit *to test the efficacy of discharge plans.*
- ▲ Arrange for ongoing home therapy.
- Assist family in arranging for even distribution of workload. Build in relief for caretakers *to prevent fatigue during performance of physically/emotionally exhausting tasks.*
- ▲ Arrange for alternate placement when family is unable to provide care.
- Provide telephone support or support in the form of home visits.
- ▲ Refer to social services for financial and homemaking concerns. Inform of community resources as appropriate (drug abuse clinic, etc).

PATIENT EDUCATION

- Ensure that family/patient has been instructed in the use of all assistive devices.
- Begin care instruction/demonstrations early enough during hospital stay *to enable patient to learn tasks.*
- Teach care measures to as many family members as possible *to provide multiple competent providers and intrafamilial support.*

By: Deidra Gradishar, RNC, BS

Hopelessness

A sustained, subjective emotional and cognitive state in which the person does not see alternatives or choices available to solve problems or to achieve what is desired. In addition, the person cannot mobilize his/her own energy to accomplish goals.

RELATED FACTORS / DEFINING CHARACTERISTICS	EXPECTED OUTCOMES AND NURSING INTERVENTIONS / *RATIONALE* (■ = INDEPENDENT; ▲ = COLLABORATIVE)

RELATED FACTORS

Chronic and/or terminal illness
Impaired body image
New and/or unexpected signs or symptoms of a previous disease
Prolonged discomfort
Impaired functional abilities
Prolonged treatments/ diagnostic studies with no positive results
Prolonged dependence on equipment
Prolonged restricted activity
Prolonged isolation
Loss of social support
Multiple stressful life events

DEFINING CHARACTERISTICS

Passivity
Decreased verbalization
Lack of initiative
Decreased response to stimuli
Apathetic
Verbalizes that life has no meaning
Feels "empty"
Poor problem-solving, decision making
Inability to set goals
Cannot recognize sources of hope
Sleep, appetite disturbances
Socially withdrawn
Sadness
Suicidal thoughts

EXPECTED OUTCOMES

Patient begins to recognize choices and alternatives.
Patient begins to mobilize energy in own behalf (i.e., making decisions).

ONGOING ASSESSMENT

- Assess role the illness plays in patient's hopelessness. *Level of physical functioning, endurance for activities, duration and course of illness, prognosis and treatments involved can contribute to hopelessness.*
- Assess physical appearance (i.e., grooming, posture, hygiene).
- Assess appetite, exercise, and sleep patterns.
- Evaluate patient's ability to set goals/make decisions, plans. *A patient who feels hopeless will feel that goal-setting is futile, and that goals cannot be met.*
- Note whether patient perceives unachieved outcomes as failures. *Repeated perceptions of failure will reinforce patient's feelings of hopelessness.*
- Note whether patient emphasizes failures instead of accomplishments.
- Assess for feelings of hopelessness, lack of self-worth, giving up, suicidal ideas.
- Assess for potential source of hope (i.e., self, significant others, religion).
- Assess person's expectations for the future.
- Assess person's social support network.
- Assess meaning of the illness and treatments to the individual and family. *Certain misconceptions (i.e., patients with cancer always die) may be corrected and hope restored.*
- Assess patient's perception and need for control in the situation.
- Assess previous coping strategies used and their effectiveness.
- Identify patterns of coping related to illness *that enhance problem-solving skills and enable patient to achieve goals.*
- Assess patient's belief in self and own abilities. See Self-esteem disturbance, p. 55.
- Assess patient's values and satisfaction with role/purpose in life.
- Assess ability for solving problems. *Problem-solving is a skill that may be taught to decrease hopelessness.*

THERAPEUTIC INTERVENTIONS

- Provide physical care patient is unable to provide for self in a manner that communicates warmth, respect, and acceptance of the patient's abilities.
- Implement individualized strategies *to resolve difficulties with diet, sleep, activity, and endurance.*
- Implement physical care routine *that enables patient to function at optimum level* and is compatible with patient/family resources.
- Assist patient to evaluate situations and accomplishments accurately.
- Help patient set realistic goals by identifying short-term goals and revising them as needed.
- Provide opportunity for the patient to express feelings of pessimism.
- Express hope for patient who feels hopeless.
- Encourage hopes that are active and reality-based.
- Support patient's relationships with significant others; involve them in patient's care as appropriate.
- Provide opportunities for patient to control environment.
- *Promote ego integrity* by:
    Encouraging patient to reminisce about past life (self-validation).
    Showing patient that he/she gives something to you as a clinician.
- Encourage patient to set realistic goals and to acknowledge all accomplishments no matter how small.
- Facilitate problem solving by identifying the problem and appropriate steps.

RELATED FACTORS / DEFINING CHARACTERISTICS	EXPECTED OUTCOMES AND NURSING INTERVENTIONS / *RATIONALE* (■ = INDEPENDENT; ▲ = COLLABORATIVE)

PATIENT EDUCATION

- Provide accurate and ongoing information about illness, treatment effects, and care needed. *Misconceptions about diagnosis and prognosis may be contributing to hopelessness.*
- Let patient/family know when situations are temporary. *The outlook may appear less hopeless when time-limited.*
- Educate patient/family on using a combination of problem-solving and emotive coping.
- Help patient/family to learn and use effective coping strategies.

By: Judith Popovich, RN, MS, CCRN

Hyperthermia

HEAT EXHAUSTION, HEAT STROKE

A state in which an individual's temperature is elevated above normal. Hyperthermia is a sustained temperature above the normal variance; usually greater than 39° C (core). Most incidents of hyperthermia are due to activity and salt and water deprivation in a hot environment. Hyperthermia may occur more readily in persons who have endocrine disorders, use alcohol, take diuretics, anticholinergics, or phototoxic agents.

RELATED FACTORS / DEFINING CHARACTERISTICS	EXPECTED OUTCOMES AND NURSING INTERVENTIONS / *RATIONALE* (■ — INDEPENDENT; ▲ = COLLABORATIVE)

RELATED FACTORS

Exposure to hot environment
Vigorous activity
Medications
Anesthesia
Increased metabolic rate
Illness/trauma
Dehydration
Inability to perspire

DEFINING CHARACTERISTICS

Body temperature >39° C
Hot, flushed skin
Diaphoresis
Increased heart rate
Increased respiratory rate
Hypotension
Irritability
Fluid/electrolyte imbalance
Convulsions

EXPECTED OUTCOMES

Patient maintains body temperature below 39° C.
Patient maintains respiratory and heart rates WNL.

ONGOING ASSESSMENT

- Obtain age and weight. *Extremes of age or weight increase the risk for inability to control body temperature.*
- Assess vital signs, especially tympanic or rectal temperature. *Provides more accurate indication of core temperature.*
- Measure I & O.
- ▲ Monitor serum electrolytes, especially serum Na.
- Determine precipitating factors.

THERAPEUTIC INTERVENTIONS

- Control environmental temperature.
- Remove excess clothing and covers.
- ▲ Provide antipyretic medications as ordered.
- ▲ Provide O$_2$ therapy in extreme cases. *Hyperthermia increases metabolic demand for O$_2$.*
- Cool with tepid bath. Do not use alcohol, *as it cools the skin too rapidly, causing shivering. Shivering increases metabolic rate and body temperature.*
- ▲ Control excessive shivering with medications such as chlorpromazine and diazepam, if necessary.
- ▲ Provide ample fluids, PO or IV. *If patient is dehydrated or diaphoretic, fluid loss contributes to fever.*
- ▲ Provide additional cooling mechanisms commensurate with significance of fever and related manifestations:
  Cooling mattress.
  Cold packs applied to major blood vessels.
  Gastric lavage.
  Evaporative cooling.
  Rectal enemas.
  Peritoneal lavage/cardiopulmonary bypass in an emergency.
- Adjust cooling measures on the basis of physical response.
- Notify physician of significant changes.

Continued.

Hyperthermia—cont'd

RELATED FACTORS / DEFINING CHARACTERISTICS	EXPECTED OUTCOMES AND NURSING INTERVENTIONS / *RATIONALE* (■ = INDEPENDENT; ▲ = COLLABORATIVE)

PATIENT EDUCATION
- Explain temperature measurement and all treatments.
- Provide information regarding normal temperature and control.
- Discuss precipitating factors and preventive measures.
- Provide instruction regarding home care and temperature measurement.

By: Michele Knoll Puzas, RN,C, MHPE

Hypothermia

COLD STRESS, COLD INJURY

The state in which an individual's body temperature is sustained at a significantly lower level than normal; usually lower than 35° C (tympanic/rectal). Hypothermia results when the body cannot produce heat at a rate equal to that lost to the environment through conduction, convection, radiation, or evaporation. Core temperature below 32°C (90°F) is severe and life threatening. Hypothermia can be classified as inadvertent (seen postoperatively), intentional (for medical purposes), and accidental (exposure related).

RELATED FACTORS / DEFINING CHARACTERISTICS	EXPECTED OUTCOMES AND NURSING INTERVENTIONS / *RATIONALE* (■ = INDEPENDENT; ▲ = COLLABORATIVE)

RELATED FACTORS

Exposure to cold environment
Illness/trauma
Inability to shiver
Poor nutrition
Inadequate clothing
Alcohol consumption
Medications: vasodilators
Excessive evaporative heat loss from skin
Decreased metabolic rate

DEFINING CHARACTERISTICS

Mild:
Shivering
Confusion/slurred speech
Staggering gait/sluggish reflexes
Muscle rigidity
Cold appearance
Cool skin
Piloerection
Hypertension
Increased heart rate
Moderate:
Mental confusion
Irritability
Pallor
Decreased heart rate
Decreased respiratory rate
Cardiac arrhythmias
Fixed pupils
Loss of reflexes
Severe:
Unconsciousness (29° C)
Hypotension
Respiratory arrest
Flat brain waves (19° C)
Cardiac standstill (15° C)

EXPECTED OUTCOMES

Patient maintains a body temperature above 35° C (core).
Patient's vital signs are WNL; skin is warm.

ONGOING ASSESSMENT
- Assess for extremes in age and weight.
- Assess vital signs.
- ▲ Monitor electrolytes and ABGs. *Acidosis may result from hypoventilation and hypoglycemia.*
- Evaluate for drug or alcohol consumption.
- Determine precipitating event and risk factors.
- Evaluate peripheral perfusion at frequent intervals.
- Monitor urinary output. *Decreased output may indicate dehydration or poor renal perfusion.*
- Monitor cardiac rate/rhythm

THERAPEUTIC INTERVENTIONS
- Provide extra covering:
  Clothing, including head covering. *Heat loss tends to be greatest from the top of the head.*
  Blankets. Cover postoperative patients with heat-retaining blankets. *A majority of these patients experience mild to moderate hypothermia.*
- Provide heated oral fluids for alert patients.
- Keep patient's linen dry. *Moisture facilitates evaporative heat loss.*
- Control environmental temperature.
- ▲ Provide extra heat source:
  Heat lamp, radiant warmer.
  Heated moisturized O_2. *Shivering increases O_2 consumption.*
  Warming mattress, pads, or blankets.
  Warmed IV fluids/lavage fluids.
  Submersion in warm bath.
- Regulate heat source according to physical response.

PATIENT EDUCATION
- Explain all procedures and treatments.
- Provide information regarding normal temperature.
- Discuss preventive measures.
- Enlist support services as appropriate.

By: Michele Knoll Puzas, RN,C, MHPE

Ineffective management of therapeutic regimen

A pattern of regulating and integrating into daily living a program for treatment of illness and the sequelae of illness that is unsatisfactory for meeting specific health goals.

| RELATED FACTORS / DEFINING CHARACTERISTICS | EXPECTED OUTCOMES AND NURSING INTERVENTIONS / *RATIONALE*
(■ = INDEPENDENT; ▲ = COLLABORATIVE) |

RELATED FACTORS

Complexity of health care
Complexity of therapeutic regimen
Decisional conflicts
Economic difficulties
Excessive demands made on individual or family
Family conflict
Family patterns of health care
Inadequate number and types of cues to action
Knowledge deficit of prescribed regimen
Perceived seriousness
Perceived susceptibility
Perceived barriers
Social support deficits
Perceived powerlessness

DEFINING CHARACTERISTICS

Choices of daily living ineffective for meeting the goals of treatment or prescription program
Increased illness
Verbalized desire to manage illness
Verbalized difficulty with prescribed regimen
Verbalization by patient that he/she did not follow prescribed regimen

EXPECTED OUTCOMES

Patient describes intention to follow prescribed regimen.
Patient describes/demonstrates required competencies.
Patient identifies appropriate resources.

ONGOING ASSESSMENT

- Assess prior efforts to follow regime.
- Assess for related factors that may negatively affect success with following regimen. *Knowledge of causative factors provides direction for subsequent intervention.*
- Assess patient's individual perceptions of health problems. *According to the Health Belief Model, patient's perceived susceptibility to and perceived seriousness and threat of disease affect his/her compliance with program.*
- Assess patient's confidence in his/her ability to perform desired behavior. *According to the self-efficacy theory, positive conviction that one can successfully execute a behavior is correlated with performance and successful outcome.*
- Assess patient's ability to learn or perform desired health-related care.

THERAPEUTIC INTERVENTIONS

- Include patient in planning the treatment regimen. *Patients who become co-managers of their care have a greater stake in achieving a positive outcome.*
- Tailor the therapy to patient's life-style (e.g., taking diuretics at dinner if working during the day).
- Inform patient of the benefits of adherence to prescribed regimen. *Increased knowledge fosters compliance.*
- Simplify the regimen. Suggest long-acting forms of medications and eliminate unnecessary PRN medication. *The more often patients have to take medications during the day, the greater the risk of not following through.*
- Eliminate unnecessary clinic visits.
- Develop a system for patient to monitor his/her own progress.
- Develop with patient a system of rewards that follow successful follow-through.
- Concentrate on the behaviors that will make the greatest contribution to the therapeutic effect.
- If negative side effects of prescribed treatment are a problem, explain that many side effects can be controlled or eliminated.
- If patient lacks adequate support in changing life-style, initiate referral to support group (e.g., American Diabetes Association, weight loss programs, Y Me, stop smoking clinics, stress management classes, social services). *Groups that come together for mutual support and information can be beneficial.*

PATIENT EDUCATION

- Use a variety of teaching methods. *Learning is enhanced.*
- Introduce complicated therapy one step at a time. *Allows learner to concentrate more completely on one topic at a time.*
- Instruct patient on the importance of reordering medications 2 to 3 days before running out.
- Include significant others in explanations and teaching *to encourage their support and assistance in following plans.*
- Allow learner to practice new skills; provide immediate feedback on performance. *This allows patient to use new information immediately, thus enhancing retention. Immediate feedback allows learner to make corrections rather than practicing the skill incorrectly.*
- Role-play scenarios when non-adherence to plan may easily occur. Demonstrate appropriate behaviors. *Helping patient expand his/her repertoire of responses to difficult situations will assist in meeting treatment goals.*

By: Meg Gulanick, RN, PhD

Infection, high risk for

The state in which an individual is at increased risk for being invaded by pathogenic organisms.

RISK FACTORS

EXPECTED OUTCOMES AND NURSING INTERVENTIONS / *RATIONALE*
(■ = INDEPENDENT; ▲ = COLLABORATIVE)

RISK FACTORS

Inadequate primary defenses: broken skin, injured tissue, body fluid stasis

Inadequate secondary defenses: immunosuppression, leukopenia

Malnutrition

Intubation

In-dwelling catheters, drains

Intravenous devices

Invasive procedures

Rupture of amniotic membranes

Chronic disease

Failure to avoid pathogens (exposure)

Inadequate acquired immunity

EXPECTED OUTCOMES

Patient remains free of infection, as evidenced by normal vital signs, absence of purulent drainage from wounds, incisions, and tubes

Infection is recognized early to allow for prompt treatment.

ONGOING ASSESSMENT

- Assess for presence/existence of/history of risk factors such as open wounds and abrasions; in-dwelling catheters (Foley, peritoneal); wound drainage tubes (T-tubes, Penrose, Jackson-Pratt); endotracheal/tracheostomy tubes; venous/arterial access devices; and orthopedic fixator pins.
- ▲ Monitor white blood count. *(Rising WBC indicates body's efforts to combat pathogens; normal values: 4000-11,000. Very low WBC (neutropenia <1000) indicates severe risk for infection because patient does not have sufficient WBCs to fight infection.)*
- Monitor for signs of infection:

  Redness, swelling, increased pain, or purulent drainage at incisions, injured sites, exit sites of tubes, drains, or catheters. *Any suspicious drainage should be cultured: antibiotic therapy is determined by pathogens identified at culture.*

  Elevated temperature. *Fever of up to 38° C for 48 hours after surgery is related to surgical stress; after 48 hours, fever above 37.7° C suggests infection; fever spikes that occur and subside are indicative of wound infection; very high fever accompanied by sweating and chills may indicate septicemia.*

  Color of respiratory secretions. *Yellow or yellow-green sputum is indicative of respiratory infection.*

  Appearance of urine. *Cloudy, foul-smelling urine with visible sediment is indicative of urinary tract or bladder infection.*

- Assess nutritional status, including weight, history of weight loss, and serum albumin. *Patients with poor nutritional status may be anergic, or unable to muster a cellular immune response to pathogens and are therefore more susceptible to infection.*
- In pregnant patients, assess intactness of amniotic membranes. *Prolonged rupture of amniotic membranes prior to delivery places the mother and infant at increased risk for infection.*
- Assess for exposure to individuals with active infections.
- Assess for history of drug use/treatment modalities that may cause immunosuppression. *Antineoplastic agents and corticosteroids reduce immunocompetence.*
- Assess immunization status. *Elderly patients and those not raised in the United States may not have completed immunizations, and therefore not have sufficient acquired immunocompetence.*

THERAPEUTIC INTERVENTIONS

- Maintain asepsis for dressing changes/wound care, catheter care/handling, and peripheral IV/central venous access management.
- Wash hand before contact with patient, and between procedures with patient. *Friction and running water effectively remove micro-organisms from hands. Washing between procedures reduces the risk of transmitting pathogens from one area of the body to another, i.e., perineal care/central line care.*
- Limit visitors *to reduce the number of organisms in patient's environment,* and restrict visitation by individuals with any type of infection *to reduce the transmission of pathogens to the patient at risk for infection. The most common modes of transmission are by direct contact (touching) and by droplet (air-borne).*
- Encourage intake of protein- and calorie-rich foods *to maintain optimal nutritional status.*
- Encourage fluid intake of 2000-3000 cc of water per day (unless contraindicated) *to promote dilute urine and frequent emptying of bladder; reducing stasis of urine reduces risk of bladder infection/UTI.*
- Encourage coughing and deep breathing; consider use of incentive spirometer. *These measures reduce stasis of secretions in the lungs and bronchial tree. When stasis occurs, pathogens can cause upper respiratory infections, including pneumonia.*
- ▲ Administer antimicrobial (antibiotic) drugs as ordered. *Antimicrobial drugs include antibacterial, antifungal, antiparasitic, and antiviral agents. Ideally, the selection of the drug is based on cultures from the infected area; this is often impossible/impractical, and in these cases, empirical management (usually with a broad-spectrum drug) is undertaken. All of these agents are either toxic to the pathogen or retard the pathogen's growth.*

RISK FACTORS	EXPECTED OUTCOMES AND NURSING INTERVENTIONS / *RATIONALE* (■ = INDEPENDENT; ▲ = COLLABORATIVE)

THERAPEUTIC INTERVENTIONS

▲ Place patient in protective isolation *to minimize risk of infection* if patient is at very high risk.

■ *Protect mucous membranes* by recommending the use of soft-bristled toothbrushes and stool softeners.

PATIENT TEACHING

■ Teach patient to wash hands frequently, especially after toileting, before meals, and before and after administering self-care. *Patients can spread infection from one part of the body to another, as well as pick up surface pathogens; handwashing reduces these risks.*

■ Teach patient the importance of avoiding contact with those who have infections, colds, etc.

■ Teach family members about protecting susceptible patient from themselves and others with infections, colds, etc.

■ Teach patient/family purpose and proper technique for maintaining isolation.

■ Teach patient to take antibiotics as prescribed. *Most antibiotics work best when a constant blood level is maintained; a constant blood level is maintained when medications are taken as prescribed. The absorption of some antibiotics is hindered by certain foods; patient should be instructed accordingly.*

■ Teach patient the signs and symptoms of infection, and when to report these to the physician/nurse.

■ Demonstrate and allow return demonstration of all high-risk procedures that patient/family will do following discharge, such as dressing changes, peripheral/central IV site care, self-catheterization *(may use clean technique; infection more related to overdistended bladder resulting from infrequent catheterization than to use of clean vs. sterile technique),* and peritoneal dialysis.

By: Audrey Klopp, RN, PhD, ET

Knowledge deficit

PATIENT TEACHING; HEALTH EDUCATION

A state in which cognitive information or psychomotor skills are lacking.

RELATED FACTORS / DEFINING CHARACTERISTICS	EXPECTED OUTCOMES AND NURSING INTERVENTIONS / *RATIONALE* (■ = INDEPENDENT; ▲ = COLLABORATIVE)

RELATED FACTORS

New condition, procedure, treatment

Cognitive/physical limitation

Misinterpretation of information

Decreased motivation to learn

Emotional state affecting learning (anxiety, denial, or depression)

Unfamiliarity with information resources

DEFINING CHARACTERISTICS

Questioning members of health care team

Verbalizing inaccurate information

Denial of need to learn

Incorrect task performance

Expressing frustration or confusion when performing task

EXPECTED OUTCOMES

Patient/verbalizes desired content, and/or performs desired skill.

ONGOING ASSESSMENT

■ Assess ability to learn or perform desired health-related care. *Cognitive or physical impairments need to be identified so an appropriate teaching plan can be designed.*

■ Identify priority of learning need within the overall plan of care. *Adults learn material that is important to them.*

■ Assess motivation and willingness of patient/significant others to learn. *Adults must see a need or purpose for learning. Some patients are ready to learn soon after they are diagnosed; others cope better by denying/delaying the need for instruction.*

■ Question patient regarding previous experience and health teaching. *Adults bring many life experiences to each learning session.*

■ Identify any existing misconceptions regarding material to be taught.

■ Determine cultural influences on health teaching. *Providing a climate of acceptance allows patients to be themselves and to hold their own beliefs as appropriate.*

THERAPEUTIC INTERVENTIONS

■ Provide physical comfort for learner. *This allows patient to concentrate on what is being discussed or demonstrated.*

■ Provide a quiet atmosphere without interruption. *This allows patient to concentrate more completely.*

Continued.

Knowledge deficit—cont'd

RELATED FACTORS / DEFINING CHARACTERISTICS	EXPECTED OUTCOMES AND NURSING INTERVENTIONS / *RATIONALE* (■ = INDEPENDENT; ▲ = COLLABORATIVE)
	THERAPEUTIC INTERVENTIONS

- Provide an atmosphere of respect, openness, trust, and collaboration.
- Establish objectives and goals for learning at the beginning of the session. *This allows learner to know what will be discussed and expected during the session. Adults tend to focus on here-and-now, problem-centered education.*
- Allow learner to identify what is most important to him/her. *This clarifies learner expectations and helps the nurse match the information to be presented to the individual's needs.*
- Explore attitudes and feelings about changes. *This assists the nurse in understanding how learner may respond to the information and possibly how compliant patient may be with the expected changes.*
- Allow for and support self-directed, self-designed learning. *Adults learn when they feel they are personally involved in the learning process.*
- Assist the learner in integrating information into daily life. *This helps learner make adjustments in daily life that will result in the desired change in behavior (or learning).*
- Allow adequate time for integration that is in direct conflict with existing values or beliefs.
- Give clear, thorough explanations and demonstrations.
- Provide information using various mediums (e.g., explanations, discussions, demonstrations, pictures, written instructions, and videotapes). *Different people take in information in different ways.*
- When presenting material, move from familiar, concrete information to less familiar or more abstract concepts. *This provides patient with the opportunity to understand new material in relation to familiar material.*
- Focus teaching sessions on a single concept or idea. *This allows learner to concentrate more completely on material being discussed.*
- Keep sessions short *to prevent fatigue.*
- Encourage questions. *Learners often feel shy or embarrassed about asking questions and often want permission to ask them.*
- Allow learner to practice new skills; provide immediate feedback on performance. *This allows patient to use new information immediately, thus enhancing retention. Immediate feedback allows learner to make corrections rather than practicing the skill incorrectly.*
- Encourage repetition of information or new skill *to assist in remembering.*
- Provide positive, constructive reinforcement of learning. *A positive approach allows learner to feel good about learning accomplishments, gain confidence, and maintain self-esteem while correcting mistakes.*
- Document progress of teaching/learning. *This allows additional teaching to be based on what learner has completed, thus enhancing learner self-esteem and encouraging most cost-effective teaching.*
- Refer patient to support groups as needed *to allow patient to interact with others who have similar problems or learning needs.*
- Include significant others whenever possible *to encourage ongoing support for patient.*

By: Meg Gulanick, RN, PhD

Noncompliance

A patient's informed decision not to adhere to a therapeutic recommendation; failure to follow prescribed treatment plan.

RELATED FACTORS / DEFINING CHARACTERISTICS	EXPECTED OUTCOMES AND NURSING INTERVENTIONS / *RATIONALE* (■ = INDEPENDENT; ▲ = COLLABORATIVE)
RELATED FACTORS	**EXPECTED OUTCOMES**
Patient's value system	Patient complies with therapeutic plan as evidenced by: appropriate pill count, appropriate amount of drug in blood/urine, evidence of therapeutic effect, kept appointments, fewer hospital admissions, patient reporting compliance, and significant other reporting compliance.
Health beliefs	
Cultural beliefs	
Spiritual values	
Client-provider relationships	

RELATED FACTORS / DEFINING CHARACTERISTICS	EXPECTED OUTCOMES AND NURSING INTERVENTIONS / *RATIONALE* (■ = INDEPENDENT; ▲ = COLLABORATIVE)

DEFINING CHARACTERISTICS

Behavior indicative of failure to adhere

Objective tests: improper pill counts or missed prescription refills; body fluid analysis inconsistent with compliance

Evidence of development of complications

Evidence of exacerbation of symptoms

"Revolving-door" hospital admissions

Missed appointments

Therapeutic effect not achieved or maintained

ONGOING ASSESSMENT

- Assess patient's individual perceptions of health problems. *According to Health Belief Model, patient's perceived susceptibility to and perceived seriousness and threat of disease affect compliance with treatment plan.*
- Determine cultural/spiritual influences on importance of health care. *Not all persons view maintenance of health the same. For example, some may place trust in God for treatment, and refuse pills/blood/surgery. Others may only want to follow the "natural/health food" regime.*
- Compare actual therapeutic effect with expected effect. *Provides information on compliance. However, if therapy is ineffective or based on a faulty diagnosis, even perfect compliance will not result in the expected therapeutic effect.*
- Plot pattern of hospitalizations and clinic appointments.
- Ask patient to bring prescription drugs to appointment; count remaining pills. *Provides some objective evidence of compliance. Technique is commonly used in drug research protocols.*
- ▲ Assess serum or urine drug level. *Therapeutic blood levels will not be achieved without consistent ingestions of medication; overdosage/overtreatment can likewise be assessed.*
- Assess beliefs about current illness. *Determining what patient thinks is causing his/her symptoms or disease, how likely it is that the symptoms may return, and any concerns about the diagnosis or symptoms will provide a basis for planning future care.*
- Assess beliefs about the treatment plan. *Understanding any worries or misconceptions patient may have about the plan or side effects will guide future interventions.*

THERAPEUTIC INTERVENTIONS

- Develop a therapeutic relationship with patient and family. *Compliance increases with a trusting relationship with a consistant caregiver.*
- Include patient in planning the treatment regimen. *Patients who become co-managers of their care have a greater stake in achieving a positive outcome.*
- Remove disincentives to compliance. *Actions such as decreasing waiting time in the clinic, suggesting medications that do not cause side effects that are unacceptable to patient, etc. can improve compliance.*
- ▲ Simplify therapy. Suggest long-acting forms of medications and eliminate unnecessary p.r.n. medication. Eliminate unnecessary clinic visits. *Compliance increases when therapy is as short and includes as few treatments as possible.*
- Tailor the therapy to patient's life-style; (e.g., diuretics may be taken with the evening meal for patients who work outside the home).
- Increase the amount of supervision provided: *home health nurses and frequent return visits/appointments can provide increased supervision.*
- As compliance improves, gradually reduce the amount of professional supervision and reinforcement.
- Develop a behavioral contact. *This helps patient understand/accept his/her role in the plan of care and clarifies what patient can expect from the health care worker/system.*
- Develop with patient a system of rewards that follow successful compliance. *Rewards can be administered by the patient or family at home.*
- Provide social support through patient's family and self-help groups. *Such groups may assist patient in gaining greater understanding of the benefits of treatment.*

PATIENT EDUCATION

- Tailor the information in terms of what the patient feels is the cause of his/her health problem and his/her concerns about therapy.
- Explore with significant others the effects of patient therapy on them.
- Teach significant others to eliminate disincentives and/or increase rewards to patient for compliance.

By: Jeff Zurlinden, RN, MS

Nutrition, altered: less than body requirements

The state in which an individual's intake of nutrients is insufficient to meet metabolic needs.

STARVATION; WEIGHT LOSS; ANOREXIA

RELATED FACTORS / DEFINING CHARACTERISTICS	EXPECTED OUTCOMES AND NURSING INTERVENTIONS / *RATIONALE* (■ = INDEPENDENT; ▲ = COLLABORATIVE)

RELATED FACTORS

Inability to ingest foods

Inability to digest foods

Inability to absorb/metabolize foods

Inability to procure adequate amounts of food

Knowledge deficit

Pica

Unwillingness to eat

Increased metabolic needs caused by disease process or therapy

DEFINING CHARACTERISTICS

Loss of weight with or without adequate caloric intake

>10%-20% below ideal body weight

Documented inadequate caloric intake

EXPECTED OUTCOMES

Patient/significant other verbalizes and demonstrates selection of foods/meals that will achieve a cessation of weight loss.

Patient weighs within 10% of ideal body weight.

ONGOING ASSESSMENT

- Document patient's actual weight on admission; do not estimate. *Patients may be unaware of their actual weight/weight loss due to estimating weight.*
- Weigh patient weekly. *During aggressive nutritional support, patient can gain up to .5 pounds/day.*
- Obtain nutritional history; include family and significant others in assessment. *Patient's perception of actual intake may differ.*
- ▲ Monitor laboratory values that indicate nutritional well-being/deterioration:
    Serum albumin. *Indicates degree of protein depletion (<2.5 g/dl indicates severe depletion; 3.8-4.5 g/dl is normal).*
    Tranferrin. *Important for iron transfer and typically decreases as serum protein decreases.*
    RBC and WBC counts. *Usually decreased in malnutrition, indicating anemia and decreased resistance to infection.*
    Serum electrolyte values. *Potassium is typically increased and sodium is typically decreased in malnutrition.*
- Monitor/explore attitudes toward eating/food. *Many psychological, psychosocial, and cultural factors determine the type, amount, and appropriateness of food consumed.*
- Document appetite. Record exact I & O (do not estimate).
- Encourage patient participation (daily log). *Determination of type, amount, and pattern of food/fluid intake is facilitated by accurate documentation by patient/nurse as the intake occurs; memory is insufficient.*

THERAPEUTIC INTERVENTIONS

- Consult dietitian *for further assessment and recommendations regarding food preferences and nutritional support.*
- Assist patient with meals as needed. Ensure a pleasant environment, a facilitative position, *(HOB elevated 30 degrees aids in swallowing and reduces risk of aspiration)*, and good oral hygiene and dentition.
- Encourage family to bring food from home as appropriate.
- Discuss possible need for enteral/parenteral nutritional support with patient, family, and physician as appropriate.
- Encourage exercise. *Metabolism and utilization of nutrients are enhanced by activity.*
- Encourage consumption of between-meal supplements as ordered.
- Discourage beverages that are caffeinated *(may decrease appetite)* and carbonated beverages *(may lead to early satiety).*

PATIENT EDUCATION

- Review and reinforce the following to patient/significant others:
    Importance of maintaining adequate caloric intake: *an average (70 kg) adult needs 1800-2200 Kcal per day; patients with burns, severe infections, or draining wounds may require 3000-4000 Kcal/day.*
    Foods high in calories/protein that will promote weight gain and nitrogen balance (e.g., small frequent meals of foods high in calories and protein).

By: Audrey Klopp, RN, PhD, ET

Nutrition, altered: more than body requirements

OBESITY; OVERWEIGHT

The state in which an individual is experiencing an intake of nutrients that exceeds metabolic demands. Obesity is present when body weight is 10-20% greater than normal for height/frame.

RELATED FACTORS / DEFINING CHARACTERISTICS	EXPECTED OUTCOMES AND NURSING INTERVENTIONS / *RATIONALE* (■ = INDEPENDENT; ▲ = COLLABORATIVE)

RELATED FACTORS

Lack of knowledge of nutritional needs, food intake, and/or food preparation
Poor dietary habits
Use of food as coping mechanism
Metabolic disorders
Diabetes
Sedentary activity level

DEFINING CHARACTERISTICS

Weight 10%-20% over ideal for height and frame
Reported or observed dysfunctional eating patterns

EXPECTED OUTCOMES

Patient verbalizes measures necessary to achieve weight reduction goals.
Patient demonstrates appropriate selection of meals/menu planning toward the goal of weight reduction.
Patient begins an appropriate program of exercise.

ONGOING ASSESSMENT

- Weigh patient; do not estimate.
- Perform nutritional assessment and obtain dietary history. *Diet history should include typical pattern/amount/type of foods eaten, and any information or thoughts patient can share about cause of obesity.*
- Assess effects/complications of obesity. *Medical complications include cardiovascular and respiratory dysfunction, higher incidence of diabetes mellitus, and aggravation of musculoskeletal disorders. Social complications and poor self-esteem may also result from obesity.*
- Assess exercise activity.
- Assess patient's knowledge regarding cause of obesity, appropriate food selection, and diet/exercise planning.
- Assess patient's desire for/interest in surgical intervention.

THERAPEUTIC INTERVENTIONS

▲ Consult dietitian *to assist patient in appropriate food selection.*
- Encourage patient in appropriate food selection.
- Encourage patient to keep a daily log of food/liquid ingestion and caloric intake *as memory is inadequate for quantification of intake. A visual record may also help patient to make more appropriate food choices and serving sizes.*
- Encourage water intake. *Water assists in the excretion of by-products of fat breakdown and helps prevent ketosis.*
- Encourage patient to be more aware of nutritional habits:
  To realize the time needed for eating (encourage putting fork down between bites).
  To focus on eating and to avoid other diversional activities (e.g., reading, television viewing, telephoning).
  To observe for cues that lead to eating (e.g., odor, time, depression, and boredom).
  To eat in the same place as often as possible.
  To identify actual need for food.
- Encourage exercise.
- Help patient set realistic weight loss goals.

PATIENT EDUCATION

- Review and reinforce teaching regarding:
  Four food groups and proper serving sizes.
  Caloric content of food.
  Methods of preparation.
- Provide family counseling as needed, being sure to identify and include the person primarily responsible for grocery shopping and food preparation.
- Encourage diabetic patients to attend diabetic classes. Review and reinforce principles of dietary management of diabetes.
- Review complications associated with obesity.
- Remind patient that significant weight loss requires a long time.

By: Audrey Klopp, RN, PhD, ET

Oral mucous membrane, altered

A state in which an individual experiences disruptions in the tissue layers of the oral cavity.

RELATED FACTORS / DEFINING CHARACTERISTICS	EXPECTED OUTCOMES AND NURSING INTERVENTIONS / *RATIONALE* (■ = INDEPENDENT; ▲ = COLLABORATIVE)

RELATED FACTORS

Pathological conditions—oral cavity (radiation to head or neck)
Dehydration
Trauma: chemical, (e.g., acidic foods, drugs, noxious agents, alcohol); mechanical (e.g., ill-fitting dentures, braces, tubes [endotracheal/ nasogastric]), surgery in oral cavity
NPO for more than 24 hours
Ineffective oral hygiene
Mouth breathing
Malnutrition
Infection
Lack of or decreased salivation
Medication

DEFINING CHARACTERISTICS

Oral pain/discomfort
Coated tongue
Xerostomia (dry mouth)
Stomatitis
Oral lesions or ulcers
Lack of or decreased salivation
Leukoplakia
Edema
Hyperemia
Oral plaque
Desquamation
Vesicles
Hemorrhagic gingivitis
Halitosis

EXPECTED OUTCOMES

Patient has intact oral mucosa.
Patient demonstrates appropriate oral hygiene.
Patient verbalizes relief from stomatitis.

ONGOING ASSESSMENT

- Assess oral hygiene practices. *Provides information on possible causative factors, and provides guidance for subsequent education.*
- Assess status of oral mucosa; include tongue, lips, mucous membranes, gums, saliva, and teeth.
  Use adequate source of light.
  Remove dental appliances.
  Use a moist, padded tongue blade to gently pull back the cheeks and tongue *in order to expose all areas of oral cavity for inspection.*
- Assess for extensiveness of ulcerations involving the intraoral soft tissues, including palate, tongue, gums, and lips. *Sloughing of mucosal membrane can progress to ulceration.*
- Observe for evidence of infection and report to physician. Severe mucositis may manifest as:
  Candidiasis: (Cottage cheese-like white or pale yellowish patches on tongue, buccal mucosa and palate).
  Herpes simplex: (Painful itching vesicle (typically on upper lips) that ruptures within 12 hours and becomes encrusted with a dried exudate).
  Gram-positive bacterial infection, specifically staphylococcal and streptococcal infections: (Dry, raised wart-like yellowish-brown, round plaques on buccal mucosa).
  Gram-negative bacterial infections: (Creamy to yellow-white shiny, nonpurulent patches often seated on painful, red, superficial, mucosal ulcers, and erosions);
  Fever, chills, rigors.
- Assess nutrition status: *Malnutrition can be a contributing cause. Oral fluids needed for moisture to membranes.*
- Assess for ability to eat and drink. *Inability to chew and swallow may occur secondary to pain of inflamed/ulcerated oral and/or oropharyngeal mucous membranes.*

THERAPEUTIC INTERVENTIONS

- Implement meticulous mouth care regime after each meal and q4h while *awake to prevent buildup of oral plaque and bacteria. Patient's with oral catheters and oxygen may require additional care.* [See Patient education below for description of oral care.]
▲ If signs of mild stomatitis occur (sensation of dryness and burning; mild erythema and edema along the mucocutaneous junction):
  Increase frequency of oral hygiene by rinsing with one of the suggested solutions between brushings and once during the night.
  Discontinue flossing if it causes pain.
  Provide systemic or topical analgesics as ordered. *Increased sensitivity/to pain is due to thinning of oral mucosal lining.*
  Instruct patient that topical analgesics can be administered as "swished and swallow" or "swish and spit" 15 to 20 minutes before meals, or painted on each lesion immediately prior to mealtime.
    Topical analgesics include:
    1. dyclone 1%
    2. viscous lidocaine (10 ml per dose up to 120 ml in 24 hours)
    3. xylocaine (viscous 2%)
    4. Benadryl elixir (12.5 mg per 5 ml) and an antacid mixed in equal proportions. *These provide a "numbing" feeling.*
  Instruct patient to hold solution for several minutes before expectorating, and not to use solution if mucosa is severely ulcerated and if drug sensitivity exists.
  Caution client to chew or swallow after each dose *as numbness of throat may be experienced.*
  Explain use of topical protective agent *to coat the lesions and promote healing* as prescribed:
    Kaolin preparations.
    Substrate of an antacid. *This substance is prepared by allowing antacid to settle. The pasty residue is swabbed onto the inflamed areas and, after 15-20 minutes, rinsed with saline or water.*

THERAPEUTIC INTERVENTIONS

- For severe mucositis infection:

    Administer local antibiotics and/or antifungal agents as ordered. *Mycostatin, nystatin, and Mycelex Troche are commonly prescribed.*

    Discontinue use of toothbrush and flossing *as this will increase damage to ulcerated tissues. A disposable foamstick ("Toothette") or sterile cotton swab are gentle ways to apply cleansing solutions.*

    Continue use of lubricating ointment on the lips.

- For eating problems:

    Encourage diet high in protein and vitamins *to promote healing and new tissue growth.*

    Serve foods and fluids lukewarm or cold *as this may feel soothing to the oral mucosa.*

    Serve frequent small meals/snacks spaced throughout the day.

    Encourage soft foods (mashed potatoes, puddings, custards, creamy cereals) *to avoid tissue trauma and pain.*

    Encourage use of a straw *to make swallowing easier.*

    Encourage peach, pear, or apricot nectars and fruit drinks instead of fruit juices *as these are not irritating and are easier to swallow.* See Fluid volume deficit, p. 25.

▲ Refer patient to dietitian for instructions on maintenance of a well-balanced diet.

PATIENT EDUCATION

Instruct patient to:

- Gently brush all surfaces of teeth, gums, and tongue with a soft nylon brush *to loosen debris.*
- Brush with a non-irritating dentifrice such as baking soda.
- Remove and brush dentures thoroughly during and after meals and as needed.
- Rinse the mouth thoroughly during and after brushing.
- Avoid alcohol-containing mouthwashes *as these may dry oral mucous membranes.*
- Use recommended mouth rinses:

    Hydrogen peroxide and saline or water (1:2 or 1:4). Peroxide solutions should be mixed immediately before use *to maintain oxydizing property* and held in mouth for 1-1½ minutes. Follow with a rinse of water or saline.

    Baking soda and water (1 tsp in 500 ml).

    Salt (½ tsp), baking soda (1 tsp), and water (100 ml).

- Keep lips moist *to prevent drying and cracking.* Use a water-soluble lubricant (K-Y jelly, Aquaphor Cream) *to minimize risk of aspirating non—water-soluble agent.*
- Include food items with each meal that require chewing *as this stimulates gingival tissue and promotes circulation.*
- Minimize trauma to mucous membranes. Avoid use of tobacco and alcohol *as these are irritating and drying to the mucosa.* Avoid extremely hot or cold foods. Avoid acidic or highly spiced foods. Note and remove any loose-fitting dentures.

By: Meg Gulanick, RN, PhD
   Christa Schroeder, RN, MS
   Marina Bautista, RN, BSN

Physical mobility, impaired

IMMOBILITY

A state in which a person has limitations of independent physical movement.

RELATED FACTORS

Activity intolerance
Perceptual/cognitive impairment

EXPECTED OUTCOMES

Patient performs physical activity independently or with assistive devices as needed.
Patient is free of complications of immobility, as evidenced by intact skin, absence of thrombophlebitis, and normal bowel pattern.

Continued.

Nursing Diagnosis Care Plans

RELATED FACTORS / DEFINING CHARACTERISTICS	EXPECTED OUTCOMES AND NURSING INTERVENTIONS / *RATIONALE* (■ = INDEPENDENT; ▲ = COLLABORATIVE)

RELATED FACTORS—cont'd

Musculoskeletal impairment
Neuromuscular impairment
Medical restrictions
Prolonged bed rest
Limited strength
Pain/discomfort
Depression/severe anxiety

DEFINING CHARACTERISTICS

Inability to move purposefully within physical environment, including bed mobility, transfers, and ambulation
Reluctance to attempt movement
Limited ROM
Decreased muscle endurance, strength, control, or mass
Imposed restrictions of movement, including mechanical, medical protocol, and impaired coordination
Inability to perform action as instructed

ONGOING ASSESSMENT

- Assess for impediments to mobility (See Related factors).
- Assess patient's ability to perform ADL effectively and safely on a daily basis.

Suggested Code for Functional Level Classification*

0 Completely independent
1 Requires use of equipment or device
2 Requires help from another person for assistance, supervision, or teaching
3 Requires help from another person and equipment or device
4 Is dependent, does not participate in activity

- Assess patient/significant others knowledge of immobility and its implications.
- Assess for developing thrombophlebitis (calf pain, Homans' sign, redness, localized swelling, and rise in temperature). *Bed rest/immobility promote clot formation.*
- Assess skin integrity. Check for signs of redness, tissue ischemia (especially over ears, shoulders, elbows, sacrum, hips, heels, ankles, and toes).
- Monitor I & O record and nutritional pattern. Assess nutritional needs as they relate to immobility (possible hypocalcemia, negative nitrogen balance). *Pressure sores develop more quickly in patients with a nutritional deficit.*
- Assess elimination status (usual pattern, present patterns, signs of constipation). *Immobility promotes constipation.*
- Assess emotional response to disability/limitation.
- Evaluate need for home assistance (physical therapy, visiting nurse, assistive device).

THERAPEUTIC INTERVENTIONS

- Encourage and facilitate early ambulation and other ADL when possible. Assist with each initial change: dangling, sitting in chair, ambulation.
- Facilitate transfer training by using appropriate assistance of persons/devices when transferring patients to bed, chair, or stretcher.
- Encourage appropriate use of assistive devices for transfer.
- Provide positive reinforcement during activity.
- Allow patient to perform tasks at his/her own rate. Do not rush patient. Encourage independent activity as able and safe. *Hospitals workers are frequently in a hurry and do more for patients than needed, thereby slowing patient's recovery and reducing his/her self-esteem.*
- Keep side rails up and bed in low position *to promote safe environment.*
- ▲ Consult rehabilitation medicine personnel as appropriate.
- Turn and position every 2 hours or as needed *to optimize circulation to all tissues and to relieve pressure.*
- Maintain limbs in functional alignment (e.g., with pillows, sandbags, wedges, or prefabricated splints). Support feet in dorsiflexed position *to prevent footdrop* and/or excessive plantar flexion or tightness. Use bed cradle *to keep heavy bed linens off feet.*
- Perform passive/active assistive ROM exercises to all extremities *to promote increased venous return, prevent stiffness, and maintain muscle strength and endurance.*
- Turn patient to prone or semiprone position once daily unless contraindicated *to drain bronchial tree.*
- Use prophylactic antipressure devices as appropriate *to prevent tissue breakdown.*
- Clean, dry, and moisturize skin as needed.
- Encourage coughing and deep breathing exercises. Use suction as needed *to prevent buildup of secretions.* Use incentive spirometer *to increase lung expansion.*
- Encourage liquid intake of 2000-3000 ml/day unless contraindicated *to optimize hydration status and prevent hardening of stool.*
- Initiate supplemental high-protein feedings as appropriate.
- ▲ Set up a bowel program (adequate fluid, foods high in bulk, physical activity, stool softeners, laxatives) as needed. Record bowel activity level.
- Assist patient in accepting limitations. Emphasize abilities.

*Code adapted by North American Nursing Diagnosis Association. Taxonomy I. (Rev. 1990). St. Louis: NANDA. p. 71. From Jones, E., et al. Patient classification for long-term care: Users' manual. HEW, Publication No. HRA-74-3107, November 1974.

RISK FACTORS	EXPECTED OUTCOMES AND NURSING INTERVENTIONS / *RATIONALE* (■ = INDEPENDENT; ▲ = COLLABORATIVE)

PATIENT EDUCATION

- Explain progressive physical activity to patient. Help patient/significant others to establish reasonable and obtainable goals.
- Instruct patient/significant others regarding hazards of immobility. Emphasize importance of position change, ROM, coughing, exercises, etc.
- Reinforce principles of progressive exercise, emphasizing that joints are to be exercised to the point of pain, not beyond. *No pain, no gain is not always true!*
- Instruct patient/family regarding need to make home environment safe.
- Encourage verbalization of feelings, strengths, weaknesses, and concerns.

By: Linda Arsenault, RN, MSN, CNRN
 Marilyn Magafas, RN,C, BSN, MBA
 John Larocco, PT
 Susan Eby, PT, MS

Pain

A highly subjective state in which a variety of unpleasant sensations and a wide range of distressing factors may be experienced by the sufferer. Pain may be acute, a symptom of injury or illness such as a myocardial infarction, or chronic, lasting longer than 6 months, the result of a long-term illness such as arthritis. Pain may also arise from emotional, psychological, cultural, or spiritual distress. Pain can be very difficult to explain, because it is unique to the individual; pain should be accepted as described by the sufferer.

RELATED FACTORS / DEFINING CHARACTERISTICS	EXPECTED OUTCOMES AND NURSING INTERVENTIONS / *RATIONALE* (■ = INDEPENDENT; ▲ = COLLABORATIVE)

RELATED FACTORS

Childbirth pain
Operative pain
Cardiovascular pain
Pain resulting from medical problems
Musculoskeletal pain
Pain resulting from diagnostic procedures or medical treatments
Pain resulting from trauma
Pain resulting from emotional, psychological, spiritual, or cultural distress.

DEFINING CHARACTERISTICS

Patient/significant others report pain
Guarding behavior, protectiveness
Self-focusing, narrowed focus (altered time perception, withdrawal from social or physical contact), depression, loss of appetite

EXPECTED OUTCOMES

Patient verbalizes adequate relief of pain or ability to cope with incompletely relieved pain.

ONGOING ASSESSMENT

- Assess pain characteristics:
  Quality (e.g., sharp, burning, shooting).
  Severity (scale 1-10, 10 most severe).
  Location (anatomical description).
  Onset (gradual or sudden).
  Duration (how long, intermittent/continuous).
  Precipitating/relieving factors.
- Observe/monitor other associated signs/symptoms, such as BP, heart rate, temperature, color and moisture of skin, restlessness, and ability to focus.
- Assess for probable cause of pain.
- Assess patient's knowledge of/preference for the array of pain-relief strategies available:
  Pharmacological methods include nonsteroidal anti-inflammatory drugs (NSAIDs) that may be administered orally or parenterally (to date, Ketorolac is the only available parenteral NSAID); use of opiates that may be administered orally, intramuscularly, subcutaneously, intravenously, systemically by patient-controlled analgesia systems (PCA), or epidurally (either by bolus or continuous infusion), and local anesthetic agents. Nonpharmacological methods include cognitive-behavioral strategies such as imagery, relaxation, education, and use of TENS (transcutaneous electrical nerve stimulation) units.

Continued.

RELATED FACTORS / DEFINING CHARACTERISTICS	EXPECTED OUTCOMES AND NURSING INTERVENTIONS / *RATIONALE* (■ = INDEPENDENT; ▲ = COLLABORATIVE)

DEFINING CHARACTERISTICS— cont'd

Relief/distraction behavior (e.g., moaning, crying, pacing, seeking out other people or activities, restlessness, irritability, alteration in sleep pattern)

Facial mask of pain

Alteration in muscle tone: listlessness/flaccidness; rigidity/tension)

Autonomic responses not seen in chronic, stable pain (e.g., diaphoresis; change in BP, pulse rate; pupillary movements; decreased respiratory rate; pallor; nausea)

ONGOING ASSESSMENT

- Evaluate patient's response to pain and medications or therapeutics aimed at abolishing/relieving pain. *It is important to help patients express as factually as possible (i.e., without the effect of mood, emotion, or anxiety) the effect of pain relief measures. Discrepancies between behavior or appearance and what patient says about pain relief (or lack of it) may be more a reflection of other methods patient is using to cope than pain relief itself.*
- Assess to what degree cultural, environmental, intrapersonal, and intrapsychic factors may contribute to pain/pain relief.
- Evaluate what the pain means to the individual. *The meaning of the pain will directly influence patient's response. Pain will influence activity, family role, self-concept, etc.*
- Assess patient's past coping mechanisms *to determine what measures worked best in the past.*
- Assess patient's expectations for pain relief. *Some patients may be content to have pain decreased; others will expect complete elimination of pain. This will impact on their perception of the effectiveness of the treatment modality and their willingness to participate in further treatments.*
- Assess patient's willingness/ability to explore a range of techniques aimed at controlling pain.
- Assess appropriateness of patient as PCA candidate: no history of substance abuse; no allergy to narcotic analgesics; clear sensorium; cooperative and motivated about use; no history of renal, hepatic, or respiratory disease; manual dexterity; and no history of major psychiatric disorder. *Patient-controlled analgesia (PCA) is the IV infusion of a narcotic (usually morphine or Demerol) via an infusion pump that is controlled by the patient. This allows the patient to manage pain relief within prescribed units.*
- Monitor for changes in general condition that may herald need for change in pain relief method. *For example, a PCA patient becomes confused and cannot manage PCA, or a successful modality ceases to provide adequate pain relief, as in relaxation breathing in early stages of labor.*
- If patient is on PCA, assess:
  Pain relief.
  Intactness of IV line. *If IV is not patent, patient will not receive pain medication.*
  The amount of pain medication patient is requesting. *If demands for medication are very frequent, patient's dosage may need to be increased. If demands are very low, patient may require further instruction to properly use PCA.*
  Possible PCA complications such as excessive sedation, respiratory distress, urinary retention, nausea/vomiting, constipation, and IV site pain, redness, or swelling.
- If patient is receiving epidural analgesia, assess:
  Pain relief.
  Intactness/length of catheter. *If the catheter becomes dislodged, and is no longer in the epidural space, patient will not receive pain medication, and may be at risk for infection.*
  Possible epidural analgesia complications such as excessive sedation, respiratory distress, urinary retention, and numbness/tingling of lower extremities.
- Assess for effects of chronic pain such as depression; guilt; hopelessness; sleep, sexual, and nutritional disturbances; and alterations in interpersonal relationships.

THERAPEUTIC INTERVENTIONS

- Anticipate need for analgesics or additional methods of pain relief. *One can most effectively deal with pain by preventing it. Early intervention may decrease the total amount of analgesic required.*
- Respond immediately to complaint of pain. *In the midst of painful experiences patient's perception of time may become distorted. Prompt responses to complaints may result in decreased anxiety in patient. Demonstrated concern for patient's welfare and comfort fosters the development of a trusting relationship.*
- Eliminate additional stressors or sources of discomfort whenever possible. *Patients may experience an exaggeration in pain or a decreased ability to tolerate painful stimuli if environmental, intrapersonal, or intrapsychic factors are further stressing them.*
- ▲ Give analgesics as ordered, evaluating effectiveness and observing for any signs and symptoms of untoward effects. *Pain medications are absorbed and metabolized differently by patients, so their effectiveness must be evaluated from patient to patient. Analgesics may cause side effects that range from mild to life-threatening.*

THERAPEUTIC INTERVENTIONS

- Notify physician if interventions are unsuccessful or if current complaint is a significant change from patient's past experience of pain. *Patients who request pain medications at intervals more frequent then prescribed may actually require higher doses of analgesia or more potent analgesia.*
- Provide rest periods to facilitate comfort, sleep, and relaxation. *The patient's experiences of pain may become exaggerated as the result of fatigue. In a cyclic fashion, pain may result in fatigue, which may result in exaggerated pain and exhaustion. A quiet environment, a darkened room, and a disconnected phone are all measures geared toward facilitating rest.*
- Whenever possible, reassure patient that pain is time-limited and that there is more than one approach to easing pain. *When pain is perceived as everlasting and unresolvable, patient may give up trying to cope with it or experience a sense of hopelessness and loss of control.*
- ▲ Apply heat or cold compresses, as ordered. *Hot moist compresses have a penetrating effect. The warmth rushes blood to the affected area to promote healing. Cold compresses may reduce local edema and promote some numbing, thereby promoting comfort.*

If patient is on PCA:
- ▲ Dedicate use of IV line for PCA only; consult pharmacist before mixing drug with narcotic being infused; *IV incompatibilities are possible.*
- Post "No additional analgesia" sign over bed *to prevent inadvertent analgesic overdosage.*
- Keep Narcan/other narcotic-reversing agent readily available.

If patient is receiving epidural analgesia:
- Post "No additional analgesia" sign over bed *to prevent inadvertent analgesic overdosage.*
- Label all tubing (epidural catheter, IV tubing to epidural catheter) clearly *to prevent inadvertent administration of inappropriate fluids or drugs into epidural space.*
- Keep Narcan/other narcotic-reversing agent readily available. *In the event of respiratory depression, these drugs reverse the narcotic effect.*
- Instruct the patient in use of one or a combination of the following techniques:
  Imagery: *The use of a mental picture or an imagined event that involves use of the five senses to distract oneself from painful stimuli.*
  Distraction techniques: *Heightening one's concentration upon nonpainful stimuli to decrease one's awareness and experience of pain. Some methods are breathing modifications and nerve stimulation.*
  Relaxation exercises: *Techniques used to bring about a state of physical and mental awareness and tranquility. The goal of these techniques is to reduce tensions, subsequently reducing pain.*
  Massage of affected area when appropriate. *Massage decreases muscle tension and can promote comfort.*

PATIENT EDUCATION

- Provide anticipatory instruction on pain causes, appropriate prevention, and relief measures.
- Explain cause of pain/discomfort, if known.
- Instruct patient to report pain *so that relief measures may be instituted.*
- Instruct patient to evaluate and report effectiveness of measures used.

For patients on PCA or those receiving epidural analgesia:
- Teach patient preoperatively *so that anesthesia effects do not obscure teaching.*
- Teach patient the purpose, benefits, techniques of use/action, need for IV line (PCA only), other alternatives for pain control, and of the need to notify nurse of machine alarm and occurrence of untoward effects.
- For all types of pain medications teach patient effective timing of dose in relation to potentially uncomfortable activities and prevention of peak pain periods.

By: Deidra Gradishar, RNC, BS
Linda Muzio, RN, MSN, PhD candidate
Ann Filipski, RN, MSN, CS, PsyD candidate
Audrey Klopp, RN, PhD, ET

Powerlessness

The state in which a person perceives an inability to influence others to think, act, or feel a certain way; one perceives a loss of personal control over events or situations.

RELATED FACTORS / DEFINING CHARACTERISTICS	EXPECTED OUTCOMES AND NURSING INTERVENTIONS / *RATIONALE* (■ = INDEPENDENT; ▲ = COLLABORATIVE)

RELATED FACTORS

Acute or chronic illness
Inability to communicate
Dependence on others for activities of daily living
Inability to perform role responsibilities
Progressive debilitating disease
Lack of knowledge

DEFINING CHARACTERISTICS

Expression of dissatisfaction over being unable to control situation
Reluctance to participate in decision making
Diminished patient-initiated interaction
Submissiveness; apathy
Withdrawal; depression
Aggressive, acting out, and/or violent behavior
Feeling of hopelessness
Decreased participation in activities of daily living

EXPECTED OUTCOMES

Patient begins to identify ways to achieve control over personal situation.

ONGOING ASSESSMENT

- Assess the role the illness plays in patient's powerlessness. *Uncertainty about events, duration and course of illness, prognosis, and dependence on others for help and treatments involved can contribute to powerlessness.*
- Assess impact of powerlessness on patient's physical condition (i.e., appearance, oral intake, hygiene, sleep habits). *Individuals may feel as though they are unable to control very basic aspects of life.*
- Note whether patient demonstrates need for information about illness, treatment plan, and procedures. *This will differentiate powerlessness from knowledge deficit.*
- Evaluate the effects of information provided on patient's behavior and feelings. *A powerless patient may ignore information.*
- Assess for feelings of anger, frustration, withdrawal, submissiveness, anxiety, and powerlessness.
- Identify situations and/or interactions that may cause the patient to feel powerless.
- Assess patient's power needs/need for control.
- Assess for feelings of hopelessness, depression, and apathy.
- Assess patient's decision-making ability. *Making a decision implies that one has power/control to change something. Patients who feel powerless may be unable to make decisions.*
- Assess impact of illness and hospitalization on patient's sense of control. *Patients do lose control of some basic aspects of living; to an extent, this is seen in many patients.*
- Assess patient's ability to set realistic goals.
- Assess patient's desires/abilities to be an active participant in self-care.

THERAPEUTIC INTERVENTIONS

- Provide physical care the patient is unable to provide for self in a manner that *communicates warmth, respect, acceptance of the patient's abilities.*
- Implement individualized strategies to resolve difficulties with hygiene, diet, and sleep. *Allowing/helping patient to decide when, etc., may ease powerlessness.*
- Provide appropriate information to patient about illness, treatment plan, and procedures.
- Provide patient with opportunities for expressing feelings of anger, anxiety, and powerlessness.
- Acknowledge patient's knowledge of self and personal situation.
- *Enhance patient's power resources* by fostering patient involvement in decision making, by giving information, and by enabling patient to control environment as appropriate.
- Avoid using coercive power when approaching patient *as this may intensify patient's feelings of powerlessness and result in decreased self-esteem.*
- Acknowledge the nurse's ability for "expert" and "reward" power; *these types of power in patient/nurse interaction may enable the patient to mobilize own power resources.*
- Assist patient with setting and achieving goals.
- Point out patient's accomplishments *to foster hope.*

By: Judith Popovich, RN, MS, CCRN

Self care deficit

State in which a person experiences difficulty in performing tasks of daily living, such as feeding self, dressing, bathing, toileting, transferring from bed, and walking.

RELATED FACTORS / DEFINING CHARACTERISTICS	EXPECTED OUTCOMES AND NURSING INTERVENTIONS / *RATIONALE* (■ = INDEPENDENT; ▲ = COLLABORATIVE)

RELATED FACTORS

Neuromuscular impairment, secondary to CVA, rheumatoid arthritis
Musculoskeletal disorder
Cognitive impairment
Energy deficit

DEFINING CHARACTERISTICS

Inability to feed self independently
Inability to dress self independently
Inability to bathe and groom self independently
Inability to perform toileting tasks independently
Inability to transfer from bed to wheelchair
Inability to ambulate independently
Inability to perform miscellaneous common tasks:
  Telephoning
  Writing

EXPECTED OUTCOMES

Patient safely performs (to maximum ability) self-care activities.

ONGOING ASSESSMENT

- Assess ability to carry out ADLs (feed, dress, groom, bathe, toilet, transfer, and ambulate) on regular basis.
- Assess specific cause of each deficit (e.g., weakness, visual problems, cognitive impairment). *Different etiologies may require more specific interventions to enable self-care.*
- Assess patient's need for assistive devices *to increase independence in ADL performance.*
- Assess for need of home health care after discharge.
- Identify preferences (food, personal care items, etc.)

THERAPEUTIC INTERVENTIONS

- Assist patient in accepting necessary amount of dependence. *If disease/injury/illness resulting in self-care deficit is recent, patient may need to grieve before accepting that dependence is possible.*
- Set short-range goals with patient *to facilitate learning and decrease frustration.*
- Encourage independence, but intervene when patient cannot perform *to decrease frustration.*
- Use consistent routines. *This helps patient to organize and carry out self-care skills.*
- Provide positive reinforcement for all activities attempted; note partial achievements.

Feeding:

- Encourage patient to feed self as soon as possible (using unaffected hand, if appropriate). Assist with setup as needed.
- Ensure that patient wears dentures and eyeglasses if needed.
- ▲ Assure that consistency of diet is appropriate for patient's level of chewing and swallowing, as assessed by speech therapist.
- Provide patient with appropriate utensils (straw, food guard, rocking knife, nonskid placemat) to aid in self-feeding. *These items increase opportunities for success.*
- Place patient in optimal position for feeding, preferably sitting up in a chair.
- Consider appropriate setting for feeding task where patient has supportive assistance yet is not embarrassed. *Embarrassment may hinder patient's attempts to feed self.*
- If patient has visual problems, carefully assess placement of food on plate. *Following CVA, patients may have unilateral neglect, and may ignore half the plate.*

Dressing/Grooming:

- Provide privacy during dressing.
- Provide frequent encouragement and assistance as needed with dressing *to reduce energy expenditure and frustration.*
- Plan daily activities so patient is rested prior to activity.
- ▲ Provide appropriate assistive devices for dressing as assessed by nurse and occupational therapist.
- Place patient in wheelchair or stationary chair *to assist with support when dressing. Dressing can be very fatiguing.*
- Encourage use of clothing one size larger *to ensure easier dressing and comfort.*
- Suggest brassiere that opens in front and half slips, *which may be easier to manage.*
- Suggest elastic shoelaces *to eliminate tying.*
- Provide make-up and mirror; assist as needed.

Bathing/Hygiene:

- Maintain privacy during bathing as appropriate.
- Ensure that needed utensils are close by *to conserve energy and optimize safety.*
- Instruct patient to select bath time when rested and unhurried.
- Provide patient with appropriate assistive devices (long-handled bath sponge *to aid in bed bathing;* shower chair; safety mats for floor; grab bars for bath/shower).
- Encourage patient to comb own hair (a one-handed task).

Continued.

Self care deficit—cont'd

RELATED FACTORS / DEFINING CHARACTERISTICS	EXPECTED OUTCOMES AND NURSING INTERVENTIONS / *RATIONALE* (■ = INDEPENDENT; ▲ = COLLABORATIVE)

Bathing/Hygiene—cont'd

- Encourage patient to perform minimum of oral-facial hygiene as soon as possible. Assist with brushing teeth and shaving, as needed.
- Assist patient with care of fingernails and toenails as required.
- Offer frequent encouragement. *Patients often have difficulty seeing progress.*
- Document increased independence in bathing.

Toileting:

- Evaluate/document previous and current patterns for toileting; institute a toileting schedule.
- Provide privacy while patient is toileting.
- Keep call light within reach and instruct patient to call as early as possible *so staff have time to assist with transfer to commode/toilet.*
- Assist patient in removing/replacing necessary clothing.
- Encourage use of commode/toilet as soon as possible.
- Offer bedpan or place patient on toilet every 1 to 1½ hours during day and 3 times during night *to eliminate incontinence. Time intervals can be lengthened as patient begins to indicate needs to void and have bowel movements.*
- Keep toilet paper within easy reach but closely monitor patient for loss of balance/fall.

Transferring/Ambulation:

- Plan teaching session for transferring/walking when patient is rested. *Tasks require energy. Fatigued patients may have more difficulty and may become unnecessarily frustrated.*
- Assist with bed mobility:
  Encourage to use the stronger side (if appropriate) as best as possible.
  Allow patient to work at own rate of speed.
  When patient is sitting up at side of bed, instruct him/her not to pull on staff. *This may cause staff to lose balance and fall.*
- When transferring to w/c, always place chair on patient's strong side at slight angle to bed and lock brakes.
- When minimal assistance is needed, stand on patient's weak side, place nurse's hand under patient's weak arm. (Nurse: Keep your feet well apart; lift with legs, not back, *to prevent back strain*).
- For moderate assistance, place nurse's arms under both armpits with nurse's hands on patient's back. *(This forces patient to keep weight forward).*
- For maximum assistance, place right knee against patient's strong knee, grasp patient around waist with both arms, and pull him/her forward; encourage patient to put weight on strong side.
- Assist with ambulation (if appropriate).
  Stand on patient's weak side *to assist with balance and support.*
  If using cane, place cane in patient's strong hand and ensure proper foot-cane sequence.
  See also Physical mobility, impaired p. 47.

Common Miscellaneous Skills:

- *Telephone:* Evaluate need for adaptive equipment through therapy department (pushbutton phone, larger numbers, increased volume).
- *Writing:* Supply patient with felt-tip pens. *These mark with little pressure and are easier to use).* Evaluate need for splint on writing hand *to assist with holding.*
- Provide supervision for each activity until patient is no longer at risk.
- Encourage maximum independence.
- Institute care plans for related problems as appropriate: Self-esteem disturbance p. 55; Activity intolerance, p. 2; Physical mobility, impaired p. 47.

PATIENT EDUCATION

- Plan teaching sessions *so patient has time to practice tasks.*
- Instruct patient in use of assistive devices as appropriate.
- Teach family/significant others to foster independence, and to intervene if the patient becomes fatigued, is unable to perform task or becomes excessively frustrated. *This demonstrates caring/concern, but does not interfere with patient's efforts to achieve independence.*

By: Margaret Gleason, RN, BSN

Self-esteem disturbance

Mild to marked alteration in an individual's view of himself or herself, including negative self-valuation/feelings about self or capabilities. One's self-esteem is affected by (and may also affect) ability to function in the larger world and relate to others within it. Self-esteem disturbance may be expressed directly or indirectly.

RELATED FACTORS / DEFINING CHARACTERISTICS	EXPECTED OUTCOMES AND NURSING INTERVENTIONS / *RATIONALE* (■ = INDEPENDENT; ▲ = COLLABORATIVE)

RELATED FACTORS

Bodily injury
Alteration in body image
Actual or anticipated loss
Change in relationships with others
Change in social roles (e.g., hospitalization, assumption of the "sick role")
Behavior out of line with personal values
Unresolved grief

DEFINING CHARACTERISTICS

Report by patient/significant other(s) of change in self-esteem
Expressions of shame/guilt
Rejection of positive feedback
Sensitivity to criticism
Change in behavior (e.g., severe or prolonged denial, refusal to participate in care or treatment withdrawal, decrease in functioning, disproportionate sense of capability)
Change in cognitive/intellectual functioning (impaired judgment/thinking, inability to make decisions, poor reality testing)
Change in affect and/or appearance (sadness, anger, irritability, decreased attention to grooming)

EXPECTED OUTCOMES

Patient begins to recognize, accept, and verbalize positive aspect of self and self-capabilities.

ONGOING ASSESSMENT

- Document past and current level of functioning: emotional, social, interpersonal, intellectual, vocational, and physical.
- Note quality/quantity of verbalizations regarding self.
- Note report by patient/significant others of changes in self-esteem.
- Assess for evidence of change in behavior.
- Assess the degree to which patient feels "in control" of own behavior.
- Assess the degree to which patient feels loved and respected by others.
- Assess whether patient feels satisfied with his/her own behavior. *Patients with self-esteem disturbance may feel as though their behavior is not in keeping with their own personal, moral, or ethical values; they may also deny these behaviors, project blame, and rationalize personal failures.*
- Assess how competent patient feels about ability to perform and/or carry out own/ other's expectations.
- Assess for unresolved grief.

THERAPEUTIC INTERVENTIONS

- Provide environment conducive to expression of feelings:
    Make frequent contact in unhurried manner.
    Avoid excessive focus on physical tasks.
    Use active listening.
    Provide privacy.
    Allow patient to personalize environment with own belongings and/or familiar persons as appropriate.
- Convey sense of respect for abilities/strengths in addition to recognizing problems/ concerns. *Assistance with problem solving and reality testing is best provided within the context of a trusting relationship.*
- Serve as role model for patient/significant others in healthy expression of feelings/ concerns.
- Discuss "normal" impact of alteration in health status (temporary or permanent) on self esteem. *Use of lay support groups/individuals may help patient with self-esteem disturbance to recognize positives even in the face of injury, disease, or loss.*
- Reassure patient that such changes frequently result in a variety of emotional/behavioral responses.
- Advise of realistic need for additional support in coping with change and stress.
- Provide anticipatory guidance *to minimize anxiety and fear of the unknown and to allow for a sense of control.*
    Explain routines and procedures in plan of treatment.
    Orient patient/significant others to environment.
    Use language and terminology patient/significant others can understand.
    Provide opportunities for questions and verbalization of feelings.
    Include patient/significant others in planning care whenever possible.
    Observe response to information, caretakers, and environment. *Anxiety (if excessive) may interfere with ability to function and test reality.*

Continued.

Nursing Diagnosis Care Plans

RELATED FACTORS / DEFINING CHARACTERISTICS	EXPECTED OUTCOMES AND NURSING INTERVENTIONS / *RATIONALE* (■ = INDEPENDENT; ▲ = COLLABORATIVE)

THERAPEUTIC INTERVENTIONS

- Assist in efforts to obtain understanding and mastery of new experiences:
    Support efforts to maintain independence, reality, positive self-esteem, sense of capability, and problem solving.
    Provide realistic appraisal of progress.
    Reinforce efforts at constructive change.
    Recognize variations in manner and pace at which each individual attempts to adjust to illness.
    Encourage involvement in varied activities and interaction with others.
    Use referral sources (other professional or lay persons) as appropriate to support coping efforts.
- Assist patient in grief work and let patient know that self-esteem disturbance is common during grief.

PATIENT EDUCATION

- Teach patient the importance of intact self-esteem as it relates to physical and emotional well-being.
- Teach patient to seek and/or plan activities likely to result in a healthy self-esteem.
- Teach patient necessary self-care measures related to primary disease. *Each success will reinforce positive self-esteem.*
- Teach patients the harmful effects of negative self-talk.

By: Ann Filipski, RN, MSN, CS, PsyD candidate
Susan R. Laub, RN, MEd, CS

Sensory/perceptual alterations: Visual

A state in which an individual experiences a change in the amount or patterning of incoming stimuli, accompanied by a diminished, exaggerated, distorted, or impaired response to such stimuli. Whereas sensory/perceptual alterations may include visual, auditory, kinesthetic, gustatory, tactile and/or olfactory disorders, this care plan addresses visual impairment only.

RELATED FACTORS / DEFINING CHARACTERISTICS	EXPECTED OUTCOMES AND NURSING INTERVENTIONS / *RATIONALE* (■ = INDEPENDENT; ▲ = COLLABORATIVE)

RELATED FACTORS

Therapeutically restricted environments:
  Isolation
  Bedrest
  Special care units
Socially restricted environments:
  Institutionalization
  Home-boundedness
  Terminal illness
  Bereavement
Pain
Sleep deprivation
Stress/anxiety (altered perceptual field)
Chemical alteration

EXPECTED OUTCOMES

Patient achieves optimal functioning within limits of visual impairment as evidenced by ability to care for self and ability to navigate environment safely.

ONGOING ASSESSMENT

- Assess age. *Cataracts, retinal detachments, and glaucoma increase in frequency as aging occurs.*
- Determine nature of visual symptoms, onset, and degree of visual loss. Ask patient about specifics, such as ability to read, see TV, falls; *visual loss may occur gradually, making quantification of loss difficult.*
- Inquire about previous visual complaints, eye injury, or ocular pain.
- Assess central vision with each eye individually and together. *Vision loss may be unilateral or bilateral, and may not affect both eyes to the same extent.*
- Assess peripheral field of vision and visual acuity. *Glaucoma affects peripheral vision; its onset is insidious, and has no associated symptoms.*
- Inquire about patient/family history of systemic or CNS disease. *Family/patient history of atherosclerosis, diabetes, thyroid disease, and hypertension should be investigated as possible etiologies for visual loss.*
- Assess eye and lid for inflammation, edema, positional defects, and deviation.
- Assess factors/aids that improve vision, such as glasses, contact lenses, or bright lights.
- Evaluate patient's ability to function within limits of visual impairment.
- Evaluate psychological response to visual loss. *Anger, depression, and withdrawal are common responses.*

RELATED FACTORS / DEFINING CHARACTERISTICS	EXPECTED OUTCOMES AND NURSING INTERVENTIONS / *RATIONALE* (■ = INDEPENDENT; ▲ = COLLABORATIVE)

RELATED FACTORS—cont'd

Disease/trauma to visual pathways/cranial nerves II, III, IV, and VI secondary to:
Stroke
Intracranial aneurysms
Brain tumor
Trauma
Myasthenia gravis
Multiple sclerosis
Glaucoma
Cataract
Advanced age

DEFINING CHARACTERISTICS

Lack of eye-to-eye contact
Abnormal eye movement
Failure to locate distant objects
Squinting, frequent blinking
Bumping into things
Clumsy behavior
Closing of one eye to see
Frequent rubbing of eye
Deviation of eye
Gray opacities in eyes
Head tilting
Disorientation
Reported/measured changes in visual acuity
Anxiety
Change in usual response to visual stimuli
Anger
Visual distortions
Incoordination

THERAPEUTIC INTERVENTIONS

- Identify self to patient, and acknowledge visual impairment *to reduce patient's anxiety.*
- Orient patient to environment *to reduce fear related to unfamiliar environment;* do not make unnecessary changes in environment *(to ensure safety).*
- Provide adequate lighting:
  Bright for patients with dimmed vision. *Improves vision.*
  Subdued for patients with photophobia. *Decreases discomfort.*
- Place meal tray, tissues, water, and call light within patient's range of vision *to ensure safety.*
- Place sign over bed indicating type and degree of impairment, and any contraindicated activities *to provide continuity of care.*
- Use visual aids (e.g., magnifying glass, large-type printed books and magazines), when appropriate.
- If patient is blind:
  Place sign in front of chart.
  Inform him/her of date and time.
  Explain arrangement of food on tray and plate, using clockwise sequence.
  Place food on tray and plate in same place each meal.
  Encourage use of sense of touch to become familiar with new objects.
  Explain sounds.
- Encourage use of radios and tapes. *Time passes slowly when one is inactive. Diversional activities should be encouraged. Radio and television increase awareness of day and time.*
- Remove environmental barriers *to ensure safety.* If furniture or waste baskets are moved, notify patient of changes.
- Encourage patient's roommate and other patients to avoid leaving doors partially open; should be fully open or closed.
- Maintain bed in low position with side rails up, if appropriate. *Side rails help remind patient not to get up without help.* Keep bed in locked position.
- Guide patient when ambulating, if appropriate. Walk ahead, with patient's arm around your elbow. Describe where you are walking; identify obstacles.
- Instruct patient to hold both arms of chair before sitting.
- ▲ Consult OT personnel for assistive devices and training in their use.
- Supervise patient when smoking *to prevent accidental fires.*

PATIENT EDUCATION

- Involve significant others in patient's care and instructions. Help them understand nature and limitations of disease. *Patient/family need information to plan strategies for coping with impairment.*
- Reinforce physician's explanation of medical management and surgical procedures, if any.
- Teach general eye care:
  Wash hands before touching eyes or eye medication.
  Maintain sterility of all eye droppers, tubes of medications, etc.
  Do not share eye make-up.
  Care for contact lenses as recommended by manufacturer.
  Do not rub eyes.
- Demonstrate proper administration of eye drops or ointments.
- Help family/significant others identify and make arrangements at home to provide for patient's safety, if indicated.
- ▲ Make appropriate referrals to home health agency for nursing and social service follow-up.
- Reinforce need to use community agencies, if indicated (e.g., American Foundation for the Blind, 15 West 16th St., New York, NY 10011).

By: Maria Dacaney, RN

Sexuality patterns, altered

IMPOTENCE; INTIMACY

The patient or significant other expresses concern regarding the means or manner of sexual expression or physical intimacy. Alterations in human sexual response may be related to genetic, physiological, emotional, cognitive, religious, and/or sociocultural factors (or some combination thereof).

RELATED FACTORS / DEFINING CHARACTERISTICS	EXPECTED OUTCOMES AND NURSING INTERVENTIONS / *RATIONALE* (■ = INDEPENDENT; ▲ = COLLABORATIVE)

RELATED FACTORS

Physical changes or limitations (may be time limited or chronic)
  Acute illness
  Pain or discomfort
  Recent surgery or trauma
  Loss of mobility or normal ROM
  Decreased activity tolerance
  Hormonal change
  Alcohol/substance abuse
  Medication effects
  Pregnancy
  Infertility
Fear/anxiety
  Concerns about pregnancy or STDs
  Religious/cultural prohibitions
  Lack of privacy
  Social stigma
  Conflicting values
Knowledge deficit
  Lack of education regarding sexuality
  Means of birth control
  "Safe"/"safer" sex practices
  Limited social skills
Emotional factors
  Change in body or self image
  Recent loss or trauma
  Affective disturbances
  Low self-esteem/poor self-concept
  Dementia
  Discomfort with sexual orientation
  Identity disturbances
  History of traumatic experiences (rape, sexual abuse, etc.)
  Psychosis or other psychiatric disorder
Situational factors
  Absence of partner
  Social isolation
  Lack of appropriate environment

EXPECTED OUTCOMES

Patient or couple verbalizes satisfaction with the way they express physical intimacy. Patient exhibits sexually appropriate behavior.

ONGOING ASSESSMENT

- Assess level of understanding regarding human sexuality and functioning.
- Explore current and past sexual patterns, practices, and degree of satisfaction *to determine realistic approach to care planning.*
- Identify level of comfort in discussion for client and/or significant other.
- Identify potential/actual factors that may contribute to current/future alteration in sexual functioning. (See list of related factors.)
- Document nature, onset, duration, and course of sexual difficulty.

THERAPEUTIC INTERVENTIONS

- Use a relaxed, accepting manner in discussing sexual issues. Convey acceptance and respect for client concerns. *Clients are often hesitant to report such concerns and/or difficulties because sexuality remains a private, uncomfortable matter for many within our culture.*
- Provide privacy and adequate time to discuss sexuality. *Respecting the individual and treating his/her concerns/questions as normal and important may foster greater self-acceptance and decrease anxiety.*
- Encourage sharing of concerns, feelings, and information between patient and current or future partner. Whenever possible, involve both in sexual health education and counseling efforts. *For some sexual problems it is the couple relationship that provides the focus for intervention.*
- Discuss the multiplicity of influences upon sexual functioning (physiological, emotional, etc.) Offer opportunities to ask questions and express feelings.
- Explore awareness of and comfort with a range of sexual expression and activities (not just sexual intercourse).
- Assist patient/other in identifying possible options to overcome situational, temporary, or long-term influences on sexual functioning.
- Encourage patients and significant others to locate and read relevant educational materials regarding sexuality. *Many excellent books are available that undo myths and errors and promote increased knowledge and communication about sexual concerns.*
- ▲ Consider referral for further work-up and or treatment. (i.e., primary health care provider, specialized physician or mental health consultant, substance abuse treatment program, or sexual dysfunction clinic, etc.). *Sexual counseling may be beyond the skill/training of the nurse.*
- Consider referral to self-help and/or support groups (i.e., Reach for Recovery, Ostomy Association, Mended Hearts, Huff and Puff, Sexual Impotence Resolved, Us Too, HIV Support Groups, Y Me, Survivors of Abuse, Resolve, etc.). *Self-help support groups are unique sources of empathy, information, and successful role models.*

RELATED FACTORS / DEFINING CHARACTERISTICS	EXPECTED OUTCOMES AND NURSING INTERVENTIONS / *RATIONALE* (■ = INDEPENDENT; ▲ = COLLABORATIVE)

DEFINING CHARACTERISTICS

Verbalized concern(s) regarding sexual functioning

Questions regarding "normal" sexual functioning

Expressed dissatisfaction with sexuality (i.e., decreased satisfaction, symptoms of sexual dysfunction, concerns about sexual preference or orientation, difficulties in accepting self/others as sexual beings, etc.)

Reported changes in relationship with partner(s)

Actual/perceived limitation secondary to diagnosis or therapy

Noncompliance with medications/treatments with associated risk of impaired or altered sexual functioning

Reported changes in previously established sexual patterns

Sexual behavior inappropriate to circumstance or setting

Frequent efforts designed to elicit affirmation of sexual desirability

PATIENT EDUCATION

- Provide accurate and timely health teaching regarding "normal" range of sexual expression and sexual practices throughout the life cycle. *Satisfying sexual functioning and practice are not automatic and need to be learned.*
- Discuss range of possibilities and consequences (both positive and negative) associated with sexual expression of all types (change in relationship, impact on physical and/or emotional health, possibility of pregnancy, sexually transmitted diseases, etc.)
- Offer information regarding birth control methods, means of safe/safer sex, etc.
- Explain the effects on sexual functioning of patient's medication(s), illness or disease process, health alteration, surgery, or therapy.
- Be specific in providing instruction to patient/other regarding any limitations on sexual activity due to illness, surgery, or other events.
- Provide role modeling in use of social skills.
- Explain alternative means/forms of expressing intimacy and/or sexual expression, such as: alternative positions for intercourse that decrease discomfort or degree of physical exertion for those with impaired mobility or cardiopulmonary disease. Consider concerns imposed by patient's/significant other's health status, illness, etc.

By: Ann Filipski, RN, MSN, CS, PsyD candidate
Jeff Zurlinden, RN, MS

Skin integrity, impaired: high risk for

A state in which an individual's skin is at risk for becoming adversely altered.

PRESSURE SORES; BED SORES; DECUBITUS CARE

RISK FACTORS	EXPECTED OUTCOMES AND NURSING INTERVENTIONS / *RATIONALE* (■ = INDEPENDENT; ▲ = COLLABORATIVE)

RISK FACTORS

Extremes of age
Immobility
Poor nutrition
Mechanical forces (pressure, shear, friction)
Pronounced bony prominences
Poor circulation
Altered sensation
Incontinence
Environmental moisture
Radiation
Hyper/hypothermia
AIDS

EXPECTED OUTCOMES

Patient's skin remains intact, as evidenced by no redness over bony prominences and capillary refill <6 seconds over areas of redness.

ONGOING ASSESSMENT

- Determine age. *Elderly patients' skin is less elastic and has less moisture, making for higher risk of skin impairment.*
- Assess general condition of skin. *Healthy skin varies from individual to individual, but should have good turgor (an indication of moisture), feel warm and dry to the touch, be free of impairment (scratches, bruises, excoriation, rashes), and have quick capillary refill (<6 seconds).*
- Specifically assess skin over bony prominences (sacrum, trochanters, scapulae, elbows, heels, inner and outer malleus, inner and outer knees, back of head). *Areas where skin is stretched tautly over bony prominences are at highest risk for breakdown because the possibility of ischemia to skin is high due to compression of skin capillaries between a hard surface (mattress, chair, OR table) and the bone.*

Continued.

Nursing Diagnosis Care Plans

RISK FACTORS	EXPECTED OUTCOMES AND NURSING INTERVENTIONS / *RATIONALE* (■ = INDEPENDENT; ▲ = COLLABORATIVE)

ONGOING ASSESMENT

- Assess patient's awareness of the sensation of pressure. *Normally, individuals shift their weight off pressure areas every few minutes; this occurs more or less automatically, even during sleep. Patients with decreased sensation are unaware of unpleasant stimuli (pressure) and do not shift weight.*
- Assess patient's ability to move (shift weight while sitting, turn over in bed, move from bed to chair). *Immobility is the major risk factor in skin breakdown.*
- Assess patient's nutritional status, including weight, weight loss, and serum albumin levels. *Albumin level <2.5 g/dl is a grave sign, indicating severe protein depletion.*
- Assess for history of radiation therapy. *Radiated skin becomes thin and friable, and is at higher risk for breakdown.*
- Assess for history/presence of AIDS. *Early manifestations of HIV-related diseases may include skin lesions (e.g., Kaposi's sarcoma); additionally, because of their immunoincompetence, patients with AIDS frequently have skin breakdown.*
- Assess for fecal and/or urinary incontinence. *The urea in urine turns into ammonia within minutes, and is caustic to the skin. Stool may contain enzymes that cause skin breakdown. Use of diapers and incontinence pads with plastic liners trap moisture and hasten breakdown.*
- Assess for environmental moisture (wound drainage, high humidity) that *may contribute to skin maceration.*
- Assess surface that patient spends majority of time on (mattress for bedridden patient, cushion for persons in wheelchairs). *Patients who spend the majority of time on one surface need a pressure reduction or pressure relief device to lessen the risk for breakdown.*
- Assess amount of shear *(pressure exerted laterally)* and friction *(rubbing)* on patient's skin. *A common cause of shear is elevating the head of the patient's bed; the body's weight is shifted downward onto the patient's sacrum. Common causes of friction include the patient rubbing heels/elbows against bed linen, and moving the patient up in bed without the use of a lift sheet.*
- Reassess skin at least every 24 hours and whenever the patient's condition or treatment plan results in an increased number of risk factors. *The incidence of skin breakdown is directly related to the number of risk factors present.*

THERAPEUTIC INTERVENTIONS

- If patient is restricted to bed:
  Implement and post a turning schedule, restricting time in one position to 2 hr or less and customizing the schedule to patient's routine and to nursing care needs. *A schedule that does not interfere with the patient's and nurses' activities is likely to be followed.*
- ▲ Implement pressure-relieving devices commensurate with degree of risk for skin impairment:
  For low-risk patients: good-quality (dense, at least 5 inches thick) foam mattress overlay.
  For moderate risk patients: water mattress, static or dynamic air mattress.
  For high-risk patients or those with existing stage III or IV pressure sores (or with stage II pressure sores *and* multiple risk factors): low-air-loss beds (Mediscus, Flexicare, Kinair) or air-fluidized therapy (Clinitron, Skytron). *Low-air-loss beds are constructed to allow elevated head of bed (HOB) and patient transfer. These should be used when pulmonary concerns necessitate elevating HOB or when getting patient up is feasible. Air-fluidized therapy supports patient's weight at well below capillary closing pressure but restricts getting patient out of bed easily.*
- Maintain functional body alignment.
- Limit chair sitting to 2 hr at any one time. *Pressure over sacrum may exceed 100 mm Hg pressure during sitting.*
- Encourage ambulation if patient is able.
- Increase tissue perfusion by massaging *around* affected area. *Massaging reddened area may damage skin further.*
- Clean, dry, and moisturize skin, especially over bony prominences, b.i.d., or as indicated by incontinence or sweating. If powder is desirable *to reduce friction,* use medical-grade cornstarch; avoid talc.

RISK FACTORS	EXPECTED OUTCOMES AND NURSING INTERVENTIONS / *RATIONALE* (■ = INDEPENDENT; ▲ = COLLABORATIVE)

THERAPEUTIC INTERVENTIONS

▲ Encourage adequate nutrition and hydration:
   2000-3000 calories/day (more if increased metabolic demands).
   Fluid intake of 2000 ml/day unless medically restricted.
   Dietitian consultation as appropriate.
   Hydrated skin is less prone to breakdown.
- Use lift sheets to move patient in bed and discourage patient from elevating HOB. *These measures reduce shearing forces on the skin.*
▲ Leave blisters intact by wrapping in gauze or applying a hydrocolloid (Duoderm, Sween-Appeal), or a vaporpermeable membrane dressing (Op-Site, Tegaderm). *Blisters are sterile natural dressings.*

PATIENT EDUCATION

- Teach patient and family the cause(s) of pressure ulcer development:
   Pressure on skin, especially over bony prominences.
   Incontinence.
   Poor nutrition.
   Shearing/friction against skin.
- Reinforce the importance of mobility/turning/ambulation in prevention of pressure ulcers.
- Teach patient/family proper use and maintenance of pressure-relieving devices to be used at home.

By: Audrey Klopp, RN, PhD, ET
   Virginia M. Storey, RN, ET
   Kathryn S. Bronstein, RN, PhD, CS

Sleep pattern disturbance

INSOMNIA

A disruption in the individual's usual diurnal pattern of sleep and wakefulness that may be temporary or chronic. Such disruptions may result in both subjective distress and apparent impairment in functional abilities.

RELATED FACTORS / DEFINING CHARACTERISTICS	EXPECTED OUTCOMES AND NURSING INTERVENTIONS / *RATIONALE*

RELATED FACTORS

Pain/discomfort
Environmental changes
Anxiety/fear
Depression
Medications
Excessive/inadequate stimulation
Abnormal physiological status/symptoms (dyspnea, hypoxia, neurological dysfunction, etc.)
Normal changes associated with aging

DEFINING CHARACTERISTICS

Patient/significant other report of alteration in "normal" sleep pattern
Difficulty in falling or remaining asleep
Complaints of not feeling rested
Early morning awakening

EXPECTED OUTCOMES

Patient achieves optimal amounts of sleep as evidenced by rested appearance, verbalization of feeling rested, and improvement in sleep pattern.

ONGOING ASSESSMENT

- Assess past patterns of sleep in normal environment: amount, bedtime rituals, depth, length, positions, aids, and interfering agents. *Sleep patterns are unique to each individual.*
- Assess patient's perception of cause of sleep difficulty and possible relief measures *to facilitate treatment.*
- Document nursing observations of sleeping and wakeful behaviors. Record number of sleep hours. Note physical (e.g., sleep apnea, pain/discomfort, urinary frequency) and/or psychological (e.g., fear, anxiety) circumstances that interrupt sleep.
- Identify factors that may facilitate or interfere with "normal patterns." *Considerable confusion and mythology about sleep exist. Knowledge of its role in health/wellness and the wide variation among individuals may allay anxiety, thereby promoting rest and sleep.*
- Evaluate timing/effects of medications that disrupt sleep.

THERAPEUTIC INTERVENTIONS

- Maintain environment conducive to sleep/rest (e.g., quiet, comfortable temperature, ventilation, closed door).
- Assist patient in observing any previous bedtime ritual *to promote relaxation.*
- Provide nursing aids (e.g., back rub, bedtime care, pain relief, comfortable position, relaxation techniques) *to promote rest, relaxation.*

Continued.

Sleep pattern disturbance—cont'd

RELATED FACTORS / DEFINING CHARACTERISTICS	EXPECTED OUTCOMES AND NURSING INTERVENTIONS / *RATIONALE* (■ = INDEPENDENT; ▲ = COLLABORATIVE)

DEFINING CHARACTERISTICS—cont'd
 	
Restlessness
Lethargy/fatigue
Insomnia
Irritability
Dozing
Yawning
Altered mental status
Difficulty in arousal
Change in activity level
Altered facial expression (e.g., blank look, fatigued appearance)
Reddened eyes
	THERAPEUTIC INTERVENTIONS
	• Organize nursing care *to promote minimal interruption in sleep/rest.*
	  Eliminate nonessential nursing activities.
	  Prepare patient for necessary anticipated interruptions/disruptions.
	• Attempt to allow for sleep cycles of at least 90 min. *Experimental studies have indicated that 60-90 min are needed to complete one sleep cycle and the completion of an entire cycle is necessary to benefit from sleep.*
	• Establish semblance of "normal" daily routine with periods of activity, rest. *Adherence to previously established patterns/routines minimizes energy required for adaptation and disruption in biological rhythms.*
	• Provide soporifics (e.g., milk, avoidance of stimulants such as caffeine or cola beverages, and decreased exercise several hours before sleep) as needed.
	▲ Administer hypnotics as ordered and evaluate effectiveness. *Use of hypnotic medications should be thoughtful and avoided if less aggressive means are effective because of their potential for cumulative effects and generally limited period of benefit.*
	• Discourage pattern of daytime naps unless deemed necessary or part of usual pattern. *Napping can disrupt normal sleep pattern.*
	• Increase daytime physical activities as indicated *to reduce stress and promote sleep.*
	• Limit fluids before bedtime *to reduce need for voiding during night.*
	
	PATIENT EDUCATION
	• Teach about possible causes of sleeping difficulties and optimal ways to treat them.
	• Instruct to avoid bedtime foods and beverages that interfere with sleep.
	• Instruct on muscle relaxation or other nonpharmacological forms of sleep inducement.

By: Sue Galanes, RN, MS, CCRN

Spiritual distress

An experience of profound disharmony in the client's belief or value system that threatens the meaning of the client's life. During spiritual distress the client loses hope, questions his/her belief system, or feels separated from his/her personal source of comfort and strength.

RELATED FACTORS / DEFINING CHARACTERISTICS	EXPECTED OUTCOMES AND NURSING INTERVENTIONS / *RATIONALE* (■ = INDEPENDENT; ▲ = COLLABORATIVE)

RELATED FACTORS
 	
Separation from religious ties
Separation from loved ones
Chronic or debilitating illness
Terminal illness
Surgery
Pain
Loss or illness of a loved one
 	
DEFINING CHARACTERISTICS
 	
Questions meaning of life/death and/or belief system
Seeks spiritual assistance
Voices guilt, loss of hope, spiritual emptiness, or feeling of being alone
Appears anxious, depressed, discouraged, fearful, or angry
	EXPECTED OUTCOMES
	Patient expresses hope in and value of his/her own belief system.
	
	ONGOING ASSESSMENT
	• Assess history of formal religious affiliation. *Information regarding specific religion and importance of rituals or practices may improve understanding of patient's needs while hospitalized.*
	• Assess other significant beliefs. *Individuals may have other important beliefs besides religion that provide strength and inspiration.*
	• Assess spiritual meaning of illness or treatment. *Questions such as the following provide a basis for future care planning:*
	  "What is the meaning of your illness?"
	  "How does your illness or treatment affect your relationship with God, your beliefs, or other sources of strength?"
	  "Does your illness or treatment interfere with expressing your spiritual beliefs?"
	• Assess hope.
	• Assess whether patients have any unfinished business. *Patients may not find peace or harmony until business is resolved.*

RELATED FACTORS / DEFINING CHARACTERISTICS	EXPECTED OUTCOMES AND NURSING INTERVENTIONS / *RATIONALE* (■ = INDEPENDENT; ▲ = COLLABORATIVE)

THERAPEUTIC INTERVENTIONS

- Display an understanding and accepting attitude. Encourage verbalization of feelings of anger or loneliness.
- Structure your interventions in terms of patient's belief system. *Patients have a right to their beliefs, even if they conflict with the nurse's beliefs.*
- Develop an ongoing relationship with patient.
- When requested by patient or family, arrange for clergy, religious rituals, or the display of religious objects.
- If requested, pray with patient. *This provides a sense of connectedness to others.*
- If patient belongs to a highly codified or ritualized religion, such as Orthodox Judaism, arrange for clergy at times of passage, such as birth or death.
- Acknowledge and support patient's hopes. *Hopes are different from denial or delusions. Supporting a hope for discharge does not mean supporting a denial of the seriousness of the patient's condition. Hope allows the patient to face the seriousness of the situation.*
- Do not provide logical solutions for spiritual dilemmas. *Spiritual beliefs are based on faith and are independent of logic.*
- See Hopelessness p. 36.

PATIENT EDUCATION

- Provide information in a way that does not interfere with patient's beliefs, faith, or hopes. *This demonstrates respect for patient's individuality.*
- Inform the patient of how to obtain religious rites or seek spiritual guidance.

By: Jeff Zurlinden, RN, MS

Swallowing, impaired

DYSPHAGIA

The state in which an individual has decreased ability to pass fluids and/or solids from the mouth to the stomach voluntarily.

RELATED FACTORS / DEFINING CHARACTERISTICS	EXPECTED OUTCOMES AND NURSING INTERVENTIONS / *RATIONALE* (■ = INDEPENDENT; ▲ = COLLABORATIVE)

RELATED FACTORS

Neuromuscular:
- Decreased or absent gag reflex
- Decreased strength or excursion of muscles involved in mastication
- Perceptual impairment
- Facial paralysis (cranial nerves VII, IX, X, XII)

Mechanical:
- Edema
- Tracheostomy tube
- Tumor

Fatigue

Limited awareness

Reddened irritated oropharyngeal cavity (stomatitis)

DEFINING CHARACTERISTICS

Observed evidence of difficulty in swallowing:
- Coughing
- Choking
- Pocketing of food along side of mouth

Verbalized difficulty

EXPECTED OUTCOMES

Patient maintains adequate nutrition, as evidenced by stable weight.

Patient does not experience aspiration.

Patient verbalizes appropriate maneuvers to prevent choking and aspiration: positioning during eating, type of food tolerated, and safe environment.

Patient/significant other verbalizes emergency measures to be enacted should choking occur.

ONGOING ASSESSMENT

- Assess presence/absence of gag and cough reflexes. *A depressed gag or cough reflex increases the risk of aspiration.*
- Assess strength of facial muscles. *Pathology of cranial nerves, especially VII, IX, X, and XII affect motor function and control.*
- Assess ability to swallow small amount of water (*if aspirated, little or no harm to patient occurs*).
- Assess for residual food in mouth after eating.
- Assess regurgitation of food/fluid through nares.
- Assess choking during eating/drinking.
- Assess breath sounds and respiratory status q4hr *for clinical evidence of aspiration.*

THERAPEUTIC INTERVENTIONS

- Before mealtime, provide adequate rest periods. *Fatigue can further contribute to swallowing impairment.*
- Remove or reduce environmental stimuli (television, radio) *so patient can concentrate on swallowing.*

Continued.

RELATED FACTORS / DEFINING CHARACTERISTICS	EXPECTED OUTCOMES AND NURSING INTERVENTIONS / *RATIONALE* (■ = INDEPENDENT; ▲ = COLLABORATIVE)
	THERAPEUTIC INTERVENTIONS

THERAPEUTIC INTERVENTIONS

- Provide oral care before feeding. Clean and insert dentures before each meal.
- Place suction equipment at bedside. Suction p.r.n. *With impaired swallowing reflexes, secretions can rapidly accumulate in posterior pharynx and upper trachea and increase risk of aspiration.*
- If decreased salivation is contributing factor:
    Before feeding, swab oral cavity with lemon-glycerin or encourage patient to suck tart-flavored hard candy. *Tart flavors stimulate salivation.*
    Use artificial saliva.
- Maintain patient in high Fowler's position with head flexed slightly forward during meals. *Upright position facilitates gravity flow of food/fluid through alimentary tract. Aspiration is less likely to occur with head tilted slightly forward (position narrows airway).*
- Encourage intake of food patient can swallow; provide frequent small meals and supplements. *Foods with consistency of pudding, hot cereal, and semisolid food are most easily swallowed because of consistency and weight. Thin foods are most difficult; gravy or sauce added to dry foods facilitates swallowing.*
- Instruct patient not to talk while eating.
- Encourage patient to chew thoroughly and eat slowly. Provide patient with direction/reinforcement until he/she has swallowed each mouthful *to keep focus on task.*
- Identify food given to patient before each spoonful.
- Proceed slowly, giving small amounts; whenever possible, alternate servings of liquids and solids *to help prevent foods from being left in the mouth.*
- Encourage high-calorie diet that includes all food groups, as appropriate. Avoid milk, milk products, and chocolate *(can lead to thickened secretions.)*
- If food is pouched, encourage patient to turn head to unaffected side and manipulate tongue to paralyzed side *to clean out residual food.*
- If patient has had a cerebrovascular accident (CVA), place food in back of mouth, on unaffected side and gently massage unaffected side of throat.
- Place whole or crushed pills in custard, gelatin, etc. (First ask pharmacist which pills should not be crushed).
- Encourage patient to feed himself/herself as soon as possible.
- If oral intake not possible or inadequate, initiate alternative feedings (e.g., nasogastric feedings, gastrostomy feedings, hyperalimentation).

Follow-up:
- ▲ Initiate dietary consultation for 72-hr calorie count and food preferences.
- ▲ Initiate speech pathology consultation for swallowing impairment evaluation and patient assistance.

PATIENT EDUCATION

- Discuss with and demonstrate to patient/significant others the following:
    Avoidance of certain foods or fluids.
    Upright position during eating.
    Allowance of time to eat slowly and chew thoroughly.
    Provision of high-calorie meals.
    Use of fluids to help facilitate passage of solid foods.
    Monitoring of patient for weight loss or dehydration. *Fluid intake should equal 2-3 L/day; weight loss of 5 lb/wk over 2 wk should be reported to physician.*
- Facilitate dietary counseling from hospital dietitian.
- Help patient/significant other set realistic goals *to prevent feelings of frustration and disappointment.*
- Provide name and telephone number of primary nurse and physician and information on when to call.
- Demonstrate to patient/significant other/family what should be done if patient aspirates (chokes, coughs, becomes short of breath): for example, use of suction if available and of the Heimlich maneuver if patient is unable to speak or breathe. If liquid aspiration, turn patient three-fourths prone with head slightly lower than chest, *(allowing drainage of secretions).* Wipe away secretions.
    If patient has difficulty breathing, call the Emergency Medical System (911).
- Encourage family members/significant other to seek out CPR instruction in hospital/community.

By: Linda Arsenaut, RN, MSN, CNRN

Thought processes, altered

CONFUSION: DISORIENTATION; INAPPROPRIATE
SOCIAL BEHAVIOR; ALTERED MOOD STATES;
DELUSIONS; IMPAIRED COGNITIVE PROCESSES

A condition in which an individual experiences a disruption in cognitive processes, defined as those mental processes by which knowledge is acquired. These mental processes include reality orientation, comprehension, awareness, and judgment. A disruption in these mental processes may lead to inaccurate interpretations of the environment and may result in an inability to evaluate reality accurately.

RELATED FACTORS / DEFINING CHARACTERISTICS	EXPECTED OUTCOMES AND NURSING INTERVENTIONS / *RATIONALE* (■ = INDEPENDENT; ▲ = COLLABORATIVE)

RELATED FACTORS

Organic mental disorders (non-substance-induced):
  Dementia
  Primary degenerative, e.g.,
   Alzheimer's disease, Pick's
   disease
  Multi-infarct, e.g., cerebral
   arteriosclerosis
  Those organic mental disor-
   ders associated with other
   physical disorders:
     Huntington's chorea
     Multiple sclerosis
     Parkinson's disease
     Cerebral hypoxia
     Hypertension
     Hepatic disease
     Epilepsy
  Adrenal, thyroid, or parathy-
   roid disorders
  Head trauma
  CNS infections (encephalitis,
   syphilis, meningitis)
  Intracranial lesions (benign
   or malignant)
  Sleep deprivation
Organic mental disorders (substance induced):
  Organic mental disorders
   attributed to the ingestion
   of alcohol (alcohol withdrawal; dementia associated with alcoholism)
  Organic mental disorders
   attributed to the ingestion
   of drugs/mood-altering
   substances
Schizophrenic disorders
Personality disorders in which
 there is evidence of altered
 thought processes
Affective disorders in which
 there is evidence of altered
 thought processes

I. For Disorientation:

EXPECTED OUTCOMES

Patient experiences reduced disorientation to time, place, person, and situation.
Patient interacts with others appropriately.

ONGOING ASSESSMENT

- Assess degree of orientation to time, place, person, and situation regularly and frequently. *This will determine the amount of orientation the patient will need to evaluate reality accurately.*

THERAPEUTIC INTERVENTIONS

- Orient to surroundings and reality as needed.
    Use patient's name when speaking to him/her.
    Speak slowly and clearly. Present information in a matter-of-fact manner *to decrease chances for misinterpretation.*
    Refer to the time of day, date, and recent events in your interactions with the patient.
    Encourage patient to check calendar and clock frequently.
    Encourage patient to have familiar personal belongings in his/her environment.
    Be matter-of-fact and respectful when correcting patient's misperceptions of reality.
- Use the words *you* and *I*, instead of *we*, to increase orientation and to encourage patient to maintain his/her sense of separateness and personal boundary. *Orientation to one's environment increases one's ability to trust others. Increased orientation assures a greater degree of safety for the patient. It also encourages the patient's cooperation in any necessary treatments or tests. Familiar personal possessions increase the patient's comfort level.*

II. For Altered Behavioral Patterns:

EXPECTED OUTCOMES

Patient demonstrates socially appropriate behavior, as evidenced by a decrease in suspiciousness, aggression, and provocative behavior.

ONGOING ASSESSMENT

- Regularly assess patient's behavior and social interactions for appropriateness.
- Evaluate ability and willingness to respond to verbal direction and limits.
- Observe for statements reflecting a desire or fantasy to inflict harm on self or others. *Patient's ability and/or willingness to respond to verbal direction and/or limits may vary with patient's mood, perceptions, degree of reality orientation, and environmental stressors. Confusion, disorientation, impaired judgment, suspiciousness, and loss of social inhibitions all may result in socially inappropriate and/or harmful behavior to self or others.*

Continued.

RELATED FACTORS / DEFINING CHARACTERISTICS	EXPECTED OUTCOMES AND NURSING INTERVENTIONS / *RATIONALE* (■ = INDEPENDENT; ▲ = COLLABORATIVE)

DEFINING CHARACTERISTICS

Disorientation to one or more of the following: time, person, place, situation
Altered behavioral patterns (regression, poor impulse control)
Altered mood states (lability, hostility, irritability, inappropriate affect)
Impaired ability to perform self-maintenance activities, (i.e., grooming, hygiene, food and fluid intake)
Altered sleep patterns
Altered perceptions of surrounding stimuli caused by impairment in the following cognitive processes:
 Memory
 Judgment
 Comprehension
 Concentration
 Ability to reason, problem solve, calculate, and conceptualize
Altered perceptions of surrounding stimuli caused by hallucinations, delusions, confabulation, and ideas of reference

THERAPEUTIC INTERVENTIONS

- Maintain routine interactions, activities, and close observation without increasing patient's suspiciousness. *Patients with impaired judgment and loss of social inhibitions require close observation to discourage inappropriate behavior and prevent harm or injury to self and others.*
- Develop an open and honest relationship in which expectations are respectfully and clearly verbalized. Make only those promises that can be kept. Verbalize acceptance of patient despite the inappropriateness of his/her behavior. *Honesty, openness, and verbalized acceptance of patient increase his/her self-respect and esteem. Keeping promises establishes a sense of trust and reliability between patient and staff.*
- Provide role modeling for patient through appropriate social and professional interactions with other patients and staff. *Role modeling provides patient an opportunity to observe socially appropriate behavior.*
- Encourage to assume responsibility for own behavior. Verbalize to patient the staff's willingness to assist in maintaining appropriate behavior when patient appears to need structure. *Encouraging patient to assume responsibility for own behavior will increase his/her sense of independence. Staff intervention will provide a feeling of security and reassurance.*
- Provide situations in which group interactions with other patients allows feedback regarding his/her behavior. *It is important for patient to learn socially appropriate behavior through group interactions. This provides an opportunity for the patient to observe the impact his/her behavior has on those around him/her. It also facilitates the development of acceptable social skills.*
- Provide positive reinforcement for efforts and appropriate behavior; confront when behavior is inappropriate, and withdraw attention. *Attention drawn to patient's inappropriate behavior may reinforce it.*

III. For Altered Mood States:

EXPECTED OUTCOMES

Patient exhibits appropriate affect and decreased lability and hostility.

ONGOING ASSESSMENT

- Assess mood and affect regularly. **Affect** *is defined as an emotion that is immediately expressed and observed. Affect is inappropriate when it is not in conjunction with the content of the patient's speech and/or ideation.* **Lability** *is defined as repeated, abrupt, and rapid changes in affect.* **Mood** *is defined as a pervasive and sustained emotion. Frequent and regular assessment of patient's mood and affect will assist in determining the predominance of a particular affect or mood and any deviations. This assessment will also determine the presence of any lability or hostility.*
- Assess for environmental and situational factors that may contribute to the change in mood or affect. *It is important to remember that patients with thought disorders may also experience fluctuations in mood and affect based on external stimuli, including environmental and situational factors.*

THERAPEUTIC INTERVENTIONS

- Demonstrate acceptance of patient as an individual. *It is important to communicate to patient one's acceptance of him/her regardless of his/her behavior.*
- Demonstrate tolerance of fluctuations in affect and mood. Address inappropriate affect and mood in a calm, yet firm, manner. *Calmness communicates self-control and tolerance of the patient and his/her affect and mood. Addressing and setting limits for inappropriate behavior communicate clear expectations for patient.*
- Identify environmental stimuli that cause increased restlessness or agitation for the patient. Remove patient when possible from external stimuli that appear to exacerbate irritable and hostile behavior. *The patient's ability to recognize irritating stimuli and remove himself/herself from the source may be impaired. Removing patient from external stimuli that exacerbate fluctuations in mood and affect encourages a sense of protection and security for patient.*
- Encourage involvement in group activities as tolerated. *Involvement in group activities is determined by various factors, including the group size, activity level, and patient's tolerance level. Remain aware that patient's fluctuations in mood and affect will affect his/her ability to respond appropriately to others and his/her capacity to handle complex and multiple stimuli.*

IV. For Impaired Ability to Perform Activities of Daily Living:

EXPECTED OUTCOMES

Patient participates in own ADL.

ONGOING ASSESSMENT

- Regularly assess patient's ability and motivation to initiate, perform, and maintain self-care activities. *Assessment will identify areas of physical care in which patient needs assistance. These areas of physical care include nutrition, elimination, sleep and rest, exercise, bathing, grooming, and dressing. It is important to distinguish between ability and motivation in the initiation, performance, and maintenance of self-care activities. Patients may present with ability and minimal motivation or motivation and minimal ability.*
- Obtain history from patient, family, and friends regarding patient's dietary habits. *Information about patient's dietary habits is important in determining the presence of food allergies. It will also determine patient's personal food preferences, cultural dietary restrictions, and ability to verbalize hunger.*
- Obtain accurate weight on admission and maintain ongoing records through patient's length of treatment. Weigh patient on a scheduled basis (e g , daily, twice weekly). *Accurate records of patient's body weight help determine significant fluctuations.*
- Maintain adequate records of the patient's intake and output, elimination patterns, and any associated concerns verbalized by patient. *The patient with impaired thought processes may be unable to self-monitor intake, output, and elimination patterns.*
- ▲ Monitor laboratory values and report any significant changes. *Laboratory data provide objective information regarding the adequacy of patient's diet.*
- Obtain information from patient's family regarding personal grooming and hygiene habits. *This information will assist in developing a specific plan for grooming and hygiene activities.*

THERAPEUTIC INTERVENTIONS

- ▲ Obtain dietary consultation and determine the number of calories patient will require to maintain adequate nutritional intake based on body weight and structure. *The patient with an altered thought process may be impaired in maintaining adequate nutritional intake.*
- Encourage adequate fluid intake and physical exercise. *Both ongoing exercise and adequate fluid intake help prevent constipation.*
- Assist patient with bathing, grooming, and dressing as needed. *The patient with impaired thought processes may be unable to perform grooming activities.*
- Provide patient with positive reinforcement for his/her efforts in maintaining self-care activities. *Positive reinforcement is perceived by patient as support.*

V. For Altered Sleep:

EXPECTED OUTCOMES

Patient achieves normal sleep pattern.

ONGOING ASSESSMENT

- Assess how sleep is altered. Establish whether patient has difficulty falling asleep, awakens during the night, early in the morning, or is experiencing insomnia. *It is important to determine an accurate baseline for planning interventions.*
- Maintain accurate records of patient's sleep patterns.

THERAPEUTIC INTERVENTIONS

- Decrease stimuli before patient goes to bed by suggesting a warm bath, turning down TV/radio, and dimming the lights. *Sleep and rest will be encouraged when loud stimuli are minimized.*
- Decrease intake of caffeinated substances (tea, colas, coffee). *Caffeine stimulates CNS and may interfere with patient's ability to rest and sleep.*
- Evaluate sedative effects of medications and schedule administration to diminish daytime sedation and promote sleep at night. *This will discourage sleeping during day and promote restful night sleep.*

Continued.

Nursing Diagnosis Care Plans

RELATED FACTORS / DEFINING CHARACTERISTICS	EXPECTED OUTCOMES AND NURSING INTERVENTIONS / *RATIONALE* (■ = INDEPENDENT; ▲ = COLLABORATIVE)

THERAPEUTIC INTERVENTIONS— cont'd

- Discourage long periods of nurse/patient contact at night. *Brief contacts as needed are less disruptive of sleep.*
- If patient is experiencing hypersomnia, discourage sleep during the day. Limit the time patient spends in his/her room and provide stimulating activities. *Structured expectations will provide a focus for activities, and contact will also provide opportunity to examine feelings the patient may be avoiding through excessive sleep.*

VI. For Altered Perceptions of Surrounding Stimuli:

EXPECTED OUTCOMES

Patient will demonstrate reality-based perceptions, as evidenced by decreased verbalizations of hallucinations and delusions and decreased threats to self and others.

ONGOING ASSESSMENT

- Assess and observe patient's ability to verbalize own needs and trust those around him/her.
- Assess patient's memory (recent and remote).
- Assess and observe patient's judgment and awareness of safety.
- Assess ability to concentrate, follow instructions, and problem solve on an ongoing basis.
- Assess patient's communication patterns. *Observe for the presence of delusions and/or hallucinations. Delusions are false beliefs that have no basis in reality. They may be fixed (persistent) or transient (episodic). Hallucinations are perceptions of external stimuli without the actual presence of those stimuli. Hallucinations may be visual, auditory, olfactory, tactile, and gustatory and are perceived by patient as real.*

THERAPEUTIC INTERVENTIONS

- Encourage patient to communicate own thoughts and perceptions with significant others in the environment. *Validation of patient's needs, thoughts, and perceptions will encourage trust and openness.*
- Clarify patient's misperceptions of events and situations that may result from memory impairment. *Clarification is necessary and more easily accepted when offered in a respectful manner.*
- Orient to time, place, person, and situation as needed. *The patient's ability to orient himself/herself may be impaired by memory loss.*
- Minimize situations that provoke anxiety. *Anxiety may impair patient's ability to communicate, problem solve, and reason.*
- Provide protective supervision. *The patient's safety is a priority. The patient may be unable to accurately assess potentially dangerous items and situations such as wet floors, electrical appliances, and verbal threats from other patients as a result of severe impairment in judgment.*
- If patient is experiencing delusional thinking, assist him/her in recognizing the delusions. Acknowledge the delusions without agreeing to the content of the delusions. *Delusions can be anxiety-provoking and distressing for patient. It is important to acknowledge this distress but to convey that one does not accept the delusions as real.*
- If patient is experiencing hallucinations, such as inappropriate gestures, laughter, talking to oneself without the presence of others:
  Communicate verbally with patient by using concrete and direct words and avoiding gesturing.
  Encourage patient to inform staff when experiencing hallucinations.
  Discuss content of the hallucinations to determine appropriate interventions.
  Determine whether the hallucinations are resulting in thoughts and/or plans to harm himself/herself or others.
  Early detection of behavior reflecting active hallucinations will encourage early response to patient's behavior. This will increase the likelihood of successful interventions for agitated and unpredictable behavior. It is important to acknowledge the presence of the hallucinations without accepting them as real.

By: Ursula Brozek, RN, MS

Tissue integrity, impaired

The state in which an individual experiences damage to integumentary or subcutaneous tissue. If untreated, impaired tissue is at risk for infection, and can lead to systemic infection (sepsis).

RELATED FACTORS / DEFINING CHARACTERISTICS	EXPECTED OUTCOMES AND NURSING INTERVENTIONS / *RATIONALE* (▪ = INDEPENDENT; ▲ = COLLABORATIVE)

RELATED FACTORS
Trauma
Infection
Altered circulation

DEFINING CHARACTERISTICS
Affected area hot, tender to touch
Skin purplish
Swelling around initial injury
Local pain
Protectiveness toward site

EXPECTED OUTCOMES

Condition of impaired tissue improves as evidenced by decreased redness, swelling, and pain.

ONGOING ASSESSMENT

- Elicit details of initial injury and treatment.
- Assess condition of tissue. *Redness, swelling, pain, burning, and itching are signs of the body's immune response to localized tissue trauma.*
- Assess for signs of infection. *Purulent drainage from the injured area is an indication of infection.*
- Assess temperature, *an indication of infection.*
- Assess patient's level of discomfort.

THERAPEUTIC INTERVENTIONS

- Apply continuous or intermittent wet dressings *to reduce intensity of inflammation.*
- Protect healthy skin from maceration when wet dressings are applied:
    Remove moisture by blotting gently; avoid friction.
    Consider use of liquid skin barriers.
- Discourage rubbing and scratching *(can cause further injury and delay healing).* Provide gloves or clip nails if necessary.
- ▲ Provide medicated soaks for open wounds, as ordered.
- ▲ Administer IV antibiotics as ordered.
- ▲ Administer antipyretics *to reduce temperature as prescribed.*
- ▲ Administer analgesics as prescribed *to reduce pain.*

PATIENT EDUCATION

- Teach patient about cause of tissue integrity impairment.
- Instruct patient in proper care of area, (i.e., cleansing, dressing, and application of topical medications).
- Teach patient signs and symptoms of infection and when to notify physician/nurse.
- Teach patient pain control measures: (i.e., soaks, use of analgesics, and distraction).

By: Sherry Adams, RN, ADN

Tissue perfusion, altered: peripheral, cardiopulmonary, cardiovascular, cerebral

Reduced arterial blood flow being delivered to body tissues, causing decreased nutrition and oxygenation at the cellular level. Management is directed at removing vasoconstricting factors, improving peripheral blood flow, and reducing metabolic demands on the body. This care plan focuses on problems in hospitalized patients.

RELATED FACTORS / DEFINING CHARACTERISTICS	EXPECTED OUTCOMES AND NURSING INTERVENTIONS / *RATIONALE* (▪ = INDEPENDENT; ▲ = COLLABORATIVE)

RELATED FACTORS

Peripheral
In-dwelling arterial catheters
Constricting cast
Compartment syndrome
Embolism/thrombus
Arterial spasm
Vasoconstriction
Positioning

EXPECTED OUTCOMES

Patient maintains optimal tissue perfusion to vital organs, as evidenced by strong peripheral pulses, normal ABGs, alert LOC, and absence of chest pain.

ONGOING ASSESSMENT

- Assess for signs of decreased tissue perfusion (see Defining characteristics for each category).

Continued.

Tissue perfusion, altered—cont'd

RELATED FACTORS / DEFINING CHARACTERISTICS	EXPECTED OUTCOMES AND NURSING INTERVENTIONS / *RATIONALE* (■ = INDEPENDENT; ▲ = COLLABORATIVE)

Cardiopulmonary
Pulmonary embolism
Low Hgb
Cardiovascular
Myocardial ischemia
Vasospasm
Hypovolemia
Cerebral
↑ ICP
Vasoconstriction
Intracranial bleeding
Cerebral edema

DEFINING CHARACTERISTICS
Peripheral
Weak/absent peripheral pulses
Edema
Numbness, pain, ache in extremities
Cool extremities
Dependent rubor
Clammy skin
Mottling
Differences in BP in opposite extremities
Prolonged capillary refill
Cardiopulmonary
Tachycardia
Dysrhythmias
Hypotension
Tachypnea
Abnormal ABGs
Cardiovascular
Angina
Cerebral
Restlessness
Confusion
Lethargy
Seizure activity
Decreased Glasgow coma scores
Pupillary changes
Decreased reaction to light

ONGOING ASSESSMENT
- Assess for possible causative factors related to temporarily impaired arterial blood flow. *Early detection of cause facilitates prompt effective treatment.*
- ▲ Monitor PT/PTT if anticoagulants used for treatment.
- Monitor quality of all pulses. *Assessment needed for ongoing comparisons; loss of pulse must be reported/treated immediately.*

THERAPEUTIC INTERVENTIONS
- Maintain optimal cardiac output *to ensure adequate perfusion of vital organs.*
- ▲ Assist with diagnostic testing as indicated. *Doppler flow studies, angiograms, etc. may be required for accurate diagnosis.*
- Anticipate need for possible embolectomy, heparinization, vasodilator therapy, thrombolytic therapy, and fluid rescue.

SPECIFIC INTERVENTIONS
Peripheral
- Keep cannulated extremity still. Use soft restraints or armboards as needed. *Movement may cause trauma to artery.*
- Do passive ROM exercises to unaffected extremity every 2 to 4 hr *to prevent venous stasis.*
- ▲ Anticipate/continue anticoagulation as ordered.
- ▲ Prepare for removal of arterial catheter as needed. *Circulation is potentially compromised with cannula—should be removed ASAP.*
- ▲ If compartment syndrome is suspected, prepare for surgical intervention (i.e., fasciotomy).
- ▲ If cast causes altered tissue perfusion, anticipate cast removal.
Cardiopulmonary
- ▲ Administer O₂ as needed.
- Position properly *to promote optimal lung ventilation and perfusion.*
- ▲ Report changes in ABGs (hypoxemia, metabolic acidosis, hypercapnea).
- ▲ Anticipate and institute anticoagulation as prescribed.
- ▲ Institute continuous pulse oximetry. *Provides information on oxygen saturation of arterial blood.*
- See Pulmonary embolus, p. 216
Cardiovascular
- ▲ Administer NTG sublingually for angina.
- ▲ Administer O₂ as ordered.
- See Angina, p. 77
Cerebral
- ▲ Ensure proper functioning of ICP catheter (if present).
- If increased ICP exists, elevate head of bed 30-45 degrees *to promote venous outflow from brain and help reduce pressure.*
- Avoid measures that may trigger increased ICP (straining, strenuous coughing, positioning with neck in flexion, head flat).
- ▲ Administer anticonvulsants as needed.
- Reorient to environment prn.

PATIENT EDUCATION
- Explain all procedures and equipment.
- Instruct to inform nurse immediately of any pain, or problems with equipment.
- Provide information on normal tissue perfusion and possible causes for impairment.

By: Margaret Norton, RN, MSN

Urinary elimination, altered patterns of (incontinence)

STRESS INCONTINENCE; URGE INCONTINENCE;
OVERFLOW INCONTINENCE; REFLEX
INCONTINENCE; CONSTANT INCONTINENCE,
FUNCTIONAL INCONTINENCE

There are several types of urinary incontinence; all are characterized by the involuntary passage of urine. Urinary incontinence is not a disease but rather a symptom. Incontinence occurs more frequently among women, and incidence increases with age. An estimated 10 million people are incontinent. This care plan addresses six types: stress, urge, overflow, reflex, constant, and functional.

RELATED FACTORS / DEFINING CHARACTERISTICS	EXPECTED OUTCOMES AND NURSING INTERVENTIONS / *RATIONALE* (■ = INDEPENDENT; ▲ = COLLABORATIVE)

STRESS INCONTINENCE

RELATED FACTORS

Multiple vaginal deliveries
Pelvic surgery
Hypoestrogenism (aging, menopause)
Diabetic neuropathy
Trauma to pelvic area
Obesity
Radial prostatectomy
Myelomeningocele
Infection

DEFINING CHARACTERISTICS

Leakage of urine during exercise
Leakage of urine during coughing, sneezing, laughing, or lifting

EXPECTED OUTCOMES

Patient is continent of urine or verbalizes satisfactory management.

ONGOING ASSESSMENT

- Ask whether urine is lost involuntarily during coughing, laughing, sneezing, lifting, or exercising. *Whenever intra-abdominal pressure increases, a weak sphincter and/or relaxed pelvic floor muscles allow urine to escape involuntarily.*
- Examine perineal area for evidence of pelvic relaxation:
  Cystourethrocele *(sagging bladder/urethra).*
  Rectocele *(relaxed, sagging rectal mucosa).*
  Uterine prolapse *(relaxed uterus).*
- Determine parity. *Childbirth trauma weakens pelvic muscles.*
- Explore menstrual history.
- Ask about previous surgical procedures.
- Weigh patient. *Obesity contributes to increased intra-abdominal pressure.*
- ▲ Culture urine. *Infection can cause incontinence.*

THERAPEUTIC INTERVENTIONS

- Teach patient to perform Kegel exercises *to strengthen the pelvic floor musculature.*
- ▲ Administer sympathomimetics and estrogens as ordered *to increase sphincter tone and improve muscle tone.*
- Teach patient to use transcutaneous electrical nerve stimulator (TENS) as indicated *to improve pelvic floor tone.*
- ▲ Teach female patient use of vaginal pessary, *a device reserved for poor surgical candidates that works by elevating the bladder neck, thereby increasing urethral resistance.*
- Prepare patient for surgery as indicated. *Many types of procedures are used to control stress incontinence; the most commonly performed are Marshall-Marchetti, Burch's colposuspension, and sling procedures.*
- Prepare patient for the implantation of an artificial urinary sphincter, *which uses a subcutaneous pumping device to deflate/inflate a cuff that controls micturition.*
- Encourage weight loss if obese.

URGE INCONTINENCE

RELATED FACTORS

Uninhibited bladder contraction
CVA
Spinal cord injury
Parkinsonism
Multiple sclerosis
Benign prostatic hypertrophy
Infections
Psychogenic

EXPECTED OUTCOMES

Patient is continent of urine or verbalizes management.

ONGOING ASSESSMENT

- Ask patient to describe episodes of incontinence; note descriptions of "feeling the need suddenly but being unable to get to the bathroom in time."
- Consider age; *this type of urinary incontinence is the most frequent type among the elderly.*
- ▲ Culture urine.

Continued.

Urinary elimination, altered patterns of (incontinence)—cont'd

RELATED FACTORS / DEFINING CHARACTERISTICS	EXPECTED OUTCOMES AND NURSING INTERVENTIONS / *RATIONALE* (■ = INDEPENDENT; ▲ = COLLABORATIVE)
DEFINING CHARACTERISTICS Sudden, "unannounced" need to void Frequent urinary accidents associated with "not getting there in time" Inability to delay voiding	**THERAPEUTIC INTERVENTIONS** ▲ Administer medications that reduce or block detrusor contractions (anticholinergics); *these inhibit smooth muscle contractions and may reduce episodes of incontinence.* ■ Prepare patient for surgical correction (sphincterotomy) as indicated; *denervation, resulting in complete incontinence, may be undertaken (rhizotomy). Urinary diversion (ileal conduit) may be performed as a last resort.* ■ Educate patient in the use of biofeedback techniques *for control of pelvic floor musculature.* ■ Facilitate access to toilet/teach patient to make scheduled trips to bathroom.

OVERFLOW INCONTINENCE

RELATED FACTORS
Bladder outlet obstruction
Prostatic hypertrophy
Extensive pelvic surgery
Myelomeningocele
Trauma
Multiple sclerosis
Diabetes mellitus
Infrequent voiding patterns
Fecal impaction
Drugs that lead to urinary retention:
    Anticholinergic
    Antispasmodics
    Tricyclic antidepressants
    Seizure medications
 	
DEFINING CHARACTERISTICS
Frequency
Urgency
Dribbling
Bladder distention
	EXPECTED OUTCOMES
	Patient is continent of urine or verbalizes management.
	
	ONGOING ASSESSMENT
	■ Assess for presence/history of related factors. *Many related factors cannot be eliminated, but can be improved with medical management.*
	■ Assess for frequency, urgency, or dribbling.
	■ Palpate bladder to determine distention. *Overflow incontinence occurs when the bladder is overfilled but the outlet is obstructed. Pressures force out small amounts of urine.*
	
	THERAPEUTIC INTERVENTIONS
	▲ Relieve urinary retention by:
	    Intermittent catheterization.
	    In-dwelling catheterization.
	■ Prepare patient for surgery *aimed at definitive repair of outlet obstruction.*
	■ Assist in management of systemic medical diseases.
	■ Teach and encourage routine voiding. *Minimizing overfilling reduces incontinent episodes.*
	■ Remove fecal impaction and normalize bowel evacuation. *This allows for normal bladder filling.*
	▲ Notify physician if prescribed drugs are possible causes of this type of urinary incontinence; adjust dosage and/or schedule according to prescription.

REFLEX INCONTINENCE

RELATED FACTORS Spinal cord injury Stimulation of perineum in presence of spinal cord injury **DEFINING CHARACTERISTICS** Loss of urine without warning	**EXPECTED OUTCOMES** Patient verbalizes/demonstrates management techniques. **ONGOING ASSESSMENT** ■ Ask whether patient feels urgency or sensation of voiding. *Spinal cord injury may have damaged sensory fibers.* ■ Document history of spinal cord injury, including level. **THERAPEUTIC INTERVENTIONS** ■ Teach patient (or perform for patient) intermittent (self-) catheterization *to empty bladder at specified intervals.* ■ Consider use of external catheter. ▲ Use in-dwelling catheter as last resort. *Although risk of infection is considerable with both external and in-dwelling catheters, in-dwelling catheters interfere with clothing, movement, and sexual activity and may result in odor or other embarrassing sensory phenomena.*

CONSTANT (OR CONTINUAL) INCONTINENCE

RELATED FACTORS

Pelvic surgery
Fistulas: iatrogenic, postoperative, and postradiation
Trauma
Exstrophy of bladder

DEFINING CHARACTERISTICS

Continual involuntary loss of urine.

EXPECTED OUTCOMES

Patient remains dry and comfortable.

ONGOING ASSESSMENT

- Assess amount of urine loss.
- Assess perineal skin condition. *The urea in urine converts to ammonia in a short period of time and is caustic to skin.*

THERAPEUTIC INTERVENTIONS

- Use diapers or external collection devices. *Most of these patients are women with fistulas; in-dwelling catheters are useless in the presence of vesicovaginal or urethrovaginal fistulae.*
- Prepare patient for surgical correction as indicated.

FUNCTIONAL INCONTINENCE

RELATED FACTORS

Unavailability of toileting facility
Inability to reach toileting facility
Untimely responses to requests for toileting
Limited physical mobility

DEFINING CHARACTERISTICS

Recognizes need to urinate, but is unable to access toileting facility

EXPECTED OUTCOMES

Patient experiences fewer episodes (or no episodes) of incontinence.

ONGOING ASSESSMENT

- Assess patient's recognition of need to urinate. *Patients with functional incontinence are incontinent because they cannot get to an appropriate place to void. Hospitalized patients are frequently labeled "incontinent" because their requests for toileting are unmet.*
- Assess availability of functional toileting facilities (working toilet, bedside commode).
- Assess patient's ability to reach toileting facility, both independently and with help.
- Assess frequency of patient's need to toilet.

THERAPEUTIC INTERVENTIONS

- Establish a toileting schedule. *A toileting schedule assures the patient of a specified time for voiding, and reduces episodes of functional incontinence.*
- Explore the benefit of placing a bedside commode near the patient's bed.
- Prophylactically care for perineal skin. *Moisture-barrier ointments are useful in protecting perineal skin from urine scalds.*
- Treat any existing perineal skin excoriation with a vitamin-enriched cream, followed by a moisture barrier.

PATIENT EDUCATION (ALL TYPES OF INCONTINENCE)

- Teach patient normal anatomy of GU tract and factors that normally control micturition and maintain continence.
- Assist patient in recognizing that any episode(s) of incontinence that pose(s) a social or hygienic problem deserve(s) investigation *so that appropriate therapy can be implemented.*
- Inform patient of the high incidence of urinary incontinence. *This information may decrease feelings of hopelessness and isolation that frequently accompany urinary incontinence.*
- Assist patients, through careful interview, to identify possible causes for urinary incontinence.
- Teach patients the necessity, purpose, and expected results of urodynamic diagnostic evaluation. *Urodynamic studies evaluate bladder filling and sphincter activity and are particularly useful in differentiating stress and urge incontinence.*
- Provide information regarding all available methods of managing urinary incontinence *so that patient can make an informed decision.* Methods include:
  Use of absorbent pads or undergarments that accommodate absorbent pads.
  Diapers.
  Linen protectors for bedridden patient.
  External collection devices such as male external catheters and female external catheters.
  In-dwelling catheters.
  Intermittent catheterization.

Continued.

■ **Urinary elimination, altered patterns of (incontinence)—cont'd**

RELATED FACTORS / DEFINING CHARACTERISTICS	EXPECTED OUTCOMES AND NURSING INTERVENTIONS / *RATIONALE* (■ = INDEPENDENT; ▲ = COLLABORATIVE)
	PATIENT EDUCATION (ALL TYPES OF INCONTINENCE)

    Surgical procedures.

    Electrical nerve stimulators.

    Pharmacotherapeutic agents. *Patients need information on drugs used to treat urinary incontinence as well as those used for other problems that may precipitate or worsen incontinence.*

    Drugs that may precipitate or worsen incontinence: diuretics, sedatives, hypnotics, anticholinergics, and alcohol.

    Drugs that may be used to treat urinary incontinence: α-blockers *(increase bladder pressures and decrease outlet pressures),* β-blockers *(increase outlet resistance),* cholinergics *(increase bladder pressures),* anticholinergics *(depresses smooth muscle activity in hypertonic bladder),* and α-adrenergics *(increase sphincter tone).*

▪ Provide information on odor control. *Vinegar and commercially prepared solutions are useful in neutralizing urinary odor.*

▪ Familiarize patient with potential risk of skin breakdown. *Urea contained in urine metabolizes to ammonia within minutes and is responsible for "urine burns" or "scalding." Spray or wipe preparations, such as Skin Prep and Bard Barrier Film, protect skin from urine.*

▪ Refer to Help for Incontinent People (HIP), PO Box 544, Union, SC 29379.

By: Audrey Klopp, RN, PhD, ET

Urinary retention

The state in which an individual experiences incomplete emptying of the bladder.

RELATED FACTORS / DEFINING CHARACTERISTICS	EXPECTED OUTCOMES AND NURSING INTERVENTIONS / *RATIONALE* (■ = INDEPENDENT; ▲ = COLLABORATIVE)

RELATED FACTORS

General anesthesia
Regional anesthesia
High ureteral pressures caused by disease, injury, or edema
Pain
Infection
Inadequate intake
Ureteral blockage

DEFINING CHARACTERISTICS

Decreased (<30 ml/hr) or absent urinary output for 2 consecutive hrs
Frequency
Hesitancy
Urgency
Lower abdominal distention
Abdominal discomfort
Dribbling

EXPECTED OUTCOMES

Patient empties bladder completely.

ONGOING ASSESSMENT

▪ Evaluate previous patterns of voiding. *There is a wide range of "normal" voiding frequency.*

▪ Visually inspect lower abdomen for distention.

▪ Palpate over bladder for distention.

▪ Evaluate time intervals between voidings.

▪ Assess amount, frequency, and character (color, odor, and specific gravity).

▪ Determine balance between I & O. *I>O may indicate retention.*

▲ Monitor urinalysis, urine culture, and sensitivity. *Urinary tract infection can cause retention, but is more likely to cause frequency.*

▪ If in-dwelling catheter is in situ, assess for patency and kinking.

▲ Monitor BUN and creatinine *to differentiate between urinary retention and renal failure.*

THERAPEUTIC INTERVENTIONS

▪ Initiate methods to facilitate voiding:

    Encourage fluids.

    Offer cranberry juice daily *to keep urine acidic. This helps prevent infection because cranberry juice contains hippicuric acid.*

    Position patient in upright position on toilet if possible.

    Place bedpan/urinal or bedside commode within reach.

    Provide privacy.

    Encourage patient to void every 4 hr.

    Have patient listen to sound of running water or place hands in warm water and/or pour warm water over perineum.

    Offer fluids before voiding.

    Perform Credé over bladder. *Credé increases bladder pressure, and this in turn may stimulate relaxation of sphincter to allow voiding.*

THERAPEUTIC INTERVENTIONS

▲ Administer bethanechol (Urecholine) as ordered *to stimulate parasympathetic nervous system to release acetylcholine at nerve endings and to increase tone and amplitude of contractions of smooth muscles of urinary bladder.* Side effects are rare after oral administration of therapeutic dose. In small subcutaneous doses side effects may include: abdominal cramps, sweating, and flushing. In larger doses they may include: malaise, headache, diarrhea, nausea, vomiting, asthmatic attacks, bradycardia, lowered BP, atrioventricular block, and cardiac arrest.

▲ Institute intermittent catheterization. *Because many causes of urinary retention are self-limited, the decision to leave an in-dwelling catheter in should be avoided.*

▲ Insert in-dwelling (Foley) catheter as ordered:
Tape catheter to abdomen (male) *to prevent ureteral fistula.*
Tape catheter to thigh (female) *to prevent inadvertent displacement.*
Cleanse insertion site every shift with soap and water and dry thoroughly.

PATIENT EDUCATION

▪ Educate patient/significant others about the importance of adequate intake, (i.e., 8 to 10 glasses of fluids daily).

▪ Instruct patient/significant others on measures to help voiding (as described).

▪ Instruct patient/significant others on signs and symptoms of overdistended bladder (e.g., decreased or absent urine, frequency, hesitancy, urgency, lower abdominal distention, or discomfort).

▪ Instruct patient/significant others on signs and symptoms of urinary tract infection (e.g., chills and fever, frequent urination or concentrated urine, and abdominal or back pain).

▪ See Urinary tract infection, p. 480.

By: Doris M. McNear, RN, MSN

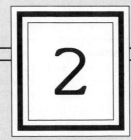

Cardiac and Vascular Care Plans

Angina pectoris, stable

CHEST PAIN

A clinical syndrome characterized by the abrupt or gradual onset of substernal discomfort caused by insufficient coronary blood flow and/or inadequate O_2 supply to the myocardial muscle. The characteristics of angina are usually constant for a given patient. The pain is precipitated by effort or emotional stress or both. Conditions such as fever, anemia, tachyarrhythmias, hypothyroidism, and polycythemia may also provoke angina. Stable angina usually persists only 3-5 minutes and subsides with cessation of the precipitating factor, rest, or use of nitroglycerin (NTG). Patients do not require hospitalization, though anginal episodes may occur during hospitalization for other medical problems.

NURSING DIAGNOSES

EXPECTED OUTCOMES AND NURSING INTERVENTIONS / *RATIONALE*
(■ = INDEPENDENT; ▲ = COLLABORATIVE)

Chest Pain

RELATED TO

Myocardial ischemia caused by:
Atherosclerosis and/or coronary spasm
Less common causes: severe aortic stenosis, cardiomyopathy, mitral valve prolapse, lupus erythematosus

DEFINING CHARACTERISTICS

No change in the frequency, duration, time of appearance, or precipitating factors during the previous 60 days
Pain characteristics:
Quality: choking, strangling, pressure, burning, tightness, ache, heaviness
Location: substernal, may radiate to arms and shoulders, neck, back, jaw
Severity: scale 1-10 (usually not at top of scale)
Duration: typically 3-5 min
Onset: episodic and usually precipitated by physical exertion, emotional stress, heavy meal, exposures to temperature extremes such as cold, smoking

EXPECTED OUTCOMES

Patient verbalizes relief of chest discomfort.
Patient appears relaxed and comfortable.

ONGOING ASSESSMENT

- Assess patient's description of pain. (See Defining characteristics). Note any exacerbating factors and measures used to relieve the pain.
- Evaluate whether this is a chronic problem (stable angina) or a new presentation (see Angina pectoris, unstable, p. 79).
- Assess for the appropriateness of performing an ECG to evaluate ST-T wave changes *to assist in differentiating between angina and myocardial infarction.*
- Monitor vital signs during chest pain and following nitrate administration. *Blood pressure and heart rate usually elevate secondary to sympathetic stimulation during pain; however, nitrates cause vasodilation and resultant drop in blood pressure.*
- Monitor effectiveness of interventions.

THERAPEUTIC INTERVENTIONS

- At first signs of pain, instruct patient to relax and/or rest *to decrease myocardial O_2 demands.*
- ▲ Instruct patient to take sublingual nitroglycerine (NTG SL).
- If pain continues after repeating dose every 5 min for total of three pills, notify physician. *Chest pain unrelieved by NTG may represent unstable angina or myocardial infarction and should be evaluated immediately.*
- ▲ Administer O_2 as ordered.
- Clarify the difference between angina and a "heart attack."
- Offer assurance and emotional support by explaining all treatments and procedures, and by encouraging questions.

Knowledge Deficit

RELATED To

Unfamiliarity with disease process and treatment

DEFINING CHARACTERISTICS

Overanxiousness
Multiple questions or lack of questioning
Inaccurate follow-through of prescribed treatment

EXPECTED OUTCOME

Patient/significant others verbalize understanding of angina pectoris, its causes, and appropriate relief measures for pain.
Patient describes own cardiac risk factors and strategies to reduce them.

ONGOING ASSESSMENT

- Assess knowledge of patient/significant others.
- Assess readiness, motivation, and interest in health/illness status.
- Evaluate compliance with previously prescribed life-style changes.

THERAPEUTIC INTERVENTIONS

- Plan teaching sessions *so patient is not overwhelmed at one time.*
- Consult cardiac rehab clinical nurse specialist about available teaching materials (hospital television, brochures, group class).

Continued.

NURSING DIAGNOSES	EXPECTED OUTCOMES AND NURSING INTERVENTIONS / *RATIONALE* (■ = INDEPENDENT; ▲ = COLLABORATIVE)

THERAPEUTIC INTERVENTIONS— cont'd

- Provide information regarding:

  Anatomy and physiology of coronary circulation.

  Need to reduce identified risk factors for atherosclerosis.

    Hypertension: lower weight, reduced salt intake, exercise programs, and medications as prescribed.

    Smoking: *Causes vasoconstriction, reduces myocardial oxygen supply. Smoking doubles the risk of heart attacks.* If patient can't quit alone, refer to American Heart Association, Lung Association, Cancer Society for support group and interventions.

    High blood cholesterol: emphasis on need to reduce intake of foods high in saturated fat, cholesterol, or both (fatty meats, organ meats, lard, butter, egg yolks, whole dairy products). Arrange for evaluation by dietitian as needed. Include spouse/ significant others in meal planning. *Treatment may require antihyperlipidemia medication.*

    Diabetes: emphasis on control through diet and medication.

    Obesity: *affects hypertension, diabetes, and cholesterol levels.*

    Stress: reference to programs for stress management as appropriate.

    Sedentary existence: emphasis on benefits of exercise in reducing risks of heart attack. *Lack of exercise contributes to elevated cholesterol and overweight.* Refer to cardiac rehab program as needed. Keep exercise intensity below angina threshold.

  Risk factors that can't be modified: family history, age, sex.

  Differentiating angina from noncardiac pain.

  Need to avoid angina-provoking situations (heavy meals, extreme temperatures, emotional stress, stimulants).

  Use of sublingual NTG to relieve attacks:

    Carry pills at all times.

    Keep pills in dark, dry container, away from heat. *NTG is volatile and inactivated by heat, moisture, light.*

    Replace pills every 3-4 mo. *Once bottle is opened, NTG begins to lose its strength. Tablets that are effective should sting in the mouth.*

    Sit or lie down when taking NTG. *NTG causes vasodilation, which can lower blood pressure and cause dizziness.*

    For chest pain, put pill under tongue and let dissolve. If not relieved in 5 min, take another. If still not relieved, take a third. If this doesn't relieve pain, call physician or go to emergency room.

    Emphasize that NTG is a safe and nonaddicting drug. Use as needed.

    Headache is a common side effect and can be treated with acetaminophen (Tylenol).

  Use of prophylactic NTG to prevent pain.

  Use of other medications for long-term management:

    Long-lasting nitrates: *cause vasodilation, which increases coronary blood flow and reduces oxygen demands of the heart.*

    Beta blockers: *reduce contractility and heart rate, thereby decreasing myocardial oxygen demand.*

    Calcium channel blockers: *cause vasodilation, which increases coronary blood flow and reduces oxygen demands of the heart.*

    Antiplatelets: *to optimize blood flow.*

  Diagnostic tests for evaluating coronary artery disease:

    ECG.

    Exercise stress test (with thallium); pharmacologic stress test.

    Cardiac catheterization and coronary angiography.

  Therapeutic procedures to relieve angina unresponsive to medications and life-style changes:

    Percutaneous transluminal coronary angioplasty/atherectomy/laser interventions.

    Coronary artery bypass graft surgery.

    Comparisons of stable vs. unstable angina and myocardial infarction.

NURSING DIAGNOSES	EXPECTED OUTCOMES AND NURSING INTERVENTIONS / *RATIONALE* (■ = INDEPENDENT; ▲ = COLLABORATIVE)

Decreased Activity Tolerance

RELATED TO

Occurrence of, or fear of chest pain
Side effects of prescribed medications

DEFINING CHARACTERISTICS

Chest pain or dyspnea during activity
Fatigue
Abnormal heart rate or BP response to activity
Dizziness during activity
Change in skin temperature from warm to cool during activity
ECG changes reflecting ischemia or arrhythmias

See also:

Anxiety, p. 5, 23;
Coping, impaired individual, p. 18;
Health-Seeking Behavior, p. 33

EXPECTED OUTCOMES

Patient performs activity within limits of ischemic disease, as evidenced by absence of chest pain/discomfort and no ECG changes reflecting ischemia.

ONGOING ASSESSMENT

- Assess patient's level of physical activity prior to experiencing angina.
- Assess for defining characteristics before, during, and after activity.
- Evaluate factors that may precipitate fatigue/discomfort.

THERAPEUTIC INTERVENTIONS

While in hospital:
- Encourage adequate rest periods in between activities *to reduce oxygen demands.*
- Assist with ADL as indicated.
- Instruct in prophylactic use of NTG prior to physical exertion as needed.
- Reinforce the need to "pace activities" (phone calls, visitors, daily hygiene).

Discharge planning:
- Assist patient in reviewing required home activities and developing an appropriate plan for accomplishing them (what to do in morning vs. afternoon; how to pace household chores throughout the week).
- Remind patient not to work with arms above shoulders for long time *for this increases myocardial demands.*
- Remind patient to continue taking medications (i.e., β-blockers), despite side effects of fatigue. *Often the body does adjust to the medications after several weeks.*
- Evaluate need for additional support at home (housekeeper, neighbor to shop, family assistance).
- Encourage a program of progressive aerobic exercise *to increase functional capacity.* Refer to cardiac rehab as appropriate.

By: Beth Manglal-Lan, RN, BSN, Meg Gulanick, RN, PhD

Angina pectoris, unstable: acute phase (CCU)

PREINFARCTION ANGINA; ACUTE CORONARY INSUFFICIENCY; CRESCENDO ANGINA

Unstable (preinfarction) angina is a clinical syndrome characterized by a changing pattern of previously stable angina, new onset of severe angina, or occurrence of angina at rest. It is intermediate between death of some heart muscle (infarction) and transient muscle ischemia, which is often caused by a combination of arterial spasm and obstruction. Patients with unstable angina have an increased risk of arrhythmia, myocardial infarction, and sudden death and should be hospitalized in CCU.

NURSING DIAGNOSES	EXPECTED OUTCOMES AND NURSING INTERVENTIONS / *RATIONALE* (■ = INDEPENDENT; ▲ = COLLABORATIVE)

Chest Pain

RELATED TO

Myocardial ischemia

DEFINING CHARACTERISTICS

New onset (<60 days) angina; or
Changing pattern of previously stable angina; or
Angina occurring at rest or with minimal exertion; or
Angina occurring during sleep
ECG changes: ST depression or elevation

EXPECTED OUTCOMES

Patient verbalizes relief of pain.
Patient appears relaxed and comfortable.

ONGOING ASSESSMENT

- Assess pain characteristics:
  Quality: as with stable angina (squeezing, tightening, choking, pressing, burning).
  Location: substernal area. May radiate to extremities (e.g., arms, shoulders).
  Severity: more intense than classic angina pectoris.
  Duration: persists longer than 20 min.
  Onset: minimal exertion or during rest or sleep.
  Relief: usually does not respond to sublingual NTG or rest. May respond to IV nitroglycerin. *In acute stages, patients presenting with unstable angina can present with a variety of pain characteristics, making diagnosis difficult. Patients are admitted to rule out MI until serial lab data provide definitive diagnosis.*
- Note time since onset of first episode of chest pain. *If less than 6 hr, patients may be candidates for thrombolytic therapy as in acute MI.*

Continued.

Cardiac and Vascular Care Plans

NURSING DIAGNOSES	EXPECTED OUTCOMES AND NURSING INTERVENTIONS / *RATIONALE* (■ = INDEPENDENT; ▲ = COLLABORATIVE)

ONGOING ASSESSMENT—cont'd

▲ Monitor serial myocardial enzymes (CK-MB). *Enzymes do not elevate with unstable angina because cellular death is not occurring. They are used to rule out infarction.*

▪ Monitor ECG immediately during and after pain:

Normal or depressed ST segment.

ST segment elevation during pain with variant Prinzmetal's angina *to evaluate ST changes (to assist in diagnosing cardiac origin of pain and site of coronary artery involvement).*

THERAPEUTIC INTERVENTIONS

▪ Maintain bed rest/quiet environment *to decrease O$_2$ demands.*

▪ Instruct patient to report pain as soon as it starts. *Important for diagnosis and easier to treat.*

▪ Respond immediately to complaint of pain. *Prompt treatment may decrease myocardial ischemia and prevent damage.*

▲ Administer O$_2$ as prescribed.

▲ Give medications as prescribed, evaluating effectiveness and observing signs/symptoms of untoward reactions:

Anticipate IV nitroglycerin drip. Titrate dose to relief of pain (usually <100 μg/min) as long as BP is stable. *Relaxes smooth muscles in vascular system, causing vasodilation that results in lower blood pressure, lower vascular resistance, and decreased work of the heart.*

Anticipate fluid challenge to treat hypotension. *Nitrates cause venous pooling, which lowers blood pressure.*

β-Blockers: *Are used to decrease myocardial oxygen demand.* Anticipate IV administration; observe for side effects: hypotension, bradycardia, heart blocks, and heart failure.

Thrombolytic therapy: *Used to dissolve thrombus that may be partially occluding vessel.* Anticipate heparin drip in patients with persistent pain and positive ECG changes.

Calcium channel blockers: *prevent vasospasm.*

▪ Anticipate intra-aortic balloon pump management if pain and ischemic changes persist despite maximal medical therapy. *It increases coronary blood flow while reducing work by left ventricle during contraction.*

▪ Anticipate cardiac catheterization and, depending on results, anticipate percutaneous transluminal coronary angioplasty or coronary artery bypass surgery.

High Risk for Decreased Cardiac Output

Risk Factors

Prolonged episodes of myocardial ischemia affecting contractility

EXPECTED OUTCOMES

Patient maintains optimum cardiac output, as evidenced by:

HR 60-100/min.

Clear breath sounds.

Urine output >30 ml/hr.

Warm, dry skin.

ONGOING ASSESSMENT

▪ Assess hemodynamic status every hour and especially during episode of pain. *Increased HR and SVR, decreased urine output, adventitious breath sounds, shortness of breath and blood pressure changes are signs of left ventricular dysfunction.*

▪ Assess for myocardial ischemia (ST changes) on ECG. *ST segments may be depressed or elevated during pain.*

▪ Monitor ECG continuously for arrhythmias, especially during episode of pain.

THERAPEUTIC INTERVENTIONS

▪ Maintain bed rest/reduced activity *to reduce O$_2$ demands.*

▲ Anticipate development of life-threatening arrhythmias. *Ischemic muscle is electrically unstable and produces arrhythmias. Tachyarrhythmias or bradyarrhythmias may occur.*

Anticipate/administer lidocaine for ventricular arrhythmias per protocol.

If high-degree atrioventricular block develops, anticipate atropine/isoproterenol IV, external pacing and/or insertion of temporary pacemaker *to increase heart rate to improve cardiac output.*

▪ If symptoms develop, institute SCP, cardiac output, decreased p. 12.

▪ Anticipate possible progression to myocardial infarction. *Prolonged/unrelieved myocardial ischemia results in infarction of ventricular muscle.*

Fear

RELATED TO

Recurrent anginal attacks
Incomplete relief from pain by usual means (nitroglycerin and rest)
Threat of MI
Threat of death

DEFINING CHARACTERISTICS

Restlessness
Increased awareness
Increased questioning
Facial tension/wide-eyed
Poor eye contact
Focus on self/repeatedly seeking assurance
Increased perspiration
Expressed concern
Trembling

EXPECTED OUTCOMES

Patient verbalizes fears or concerns.
Patient appears calm and expresses trust in medical management.

ONGOING ASSESSMENT

- Assess level of fear (mild to severe). *Controlling fear and anxiety will help decrease the physiologic reactions that can aggravate their condition.*
- Assess cause of fear. *Patient may be afraid of the pain experience itself, of MI, or of dying.*

THERAPEUTIC INTERVENTIONS

- Encourage patient to call for nurse when pain or fear develops. *Fear increases heart rate and blood pressure and causes release of epinephrine, which may produce an arrhythmia.*
- Immediately respond to any complaint of pain. *Prompt treatment reassures patient that he/she is in a safe environment.*
- Make every effort to remain at bedside throughout episode of pain.
- Check on patient frequently *to provide reassurance.*
- ▲ Administer mild tranquilizer as needed *to reduce stress.*
- Establish rest periods between care and procedures *to assist in relaxation and regaining of emotional balance.*
- Assure patient that close monitoring will ensure prompt treatment. *Promotes a feeling of security.*

Knowledge Deficit

RELATED TO

Unfamiliarity with disease process, treatment, recovery

DEFINING CHARACTERISTICS

Multiple questions or lack of questioning
Verbalized misconceptions

EXPECTED OUTCOMES

Patient/significant others verbalizes understanding of anatomy/physiology of unstable angina, causes, and appropriate relief measures for pain.

ONGOING ASSESSMENT

- Assess present level of understanding of "unstable" angina.

THERAPEUTIC INTERVENTIONS

- Teach patient/significant others:
    Anatomy and physiology of the coronary condition.
    Atherosclerotic process and implications of angina pectoris.
    Use of nitroglycerin and its side effects when chest pain occurs.
    Use of calcium channel blockers. *Unstable angina has a spasm component.*
    Use of antiplatelet medicines. *Reduces risk of thrombosis.*
    Angina vs unstable angina vs MI.
    Diagnostic procedures (stress test/echocardiogram/angiogram).
    Return to prior life-style.
- Explain that symptoms may exacerbate over next few months, and close monitoring is important. *Unstable angina may progress to infarction secondary to progression of disease.*

See also:
Activity intolerance, p. 2
Cardiac rehabilitation, p. 87
Health-seeking behaviors, p. 33

By: Meg Gulanick, RN, PhD

Aortic aneurysm

DISSECTING ANEURYSM, THORACIC ANEURYSM,
ABDOMINAL ANEURYSM

A localized circumscribed abnormal dilatation of an artery, or a blood-containing tumor connecting directly with the lumen of an artery. True aneurysms result when one or all three layers of the vessel wall are involved, but the arterial wall remains as a barrier to the periarterial tissues. There are three types of true aneurysms: (1) saccular—characterized by bulbous outpouching of one side of the artery resulting in a localized thinning and stretching of the arterial wall; (2) fusiform—characterized by a uniform spindle-shaped circumferential dilatation of a segment of the artery; and (3) dissecting—in which the inner layer of the vessel wall tears and splits, creating a false channel and cavity of blood between the intimal and adventitial layers. False aneurysms (pseudoaneurysms) result from rupture or complete tear of all three layers of an arterial wall with the blood clot retained in an outpouching of tissue from the vessel wall.

Aneurysms occur as thoracic (33%), thoraco-abdominal (2%) and abdominal (65%). The natural history of an aneurysm is enlargement and rupture. As a rule, the larger the aneurysm the greater the chance of rupture. Dissection of the aorta is commonly classified according to location. Type I and type II involve the ascending aorta; type III involves the descending aorta. Dissecting aortic aneurysm is the most common catastrophe involving the aorta and has a high mortality rate if not detected early and treated appropriately. It can be treated through surgical intervention or with medical therapy.

NURSING DIAGNOSES	EXPECTED OUTCOMES AND NURSING INTERVENTIONS / *RATIONALE* (■ = INDEPENDENT; ▲ = COLLABORATIVE)

High Risk for Injury:
**Altered tissue perfusion/
dissection**

RISK FACTORS

Conditions that increase stress
on the arterial wall:
  Hypertension
  Pregnancy with hypervol-
    emia
  Coarctation of the aorta
Defect in the vessel wall:
  Marfan's syndrome
  Cystic degeneration in the
    media
Iatrogenic causes

EXPECTED OUTCOMES

Patient has reduced risk of complications from progressive dissection or rupture due to early detection of symptoms and appropriate intervention.

ONGOING ASSESSMENT

- Obtain a thorough history regarding present complaint. *Aids in ruling out cerebrovascular, cardiac, vascular occlusive, and/or renal disease. Aneurysms are commonly secondary to other factors. Research suggests a familial tendency for aneurysmal formation occurring more frequently in males.*
- Assess and monitor location and characteristics of pain:
    Thoracic: pain in neck, low back pain, shoulders, or abdomen.
    Abdominal: abdomen or back, flank or groin pain *caused by pressure on adjacent structures.*

For thoracic aneurysms:
- Monitor BP for hypertension. Also note that differential arm BP may be present *due to compression of subclavian artery.*
- Monitor for aortic murmur *secondary to aortic insufficiency.*
- Auscultate for presence for bruits over palpable pulsatile mass.
- ▲ Obtain chest x-ray to monitor for mediastinal widening, pleural effusions, and progressive enlargement of aneurysm.
- Monitor quality of peripheral pulses. *A suggested grading system is: 0 = absent, 1+ = present; 2+ = strong.*
- Assess for respiratory compromise *due to compression of the trachea or bronchus.*
- Assess for hoarseness and brashy cough. *Results from pressure on the laryngeal nerve.*
- Assess for dysphagia. *May be caused by esophageal compression.*
- Observe for upper-extremity and head swelling with cyanosis. *Can be caused by superior vena cava obstruction.*
- Monitor for neurologic deficit.
- Assess for hemoptysis *resulting from compression of the trachea or lung.*

For abdominal aneurysms:
- Palpate for abdominal tenderness and presence of pulsatile mass (4-7 cm in diameter). *Presence of abdominal aortic aneurysm greater than 4 cm in diameter is an indication for elective surgical repair, even if asymptomatic. Surgery for high-risk patients may be deferred until aneurysm shows progressive enlargement (>6 cm) or until it becomes tender or symptomatic.*

Continued.

Ongoing Assessment—cont'd

- Monitor urine output. *Reduction may result from compression of the renal arteries from infrarenal abdominal aneurysm, cross-clamping of aorta during surgery, or embolization. However, most aneurysms are located below the renal artery.*
- Assess for GI bleeding. *Caused by erosion of the duodenum.*
- Assess for lower leg edema. *Caused by erosion of the inferior vena cava.*
- Observe for retroperitoneal cyanosis. *Caused by leak or acute rupture of aneurysm.*
- Monitor for abnormal bowel function. *Caused by partial intestinal obstruction.*
- Evaluate for sexual dysfunction. *Caused by aorto-iliac occlusive disease.*
- Assess lower extremities for signs of peripheral ischemia/insufficiency: These include pain, pallor, pulselessness, paresthesia, poikilothermia (decreased temperature, coolness), and paralysis.
- Observe for abdominal distention, diarrhea, or severe abdominal pain and/or fever. *To R/O embolization or decreased perfusion to the mesenteric artery.*
- Monitor for signs and symptoms indicating progressive dissection. *A high index of suspicion is key to the treatment to reduce mortality. Clinical signs and symptoms indicate the site and progression of dissection:*
    Type I dissection may affect brachiocephalic vessel, resulting in ischemia of brain and arm.
    Dissection extending proximally to the aortic annulus may produce direct loss of the support of the aortic cusps and acute aortic regurgitation (type II).
    Types I and III dissection may cause ischemia of intestines, kidneys, or legs.

Therapeutic Interventions

- ▲ Administer pain medicines as prescribed.
- Provide nursing measures that alleviate pain:
    Position of comfort:
        Side lying may be more comfortable for patients exhibiting back pain.
        Elevate head of bed for patients who are short of breath *to promote maximum lung expansion.*
    Physical comfort: *hand holding provides emotional support.*
    Physiologic intervention: application of cold towel to forehead.
    Relaxation techniques.
- ▲ Administer potent vasodilator (Nipride) medication. *Goal is to maintain systolic BP <130 mm Hg.*
    Use infusion pump.
    Infuse the drug in a separate line, preferably a central line, *to minimize infiltration and prevent tissue damage, as well as prevent inaccurate absorption of the drug.*
- ▲ Administer β-blockers *to decrease heart rate and decrease myocardial contractility, thus reducing the stress applied to the arterial walls during each heart beat. The goal is to maintain heart rate <70 beats per minute.*
- For type I and II dissections, anticipate surgical treatment and prepare patient.
- For type III dissection, anticipate chronic medical treatment, which consists of the following long-term measures:
    Decrease or eliminate identified factors that will increase blood pressure, heart rate. *Anxiety, stress, fear, pain all elicit sympathetic responses that potentiate further dissection.*
    Provide a quiet environment as much as possible.
    Regulate staff rounds to provide patient rest periods.
    Pace activities (eating, personal hygiene, visitors) appropriately.
    Limit visitors and phone calls.
    Provide continuity of nursing staff if possible.
    Administer sedatives as prescribed.
- Prepare patient for angiography/aortography *to confirm diagnosis and delineate anatomy (if test is prescribed).*
- Prepare patient for abdominal ultrasound and/or CT scan *to confirm diagnosis.*

Continued.

NURSING DIAGNOSES	EXPECTED OUTCOMES AND NURSING INTERVENTIONS / *RATIONALE* (■ = INDEPENDENT; ▲ = COLLABORATIVE)

High Risk for Decreased Cardiac Output

RISK FACTORS

Side effects of medications
Progressive dissection
Rupture of the aorta

EXPECTED OUTCOMES

Patient maintains adequate cardiac output, as evidenced by HR <100/min, clear breath sounds, urine output >30 ml/hr, and alert mentation.

ONGOING ASSESSMENT

- Assess hemodynamic status. Monitor for signs of decreasing cardiac output, such as tachycardia, decreased urine output, and restlessness.
- Assess for signs of myocardial ischemia: chest pain, tachycardia, ST-T wave changes on ECG.

THERAPEUTIC INTERVENTIONS

▲ If decreased cardiac output is drug-induced, anticipate the following:
  For sodium nitroprusside (Nipride):
    Stop the drug.
    Administer isotonic solution (0.9 NSS) or plasma expanders *to maintain increased intravascular volume.*
  For β-blocker:
    May stop the drug or reduce dose. *β-blocker has a negative inotropic effect, which can potentiate heart failure. Presence of rales and S_3 indicates heart failure.*
▲ If decreased cardiac output is related to further dissection (severe aortic insufficiency) or ruptured aorta, anticipate emergency angiography and surgery:
    Send blood specimen for type and cross match, and other routine preop blood work.
    Stay with patient to provide emotional support.
    Assist primary physician in discussing surgery with both patient and family.
    Administer medications, IV fluids, and blood as ordered *to maintain adequate cardiac output prior to surgery.*
    Prepare patient for surgery per hospital policy and procedure.
- For immediate postop course, see Cardiac surgery, adult: immediate postoperative care, p. 108.

Anxiety

RELATED TO

Sudden onset
Impending surgery
Close monitoring by medical/ nursing staff
Fear of death
Multiple tests and procedures

DEFINING CHARACTERISTICS

Tense, anxious appearance
Request to have family at bed- side all the time
Restlessness
Increased questioning
Constant demands
Glancing about/increased alert- ness

EXPECTED OUTCOMES

Patient verbalizes reduced anxiety.
Patient demonstrates positive coping method.

ONGOING ASSESSMENT

- Assess level of anxiety.
- Assess usual coping strategies.

THERAPEUTIC INTERVENTIONS

- Encourage verbalization of fear/anxiety. *Identifying patient's fear/anxiety will facilitate staff's planning of strategies to reinforce patient's usual coping mechanisms.*
- Provide emotional support and reassurance that he/she is being observed carefully and help is available when needed.
- Ensure that call light is within reach at all times.
- Explain tests and procedures being done. Emphasize their importance in diagnosing and treating the problem.
- Update patient with test results.
- Provide adequate time for rest and some quiet time *to allow patient to sort out feelings.*
- Allow family to stay with patient as much as possible.

Knowledge Deficit: Follow-up Care

RELATED TO

New medical problem
Unfamiliarity with surgical pro- cedure and hospital care

EXPECTED OUTCOMES

Patient/family verbalizes understanding of disease process, treatment options, and goals of therapy.

ONGOING ASSESSMENT

- Assess knowledge of the disease.
- Assess understanding of medical versus surgical treatment.

THERAPEUTIC INTERVENTIONS

- Instruct patient about the following:
    Cause of aneurysm.
    Medical vs surgical treatment.
    Preoperative preparation.

NURSING DIAGNOSES	EXPECTED OUTCOMES AND NURSING INTERVENTIONS / *RATIONALE* (■ = INDEPENDENT; ▲ = COLLABORATIVE)

See also:

Fluid volume deficit, p. 25
Altered tissue perfusion,
  p. 69
Impaired skin integrity, p. 59
Pain, p. 49
Altered sexuality pattern,
  p. 58

THERAPEUTIC INTERVENTIONS—cont'd

Goals of the therapy *(avoid excess blood pressure and strain to the diseased thoracic arterial wall or over the graft site).*

Use of antihypertensive medications as prescribed. Importance of compliance.

Side effects of medicines.

Dietary restrictions. *Low-salt diet usually indicated for maintaining normotensive blood pressure.*

Relationship of obesity and high blood pressure.

Avoiding activities that are isometric or abruptly raise blood pressure (e.g., lifting and carrying of heavy objects, straining for bowel movement).

Methods for coping with stress and appropriate life-style changes.

By: Gail Smith-Jaros, RN, MSN
    Lumie Perez, RN, BSN, CCRN

Cardiac catheterization

CORONARY ANGIOGRAPHY

Cardiac catheterization and coronary angiography are specialized diagnostic procedures in which the internal structure of the heart and coronary arteries can be viewed to determine myocardial function, valvular competency, presence or absence of coronary artery disease, location and severity of coronary artery disease, and to assess the effects of prior percutaneous or surgical interventions. Cardiac catheterization may be an elective or emergency procedure, depending on the patient's clinical status. It is frequently performed on an outpatient basis.

NURSING DIAGNOSES	EXPECTED OUTCOMES AND NURSING INTERVENTIONS / *RATIONALE* (■ = INDEPENDENT; ▲ = COLLABORATIVE)

Knowledge Deficit

RELATED TO
Unfamiliarity with procedure

DEFINING CHARACTERISTICS
Expressed need for information
Multiple questions
Lack of questions
Increase in anxiety level
Statements revealing misconceptions

EXPECTED OUTCOMES

The patient verbalizes a basic understanding of heart anatomy, disease, and cardiac catheterization procedure.

ONGOING ASSESSMENT

- Assess knowledge of heart disease and catheterization.

THERAPEUTIC INTERVENTIONS

- Provide information about the specific heart problem (valve disease, coronary artery disease).
- Be in the room when the catheterization team evaluates patient (as appropriate). Interpret the information *to clarify and reinforce as necessary. Patients are very anxious about the procedure and the possible outcomes and may have difficulty asking questions and interpreting information.*
- Encourage patient to verbalize concerns *so that misunderstandings can be identified and clarified.*
- Provide a tour/description of the lab environment *to prepare patient for the appearance of the room, complexity of the equipment, and staff.*
- Explain the sensations that may be experienced during the procedure:
    Warm, flushing, nauseous feeling when dye is injected.
    Pressure or skipped heart beats as the catheter is advanced.
    Slow heart rate or low blood pressure *caused by vasovagal response or injection of contrast medium. It is treated by vigorous cough, atropine, and/or IV fluids.*
- Determine if patient has allergy to iodine-containing substances. *Patients may be allergic to the contrast dye used during injections and require premedication with antihistamines and/or steroids.*
- Explain that patient will be awake during the procedure *so they can report any chest pain should it occur, and to vigorously cough and breathe deeply at designated times to circulate dye, position catheter, and increase heart rate and blood pressure.*
- Inform of precatheterization procedures:
    NPO *to prevent nausea.* Clear liquids may be allowed if procedure is scheduled for later in the day.

Continued.

Cardiac catheterization—cont'd

NURSING DIAGNOSES	EXPECTED OUTCOMES AND NURSING INTERVENTIONS / *RATIONALE* (■ = INDEPENDENT; ▲ = COLLABORATIVE)

THERAPEUTIC INTERVENTIONS

Premedication with antihistamine and anti-anxiety medicines.
Need to empty bladder *for comfort. Test may take 2-4 hours; dye has diuretic effect.*
IV insertion *for access for medicines and fluids.*
- Explain that patient will be positioned on hard x-ray table, and either it or fluoroscopy camera can be tilted for optimal visualization of the heart.
- Prepare patient for postcatheterization procedures:
  Frequent vital sign checks.
  Assessment of peripheral pulses and dressing *to check for occlusion or bleeding.*
  With femoral cannulation: bed rest flat in bed for 6-8 hrs, and need to keep extremity immobile (log roll) *to promote homeostasis.*
  With brachial cannulation: need to sit in bed for 3-4 hours.
  Importance of drinking fluids *to flush dye from the system, reduce risk of renal complications, and promote hydration.*
  Some patients may be discharged on the same day.

High Risk for Altered Tissue Perfusion to Catheterized Extremity

RISK FACTORS

Arterial or venous spasm
Thrombus formation

EXPECTED OUTCOMES

Patient maintains tissue perfusion in affected extremity as evidenced by baseline pulse quality and warm extremity.

ONGOING ASSESSMENT

Precatheterization:
- Assess and record presence of peripheral pulses; mark pedal pulses with an *X. More than one site may be needed for cannulation during the procedure. Accurate assessment of baseline is important for comparison.*
- If pulses are markedly decreased, obtain Doppler reading *to check for pulse quality or absence.*
- Assess and record skin temperature, color, and capillary refill of all extremities.
- Assess and record movement and sensation of all extremities.
Postcatheterization:
- Assess and monitor affected extremities for pulse, skin color, temperature, and sensation according to institutional policy. *Decreased peripheral pulse, coolness, mottling, pallor, presence of pain, numbness, and tingling in affected extremity are signs of decreased tissue perfusion.*
- Check cannulation site for swelling and hematoma. *Severe edema can hinder peripheral circulation by constricting the vessels.*

THERAPEUTIC INTERVENTIONS

- Instruct patient to report signs of reduced tissue perfusion *so assessment, diagnosis, and treatment can be initiated quickly.*
- Report to physician immediately any decrease or change in the characteristics of affected extremity.
- Prepare for possible thrombectomy or embolectomy *to remove blood clot that may be compromising or obstructing circulation in affected extremity.*
▲ Prepare to heparinize if prescribed.

High Risk for Bleeding

RISK FACTORS

Disruption of vessel integrity
Heparin administration during procedure

EXPECTED OUTCOMES

Patient experiences no significant bleeding.

ONGOING ASSESSMENT

- Assess insertion site and dressing for evidence of bleeding per protocol.
- Assess for restlessness, apprehension, and change in vital signs. *These are early signs of bleeding.*
▲ Monitor vital signs, Hgb, and HcT. *Changes from baseline may represent bleeding.*

THERAPEUTIC INTERVENTIONS

▲ Maintain bed rest with affected extremity straight for 6-8 hr *to minimize risk of bleeding.* If needed, apply soft restraints to affected extremity *to remind patient not to move.*
- If femoral site is used, do not elevate head of bed >30 degrees for 6-8 hr.
▲ Maintain occlusive pressure dressing to cannulation site *to facilitate clot formation.*
- Avoid sudden movements with affected extremity *to facilitate clot formation and wound closure at insertion site.*

Continued.

NURSING DIAGNOSES	EXPECTED OUTCOMES AND NURSING INTERVENTIONS / *RATIONALE* (■ = INDEPENDENT; ▲ = COLLABORATIVE)

THERAPEUTIC INTERVENTIONS— cont'd

If bleeding is noted:
- Circle, date, and time amount of drainage or size of hematoma.
- Estimate blood loss.
- Reinforce dressing; apply pressure, sandbag (10 pounds) to bleeding site.
- Notify physician if bleeding is significant.

Fluid Volume Deficit

RELATED TO

Dye-induced diuresis
Restricted intake before procedure

DEFINING CHARACTERISTICS

Decrease in urine output
Specific gravity changes
Decrease in BP; increase in heart rate

See also:
Anxiety, p. 5; Fear, p. 23; Pain, p. 49.

EXPECTED OUTCOMES

Patient maintains adequate fluid volume, as evidenced by balanced intake and output, good skin turgor, normal blood pressure.

ONGOING ASSESSMENT

- Assess and monitor hydration status: urine output, mental status, skin, and hemodynamic parameters.
- Obtain urine specific gravity q. 4 hr until normal. *Concentrated urine with high specific gravity may indicate presence of dye in system and/or hypovolemia.*
- If patient requires nitrates, monitor BP closely, anticipating drop in BP and need for additional fluids *secondary to hypovolemic state.*

THERAPEUTIC INTERVENTIONS

- Maintain strict I & O for several hours after catheterization.
- Anticipate frequent use of urinal/bedpan for several hours after catheterization. Keep urinal within reach. *Radiographic dye causes diuresis.*
- Give oral fluids as tolerated.
- Keep water pitcher/juices at bedside. *Patient has restricted activity.*
- ▲ Institute IV fluids as prescribed, monitoring flow rate *to prevent accidental fluid overload.*

By: Maureen Kangleon, RN
Meg Gulanick, RN, PhD

Cardiac rehabilitation

POST MI AND POST CARDIAC SURGERY

Cardiac rehabilitation is the process of actively assisting patients with known heart disease to achieve and maintain optimal physical and emotional wellness. This care plan describes inpatient rehabilitation after patients are transferred from the intensive care unit. It focuses on the physical, psychosocial, and educational aspects of care to promote a smooth transition from hospital to home.

NURSING DIAGNOSES	EXPECTED OUTCOMES AND NURSING INTERVENTIONS / *RATIONALE* (■ = INDEPENDENT; ▲ = COLLABORATIVE)

Activity Intolerance

RELATED TO

Imposed activity restrictions secondary to medical condition or high-tech therapies/procedures
Pain (ischemic, postsurgery incisional)
Generalized weakness/fatigue (sedentary life-style prior to event, lack of sleep, decreased caloric intake post surgery)
Reduced cardiac output (secondary to myocardial dysfunction, dysrhythmias, postural hypotension

EXPECTED OUTCOMES

Patient verbalizes increased confidence with progressive activity.
Patient participates in prescribed activity programs without complications.
Patient describes readiness to perform ADL and routine home activities.

ONGOING ASSESSMENT

- Assess patient's activity tolerance prior to current illness. *Will serve as basis for formulating short/long term goals. NOTE: Some patients may have participated in regular exercise programs and be quite fit while others may have been incapacitated by chronic angina or valve disease.*
- Assess patient's physical status prior to exercise. Note HR, BP, need for supplemental oxygen, dysrhythmia status. *Complicated patients need closer observation and even the assistance of two nurses.*
- Assess patient's emotional readiness to increase activity. *Many MI patients may still be denying they even **had** a heart attack, and want to do **more** than prescribed; some post MI and surgical patients can be quite fearful of overexerting their hearts or causing discomfort.*

Continued.

NURSING DIAGNOSES	EXPECTED OUTCOMES AND NURSING INTERVENTIONS / *RATIONALE* (■ = INDEPENDENT; ▲ = COLLABORATIVE)

Activity Intolerance

RELATED TO— cont'd

Fear/anxiety (of overexerting heart, of experiencing angina or incisional pain)

DEFINING CHARACTERISTICS

Report of fatigue/weakness

Abnormal HR or BP response to activity

Exertional dyspnea

Chest pain

ECG changes reflecting ischemia

Dysrhythmias precipitated by activity

ONGOING ASSESSMENT— cont'd

- Monitor response to progressive activities. Report and modify regimen if the following abnormal responses are noted:

  Pulse >20 beats over baseline, or over 120 BPM.

  Chest pain/discomfort; dyspnea.

  Occurrence or increase in dysrhythmias.

  Excessive fatigue.

  ST segment displacement on ECG *(suggestive of myocardial ischemia).*

  Decrease of 10-15 mm Hg in systolic BP *(suggestive of ventricular dysfunction; excessive vasodilator drug effect, hypovolemia).*

  Systolic BP of 180 mm Hg or more, or diastolic BP >110 mm Hg *(suggestive of need for antihypertensive drug therapy). Physical activities increase demands on the healing heart. Close monitoring of patient's response provides guidelines for optimal activity progression.*

- Monitor SVO$_2$. *A saturation of >90 mm Hg is recommended. Lower values require supplemental O$_2$ during activity, and need for slower progression.*

- Assess patient's perception of effort required to perform each activity. *Borg scale uses ratings from 6-20 to determine rating of perceived exertion. A rating of 11 (fairly light) to 13 (somewhat hard) is an acceptable level for most patients.*

THERAPEUTIC INTERVENTIONS

- Encourage adequate rest periods before and after activity. *Rest decreases cardiac workload.*

- Assist and provide emotional support when increasing activity. *Patients are frequently afraid of overexerting their heart.*

- ▲ Provide pain medications as needed prior to activity. *This will facilitate patient cooperation.*

- ▲ Maintain progression of activities as ordered by cardiac rehabilitation team or physician, and as tolerated by patient. *Not everyone progresses at the same rate. Some patients progress slowly because of complicated MI, lack of motivation, inadequate sleep, fear of "overexertion," related medical problems, and previous sedentary life-style. In contrast, others who experience small infarcts and who had high fitness and activity levels before hospitalization may progress very rapidly; therefore, the following cardiac rehabilitation walking distances are only meant to be a guide.*

Cardiac Rehabilitation Stages:

Stage 1:

  Self-care activities at bedside.

  Selected ROM exercises in bed *(to reduce risk of thromboembolism).*

  Dangle 15-30 min at bedside TID *(to minimize occurrences of postural hypotension).*

Stage 2:

  Up in chair for 30-60 min TID.

  Partial bath in chair.

  Continue ROM exercises in chair *(to maintain flexibility. Postsurgical patients are usually afraid to move upper arms due to chest incision; this can result in frozen shoulder.)*

  Use incentive spirometer, cough and deep breathing exercises *(especially after cardiac surgery to prevent atelectasis. Recommended frequency is 10 times every hour while awake.)*

Stage 3:

  Continue with ROM exercises and low-intensity calisthenics *(exercises should be primarily dynamic of 1-2 METs intensity).*

  Partial bath at sink.

  Up in room as tolerated *(chair rest will reduce postural hypotension and promote better lung function).*

  Walk 75-100 feet in hall 2-3 times a day.

Stage 4:

  Continue with calisthenic exercises.

  Walk in hall 300 feet BID.

NURSING DIAGNOSES	EXPECTED OUTCOMES AND NURSING INTERVENTIONS / *RATIONALE* (■ = INDEPENDENT; ▲ = COLLABORATIVE)

THERAPEUTIC INTERVENTIONS— cont'd

Stage 5:

Continue with calisthenic exercises.

Ambulate ad lib.

Climb stairs (5-10 steps).

Perform discharge submaximal exercise stress test as prescribed (for most post MI patients). *Progression of activities can be by either increasing distance or time walked as patient tolerates or prefers. In the past, patients often exercised 1-2 times in cardiac rehabilitation center prior to discharge. However, today's early discharges do not allow that.*

▲ For patients with neurological or musculoskeletal problems, refer to Physical Therapy for assessment of ambulatory assistive device. *Assistive aids help to reduce energy consumption during physical activity.*

· Instruct patient of signs and symptoms of overexertion to use in progressing activity at home.

· Teach appropriate patients how to monitor own pulse rate. *Heart rate is a guide for monitoring intensity/duration of exercise.*

Knowledge Deficit

RELATED TO:

Unfamiliarity with disease process (MI, angina, CAD, valve disease), treatments, recovery process, follow-up care

DEFINING CHARACTERISTICS

Questioning
Verbalized misconceptions
Lack of questions

EXPECTED OUTCOMES

Patient verbalizes understanding of disease state, recovery process, and follow-up care.

Patient identifies available resources for life-style changes.

Patient verbalizes reduced fear/anxiety regarding cardiac event and pending discharge.

ONGOING ASSESSMENT

· Assess understanding of disease process, specific cardiac event, treatments, recovery, and follow-up care. *Teaching standardized content patient already knows wastes valuable time and hinders critical learning.*

· Identify specific learning needs and goals prior to discharge. *Shortened hospital stays and complex risk factor reduction programs provide challenges to the nurse and patient. Priority needs must be identified and satisfied first.*

THERAPEUTIC INTERVENTIONS

· Designate one nurse to be primarily responsible for patient education if cardiac rehabilitation nurse is not following patient. *Consistency of staff will promote consistency and completeness of information provided.*

· Provide information on needed topics:

Basic anatomy and physiology of the heart.

Pathophysiology of cardiac event (MI, CHF, CAD, valve disease).

Healing process after MI/cardiac surgery.

Angina versus heart attack.

Incisional pain versus angina.

Cardiac risk factor reduction.

Resumption of activities of daily living, such as lifting, household chores, driving a car, climbing stairs, social activities, sexual activity, and recreational activity.

Return to work.

Dietary regime.

Medications.

Immediate treatment for recurrence of chest pain/shortness of breath.

Incisional care.

Prophylactic antibiotics post valve surgery.

Follow-up medical care.

Coping mechanisms to help adjustment to new life-style.

Specific instructions, especially in written form, will help reduce patient's fears post discharge and reduce risks of either overexertion or "cardiac invalidism."

· Encourage meetings/conferences with family to discuss home treatment plan. *This will enhance smooth transition to the home.*

· Provide information on available educational/support resources: American Heart Association, Mended Hearts Groups, cardiac rehabilitation programs, stress management programs, and smoking cessation programs. *Many life-style changes require the assistance of professionals. Contact with another individual in support groups "who has been there" can be beneficial in reducing anxiety and dealing with impact of cardiac event.*

· Stress the importance of the patient's own role in maximizing their health status. *Patients need to understand that reduction of cardiac risk factors and health maintenance depends on them. Health professionals and family can only provide information and support.*

Continued.

NURSING DIAGNOSES	EXPECTED OUTCOMES AND NURSING INTERVENTIONS / *RATIONALE* (■ = INDEPENDENT; ▲ = COLLABORATIVE)

Fear

RELATED FACTORS

Anticipation of pain
Anticipation of complications
Anticipation of treatment failure
Perceived change in future health status
Perceived change in social status and life-style
Threat of death

DEFINING CHARACTERISTICS

Identifies object of fear
Increased tension
Apprehension
Increased alertness
Insomnia/nightmares
Excessive worry
Restlessness

See also:
- Ineffective breathing pattern (postsurgical), p. 10
- Pain, p. 49
- Sleep pattern disturbance, p. 61
- Nutrition, altered: less than body requirements (postsurgical), p. 44
- High-risk for decreased cardiac output, p. 12
- Body image disturbance, p. 7
- High-risk for altered sexuality pattern, p. 58

EXPECTED OUTCOMES

Patient identifies source of fear.
Patient implements a positive coping mechanism.
Patient verbalizes reduction/absence of fear.

ONGOING ASSESSMENT

- Determine what the patient is fearful of by careful, thoughtful questioning. *Accurate assessment guides appropriate intervention. Patient's concerns may range from overexerting the heart with activity, becoming a cardiac invalid, having the chest incision "pop open," vessel restenosing after PTCA or bypass surgery, or inability to resume satisfying sexual activity.*
- Assess the amount of fear experienced and measures patient is using to cope with it. *Symptoms will provide information regarding the degree of fear.*

THERAPEUTIC INTERVENTIONS

- Encourage verbalization of fears. Acknowledge your awareness of patient's fear. *This will validate the feelings the patient is having.*
- Provide anticipatory guidance to reduce fears. For example:
    Assist patient in distinguishing anginal pain from incisional pain. *Angina is usually related to exertion, not affected by muscular movement, and relieved with rest or NTG. Surgical incisional pain is aggravated by deep breathing and upper-extremity movement.*
    Explain the signs and symptoms of overexertion and how progressive resumption of activity prevents overexertion.
- Provide reliable information about future limitations (if any) in physical activity and role performance. *At least 85% of patients can resume a normal life-style. More complicated patients need guidance in understanding which limitations are temporary during recovery, and which may be more permanent.*
- Provide information about the healing process *so misconceptions can be clarified.*
- Refer to famous people (politicians, athletes, movie stars) who had similar cardiac problems or procedures and are now leading a productive life. *Examples such as Lyndon Johnson serving as President after a heart attack can provide reassurance and confidence about resuming activities.*
- Explain that patients are often "healthier" after cardiac events. *Their blocked artery may have "been fixed," they are more knowledgeable of their specific risk factors and treatment plan, and they may be taking medication to improve their health.*
- Encourage referral to a cardiac rehabilitation program and/or "coronary club." *These programs provide opportunities to discuss fears with specialists and patients experiencing similar concerns.*
- When patients become overly fearful, instruct them in performance of self-calming measures that may reduce fear or make it more manageable:
    Breathing modifications.
    Relaxation exercises.
    Calming music.
    Exercises in the use of affirmations and calming self-talk *to enhance the patient's sense of confidence.*

By: Meg Gulanick, RN, PhD
Lumie Perez, BSN, RN

Cardiac transplantation

HEART TRANSPLANT

Cardiac transplantation is a treatment option for persons with end-stage cardiac disease for whom all possible modes of surgical and medical treatment have been exhausted. Transplant candidates must meet certain criteria, including age, other disease processes, renal function, social supports, and psychological stability, to maximize the potential for success. The surgical procedure entails the excision of both donor and recipient hearts and transplantation of the donor heart into the recipient (orthotopically transplanted). With ongoing compliance to medical therapy and adherence to life-style changes, the transplant patient can live an active and productive life.

NURSING DIAGNOSES	EXPECTED OUTCOMES AND NURSING INTERVENTIONS / *RATIONALE* (■ = INDEPENDENT; ▲ = COLLABORATIVE)

Decreased Cardiac Output

RELATED TO

Arrhythmias induced by edema of conductive tissue in the donor heart secondary to manipulation of the nodal tissue at time of transplantation

Ischemia occurring during transport of donor graft or secondary to surgical procedure

Electrolyte/acid-base imbalance

DEFINING CHARACTERISTICS

Cardiac dysrhythmias:
  Junctional rhythms
  Symptomatic bradycardia
  Ventricular ectopy
Rapid/slow pulse
Shortness of breath
Dizziness
Change in mental status
Decreased BP
Cool, clammy skin

EXPECTED OUTCOMES

Patient maintains optimal cardiac output, as evidenced by regular cardiac rate and rhythm, clear breath sounds, BP within normal limits for patient, and warm, dry skin.

ONGOING ASSESSMENT

- Monitor ECG continuously, documenting any signs of inadequate heart rate (sinus pause, sinus arrest, junctional rhythm, heart blocks, and bradycardias) or ventricular ectopy. *The rate and rhythm of the transplanted heart depend on the sinus node impulse in the donor heart. Remnant P waves from native heart are of no clinical significance because these electrical impulses do not cross the suture line. Junctional rhythms are secondary to suture line edema in the atrium and generally resolve within 2 weeks.*
- Assess for signs of decreased cardiac output. *Transplanted hearts are denervated; therefore, heart rate changes gradually in response to altered metabolic needs via circulating catecholamines secreted from the adrenal medulla (i.e., there may be no compensatory tachycardia indicating hypovolemia or pump failure).*
- ▲ Monitor electrolyte and acid-base balance.

THERAPEUTIC INTERVENTIONS

- ▲ Initiate and maintain isoproterenol hydrochloride (Isuprel) drip as prescribed *to increase heart rate.*
- ▲ Use temporary epicardial pacing wires *to maintain an adequate heart rate* as needed. Check rate, mA, mode, and connections frequently. Keep pacer wires grounded (e.g., wrapped in rubber gloves) and taped securely to chest wall.
- ▲ If ventricular ectopy occurs, administer lidocaine bolus followed by drip as ordered (1 mg/kg for initial bolus, rebolus 10 min later, followed with a lidocaine drip at 2-4 mg/min).
- ▲ Give potassium replacement as ordered *to maintain serum K+ level greater than 4.0. Hypokalemia causes ventricular irritability.*
- ▲ Correct uncompensated metabolic acidosis with $NaHCO_3$ as ordered. *Acidosis precipitates ventricular ectopy.*
- See Cardiac output, decreased, p. 12; Cardiac dysrhythmias, p. 114.

High Risk for Decreased Cardiac Output

RISK FACTORS

Biventricular failure secondary to preexisting pulmonary hypertension
Global ischemia of donor heart before transplantation
Cardiac tamponade

EXPECTED OUTCOMES

Patient maintains optimal cardiac output, as evidenced by regular cardiac rate and rhythm, clear breath sounds, BP within normal limits for patient, and warm, dry skin.

ONGOING ASSESSMENT

- ▲ Monitor cardiac output by thermodilution on admission and prn.
- ▲ Assess right side of heart performance by documentation of central venous pressure (CVP).
- ▲ Assess left side of heart performance by documentation of pulmonary artery pressure (PAP), pulmonary capillary wedge pressure (PCWP), left arterial pressure (LAP), SVR, and arterial BP.
- Monitor intake and output hourly.
- Assess for signs of cardiac tamponade.
- Monitor MCT drainage.
- Assess for signs of decreased systemic perfusion, pulmonary venous congestion, and systemic venous congestion.

Continued.

Cardiac transplantation—cont'd

NURSING DIAGNOSES	EXPECTED OUTCOMES AND NURSING INTERVENTIONS / *RATIONALE* (■ = INDEPENDENT; ▲ = COLLABORATIVE)

THERAPEUTIC INTERVENTIONS

▲ Administer parenteral fluids as ordered *to maintain adequate filling pressures and optimize cardiac output.*

■ Institute measures *to reduce workload of heart* by maintaining normothermia, quiet environment, and placing patient in semi-Fowler's position.

▲ Administer inotropes (dopamine, dobutamine, calcium) as ordered *to increase myocardial contractility.*

▲ Administer vasodilators (Nipride, Tridil) as ordered *to control systemic vascular resistance, thereby reducing heart workload.*

▲ Maintain adequate oxygenation *to optimize cardiac function and reduce pulmonary vascular resistance.*

▲ Administer Isuprel as ordered *to reduce pulmonary vascular resistance and increase heart rate.*

■ See Cardiac output, decreased, p. 12.

High Risk for Injury: Bleeding/Hemorrhage

RISK FACTORS

Pericardial sac is larger than normal after transplant; therefore, a small new heart leaves an area that may conceal postoperative bleeding

Nonsurgical bleeding may be enhanced by preoperative anticoagulation or intraoperative cardiopulmonary bypass and heparinization

Surgical bleeding may be enhanced by elaborate suture lines and cannulation sites, as well as coagulopathy

EXPECTED OUTCOMES

Patient does not exhibit signs of hemorrhage, as evidenced by stable Hgb/Hct, and BP/HR within normal limits.

ONGOING ASSESSMENT

■ Assess pulse, BP, hemodynamic measurements.

■ Assess peripheral pulses, capillary refill.

■ Monitor I & O.

■ Assess MCT drainage for significant cessation (i.e., tamponade) and/or increase (i.e., hemorrhage). *Greater than 100 cc/hr for 4 hrs is significant.*

▲ Monitor Hgb/Hct.

▲ Monitor PT/PTT, platelet count; check ACT prn.

■ Observe amplitude of ECG configuration. *Decreased QRS voltage indicates tamponade.*

■ Assess heart tones. *Muffled heart sounds indicate tamponade.*

▲ Evaluate CXR for widening of mediastinal shadow. *Seen with cardiac tamponade.*

THERAPEUTIC INTERVENTIONS

■ Raise head of bed to 30 degrees and turn patient hourly *to prevent impedance of mediastinal drainage.*

■ Milk chest tubes q30 min for 12 hr, then hourly. Note amount and type of drainage (with or without clots); document output. *Current practice is not to strip chest tubes unless they are clotted.*

▲ Maintain 20 cm H_2O suction to MCT *to facilitate drainage.*

▲ Maintain current type and cross to keep 2 units packed red blood cells (PRBCs) available at all times during ICU stay. *Cells should be washed because of patient's suppressed immune system.*

▲ Use cytomegalovirus (CMV) negative blood if the recipient is CMV negative.

▲ Replace volume losses with colloids or crystalloids as ordered. Consider autotransfusion. If patient is bleeding rapidly, anticipate return to operating room.

Knowledge Deficit

RELATED TO

Unfamiliarity with:
Surgical procedure
Long-term care

DEFINING CHARACTERISTICS

Questioning
Verbalizing misconceptions
Lack of questioning

EXPECTED OUTCOMES

Patient and significant others demonstrate and communicate understanding of disease state, surgical procedures, recovery phase, activities, medications, and preventive care by date of discharge.

ONGOING ASSESSMENT

■ Assess patient/significant other's understanding of surgical procedure, follow-up care, diet, medications, activity progression, special precautions for avoiding infections, and risk factor modification.

THERAPEUTIC INTERVENTIONS

■ Describe surgical procedure, including ICU regimen and expected length of stay.

■ Provide opportunity for patient/family to ask questions and verbalize anxieties, fears about discharge planning.

▲ Coordinate discharge teaching with cardiac rehabilitation program, diet, occupational and physical therapy, respiratory therapy, social work, and any other significant departments *to ensure adequate understanding of care.*

THERAPEUTIC INTERVENTIONS— cont'd

- Inform patient/family that patient will have periodic endomyocardial biopsy *to assess for heart rejection. Biopsy is an outpatient procedure; frequency tapers significantly 6 months after surgery.*
- Inform patient he/she cannot rely on pulse rate to reflect tolerance or effects of activity accurately *because transplanted heart is denervated.*
- Instruct patient on low-salt and low-cholesterol diet. *Low-salt diet will help decrease amount of steroid-induced fluid retention. Low-cholesterol diet will decrease risk of future heart disease.*
- Instruct patient in medication regimen by using a flow chart specific for medications to be taken at home:
  Advise patient to store Cyclosporine capsules in the blister pack in which they are packaged. *Potency of the drug cannot be guaranteed more than 5 days after the package is opened.*
  Because cyclosporine A is in an oil base, administer in a glass *to prevent adherence to the container walls* and with juice or milk *to enhance palatability.*
  Cyclosporine A should be given on an empty stomach *to facilitate absorption;* steroids should be given with food.
- Caution patients of increased potential for bone "brittleness" related to steroids. Suggest wearing comfortable flat shoes *to decrease possible falls and injury.*
- Discuss possibility of emotional lability and mood alteration, *partly related to steroids, cyclosporine A, and stress of surgery and postoperative phase.*
- Instruct patient that chest movements associated with coughing, doing housework, climbing stairs, and driving may cause some discomfort for several weeks at home. No driving for at least 6-8 wk or as advised by physician. Depending on patient's occupation, return to work is not suggested for at least 3-6 mo; sometimes patient will need to change jobs.
- Instruct on importance of practicing good hygiene measures *to decrease incidence of infection from skin irritations and sores.*
- Review signs/symptoms of sternal wound complications, such as dehiscence, wound drainage, redness or swelling, or sternal instability, which may occur up to 1 mo postoperatively.
- Discuss modification of risk factors *to decrease possibility of future heart disease.*

High Risk for Ineffective Coping

RISK FACTORS

Fear of dying
Stress of waiting for surgery
Perceived body image changes
Fear of possibility of heart rejection after transplantation

EXPECTED OUTCOMES

Patient displays feelings appropriate to initial stage of coping.
Patient displays beginning signs of effective coping: relaxed appearance, sleeping well, ability to concentrate, interest in surroundings and activities.

ONGOING ASSESSMENT

- Assess patient's feelings about self, body, appearance.
- Assess patient's usual coping mechanisms and their previous effectiveness.
- Assess for signs of ineffective coping such as fears of being alone, insomnia, indifference, lack of concentration, crying. *Ineffective coping mechanisms must be identified to promote constructive behaviors.*

THERAPEUTIC INTERVENTIONS

- Encourage patient and family to express feelings. *Verbalization of feelings and sharing of emotions facilitate effective coping.*
- Establish open lines of communication:
  Initiate brief visits to patient.
  Define your role as patient informant and advocate.
  Understand the grieving process.
- Involve social services and pastoral care for additional and ongoing support resources for patient and significant others.
- Provide reading materials and resource persons as needed. *Sometimes it decreases anxiety to have a person who has had a heart transplant talk with and answer questions of the patient or family.*
- Introduce new information, using simple terms, and reinforce instructions or repeat information as necessary. *Depending on degree of anxiety, patient and/or family may not be able to absorb all information at one time.*

Continued.

Cardiac transplantation—cont'd

NURSING DIAGNOSES	EXPECTED OUTCOMES AND NURSING INTERVENTIONS / *RATIONALE* (■ = INDEPENDENT; ▲ = COLLABORATIVE)

High Risk for Infection

RISK FACTORS

Immunosuppressive drug therapy

Disruption of skin and iatrogenic sources of infection

EXPECTED OUTCOMES

Patient/family states understanding of need for strict infection control precautions. Patient/family complies with infection control measures.

ONGOING ASSESSMENT

- Observe wound healing process q8hr, prn for drainage, wound edge approximation, edema, sensitivity, andtemperature of srrounding tissue.
- ▲ Monitor WBC and cyclosporine A (CSA) levels daily. Expect adjustments of CSA and steroids, depending on results.
- Monitor vital signs routinely. Monitor temperature q2hr if elevated.
- ▲ Monitor cultures, sensitivities, and viral titers of blood, sputum, and urine.
- ▲ Culture any suspicious drainage from wound sites.

THERAPEUTIC INTERVENTIONS

- ▲ Keep patient in private room with high-efficiency particulate air filter (HEPA) capability throughout hospitalization.
- Maintain strict handwashing throughout patient's hospitalization. *In ICU, immunosuppression is greatest and ICU environment is classically known to harbor many bacteria and viruses in light of its patient population.*
- When patient is transferred to step-down unit, keep in private room or with a roommate *without infections to prevent cross contamination and infection. CDC research does not support need for protective/modified protective isolation.*
- Exclude personnel and visitors with infectious diseases (e.g., colds, flu) from patient care *because of patient's suppressed immune system.*
- Control environmental traffic (i.e., limit visitors and staff members into patient's room) *to protect patient from exposure to potential environmental organisms.*
- When entering room, wash all equipment with germicidal detergent (Staphene/ hexachlorophene).
- Change all dressings, ECG patches, and taping (i.e., endotracheal tube) daily *to decrease skin irritation and ensure close monitoring of invasive line sites. A primary cause of infection is directly related to interruption of skin barrier.*
- Change all respiratory equipment q24hr and encourage aggressive pulmonary toiletry *because pulmonary infections are second most common source of infection caused by effects of steroids and CSA.*
- Change all tubings and IV solutions per hospital policy *to decrease incidence of contamination from equipment.* Maintain aseptic technique.
- Ensure adequate diet high in calories and protein. *Infection risk greater in patients with end-stage heart disease because of their presurgical debilitated state.*

High Risk for Injury

RISK FACTORS

Steroids and immunosuppressant drug therapy

EXPECTED OUTCOMES

Injury resulting from immunosuppressive therapy is reduced, or detected early and treated.

ONGOING ASSESSMENT

- ▲ Assess patient for signs and symptoms of diabetes:
    Check urine dipsticks for glucose and ketones.
    Observe for polyuria.
    Note excessive thirst.
    Check serum glucose prn until maintenance dose of steroid is established.
- Assess gastric pH. *Increased hydrochloric acid causes development of gastric ulcers.*
- Monitor I & O, daily weight, BP. *Steroids can induce hypertension, generalized edema, and weight gain.*
- Assess for peripheral, sacral, periorbital, facial edema.
- Assess skin integrity.
- Assess for bruising, possible fractures, and vague complaints of bone pain. *Steroids cause calcium and phosphorus depletion.*
- ▲ Monitor renal functioning by checking BUN, creatinine, and CSA levels. *CSA is nephrotoxic.*

THERAPEUTIC INTERVENTIONS

▲ Administer antacids as prescribed.
▲ Place on low-sodium diet *to decrease fluid retention.*
▪ Apply support hose and elevate extremities *to reduce peripheral edema.*
▪ Keep skin well moistened with lotions *to prevent unnecessary itching from dry skin, secondary to CSA, dryness of environment and bed linens.*
▪ Reposition q2hr *to minimize potential for skin breakdown.*
▪ Pad bed rails *to decrease incidence of bruising from hitting rails.*

High Risk for Injury: Allograft Rejection

RISK FACTORS

Acute rejection:
Characterized by perivascular and interstitial mononuclear cell infiltration; progresses to necrosis if untreated.

EXPECTED OUTCOMES

Patient describes early signs of rejection.
Early detection of rejection is achieved.

ONGOING ASSESSMENT

▪ Assess overall status for increasing malaise, decreasing exercise tolerance.
▪ Evaluate ECG daily for:
Decreased QRS voltage *(may be seen with conventional immunosuppressants).*
Atrial arrhythmias.
Conduction defects. *These represent signs of rejection.*
▲ Monitor CSA trough level (drawn 1 hr before dose). *Nontherapeutic levels increase risk of rejection.*
▲ Monitor WBC and T-cell counts. *Elevated circulating T lymphocyte counts detect early rejection.*
▪ Assess peripheral circulation.
▪ Assess I&O hourly; weigh daily.
▪ Assess for signs of biventricular failure: ↓ pulses, diaphoresis, ↓ urine output, tachycardia, JVD, ascites, edema, ↓ or normalized BP.

THERAPEUTIC INTERVENTIONS

▲ Administer immunosuppressive agents daily, as prescribed.
▪ Keep right internal jugular site clean for future biopsies. (Note: Swan-Ganz catheters are in left internal jugular.) *Endomyocardial biopsy is definitive procedure to confirm rejection.*
▪ Describe to patient procedure of the endocardial biopsy, including use of local anesthesia at biopsy catheter insertion site.
▪ Teach patient about signs and symptoms of acute rejection. These are increased fatigue, irregular pulse, normalizing or lower than normal BP, increased weight, swelling, and shortness of breath.

See also:
Decreased activity intolerance, p. 2
Nutrition, altered: less than body requirements, p. 44
Powerlessness, p. 52.

By: Carol Ruback, RN, MSN, CCRN
Meg Gulanick, RN, PhD
Eileen Collins, RN, PhD

Cardiac Transplantation

Cardioverter defibrillator, implantable

A battery-powered device that delivers a series of one or more countershocks (depending upon device model) directly to the heart after it recognizes an arrhythmia through its sensing channels [via electrogram morphology shape detection algorithm and/or rate detection counter]). It is a life-prolonging therapy for patients with serious ventricular arrhythmias and is indicated for those: (1) who have survived at least one episode of sudden cardiac death caused by tachyarrhythmias not associated with acute myocardial infarction; (2) who have experienced recurrent tachyarrhythmias without cardiac arrest and who can be induced into sustained hypotensive V-tach or V-fib, or both, despite conventional antiarrhythmic drug therapy. The shock delivered (usually 0.1-35 Joules) is often described as a hard thump or as a kick on the chest. The device is implanted into the left abdominal wall pocket. On the earlier ICDs the sensing leads and defibrillator patches were implanted epicardially: the two sensing leads on the left ventricle and the defibrillator patches on the left and right ventricles. In the newer approaches the sensing lead is implanted transvenously, and the defibrillator lead is either implanted transvenously or subcutaneously on the left upper abdomen.

NURSING DIAGNOSES

EXPECTED OUTCOMES AND NURSING INTERVENTIONS / *RATIONALE*
(■ = INDEPENDENT; ▲ = COLLABORATIVE)

High Risk for Decreased Cardiac Output

RISK FACTORS

Intrinsic ventricular arrhythmias caused by:
  Ventricular aneurysm, Wolff-Parkinson-White syndrome, myocardial ischemia, refractoriness to anti-arrhythmic drug, prolonged QT syndrome, electrolyte imbalance, hypoxia, hypercapnia, or drug toxicity
System malfunction caused by:
  Improper placement of epicardial sensing leads and defibrillator patches
  Incorrect attachment of both the leads and the patches to the pulse generator
  Faulty lead system: e.g., insulation break, fracture, and overlooped leads
  Increased myocardial thresholds caused by anti-arrhythmic drug
  Pulse generator circuitry malfunction
  Difficulty determining defibrillation thresholds during electrophysiology study/implant procedure
  Failure to sense and/or emit charge to break tachyarrhythmias

EXPECTED OUTCOMES
Patient will maintain optimal cardiac output, as evidenced by warm dry skin, cardiac rhythm within normal limits for patient, adequate blood pressure for systemic perfusion, lungs clear to auscultation, and strong bilateral peripheral pulses.

ONGOING ASSESSMENT
- Observe/monitor closely for:
  Presence of sustained ventricular arrhythmias.
  Symptomatic bradycardia, asystole, or atrial tachyarrhythmias. *Such arrhythmias significantly reduce cardiac output.*
  Prolongation of QT interval if patient is on antiarrhythmic therapy. *Prolonged refractory period can precipitate arrhythmias.*
- Assess for improper function of implantable defibrillator:
  Failure to sense ventricular arrhythmia.
  Failure to emit energy charge.
  Failure to terminate ventricular arrhythmia.
  Improper sensing of tachyarrhythmias and inappropriate shocks.
- Assess for signs of pericardial effusions, myocardial perforation, and other postcardiac surgery complications.

THERAPEUTIC INTERVENTIONS
- Keep monitor alarm on at all times.
- Record rhythm strips/measure QT interval routinely q 4-8 hr and during tachyarrhythmias.
▲ Get information from the electrophysiologist on the functions of the implantable defibrillator and how it is programmed. Ask if the device is activated (on) or deactivated (off).
▲ Ensure that a special ring-type magnet is available on the nursing unit. *The magnet is to be used only by qualified personnel to check for proper lead signal (synchronous pulse tone means proper R-wave sensing). Applying magnet for 30 sec or more will deactivate the device (constant tone).*
  See below for proper technique on how to apply magnet over the pulse generator.
  Use magnet only during an emergency for activation or deactivation of the implantable defibrillator if required.
  Do not wave the magnet over the pulse generator. *Inadvertent application of the magnet may deplete the battery or may render the device unresponsive.*

NURSING DIAGNOSES	EXPECTED OUTCOMES AND NURSING INTERVENTIONS / *RATIONALE* (■ = INDEPENDENT; ▲ = COLLABORATIVE)

RISK FACTORS— cont'd

Failure of myocardium to respond to the charged energy delivered due to low energy output

Improper application of magnet

Inappropriate sensing of atrial tachyarrhythmias

Postoperative complications due to concomitant cardiac surgery (pericardial effusion; cardiac tamponade)

Extreme bradycardia/asystole following defibrillation

THERAPEUTIC INTERVENTIONS— cont'd

If V-tach/V-fib occurs:
▲ Check if patient received internal shock(s). If patient received internal shock/s:
  Notify physician and electrophysiologist.
  Document total number of shock(s) patient had received prior to conversion.
  Save rhythm strips in the chart.
  Check electrolyte level or other factors that predispose to ventricular arrhythmia.
▪ If patient did not receive internal shock and is decompensating:
  Initiate basic life support measures. Proceed with external defibrillation protocol. Do not wait for the device to emit charges. *Prompt intervention is essential to control life-threatening arrhythmias. Never assume that internal defibrillator is functioning normally.*
  Apply defibrillation paddles 3 to 4 inches away from the pulse generator. *This is to prevent the occurrence of circuit failure and muscle tissue burns.* If antero-lateral positioning is unsuccessful, try antero-posterior.
  Have oral airway available at the bedside at all times. *Allows airway clearance for proper ventilation during cardiopulmonary arrest.*

For sustained nonsymptomatic ventricular tachycardia: *Implantable defibrillator will not sense V-tach with rate slower than the programmed cut-off rate, e.g., <150 bpm.*
▲ Notify physician.
▲ Administer antiarrhythmic drug as ordered.
▲ Check potassium blood level or other factors that predispose to ventricular arrhythmia.
▪ Re-evaluate patient's hemodynamic status for V-Tach of longer duration.

If implantable defibrillator malfunction is noted:
▲ Notify electrophysiologist and the surgeon at once.
▲ Prepare lidocaine bolus and lidocaine drip (standby). *This enables suppression of abnormal ventricular activity.*
▪ Have emergency cart and defibrillator ready within reach. *This will be available for emergency use should defibrillation be needed to stabilize patient's rhythm and to support life.*
▲ If implantable defibrillator exhibits false emission of multiple shocks and is activated:
  Deactivate the device by applying a magnet over upper right corner of the device for 30 secs. *This will prevent inappropriate shocks that could worsen arrhythmias and may further damage the myocardium. Note: when deactivated a constant tone is heard instead of pulse tone (activated).*
  Anticipate return to the operating room for possible pulse generator replacement or lead reconfiguration.
  Document implantable defibrillator malfunction.

If symptomatic extreme bradycardia or asystole occurs following defibrillation:
▲ Initiate routine emergency procedure.
▲ Notify physician at once.
▲ Prepare Isuprel drip, epinephrine or atropine sulfate. Administer as ordered *to accelerate the heart rate.*
▲ Prepare for temporary pacemaker insertion.
▪ Instruct inpatient to report any complaints of palpitation, chest pain, dizziness, diaphoresis, etc. *for proper management of arrhythmia and control of impending arrest.*
▪ Instruct outpatient:
  To report to staff the delivery of any internal shock/s and total number of shocks received.
  To report to the nearest hospital emergency room if multiple discharges occur in rapid succession.
  Regarding the possibility of hospital admission following clusters of closely spaced discharges.
  To report physical symptoms felt such as chest pain, palpitation, diaphoresis, fainting, dizziness, etc. prior to receiving shock/s.
  Regarding routine evaluation after receiving shock/s including serum electrolytes, digitalis and antiarrhythmic blood levels and ECG analysis.

Continued.

Cardioverter defibrillator, implantable—cont'd

NURSING DIAGNOSES	EXPECTED OUTCOMES AND NURSING INTERVENTIONS / *RATIONALE* (■ = INDEPENDENT; ▲ = COLLABORATIVE)

Pain

RELATED FACTORS

Insertion of implantable defibrillator
Concomitant cardiac surgery
"Frozen" shoulder
Restriction of movement on affected side
Imposed restrictions of activity

DEFINING CHARACTERISTICS

Restlessness, irritability
Withdrawn behavior
Complaints of incisional pain or other discomforts
Reluctance to move
Limited range of motion of affected extremity on operative side
Patient splints chest and abdomen with hands
Pallor, diaphoresis, and increase in blood pressure

EXPECTED OUTCOMES

Patient verbalizes relief of pain, or ability to tolerate discomfort.
Patient appears comfortable and relaxed.

ONGOING ASSESSMENT

- Assess characteristics of pain.
- Observe for objective signs of discomfort.
- Evaluate source of pain (operative, musculoskeletal, or other medical problem).
- Assess patient's expectations for pain relief.
- Assess for effectiveness of pain relief measures.

THERAPEUTIC INTERVENTIONS

- Respond immediately to complaint of pain.
▲ Administer pain medications as ordered.
- Provide comfort measures. *This may decrease total amount of analgesics required.*
  Massage shoulder muscle gently.
  Give light back rub.
  Use relaxation techniques. *This will minimize muscle tension.*
- Explain to patient reasons for self-imposed restrictions of activity.
- Encourage patient to report effectiveness of interventions.
- Prior to discharge teach patient:
  How to handle routines at home, (e.g., reaching, picking up articles from the floor, lying down, etc). *This will eliminate other factors causing pain.*
  Type of clothing to wear. *Tight restrictive clothing could worsen discomfort.*

High Risk for Infection (Immediate Postsurgery/Early Recovery).

RISK FACTORS

Insertion of implantable defibrillator through the abdominal wall pocket
Median sternotomy, left lateral thoracotomy, subcostal/subxiphoid approaches for the placement of the epicardial and patch leads

EXPECTED OUTCOMES

Patient verbalizes early signs of infection to be reported.
Patient describes preventive care to reduce risk of infection.

ONGOING ASSESSMENT

- Assess operative sites for signs of infection.
- Check type and amount of any drainage from the incision sites.
- Monitor chest tube drainage for color and amount.
▲ Monitor elevated WBC and fever.
▲ If infection is suspected, assess blood/fluid cultures.

THERAPEUTIC INTERVENTIONS

- Ensure sterile technique when changing dressing. *This will reduce risk of infection to open wounds.*
- Keep dressing dry and intact. *This will reduce chance of pathogens migrating.*
- Avoid frequent contact with the incision sites.
- Suggest high-caloric, high-protein diet if necessary. *This will enhance wound healing process.*
- Notify physician if infection is suspected and report excessive drainage if present.
▲ Administer antibiotics as prescribed. *Staphylococcus can be treated successfully with intravenous erythromycin without removal of the implantable defibrillator.*
- Prior to discharge, teach patient and family:
  Signs and symptoms of infection.
  Proper technique on dressing change.
  Avoidance of shower or full bath for a week or while wound is still open.
  Avoidance of frequent contact with the affected site.
  Importance of reporting signs and symptoms of infection.

Impaired Physical Mobility

RELATED FACTORS

Medical restrictions due to concomitant heart surgery, present illness, prolonged hospitalization, and multiple diagnostic studies
Reluctance to attempt movement for fear of recurrent ventricular arrhythmias

EXPECTED OUTCOMES

Patient moves within limits of restrictions.
Patient prevents/reduces complications of immobility by performing ROM exercises, incentive spirometry, and coughing/deep breathing exercises.

ONGOING ASSESSMENT

- Assess for ability to carry out ADL. *Medical restrictions and location of implanted device interfere with many physical activities.*
- Assess skin integrity for signs of redness or tissue ischemia. *Prolonged bedrest can cause reduced circulation to skin and tissue.*
▲ Assess for signs of pulmonary compromise: ↑ respiratory rate, abnormal breath sounds, and abnormal ABGs.
- Observe for signs of thrombophlebitis.

Related Factors—cont'd

Difficulty moving about due to the size and location of the implanted device

Actual pain and fear of injury

Defining Characteristics

Generalized weakness

Muscle weakness of upper extremity on operative side

Verbalized complaints of inability to perform

Limited range of motion

Increased dependency on others

Therapeutic Interventions

- Encourage use of incentive spirometry, and to cough and deep breathe q 1 hr while awake. *Maintenance of optimal lung function will prevent atelectasis.*
- ▲ Administer pain medication as prescribed; provide comfort measures. *Promotion of pain facilitates movement.*
- Provide passive range of motion to upper extremities. *This will prevent muscle or joint stiffness and minimize discomfort.*
- Assist with active ROM exercises to nonaffected extremities.
- Encourage patient to turn q 1-2 hr. *Caution should be used when turning to the left side to avoid pain and pressure on the generator site.*
- Provide prophylactic antipressure device if indicated.
- Encourage progressive ambulation 24 hr postimplant for patient without concomitant cardiac surgery.

Risk for Body Image Disturbance

Risk Factors

Size and site of implantable defibrillator

Chest and abdominal incisions

Loss of normal cardiac function

Expected Outcomes

Patient verbalizes at least beginning acceptance of body image.

Ongoing Assessment

- Evaluate patient's behavior toward change in body appearance. *Because of the size of the device in the abdomen, the abdominal girth is larger, which makes the patient appear pregnant.*
- Assess perception of change in body structure. *Extent of response is based more on the importance of the patient's perception of his/her image than the actual value.*
- Assess perceived impact of change in ADL, social behavior, personal relationships, and occupational activities.

Therapeutic Interventions

- Encourage verbalization of feelings about actual or perceived changes.
- Acknowledge normal response to actual or perceived change in body image.
- Assist patient in incorporating actual changes in ADL. Provide tips on tying shoes, picking up and lifting heavy objects, reaching, etc.
- Support patient with positive reinforcements.
- Encourage use of support groups. *Groups that come together for mutual support and information exchange can assist patient in coping with perceived/actual changes.*
- Provide information about benefits of wearing loose clothing. For male patients suggest suspenders instead of belts.

Fear

Related Factors

Diagnosis of inducible life-threatening arrhythmia

Past history of sudden cardiac death, syncope, long history of hospitalization, and multiple diagnostic studies

Anticipation of perceived threat/danger/death

Insertion of implantable defibrillator

Anticipation of how receiving a shock will feel

Potential for defibrillator system malfunction

Loss of independence caused by change in role functions/routines

Threat/change of socioeconomic status

Interpersonal conflicts

Expected Outcomes

Patient will verbalize his/her fears openly.

Ongoing Assessment

- Assess level of fear.
- Evaluate past coping mechanisms and their effectiveness.
- Assess effectiveness of current interventions.

Therapeutic Interventions

Inpatient:

- Encourage patient to talk about fears. *Allows ventilation of repressed feelings and promotes nurse-patient relationship.*
- Avoid false reassurances. Be honest. *Assures the patient of his/her security and safety during periods of anxiety.*
- Explain electrophysiology and surgical procedures ahead of time. *Answering all concerned questions will reduce patient's anxiety level. He/she will be able to use problem-solving abilities effectively if anxiety level is low.*
- Institute measures for adequate sleep. *Improves patient's well-being and helps him/her prepare for surgery better.*
- ▲ Administer medication as prescribed for relief of anxiety.
- Provide emotional support to patient by expressing concerns in a calm, reassuring manner. *The presence of a trusted person makes patient feel secure.*

Continued.

Cardioverter defibrillator, implantable—cont'd

NURSING DIAGNOSES	EXPECTED OUTCOMES AND NURSING INTERVENTIONS / *RATIONALE* (■ = INDEPENDENT; ▲ = COLLABORATIVE)

DEFINING CHARACTERISTICS

Restlessness, irritability
Insomnia
Increased questioning
Expressed concerns
Expressed feelings of loss of control

See also:
SCPs for anxiety and fear.
Assist patient in recognizing symptoms of increased anxiety/fear and explore alternatives he/she may use to prevent being immobilized by it.

THERAPEUTIC INTERVENTIONS— cont'd

- Suggest need for counseling. Request referrals to social worker, nurse liaison, or clergy.
- Rehearse with patient what it feels like when device "goes off." *Talking through the event may help patients cope with their fears.*
Outpatient:
- Assist patient in developing his/her problem-solving abilities. *Guidance with less stressful problem-solving situation will provide base for more complex situations.*
- Encourage use of support groups. *Knowing what changes in lifestyle might occur helps to prepare for such situations; facilitates problem solving.*
- Assist/encourage family in providing emotional support to patient.

Knowledge Deficit: Individual/Family

RELATED FACTORS

Lack of exposure
Misinterpretation of information
Lack of interest to learn due to physical condition or emotional state
Overprotection
Unfamiliarity with information resources

DEFINING CHARACTERISTICS

Increased questioning
Verbalized misinformation
Inappropriate behavior
Lack of questions

EXPECTED OUTCOMES

Patient and family verbalizes understanding of the importance of implantable defibrillator, its function, and follow-up care.
Patient verbalizes acceptance of activity limitations.

ONGOING ASSESSMENT

- Assess patient's knowledge about illness, implantable defibrillator, and electrophysiology study.
- Assess family's understanding of patient's present condition, expected outcome, implantable defibrillator functions, risks of surgery, and dependence on an electronic device.
- Determine what teaching methods are most effective to both patient and family.
- Prior to discharge, assess the family's interest in the care of the patient at home.

THERAPEUTIC INTERVENTIONS

Preoperative:
- Provide information regarding patient's illness, electrical conduction system of the heart, implantable defibrillator functions, need for an implant, surgical procedures and the risks involved, dependence on electronic device, discomfort of shocks, and unpredictability of arrhythmias. *Accurate information lessens fear and anxiety.*
- Discuss positive outcome of implanted defibrillator and its advantages over other therapies.
Postoperative:
- Instruct patient to anticipate chest tube catheters and possible intubation immediately following surgery.
- Instruct patient regarding activity restrictions:
  Bedrest for 24 hr for patient without concomitant heart surgery.
  Avoid turning to the left side, hyperextension of arms, and bending over until incisions have completely healed. *This will eliminate pressures that can cause pain and discomfort at operative site.*
  Discuss the importance of deep breathing, coughing exercises, and use of incentive spirometer. *This will prevent pulmonary atelectasis.*
  Inform patient to notify nurse of:
    Any physical complaints of chest pain, palpitation, dizziness, shortness of breath, and other signs of arrhythmias and possible malfunction of implantable defibrillator malfunction.
    Loose, wet dressing or excessive drainage from the dressing.
    Total number of shock/s received.
  Inform patient of importance of early ambulation following bedrest.
- Prior to discharge: instruct patient/family regarding:
  Need to carry ID card at all times.
  Need to apply for medic alert bracelet and to wear it at all times.
  Need for regular follow-up care (every 2 mo for a period of 1 year, then monthly until the end of life of battery) and the longevity of the device (2-3 yr).

NURSING DIAGNOSES	EXPECTED OUTCOMES AND NURSING INTERVENTIONS / *RATIONALE* (■ = INDEPENDENT; ▲ = COLLABORATIVE)

THERAPEUTIC INTERVENTIONS— cont'd

How to enroll family for CPR course.
Procedure for taking pulse.
How patient can do cough CPR.
Chest and abdominal wound care.
Signs and symptoms of infection.
Signs and symptoms of tachyarrhythmias and implantable defibrillator malfunction.
Anticipating shock when symptoms occur.
Tingling sensation by person who touches patient being shocked.
Wearing support abdominal band for a short period *to prevent swelling and minimize discomfort.*
Wearing loose clothing.
Avoiding strong magnetic field. *It may cause the defibrillator to deactivate or deplete battery and may become unresponsive: diathermy, CT scans, lithotripsy, electrocautery equipment, stimulator, NMR, laser, and current industrial machinery. Newer-model microwave ovens have no reported effect. For radiation therapy, the device should be shielded.*
Device will emit "beeping noise" when near magnetic field.
Notifying physician/pacemaker lab for shock/s received immediately.
Alerting dentists or other physicians for presence of implantable defibrillator.
Alerting airport personnel regarding implantable defibrillator.
Restriction of driving. Alternate methods of transportation need to be arranged.
Avoiding contact sports like baseball, basketball, tennis, football, etc.
Magnet testing during scheduled follow-up care.

See also:
- Powerlessness, p. 52
- Coping, impaired family, p. 17
- Coping, impaired individual, p. 18.

- Utilize a variety of teaching materials:
  Videotaped cassette of patients with implantable defibrillator.
  Implantable defibrillator (demo) and equipment.
  Handout materials.
- Review implantable defibrillator manual with patient and family.
- Refer to support group. *This will allow interactions with other patients and family.*

By: Marilyn Samson-Hinton, RN, BNS

Carotid endarterectomy

VASCULAR SURGERY

Surgical procedure to remove atherosclerotic plaque from the inner wall of the carotid artery.

NURSING DIAGNOSES	EXPECTED OUTCOMES AND NURSING INTERVENTIONS / *RATIONALE* (■ = INDEPENDENT; ▲ = COLLABORATIVE)

High Risk For Altered Cerebral Tissue Perfusion

RISK FACTORS
Edema from surgery
Clot formation
Hemorrhage
Hematoma formation
Hypotension

EXPECTED OUTCOMES

Patient's optimal cerebral perfusion is maintained as evidenced by alert responsive mentation/or no further reduction in mental status and absence of progression of neurologic deficits.

ONGOING ASSESSMENT

- Assess responsiveness/level of consciousness (LOC) as indicated.
- Assess speech, symmetry of face, intellectual ability as compared to baseline (assessing for impairment of mental ability), and visual ability. *The blood supply of the brain may be altered from a decrease in carotid blood flow that can occur from excessive edema, hematoma of the operative site, or from embolization. The changes could result in neurologic deficits (stroke).* Refer to SCP Stroke, p. 248 if deficits occur.
- Assess motor responses, noting for weakness, paresis of an extremity.
- Assess pupillary reaction.
- Monitor BP q1h.
- Check dressing and incision line for bleeding.
- Check for symmetry of neck. Check behind neck of supine patient. *Blood may pool; hematoma formation posterior from incision line is possible.*
- Assess quality of pulse proximal and distal to incision.

Continued.

Carotid endarterectomy—cont'd

NURSING DIAGNOSES	EXPECTED OUTCOMES AND NURSING INTERVENTIONS / *RATIONALE* (■ = INDEPENDENT; ▲ = COLLABORATIVE)

THERAPEUTIC INTERVENTIONS
- Maintain bed rest.
- Keep side rails up and call light within reach.
- Reorient as necessary.
- Report sudden or progressive deterioration in neurologic status *to minimize damage from inadequate cerebral blood flow.*
- ▲ Administer antihypertensives as ordered *to prevent extreme elevations in BP.* Keep BP at 120-150 mm Hg systolic and 70-90 mm Hg diastolic or 86-110 mm Hg mean arterial pressure (MAP). Notify physician if out of this range. *Hypertension could result in increased edema at the operative site, hemorrhage of the incisional area, or even carotid artery disruption. However, avoid hypotension to prevent cerebral ischemia and thrombosis.*

Pain

RELATED TO
Surgical incision

DEFINING CHARACTERISTICS
Patient verbalizes pain
Decreased activity or guarding behavior
Restlessness, irritability
Altered sleep pattern
Facial mask of pain
Autonomic responses

EXPECTED OUTCOMES
Patient's pain is relieved as evidenced by verbalization of pain relief and relaxed facial expression.

ONGOING ASSESSMENT
- Assess patient's description of pain.
- Assess characteristics of pain:
- Assess autonomic responses to pain. *May include diaphoresis, altered BP, pulse, respiration rate, pallor, and pupil dilation.*

THERAPEUTIC INTERVENTIONS
- Instruct patient to report pain.
- Anticipate need for analgesics *to prevent occurrence of severe, intractable pain.*
- ▲ Administer analgesics as needed.
- Encourage rest periods.
- Offer additional comfort measures.

Ineffective Breathing Pattern

RELATED TO
Edema
Hematoma formation
Postop state

DEFINING CHARACTERISTICS
Tachypnea
Change in depth of breathing
Complaint of shortness of breath
Use of accessory muscles

EXPECTED OUTCOMES
Patient's breathing pattern is maintained as evidenced by eupnea, regular respiratory rate/pattern, and verbalization of comfort with breathing.

ONGOING ASSESSMENT
- Assess respiratory rate, rhythm, and depth.
- Assess for any increase in work of breathing such as shortness of breath and use of accessory muscles.
- Auscultate lungs for presence of breath sounds. *Routine assessment of breath sounds allows for early detection and correction of abnormalities.*
- Assess cough for effectiveness and productivity.
- Assess trachea for midline position and assess neck for symmetry *to readily detect swelling or hematoma that can obstruct airway.*
- ▲ Monitor ABGs and note changes.

THERAPEUTIC INTERVENTIONS
- Position patient with proper body alignment *for optimal lung expansion.*
- Elevate head of bed 30-40 degrees *to reduce neck edema, as patient's condition allows.*
- Maintain patient's head in straight position *to decrease stress/pulling of the operative site.*
- Change position q2h *to facilitate movement and drainage of secretions.*
- Assist patient with deep breathing q1h. If abnormal breath sounds are present, assist patient with coughing.
- Suction as needed *to clear secretions.*
- Provide reassurance and allay anxiety by staying with patient during acute episodes of respiratory distress. *Air hunger can produce extreme anxiety.*
- ▲ Maintain O₂ delivery system *so that the appropriate amount of oxygen is applied continuously and the patient does not desaturate.*
- Notify physician immediately of any abnormalities. *An expanding hematoma in the neck can be a life-threatening emergency.*

See also:
Knowledge deficit, p. 41.
Infection, high risk for, p. 40.

By: Sue Galanes RN, MS, CCRN

Chronic heart failure

CONGESTIVE HEART FAILURE (CHF);
CARDIOMYOPATHY; LEFT SIDED FAILURE; RIGHT
SIDED FAILURE; PUMP FAILURE

Heart failure is the inability of the heart to pump sufficient blood to meet the oxygen demands of the tissues. Myocardial ischemia and viral infections are the most common etiologies. Patients are classified according to the New York Heart Association standards based on severity of symptoms. Class 1 patients have no symptoms. Class 2 patients experience slight limitations in their physical activity. They can usually perform most ordinary physical activities without problem; however, they may experience fatigue, palpitations, dyspnea, or angina. Class 3 patients experience marked limitations of their activity. They are usually fairly comfortable at rest, but less than ordinary activity can cause fatigue, palpitations, dyspnea, or anginal pain. Class 4 patients experience dyspnea even at rest; activity is extremely limited. The goals of therapy for heart failure are to improve cardiac output, reduce cardiac workload, prevent complications, recognize early signs of decompensation, and provide patient education so as to reduce the frequency of readmissions and improve quality of life.

NURSING DIAGNOSES	EXPECTED OUTCOMES AND NURSING INTERVENTIONS / *RATIONALE* (■ = INDEPENDENT; ▲ = COLLABORATIVE)

Decreased Cardiac Output

RELATED TO:

Increased or decreased pre-load
Increased afterload
Decreased contractility
Tachy- or bradydysrhythmia

DEFINING CHARACTERISTICS

Decreased BP
Increased HR
Decreased urine output
Decreased peripheral pulses
Cold clammy skin
Rales
Dyspnea
Restlessness
Dysrhythmias
Abnormal heart sounds (S_3)
Decreased activity tolerance
Orthopnea
PND

EXPECTED OUTCOMES

Patient maintains optimal cardiac output, as evidenced by normal BP and HR, clear breath sounds, strong peripheral pulses, urine output >30 ml/hr, and no shortness of breath.

ONGOING ASSESSMENT

■ Assess for signs and symptoms of decreased cardiac output (see Defining characteristics).
▲ Monitor serum electrolytes *as possible causative factor for arrhythmias.*
▲ Monitor serum creatinine. *Rising creatinine is an adverse effect of diuretic therapy and ACE inhibitors.*

THERAPEUTIC INTERVENTIONS

■ Weigh daily and keep record of I & O. *This provides evidence of fluid status.*
▲ If increased preload is a problem, restrict fluids and sodium as ordered *to decrease extracellular fluid volume.*
▲ If decreased preload is a problem, increase IV fluids and closely monitor *to increase extracellular fluid volume.*
▲ Administer the following medication as ordered:
  Diuretics *to reduce volume and enhance sodium and H_2O excretion.*
  Inotropes *to improve myocardial contractility.*
  Vasodilators *to reduce preload and afterload.*
  Ace inhibitors *to decrease peripheral vascular resistance and venous tone and suppress aldosterone output.*
  Antiarrhythmics *to correct tachy- or bradydysrhythmias. Note: Frequently patients with heart failure have chronic arrhythmias that do not respond to medical therapy. Some antiarrhythmics have a negative inotropic effect, which may exacerbate heart failure.*
▲ Provide O_2 as indicated by patient's condition and saturation levels. *The failing heart may not be able to respond to increased O_2 demand. O_2 supply may be inadequate when there is fluid accumulation in the lungs. Also, the vasodilating effect of O_2 decreases pulmonary hypertension, thereby reducing the work of the right heart.*
■ If the condition becomes acute or does not respond to therapy, anticipate the need for invasive hemodynamic monitoring, intra-aortic balloon pump, right or left ventricular assist device, investigational medications, or heart transplant.

Continued.

NURSING DIAGNOSES	EXPECTED OUTCOMES AND NURSING INTERVENTIONS / *RATIONALE* (■ = INDEPENDENT; ▲ = COLLABORATIVE)

Fluid Volume Excess

RELATED TO

Decreased cardiac output causing:
  Decreased renal perfusion, which stimulates the renin-angiotensin-aldosterone system and causes release of ADH
  Altered renal hemodynamics (diminished medullary blood flow), which results in decreased capacity of nephron to excrete water

DEFINING CHARACTERISTICS

Weight gain
Edema
Crackles
Jugular venous distention (JVD)
Elevated CVP and PCWP
Ascites/HJR
Decreased urine output

EXPECTED OUTCOMES

The patient maintains optimal fluid balance, as evidenced by maintainence of normal weight, no edema, and clear breath sounds.

ONGOING ASSESSMENT

- Assess weight daily and consistently: before breakfast on the same scale, after voiding, in the same amount of clothing, without shoes. *This facilitates accurate measurement.*
- Monitor for a significant (>2 lb) weight change in 1 day or trend over several days.
- Evaluate weight in relation to nutritional status. *In some heart failure patients weight may be a poor indicator of fluid volume status. Poor nutrition and decreased appetite over time result in a decrease in weight, which may be accompanied by fluid retention though the net weight remains unchanged.*
- Evaluate urine output in response to oral diuretics. *Fluid volume excess in abdomen may interfere with absorption of oral medications. Medications may need to be given IV.*
- Monitor for excessive response to diuretics: >2 lb loss in 1 day, hypotension, weakness, BUN elevated out of proportion to serum creatinine level.
▲ Monitor for potential side effects of diuretics: hypokalemia, hyponatremia, hypomagnesemia, ↑ serum creatinine and hyperuricemia. *Long-term administration of spironolactone (Aldactone) may cause endocrine dysfunction. Carbohydrate intolerance may occur in patients with latent diabetes mellitus, especially if they are receiving thiazides.*
- Assess for presence of edema by palpating area over tibia, ankles, feet, and sacrum. *Pitting edema is manifested by a depression that remains after one's finger is pressed over an edematous area and then removed. Grade edema 1+, indicating barely perceptible, to 4+, indicating severe.*
- Auscultate breath sounds and assess for labored breathing.
- Assess for JVD and ascites. Monitor abdominal girth *to follow ascites accurately.*
- Measure intake. Include items that are liquid at room temperature such as Jello, sherbet, and Popsicles.

THERAPEUTIC INTERVENTIONS

▲ Restrict fluid and sodium as prescribed. *This will help to decrease extracellular volume.*
▲ Give diuretics as prescribed.
- Instruct patient to avoid medications that may cause fluid retention, such as nonsteroidal anti-inflammatory agents, certain vasodilators, and steroids.
- In preparation for discharge, instruct patient in how to weigh self daily and monitor intake and output at home (if indicated); emphasize that significant change in weight, leg swelling, or breathing changes should be reported.

High Risk for Alteration in Electrolyte Balance

RISK FACTORS:

Increased total body fluid (dilutes electrolyte concentration)
Decreased renal perfusion (results in greater reabsorption of sodium and K^+)
Diuretic therapy (enhances renal excretion of total body water and sodium and K^+)
Low-sodium diet

EXPECTED OUTCOMES

Patient maintains electrolytes within normal range when therapy is stable.
Nonacute variation in electrolyte balance is recognized and treated early to prevent complications.
Patient receives medication adjustments as needed if electrolyte imbalance is noted.

ONGOING ASSESSMENT

▲ Monitor serum electrolytes when administering diuretics, ACE inhibitors, and digoxin, especially in the event of large weight gain or loss, or in the presence of renal insufficiency.
  Hyponatremia: Na <136 mEq/L: may be accompanied by headache, apathy, tachycardia, and generalized weakness.
  Hypokalemia: K <3.8 mEq/L: may have fatigue; GI distress; increased sensitivity to digoxin; atrial and ventricular arrhythmia; ST segment depression; broad, sometimes inverted, progressively flatter T wave and enlarging U wave.
  Hypernatremia: Na >147 mEq/L: may be accompanied by thirst, dry mucous membranes, fever, and neurologic changes if severe.
  Hyperkalemia: K >5.1 mEq/L: may be accompanied by muscular weakness, diarrhea, and the following ECG changes: tall, peaked T waves; widened QRS; prolonged PR interval; decreased amplitude and disappearance of P wave; or ventricular arrhythmia.
- Monitor fluid losses and gains.
▲ Monitor digoxin level and effects in presence of hypokalemia.

Continued.

THERAPEUTIC INTERVENTIONS

For hyponatremia:

▲ Encourage sodium restriction as prescribed. Provide dietary instruction. *Sodium promotes water retention. In chronic heart failure, hyponatremia is usually dilutional; it is caused by a greater concentration of water than sodium.*

▲ Administer diuretics as prescribed and monitor response. *This will help restore water/ sodium balance.* Monitor effectiveness of diuretics.

▲ Encourage fluid restriction as prescribed. Use ice chips, hard candy, or frozen juice sticks to quench thirst. *Restriction of intake will reduce the work of the heart and reduce requirement for diuretic therapy.*

■ Instruct patient to avoid salt contained in over-the-counter preparations such as antacids (Alka-Seltzer).

For hypokalemia (commonly caused by prolonged use of thiazide or loop diuretics):

▲ Administer oral or IV supplement as prescribed. Oral supplements should be given directly after meals or with food *to minimize GI irritation.*

■ Encourage daily intake of potassium-rich foods (raisins, bananas, cantaloupe, dates, and potatoes).

For hypernatremia:

▲ Carefully replace water orally or IV. *Hypernatremia is commonly caused by large loss of water. Heart failure patients have a precarious fluid balance status.*

■ Anticipate reduction in diuretic dosage.

For nonacute hyperkalemia:

■ Anticipate reduction in potassium supplement.

▲ Provide diet with potassium restriction as prescribed.

▲ Discontinue potassium-sparing diuretics as prescribed.

■ Instruct patient to avoid salt substitutes containing potassium.

In emergency situations (serum K >6.0 mEq/L):

■ Place patient on ECG monitor.

▲ Administer the following temporary measures as ordered:

Regular insulin and hypertonic dextrose IV: *This causes a shift of K^+ into the cells. Onset of action is 30 min and duration is several hours.*

$NaHCO_3$: *This causes rapid movement of K^+ into the cells. The onset is within 15 min and the duration of action is 1-2 hr.*

Cation-exchange resins: *These reduce the serum K^+ slowly but have the advantage of actually removing K^+ from the body. Frequently they are given with one of the other measures.*

CaCl given IV: *Duration of action is 1 hr; immediately antagonizes the cardiac and neuromuscular toxicity of hyperkalemia.*

Dialysis: *An effective method of removing potassium but is reserved for situations in which more conservative measures fail.*

High Risk for Activity Intolerance

RISK FACTORS

Decreased cardiac output
Deconditioned state

EXPECTED OUTCOMES

Patient reports improved activity tolerance.
Patient reports ability to perform required ADL.

ONGOING ASSESSMENT

■ Assess patient's current level of activity. Determine reasons for limiting activity: physical symptoms vs. fear of overexertion.

■ Evaluate need for O_2 during increased activity. *Supplemental O_2 may help compensate for the increased O_2 demand.*

THERAPEUTIC INTERVENTIONS

■ Establish guidelines and goals of activity with patient and significant others. *Motivation is enhanced if the patient participates in goal setting.*

■ Use slow progression of activity *to prevent sudden increase in cardiac workload:*
Dangling 10-15 min tid, active ROM exercise tid, walking in room, walking in hall short distances, and then progressively increasing distances (saving energy for return trip).

■ Teach appropriate use of environmental aides (e.g., bedside commode, chair in bathroom, hall rails). *Appropriate aides will enable the patient to achieve optimal independence for self-care.*

▲ Consult cardiac rehabilitation or physical therapy for assistance in increasing activity tolerance. *Specialized therapy or cardiac monitoring may be necessary when initially increasing activity. Structured program may increase self-confidence and success.*

Continued.

Cardiac and Vascular Care Plans

NURSING DIAGNOSES	EXPECTED OUTCOMES AND NURSING INTERVENTIONS / *RATIONALE* (■ = INDEPENDENT; ▲ = COLLABORATIVE)

THERAPEUTIC INTERVENTIONS— cont'd

- Adjust medication schedule to provide optimal times for activity. *Timing nitrate and vasodilator therapy may allow exercise without development of symptoms.*
- Instruct patient in energy conservation techniques.
- Instruct patient to stop activity that causes chest pain and increased dyspnea. *This will minimize the potential for physical injury.*
- Provide emotional support while increasing activity levels *to minimize feelings of fear and anxiety.*

Sleep Pattern Disturbance

RELATED TO

Anxiety/fear
Physical discomfort/shortness of breath
Medical schedule and effects

DEFINING CHARACTERISTICS

Fatigue
Frequent daytime dozing
Irritability
Inability to concentrate
C/O difficulty falling asleep
Interrupted sleep

EXPECTED OUTCOMES

Patient verbalizes improvement in hours of sleep.
Patient appears rested.

ONGOING ASSESSMENT

- Assess current sleep pattern and sleep history.
- Assess for possible deterrents to sleep:
  Nocturia.
  Volume excess: causing dyspnea (PND), paroxysmal nocturnal dyspnea, orthopnea. *When supine the fluid returning to the heart from the extremities may cause pulmonary congestion.*
  Fear of PND.

THERAPEUTIC INTERVENTIONS

- Discourage daytime napping and increase daytime activity. *This will help the patient be tired enough to sleep at bedtime.*
- Decrease fluid intake before bedtime *to decrease need to awaken to void.*
- Avoid evening or bedtime diuretic. If needed, diuretic should be given early morning and afternoon.
- Adjust medication schedule *to provide for undisturbed night, if possible.*
- Adhere to patient's bedtime rituals *to promote relaxation.*
- Encourage verbalization of fears.
- Review measures patient can take in the event of PND, chest pain, or palpitations.
- Review how patient can summon help in nighttime. *This will help relieve anxiety.*

Altered Nutrition: Less than Body Requirements

RELATED FACTORS

Decreased appetite
Nausea
GI irritability
Medication side effects
Fatigue
Dietary restrictions
Decreased absorption secondary to hepatic venous congestion or decreased perfusion of GI organs

DEFINING CHARACTERISTICS

Calorie count less than minimal daily requirement
Observed or expressed lack of appetite or dissatisfaction with dietary restrictions
Dry weight loss (below ideal for body build and age)

EXPECTED OUTCOMES

Patient maintains optimal nutritional status, as evidenced by improved appetite, stable body weight and composition, and report of improved food tolerance.

ONGOING ASSESSMENT

- Assess eating habits and caloric intake.
- Assess:
  Knowledge about Na, cholesterol, fluid restrictions, and dietary substitutes.
  Ability to adhere to restrictions. *Financial resources and food shopping, storage, and preparation can affect compliance.*
- Monitor weight and skin turgor.
- Assess GI status. *Nausea and vomiting and hepatic congestion can impair absorption.*
- Assess emotional status. *Depression over long-term illness can contribute to anorexia.*

THERAPEUTIC INTERVENTIONS

- ▲ Collaborate with dietitian *to provide complete assessment and consistent teaching.*
- If patient is experiencing decreased appetite and nausea, alter medication schedule when possible *to decrease gastric irritation and promote absorption (e.g., some medications are better tolerated with food).*
- ▲ If dietary intake is inadequate because of symptoms related to low cardiac output:
  Administer medications ordered for decreased or increased GI motility and irritation *to provide symptomatic relief.*
  Suggest small frequent meals with rest periods before and after *to decrease feeling of fullness (hepatic venous congestion) and to minimize fatigue associated with eating and digestion.*
  See other interventions to improve cardiac output and decrease fluid excess.
- Assist the patient/family in adjustment to dietary restrictions.

THERAPEUTIC INTERVENTIONS— cont'd

- Provide simple written as well as verbal instructions. *Visual aids improve comprehension and retention and are a readily available reference.*
  Include in diet teaching:
    Reason for sodium restriction. *Increased knowledge may improve compliance.*
    Alternate seasonings *to improve palatability of food prepared without salt. Lack of food intake may be related to absence of accustomed flavor.*
    Foods to avoid generally (e.g., canned soup and vegetables, prepared frozen dinners, fast-food restaurant meals) and ways to recognize hidden sodium (preservatives, labels, consumer information service).
- Provide emotional support and understanding to patient and family. *Response to the multiple stressors of chronic illness may include depression, lack of appetite, noncompliance.*

Knowledge Deficit

RELATED TO:

Unfamiliarity with pathology and treatment
Information misinterpretation
New medications
Chronicity of disease
Ineffective teaching/learning in past
Cognitive limitation

DEFINING CHARACTERISTICS

Questioning members of health care team
Denial of need to learn
Verbalizes incorrect/inaccurate information
Development of avoidable complications

See also:
Self-esteem disturbance, p. 55
Ineffective management of therapeutic regimen, p. 39
Powerlessness, p. 52
Gas exchange, impaired, p. 27

EXPECTED OUTCOMES

Patient/significant others understand and verbalize causes, treatment, and follow-up care related to chronic heart failure.

ONGOING ASSESSMENT

- Assess knowledge of causes, treatment, follow-up care related to CHF.
- Identify existing misconceptions regarding care.

THERAPEUTIC INTERVENTIONS

- Educate patient/significant others about the following:
    Normal heart and circulation: *This is helpful in understanding the disease process.*
    CHF disease process: *Knowledge of disease and disease process will promote adherence to suggested medical therapy.*
    Factors that increase risk of progression of disease process: infection, substance abuse, ischemia. *Identification of risk factors enables patient to prevent or minimize their effects.*
    Importance of adhering to therapy. *This will point out possible consequences of noncompliance and promote adherence.*
    Symptoms to be aware of and when to report to physician, e.g., weight gain, edema, fatigue, dyspnea. *When the patient can identify symptoms that require prompt medical attention, complications can be minimized or possibly prevented.*
    Dietary modification to limit sodium ingestion. *Understanding rationale behind dietary restrictions may establish motivation necessary for making this adjustment in lifestyle.* (See previous nutrition intervention, p. 106).
    Activity guidelines (see specific information in decreased activity tolerance guidelines, p. 105). *Providing specific information lessens uncertainty and promotes adjustment to recommended activity levels.*
    Medications: instruct on action, use, side effects, and administration. *Prompt reporting of side effects can prevent drug-related complications.* Diuretics: need for potassium supplement; digoxin: heart rate, GI symptoms; ACE inhibitors: hypotension, cough; nitrates: headache, hypotension; Coumadin: signs of bleeding; Other inotropes, such as prostaglandin E inhibitors.
    Psychological aspects of chronic illness. *This will encourage patient to verbalize fears and anxiety.*
    Overall goals of medical therapy. *This will help clarify misconceptions and may promote compliance.*
    Community resources. *Referral may be helpful for financial and emotional support.*
- Encourage questions from patient/significant others. *Allows verification of understanding of information given.*

By: Carol Keeler, RN, MSN
    Lorraine M. Heaney, RN
    Jean M. Hughes, RN

Coronary bypass/valve surgery, immediate postoperative care

BYPASS (CABG); VALVE REPLACEMENT

Coronary artery bypass grafting (CABG): The surgical approach to coronary artery disease is coronary artery bypass grafting. An artery from the chest wall (internal mammary) or a vein from the leg (saphenous) is used to supply blood distal to the area of stenosis. Bleeding and myocardial ischemia are potential postoperative complications.

Valvular heart surgery: Rheumatic fever, infection, calcification, or degeneration can cause the valve to become stenotic (incomplete opening) or regurgitant (incomplete closure). Whenever possible, the native valve is repaired. If the valve is beyond repair, it is replaced. Replacement valves can be tissue or mechanical. Tissue valves have a short longevity; mechanical valves last longer, but the patient must be continuously anticoagulated. Valve surgery involves intracardiac suture lines; therefore these patients are at high risk for conduction defects and postoperative bleeding.

A still heart and bloodless field are required for cardiac surgery. Extracorporeal circulation (ECC)—the heart-lung machine—is used to divert blood from the heart and lungs, to oxygenate it, and to provide flow to the vital organs while the heart is stopped.

NURSING DIAGNOSES	EXPECTED OUTCOMES AND NURSING INTERVENTIONS / *RATIONALE* (■ = INDEPENDENT; ▲ = COLLABORATIVE)

Decreased Cardiac Output

RELATED TO

Low cardiac output syndrome *(occurs to some extent in all patients after ECC)*

DEFINING CHARACTERISTICS

Left ventricular failure:
Increased LAP, PCWP, and PAD
Tachycardia
Decreased BP, decreased CO
Sluggish capillary refill
Diminished peripheral pulses
Changes in chest x-ray (CXR)
Crackles
Decreased arterial and venous oxygen
Acidosis
Falling urine output
Right ventricular failure:
Increased RAP, CVP, and HR
Decreased LAP, PCWP, and PAD (unless biventricular failure present)
Jugular venous distention
Decreased BP, decreased perfusion, decreased CO

EXPECTED OUTCOMES

Patient maintains sufficient cardiac output to maintain vital organ perfusion, as evidenced by strong pulses, urine output >30 ml/hr, adequate B/P, and skin warm and dry.

ONGOING ASSESSMENT

▲ Continuously monitor hemodynamic parameters using invasive catheters: BP, MAP, PAD, LAP, PCWP, CO. *Arterial, venous, and S/G catheters provide information on both right and left heart function.*
▲ Monitor oxygen saturation.
■ Auscultate breath sounds for signs of right vs. left ventricular failure. *Crackles are evident in LVF but not in RVF.*
▲ Monitor serial chest x-rays. *Provide information on enlarged heart, increased pulmonary vascular markings, and pulmonary edema.*
■ Assess peripheral pulses, and skin temperature and color.
■ Document the pump time during surgery. *The more prolonged the pump run, the more profound the ventricular dysfunction.*

THERAPEUTIC INTERVENTIONS

▲ Maintain hemodynamics within parameters set by surgeon by titration of vasoactive drugs, most commonly:
IV nitroglycerin: *dilates coronary vasculature, decreases spasm of mammary grafts, dilates venous system.*
Nipride: *lowers systemic vascular resistance, decreases BP. Elevated pressure on new grafts may cause bleeding.*
Dopamine: *increases contractility, vasopressor effect, increases renal blood flow in low doses.*
Dobutrex: *increases contractility without vasopressor effect. May slightly vasodilate.*
Inocor: *increases contractility and vasodilation.*
Isuprel: *increases HR, contractility; decreases pulmonary resistance for RV failure.*
▲ Maintain oxygen therapy as prescribed.
■ If unresponsive to usual treatment, anticipate use of mechanical assistance. See IABP and ventricular assist device, p. 127 and p. 177.

NURSING DIAGNOSES	EXPECTED OUTCOMES AND NURSING INTERVENTIONS / *RATIONALE* (■ = INDEPENDENT; ▲ = COLLABORATIVE)

Fluid Volume Deficit

RELATED TO

Fluid leaks into extravascular spaces
Diuresis
Blood loss/altered coagulation factors

DEFINING CHARACTERISTICS

Decreased filling pressures (CVP, RA, PAD, PCWP, LA)
Decreased BP; tachycardia
Decreased cardiac output/ cardiac index
Decreased urine output with increased specific gravity
If blood loss occurs:
  Decreased Hgb/Hct
  Increased chest tube drainage

EXPECTED OUTCOMES

Patient maintains adequate circulating blood volume to meet metabolic demands, as evidenced by normal filling pressures, adequate BP, and urine output at 30 ml/hr.

ONGOING ASSESSMENT

▲ Assess hemodynamic parameters. See Defining Characteristics.
■ Monitor fluid status: I and O, urine specific gravity. *During ECC the blood is diluted to prevent sludging in the microcirculation. Total fluid volume may be normal or increased but because of ECC changes in membrane integrity causes fluid leaks into extravascular spaces.*
▲ Monitor coagulation factors/CBC. *Heparin is used with ECC to prevent clots from forming. Clotting derangements and bleeding are common postoperative problems.*
■ Obtain report of blood loss from OR and type and amount of fluid replacement.
■ Assess chest tube drainage and report excess.

THERAPEUTIC INTERVENTIONS

▲ Administer volume as prescribed *to maintain filling pressures within set parameters.*
■ If clots are present, milk chest tubes *to maintain patency. Clotted tubes may precipitate cardiac tamponade; see p. 169.*
▲ Keep cross-matched blood available in case major bleeding occurs.
▲ Administer coagulation drugs as prescribed: vitamin K, Protamine.
▲ Administer blood products (PRBC, FFP, platelets, Cryoprecipitate) *to correct deficiencies.*

High Risk for Decreased Cardiac Output

RISK FACTORS

Dysrhythmias resulting from:
  Ectopy (ischemia, electrolyte imbalance, and mechanical irritation)
  Bradydysrhythmias and heart block (edema/sutures in area of specialized conduction system)
  Supraventricular tachyarrhythmias (atrial stretching, mechanical irritability secondary to cannulation, or rebound from preoperative β-blockers)

EXPECTED OUTCOMES

Patient maintains normal cardiac output as evidenced by baseline cardiac rhythm, heart rate between 60-100/min, and adequate B/P to meet metabolic needs.

ONGOING ASSESSMENT

■ Continuously monitor cardiac rhythm. Document rhythm strip once per shift or prn.
▲ Monitor 12-lead ECG as prescribed.
▲ Assess electrolytes, especially potassium, magnesium, and calcium. *Electrolyte imbalances are common causes of dysrhythmias.*

THERAPEUTIC INTERVENTIONS

■ Maintain temporary pacemaker at bedside. *Temporary epicardial pacing wires are often placed prophylactically because dysrhythmias are common. During the first 24 hr the wires may be connected to a pulse generator kept on standby. See also Transvenous pacemaker, temporary, p. 138.*
▲ Administer potassium as prescribed *to keep serum level at 4-5 mEq.*
▲ Administer magnesium as prescribed *to keep level >2.0 mg.*
▲ Administer calcium as prescribed *to keep level at 8-10 mg.*
▲ Reassess electrolyte levels if brisk diuresis occurs.
▲ Treat dysrhythmias according to unit protocol. See Cardiac dysrhythmias, p. 114.
▲ If arrhythmias are unresponsive to medical treatment, avoid precordial thump. Use countershock instead to reduce risk of trauma to vascular suture lines.

High Risk for Injury: Cardiac Tamponade

RISK FACTORS

Bleeding from cannula sites
Bleeding at suture sites
Persistent coagulapathy

EXPECTED OUTCOMES

Patient experiences no signs of cardiac tamponade. If tamponade occurs, complications are reduced through early assessment and intervention.

ONGOING ASSESSMENT

■ Evaluate status of chest tube drainage every hour *to ensure patency of tubes.* Notify physician if drainage is greater than 100 cc for consecutive 3 hr.
▲ Assess hemodynamic profile using PA catheter/LAP. Assess for equalization of pressures. *The RAP, RVDP, PADP, and PCWP pressures are all elevated in tamponade, and within 2-3 mm Hg of each other. These pressures confirm diagnosis.*
■ Assess for classic signs associated with acute cardiac tamponade:
  Low arterial B/P.
  Tachypnea.
  Pulsus paradoxus (accentuation of normal drop in arterial BP during inspiration).
  Distant muffled heart sounds.
  Sinus tachycardia. *Caused by compensatory catecholamine release.*
  Jugular vein distention.
▲ Monitor Hgb/Hct, and coagulation factors.

Continued.

Coronary bypass/valve surgery—cont'd

NURSING DIAGNOSES	EXPECTED OUTCOMES AND NURSING INTERVENTIONS / *RATIONALE* (■ = INDEPENDENT; ▲ = COLLABORATIVE)

THERAPEUTIC INTERVENTIONS

- Milk chest tubes if clots are present. *Impaired drainage can cause build-up of blood in pericardial sac or mediastinum, resulting in tamponade.*
- ▲ If cardiac tamponade is rapidly developing with cardiovascular decompensation and collapse:
  Maintain aggressive fluid resuscitation, which may be required as tamponade is evacuated.
  Administer vasopressor agents (dopamine, norepinephrine) as prescribed *to maximize systemic perfusion pressure to vital organs.*
  Assemble open chest tray for bedside intervention; prepare patient for transport to surgery. *Acute tamponade is a life-threatening complication, but immediate prognosis is good with fast effective treatment.*
- See Cardiac tamponade, p. 169.

High Risk for Alteration in Myocardial Tissue Perfusion

RISK FACTORS

Spasm of native coronary or of internal mammary artery graft
Low flow or thrombosis of vein grafts
Coronary embolus
Perioperative ischemia

EXPECTED OUTCOMES

Risk of perioperative ischemia and/or infarction is reduced through early assessment and treatment.

ONGOING ASSESSMENT

- Continuously monitor ECG.
- ▲ Obtain 12 lead upon admission and prn. Compare to preoperative ECG. Note new T wave inversions, ST segment elevation or depression. *Primary nurse must know which vessels were bypassed and carefully evaluate the corresponding areas on the 12-lead ECG.*
  Right coronary artery (RCA): leads II, III, AVF.
  Posterior descending: R waves in V_1 and V_2.
  Left anterior descending: V_1 to V_4.
  Diagonals: V_5 to V_6.
  Circumflex, obtuse marginal: I, AVL, V_5.
- ▲ Monitor CPK, LDH, and isoenzymes for signs of perioperative ischemia/infarct. *Patients will be under the effects of general anesthesia and, therefore, unable to verbalize/express chest pain if myocardial ischemia is present. Lab data aids in diagnosis.*

THERAPEUTIC INTERVENTIONS

- ▲ Maintain adequate diastolic BP with vasopressors. *Coronary artery flow occurs during diastole. Adequate pressures of at least 40 mm Hg are needed to drive coronary flow and prevent graft thrombosis.*
- ▲ Maintain arterial saturation >95%.
- ▲ If signs of ischemia are noted, titrate IV nitroglycerin *to increase coronary perfusion and alleviate possible coronary spasm.*

High Risk for Altered Fluid Composition, Electrolyte Imbalance

RISK FACTORS
Fluid shifts
Diuretics

EXPECTED OUTCOMES

Patient maintains normal electrolyte balance, as evidenced by Na within 130-142; K 4-5; Cl 98-115; Ca 9-11.

ONGOING ASSESSMENT

- ▲ Observe and document serial laboratory data: Na, K, Cl, and Ca. *Hemodilution from ECC and resultant fluid shifts cause changes in fluid composition.*
- Monitor ECG for changes. *Widening QRS, ST changes, and atrioventricular blocks are seen with electrolyte imbalance.*

THERAPEUTIC INTERVENTIONS

- ▲ Maintain adequate electrolyte balance by administering desired electrolytes as prescribed. *Hypertonic solutions may be used to correct Na and Cl deficiencies. K and Ca may be corrected by administration of K^+ or CaCl. (Note: K and CaCl are given via central IV over 1 hr).*

NURSING DIAGNOSES	EXPECTED OUTCOMES AND NURSING INTERVENTIONS / *RATIONALE* (■ = INDEPENDENT; ▲ = COLLABORATIVE)

High Risk for Impaired Gas Exchange

RISK FACTORS

Retraction and compression of lungs during surgery
Surgical incision making coughing difficult.
Secretions
Pulmonary vascular congestion
Incorrect placement of ET tube

EXPECTED OUTCOMES

Patient maintains optimal gas exchange as evidenced by clear breath sounds, normal respiratory pattern, and normal ABGs.

ONGOING ASSESSMENT

- Auscultate lung fields.
▲ Monitor serial ABGs and O_2 saturation for hypoxemia.
- Assess for restlessness or changes in mental status. *Hypoxemia results in cerebral hypoxia.*
▲ Monitor serial x-rays for evidence of pleural effusions, pulmonary edema, or infiltrates on CXR.
▲ Verify that ventilator settings are maintained as prescribed:
  Tidal volume (TV) 10-15 cc/kg.
  Rate 10-14/min.
  FiO_2 to keep Po_2 greater than 80.
  PEEP + 5 cm. *Considered physiologically equal to upper airway resistance.*
- Monitor respiratory rate/pattern.

THERAPEUTIC INTERVENTIONS

▲ Change ventilator settings as ordered *to maintain ABGs within accepted limits. (Note: Patients with preexisting pulmonary dysfunction will have lower Po_2 and higher Pco_2 values). PEEP may be increased in increments of 2.5 cm to maintain adequate oxygenation on FiO_2 of 50%. Patients can usually tolerate up to 20 cm H_2O of PEEP if not hypovolemic or hypotensive.*
- Suction PRN. *During surgery the lungs are kept deflated and atelectasis as well as mucous plugs may result.*
- Hyperventilate and hyperoxygenate during suctioning *to prevent desaturation.*
- Initiate calming techniques if patient is "fighting" ventilator.
- Instruct patient/family of rationale and expected sensations associated with use of mechanical ventilation.
▲ Administer sedation as needed:
  Morphine sulfate.
  Versed: short-acting central nervous system depressant.
  Pavulon: skeletal muscle relaxant.
  Sedation helps to decrease anxiety, which may reduce myocardial O_2 consumption.
▲ Wean from ventilator and extubate as soon as possible. *Initially the cardiac surgical patient will require mechanical ventilation because of use of general anesthesia. Weaning and extubation occur as soon as anesthetic agents wear off in most patients.*
- Encourage coughing and deep breathing. Use pillow to splint incision. *Surgical incision may cause chest discomfort and inhibit deep breathing and coughing.*
▲ Provide supplemental O_2 as indicated.
- Encourage dangling/progressive activity as tolerated. *Increases lung volume and ventilation.*
- Instruct in need to use incentive spirometer.
▲ Use pain medications *to decrease incisional discomfort so that patient will cough and deep breathe.*
- Consider chest physiotherapy.
- See also Mechanical ventilation, p. 202.

Fear

RELATED TO

ICU environment
Unfamiliarity with postoperative care
Altered communication secondary to intubation
Threat of pain related to major surgery
Threat of death

EXPECTED OUTCOMES

Patient appears calm, and trusting of medical care.
Patient verbalizes fears and concerns.

ONGOING ASSESSMENT

- Recognize patient's level of fear. Note signs and symptoms, especially nonverbal communication. *Controlling fear will help reduce physiological reactions that can aggravate condition.*
- Assess patient's normal coping patterns by talking with family and significant others.

THERAPEUTIC INTERVENTIONS

- Orient to environment.
- Display calm, confident manner *to increase feeling of security.*
- Assist patient to understand that emotional responses are normal, anticipated responses to cardiac surgery.

Continued.

Cardiac and Vascular Care Plans

NURSING DIAGNOSES	EXPECTED OUTCOMES AND NURSING INTERVENTIONS / *RATIONALE* (■ = INDEPENDENT; ▲ = COLLABORATIVE)

DEFINING CHARACTERISTICS

Restlessness
Increased awareness
Glancing about
Trembling/fidgetiness
Constant demands
Facial tension
Insomnia
Wide-eyed appearance
Tense appearance

THERAPEUTIC INTERVENTIONS— cont'd

- Prepare for and explain common postoperative sensations (coldness, fatigue, discomfort, coughing, uncomfortable endotracheal tube). Clarify misconceptions *to allay fear.*
- Explain each procedure before doing it, even if previously described. *High anxiety levels can reduce attention level and retention of information. Information can promote trust/confidence in medical management.*
- Avoid unnecessary conversations between team members in front of patients. *This will reduce patient's misconceptions and fear/anxiety.*
- ▲ Provide pain medication at first sign of discomfort *to minimize discomfort and reduce fear.*
- Provide nonverbal means of communication (slate, paper and pencil, gestures). Be patient with attempts to communicate. Know and anticipate usual patient concerns.
- Ensure continuity of staff *to facilitate communication efforts and provide stability in care.*
- Encourage visiting by family or significant others *so patient doesn't feel alone. This promotes a feeling of security.*

Altered Body Temperature

RELATED TO

Hypothermia used in conjunction with ECC

DEFINING CHARACTERISTICS

Rectal temperature <37° C
Skin cool with decreased perfusion
Tachycardia or heart block

See also:

Altered level of consciousness, p. 252
High risk for infection, p. 40
Pain, p. 49
Sleep pattern disturbance, p. 61
Impaired mobility, p. 47
Hypothermia, p. 38
Cardiac rehabilitation, p. 87.

EXPECTED OUTCOMES

Patient maintains adequate body temperature (37° C).

ONGOING ASSESSMENT

- Monitor and document changes in skin temperature, perfusion, and capillary refill every hour; notify physician of changes.
- Monitor rectal temperature continuously by rectal probe. Ensure accuracy of rectal probe by checking manual temperature q4h.
- Continuously monitor ECG.
- Observe for complications of hypothermia. *May cause increased bleeding and arrhythmias.*

THERAPEUTIC INTERVENTIONS

- Use extra blanket, mattress, or warm packs *to increase temperature slowly.*
- *Protect skin against burns* by providing layer of protection between patient's skin and warming apparatus.
- Keep pacemaker on standby. *Heart block may occur, requiring pacemaker treatment.*

By: Donna MacDonald, RN, BS, CCRN
   Marian D. Cachero, RN, BSN, CCRN

Digitalis toxicity

A condition wherein the serum digitalis level is two to three times higher than therapeutic level. The margin between therapeutic and toxic doses is relatively narrow. Patients with therapeutic levels may develop digitalis toxicity and patients with toxic levels (digoxin level over 2.5 ng/ml) may not demonstrate any manifestations of toxicity. The margin is further reduced in elderly patients, in conditions such as hypokalemia, myxedema, electrolyte imbalance, hypoxia, CHF, renal insufficiency, pulmonary disease, and with administration of drugs that increase the digoxin stored by the body.

NURSING DIAGNOSES	EXPECTED OUTCOMES AND NURSING INTERVENTIONS / *RATIONALE* (■ = INDEPENDENT; ▲ = COLLABORATIVE)

High-risk for Decreased Cardiac Output

RISK FACTORS

Cardiac arrhythmia:
Unexplained sinus bradycardia; SA block
AV dissociation; 1° and 2° block
Junctional rhythm
Atrial fibrillation with ventricular response less than 50
PVCs, particularly bigeminy
Atrial tachycardia/junctional tachycardia
Ventricular tachycardia/ fibrillation

EXPECTED OUTCOMES

Patient will maintain optimal cardiac output as evidenced by normal cardiac rhythm for patient, absence of ectopy, blood pressure WNL, and warm and dry skin.

ONGOING ASSESSMENT

▲ Monitor serum digoxin levels as ordered. Note: Blood should be drawn 6 or more hours after prior dose of digoxin. *Measurement is meaningful only after equilibration of drug distribution to the tissues. A level between 1.5 and 2.5 ng/dl suggests toxicity; a level of 2.5-3 ng/dl usually confirms the diagnosis.*

- Evaluate baseline cardiac rhythm. Note and document any change in rate, rhythm, and ectopy. *Clinically overt toxicity is usually defined by characteristic cardiac arrhythmias.*

- If arrhythmia occurs, determine hemodynamic response of patient and notify physician immediately if significant or symptomatic. *Treatment is affected by many factors: total amount of digitalis, timing of last dose, physical status of patient, and nature of cardiac arrhythmias.*

▲ Observe for abnormalities in electrolytes. *Hypokalemia, hypomagnesia, and hypercalcemia can predispose to digitalis toxicity.*

THERAPEUTIC INTERVENTIONS

- Ensure that digitalis has been discontinued. *In many instances withdrawal of digitalis may be the only treatment required.*

▲ If arrhythmia occurs, anticipate use of any of the following:
Potassium supplement. Note: Administer with caution to patients with heart block. *K+ can cause further heart block if underlying hypokalemia is not present.*
Temporary external pacemaker. *In rare cases of high-degree or complete A-V block, especially when the underlying rhythm is atrial fibrillation, a temporary pacer may be required.*
Diphenylhydantoin (Dilantin): *Used to treat digitalis-induced atrial, junctional, or ventricular tachycardia.*
Lidocaine (Xylocaine): *Used for ventricular ectopy.*
Procainamide (Pronestyl): *Useful for decreasing atrial and ventricular automaticity.* Note: *Quinidine should be avoided because it displaces digoxin from binding sites and can raise digoxin levels.*
Digibind: Digoxin immune fab fragments: *used for massive digitalis overdose. The fab fragments bind to digoxin, causing rapid removal from cellular membranes.*

High-risk for Altered Nutrition: Less than Body Requirements.

RISK FACTORS

Common GI side effects of digitalis toxicity: anorexia, nausea, vomiting, and diarrhea.

EXPECTED OUTCOMES

Patient tolerates food intake without adverse effects.

ONGOING ASSESSMENT

- Assess for signs and symptoms of epigastric distress.
- Monitor actual food intake.
- Assess hydration status: skin turgor, mucous membranes, I and O, weight.
- Record and report contents, color, and amount of emesis.

THERAPEUTIC INTERVENTIONS

▲ Administer antiemetics as prescribed.
- Offer small but frequent meals as tolerated.
- Offer general liquid to soft diet as tolerated.
- Anticipate parenteral fluid replacement if nausea and vomiting persist.
- See Nutrition, altered: less than body requirements, p. 44.

Continued.

Digitalis toxicity—cont'd

NURSING DIAGNOSES	EXPECTED OUTCOMES AND NURSING INTERVENTIONS / *RATIONALE* (■ = INDEPENDENT; ▲ = COLLABORATIVE)
Knowledge Deficit **RELATED FACTORS** Unfamiliarity with therapeutic regimen. **DEFINING CHARACTERISTICS** Inability to describe therapeutic regimen. Verbalization of misconceptions Noncompliance	**EXPECTED OUTCOMES** Patient and significant others verbalize/demonstrate understanding of digitalis therapy. **ONGOING ASSESSMENT** ▪ Assess current knowledge regarding digitalis use. ▪ Assess readiness, motivation, and interest in health/illness status. **THERAPEUTIC INTERVENTIONS** ▪ Instruct patient/significant others about: Purpose of digitalis therapy: to treat congestive heart failure or to prevent/treat supraventricular arrhythmias. Dosage, frequency, administration, and actions of digitalis: *Important for patient to understand prescribed regimen because the balance between therapeutic and toxic doses is so narrow.* Side effects and toxic manifestations of digitalis: GI symptoms: anorexia, nausea, vomiting. CNS symptoms: fatigue, mental confusion, color vision (green or yellow) with haloes. Cardiac effects: skipped heart beats, irregular pulse, increased or decreased heartbeat. Patients may experience only one or two side effects. Pulse taking: should notify physician if pulse becomes irregular, <60 or >120 beats/min. ▪ Utilize informational sources such as pamphlets, time schedule of medications, or medication charts.

By: Meg Gulanick, RN, PhD

Dysrhythmias

ARRHYTHMIAS; TACHYCARDIA; BRADYCARDIA; FLUTTER; FIBRILLATION

Any disturbance in rhythm, rate, or conduction of the heart beat. Dysrhythmia may be categorized in many ways: by origin (atrial, junctional, ventricular, etc.), by rate (tachyarrhythmias, bradyarrhythmias), by chronicity (acute, chronic). In this care plan, dysrhythmias are categorized by rate.

NURSING DIAGNOSES	EXPECTED OUTCOMES AND NURSING INTERVENTIONS / *RATIONALE* (■ = INDEPENDENT; ▲ = COLLABORATIVE)
High Risk for Decreased Cardiac Output **RISK FACTORS** Rapid heart rate/rhythm secondary to ischemia Electrolyte imbalance (especially hypokalemia) Anxiety/emotional factors Drug induced (e.g., aminophylline, isoproterenol, dopamine, digoxin toxicity) Substance abuse (e.g., cocaine, alcohol) Physical activity Heart failure Pulmonary embolism Hypoxemia Stimulant intake (coffee, alcohol) Chronic lung disease	**EXPECTED OUTCOMES** Patient maintains optimal cardiac output, as evidenced by strong peripheral pulses, BP within normal limits for patient, skin warm and dry, lungs clear bilaterally, and regular cardiac rhythm. **ONGOING ASSESSMENT** ▪ Monitor heart for tachycardia (rate >100/min). ▪ If ECG monitored, observe for specific type of dysrhythmia: atrial tachycardia, atrial flutter/fibrillation with fast ventricular response, junctional tachycardia, ventricular tachycardia, paroxysmal supraventricular tachycardia (PVST). ▪ Evaluate monitor leads that show the most prominent "p" waves, such as lead II, V_1, or MCL_1. *These leads aid in differentiating atrial from ventricular dysrhythmias.* ▪ Assess for signs of reduced cardiac output that may accompany tachycardia: rapid pulse, reduced BP, dizziness, SOB, chest pain, fatigue, restlessness. *Not all patients are symptomatic with each episode. Several factors can influence response to the tachycardia: actual heart rate, duration, associated medical problems, etc.* ▪ Assess for causative factors. *Dysrhythmias are best suppressed when precipitating factors are eliminated or corrected.* ▪ Evaluate patient's emotional response to acute/chronic episodes of tachycardia.

Continued.

THERAPEUTIC INTERVENTIONS

- If patient is asymptomatic, provide reassurance that this is not a life-threatening dysrhythmia.
▲ Provide oxygen therapy as ordered *to decrease tissue irritability.*
- Anticipate need for Holter monitoring for transient dysrhythmia. *Holter monitoring provides 24-hr recording of cardiac rhythm for patients not being continuously monitored by ECG.*
▲ If acute dysrhythmia, order/perform stat ECG as appropriate to document. *ECGs provide the necessary information for diagnosing the type of dysrhythmia. It should be performed before the patient reverts to baseline rhythm.*
▲ Determine specific type of dysrhythmia *to anticipate appropriate treatment.*

For atrial or junctional dysrhythmias:
Anticipate use of vasotonic measures such as carotid sinus massage (compression) or Valsalva maneuver. *These stimulate the vagus nerve, which may slow the heart. They may also be used to help diagnose the underlying dysrhythmia.*
Anticipate/prepare medications to reduce ventricular response: digoxin, calcium channel blockers, β-blockers, adenosine. *Type of medication to be given and the route of administration (PO/IV) depends on patient's hemodynamic status, underlying medical condition, and acute/chronicity of dysrhythmia.*
After ventricular response is reduced, anticipate use of quinidine *to reduce atrial irritability. This is not recommended for patients with sick sinus syndrome, tachy-brady syndrome.*
Instruct patient to avoid intake of stimulants: caffeine, alcohol, tobacco, amphetamines.
Anticipate electrical cardioversion if dysrhythmia is chronic and unresponsive to medical therapy. *During cardioversion, low levels of energy are used to reset the natural cardiac cycle by electrically interfering with existing dysrhythmia. In nonemergencies, the patient should be sedated prior to the procedure.*

For ventricular tachycardia:
Recognize that this is a potentially life-threatening dysrhythmia.
Administer medications as ordered, noting effectiveness. Lidocaine (IV), procainamide (IV or oral), and quinidine (oral) may be used, depending on the clinical setting.
If the patient has not lost consciousness, have the patient cough very hard every few seconds. *"Cough CPR" procedures mechanically cardiovert dysrhythmia. A backup defibrillator should be ready in case the patient converts to ventricular fibrillation.*
Anticipate use of adjunct therapies (precordial thump, defibrillation, overdrive pacing) by trained personnel.

For torsades de pointes (*a specific type of multidirectional ventricular tachycardia that alternates in amplitude and direction of electrical activity; the dysrhythmia often requires no immediate intervention but may be life-threatening. Generally this dysrhythmia is associated with a prolonged QT interval on the ECG*):
Evaluate QT interval on 12-lead ECG. Be especially alert for a 25% or greater increase from the normal QT adjusted for heart rate and sex.
Anticipate the need to obtain serum antidysrhythmic drug levels and/or electrolyte levels (potassium, calcium, magnesium).
Anticipate medical therapies assistive to the treatment of torsades de pointes:
Isoproterenol: *helps to shorten the QT interval. A prolonged QT interval is a precursor to torsades de pointes, though not exclusively.*
Magnesium sulfate.
Lidocaine.
Anticipate/prepare for emergency cardioversion/defibrillation or overdrive pacing.

For ventricular fibrillation:
Initiate basic CPR.
Assist with further advanced life support measures as ordered (defibrillation, medications).

See also:
Cardioverter/Defibrillator, implantable, p. 96.

Continued.

Dysrhythmias—cont'd

NURSING DIAGNOSES	EXPECTED OUTCOMES AND NURSING INTERVENTIONS / *RATIONALE* (■ = INDEPENDENT; ▲ = COLLABORATIVE)

High Risk for Decreased Cardiac Output

RISK FACTORS

Slow heart rate/rhythm secondary to:
Ischemia
Drug-induced (e.g., digoxin toxicity, β-blockers)
Excessive parasympathetic stimulation (e.g., sensitive carotid sinus artery, inferior MI)
Diseases of the conduction system
Cardiomyopathy

EXPECTED OUTCOMES

Patient maintains optimal cardiac output, as evidenced by strong peripheral pulses, BP within normal limits for patient, skin warm and dry, lungs clear bilaterally, and cardiac rhythm regular.

ONGOING ASSESSMENT

- Monitor heart for bradycardia (rate <60/min).
- If ECG monitored, observe for specific type of dysrhythmia (e.g., sinus bradycardia, atrial fibrillation/flutter with slow ventricular response, second- and third-degree heart block). *Ability to recognize dysrhythmia is essential to early treatment.*
- Evaluate monitor leads that show most prominent "p" waves, such as lead II, V_1, or MCL_1. *These leads aid in differentiating atrial from ventricular dysrhythmias.*
- Assess for signs of reduced cardiac output that may accompany bradycardia: weak pulse, dizziness, syncope, SOB, chest pain. *Not all patients are symptomatic with each episode. Several factors can influence patient's response to the bradycardia: actual heart rate, duration, associated medical problems, etc.*
- Assess for causative factors. *Dysrhythmias are best suppressed when precipitating factors are eliminated or corrected.*
- Evaluate patient's emotional response to acute/chronic episodes of bradycardia.
- Assess need for parenteral IV line, *in case IV medications are subsequently prescribed.*
- Carefully monitor patient's response to activity. *It may increase or further decrease heart rate.*
- Monitor for side effects of medication therapy.

THERAPEUTIC INTERVENTIONS

- Anticipate need for additional testing to aid diagnosis and evaluate treatment (e.g., electrophysiology testing, Holter monitoring).
- ▲ If patient is asymptomatic, consult physician about further medical treatment. *Assessment of patient's hemodynamic status provides guidance for treatment. The patient, not the dysrhythmia, should be treated. No treatment may be indicated. Many patients have heart rates below 50-60 secondary to medication therapy. Current medications may simply be discontinued.*
- Instruct patient to avoid Valsalva maneuver (e.g., straining for stool) and vagal stimulating activities (e.g., vomiting). *Vagal stimulation reduces heart rate.*
- Be cautious when performing nasotracheal suctioning *to prevent vagal stimulation.*
- ▲ If patient is symptomatic, administer atropine IV push, as per protocol. *Atropine decreases vagal tone and increases conduction through the AV node.*
- ▲ If unresponsive to atropine, administer isoproterenol as per protocol. *Isoproterenol increases cardiac output and increases myocardial workload and thus is not indicated for patients with ischemic heart disease.*
- Anticipate temporary pacemaker insertion. *Pacemakers supplement the body's natural pacemaker to maintain a preset heart rate.* See Transvenous pacemaker, temporary, p. 138.
- ▲ If bradyarrhythmia is unresponsive to medical therapy and deteriorates to asystole:
  Initiate basic CPR.
  Assist with further advanced life support measures as prescribed (e.g., pacemaker).

Knowledge Deficit: Cause and Treatment of Dysrhythmia

RELATED TO

Anxiety
Misinformation
Lack of information
Misunderstanding of information

DEFINING CHARACTERISTICS

Noncompliance
Verbalized knowledge deficit
Verbalized inaccurate information

EXPECTED OUTCOMES

Patient verbalizes cause and treatment regimen for dysrhythmia.

ONGOING ASSESSMENT

- Assess current knowledge of dysrhythmia, medications, treatments, procedures.

THERAPEUTIC INTERVENTIONS

- Instruct patient of the side effects of medications.
- If patient is on medication that requires potassium level maintenance, inform patient of foods high in potassium. Remind patients on Quinidine that diarrhea is a common side effect and that this is a cause of potassium depletion.
- If patient is having a procedure to treat dysrhythmias, show patient equipment and/or procedure room *to enhance explanation and reduce anxiety.*
- Instruct patient with tachydysrhythmias to avoid stimulant intake: caffeine, tobacco, alcohol, amphetamines.

Continued.

NURSING DIAGNOSES	EXPECTED OUTCOMES AND NURSING INTERVENTIONS / *RATIONALE* (■ = INDEPENDENT; ▲ = COLLABORATIVE)

DEFINING CHARACTERISTICS— cont'd

Inappropriate/inaccurate self-treatment

Questioning of staff about medication and/or management

Denial of need for information, yet is unable to describe therapy accurately

THERAPEUTIC INTERVENTIONS— cont'd

- Instruct patient and/or family member(s) of method for checking pulse. State patient's normal rate, and rate that should be reported to the physician. Explain any medications that are to be withheld or administered on the basis of pulse rate finding. *Eliciting patient as "co-manager" of care increases self-esteem and ensures more appropriate treatment.*

▲ By physician's order and hospital protocol, instruct patient of methods to assist with controlling tachyarrhythmias (e.g., Valsalva maneuver, carotid sinus massage). *Increases patient's sense of control and ensures prompt treatment.*

- Instruct patients with bradyarrhythmias to avoid straining for bowel movements. Provide information on natural laxatives prn.
- Inform patient of proper procedure to follow should dysrhythmia recur (as evidenced by specific signs and symptoms). *Developing a specific plan of care provides reassurance in ability to care for self at home.*
- Instruct patient that fluid volume deficits caused by GI flu, diarrhea, and dehydration may lead to subsequent electrolyte imbalances and dysrhythmias.
- Instruct patient's family of sources for learning CPR. *Knowledge of life-saving skills may reduce anxiety related to "life-threatening" arrhythmias.*

High Risk for Ineffective Individual Coping

RISK FACTORS

Misinterpretation of condition/treatment

Situational crisis

Disturbances in self-concept/body image

Disturbances in life-style/role

Inadequate coping methods

Prolonged hospitalization

History of ineffective medical treatments

Perceived personal stress resulting from chronic condition/treatment

Lack of support system

EXPECTED OUTCOMES

Patient verbalizes acceptance of possibly chronic medical problem.

Patient describes positive actions he/she can initiate to control/treat dysrhythmia.

ONGOING ASSESSMENT

- Assess for signs of coping difficulties.
- Assess patient's specific stressors. *Depending on the cause, a variety of strategies may be required.*
- Evaluate patient's available resources/support systems. *An effective support network facilitates coping.*

THERAPEUTIC INTERVENTIONS

- Encourage patient and family to verbalize feelings about arrhythmia, procedures and changes imposed by such.
- Explain dysrhythmias, procedures, and medications in a clear concise manner to patient and family. *Assists patient to gain understanding of current situation.*
- Encourage patient to identify/use previously effective coping mechanisms.
- Maintain appropriate level of intensity of action when responding to current dysrhythmia. *Overreaction or excessive response to a patient's dysrhythmia may encourage or increase feelings of anxiety.*
- As necessary, remain with the patient during episodes of dysrhythmia or during treatments. *Staff's presence is reassuring to the patient.*

By: Maureen Weber, RN, BSN

■

Endocarditis

INFECTIVE ENDOCARDITIS, SUBACUTE BACTERIAL
ENDOCARDITIS [SBE], PROSTHETIC VALVE
ENDOCARDITIS [PVE]

An inflammatory process that affects the heart's inner lining and usually the valves. Ineffective endocarditis usually is caused by direct invasion of bacteria such as streptococci, pneumococci, and staphylococci. However, gram-negative bacilli and fungi may also be the causative agent. Persons at risk for developing endocarditis include patients with history of valve disease who undergo dental, genitourinary, surgical, or other invasive procedure; patients with prosthetic valves; immunosuppressed patients; IV drug users; patients with mitral valve prolapse or dialysis shunts. Common complications include congestive heart failure and arterial embolization of endocardial vegetations.

NURSING DIAGNOSES	EXPECTED OUTCOMES AND NURSING INTERVENTIONS / *RATIONALE* (■ = INDEPENDENT; ▲ = COLLABORATIVE)

Infection

RELATED TO

Causative organism

DEFINING CHARACTERISTICS

Increase in body temperature
  >37° C
Tachycardia
Malaise
Chills
Positive blood cultures
Elevated WBC and ESR

EXPECTED OUTCOMES

Patient demonstrates improvement in infection, as evidenced by normal temperature, increased activity level, and negative blood cultures.

ONGOING ASSESSMENT

- Assess contributory factors for illness:
  Possible port of entry (i.e., dental work, invasive procedure or treatment, prosthetic valve, IV drug use).
- Assess for history of endocarditis. *Reinfection is common.*
- Assess for fever of unknown origin *(common presenting symptom)* and chills/night sweats *(seen in acute phase).*
- Assess vital signs. *Acute endocarditis results in sudden hemodynamic decompensation; patients with subacute endocarditis are more stable.*
- Monitor temperature q4h. *Subacute endocarditis is characterized by low-grade fever; acute endocarditis is characterized by high-grade fever. Continued fever may be caused by drug allergy, drug-resistant bacteria, or superinfection.*
- ▲ Obtain three sets of blood cultures at least 1 hour apart *to determine infective organisms so appropriate antimicrobial therapy can be selected.*
- ▲ Monitor ongoing blood cultures *to evaluate adequacy of antibiotic therapy.*
- ▲ Monitor antibiotic blood levels *to ensure adequate serum concentrations.*
- ▲ Monitor CBC for increased leukocytes and ESR.

THERAPEUTIC INTERVENTIONS

- ▲ Administer prescribed IV antibiotic agent(s) as ordered *to suppress invading organisms.*
- ▲ Use appropriate therapy for elevated temperature: antipyretics, cold therapy.
- Instruct of need for extended period of IV therapy; *4-6 weeks is required to eradicate infection and prevent relapse/reinfection.*
- Discuss possibility of IV therapy at home for selected patients who demonstrate a positive response to therapy without complications, and who are interested, able, and have a support system in place.

High Risk for Decreased Cardiac Output

RISK FACTORS

Damage to valve leaflets resulting in valvular insufficiency

EXPECTED OUTCOMES

Patient maintains adequate cardiac output, as evidenced by strong peripheral pulses, blood pressure normal for patient, skin warm and dry, and clear mentation.

ONGOING ASSESSMENT

- Assess heart rate, rhythm, and BP.
- Assess for new onset or change in heart murmur, especially regurgitant. *Usually caused by damage to mitral or aortic valve.*
- Auscultate lungs every shift and prn for crackles and wheezes. *Congestive heart failure is the most common complication, and requires aggressive treatment.*
- Monitor fluid balance closely. *Oliguria is an early sign of reduced cardiac output.*
- Assess for restlessness, fatigue, change in mental status. *These are early signs of cerebral hypoxia.*
- ▲ Monitor ABGs.

| NURSING DIAGNOSES | EXPECTED OUTCOMES AND NURSING INTERVENTIONS / *RATIONALE*
 (■ = INDEPENDENT; ▲ = COLLABORATIVE) |

THERAPEUTIC INTERVENTIONS

If signs of valvular insufficiency occur:
- ▲ Initiate O₂ therapy as needed.
- ■ See Cardiac output, decreased, p. 12.
- ■ Anticipate need for valve replacement if hemodynamic status does not improve. *Patients who undergo valve replacement at first signs of heart failure have best prognosis.*

High Risk for Altered Tissue Perfusion

RISK FACTOR

Emboli from infective vegetations in the heart

EXPECTED OUTCOMES

Risk for embolic complications is reduced through early assessment and treatment.

ONGOING ASSESSMENT

- ■ Assess for signs of embolic manifestations: *Embolic fragments are released from vegetations on valves and frequently migrate to other organs and tissues.*
    Cerebral emboli: restlessness, change in mental status, stroke. *Cerebral emboli are most common manifestations.*
    Mesenteric ischemia: auscultate bowel sounds and evaluate for abdominal tenderness.
    Renal ischemia: monitor urine output, hematest urine every shift, urine specific gravity q4h.
    Peripheral embolization: petechiae, splinter hemorrhages in nail beds, Osler nodes (painful red nodes on pads of fingers and toes).
    Embolization to joints: ROM, joint tenderness.

THERAPEUTIC INTERVENTIONS

- ■ If signs and symptoms of embolization and decreased tissue perfusion occur, record and report to physician.

Knowledge Deficit

RELATED TO

New condition
Requiring information for self-management

DEFINING CHARACTERISTICS

Questioning
Verbalized misconceptions
Lack of questions

See also:

Physical mobility, impaired, p. 47
Fear, p. 23
Coping, impaired individual, p. 18

EXPECTED OUTCOMES

Patient verbalizes cause, treatment, follow-up, and prophylactic care for endocarditis.

ONGOING ASSESSMENT

- ■ Assess level of understanding of disease, treatment, and followup care.

THERAPEUTIC INTERVENTIONS

- ■ Provide information on the following:
    Basic cardiac anatomy and physiology with attention to valve structure and function.
    Sources of infection/bacteremia.
    Signs and symptoms of infection/bacteremia.
- ■ Discuss the purpose and method of administration of long-term antibiotic agent(s). *Knowledge will facilitate compliance with prolonged therapy.*
- ■ If patient is a suitable candidate, teach techniques necessary for home infusion. Include support person.
- ■ Provide information on the side effects of antibiotic agent(s). Encourage patient to seek prompt medical attention if side effects occur. *Early detection will reduce complications.*
- ■ Educate patient to inform all physicians and dentists of history of infective endocarditis. *Previous episode of infective endocarditis increases risk of subsequent episodes.*
- ■ Explain importance of prophylactic antibiotics before and after dental work and invasive surgical procedures.

By: Carol Ruback, RN, MSN, CCRN
    Meg Gulanick, RN, PhD

Femoral-popliteal bypass: Immediate postoperative care

A revascularization procedure of the femoral artery by surgical bypass graft to the popliteal artery.

REVASCULARIZATION

NURSING DIAGNOSES	EXPECTED OUTCOMES AND NURSING INTERVENTIONS / *RATIONALE* (■ = INDEPENDENT; ▲ = COLLABORATIVE)
High Risk for Altered Peripheral Perfusion **RISK FACTORS** Graft occlusion Coagulopathy Edema Hypotension Hematoma	**EXPECTED OUTCOMES** Patient's peripheral circulation is optimized as evidenced by warm skin to extremities and adequate arterial pulsation distal to the graft. **ONGOING ASSESSMENT** • Mark distal pulses (pedal and posterior tibial) with skin marker and check every hour. Use Doppler ultrasound if needed. Note pulse presence and strength, color, temperature, sensation, and movement of extremities. Compare with the unoperated side. *Graft closure is a high-risk problem.* • Assess patient's level of pain at surgical site and distally. Signs of occlusion include: burning, itching, pain in tissues distal to site of occlusion; pain aggravated with passive/active movement of limb; numbness/coldness of limb; arterial pulsation weak/absent distal to the occlusion. • During dressing changes, assess for presence of hematoma. Notify the physician immediately if present. • Check for Homan's sign. • Monitor BP. *Hypotension can reduce blood flow to periphery; ↑ B/P can cause bleeding or hematoma.* **THERAPEUTIC INTERVENTIONS** • Maintain lower extremities slightly higher than heart level *to aid in venous return and prevent edema formation. Edema formation could further add to a decrease in peripheral perfusion to the operative leg.* • Instruct on importance of keeping affected extremity straight *to prevent kinking in graft, which may precipitate clot formation.* • Gently reposition patient every 1-2 hr with knee gatch flat *to maintain optimal blood flow.* ▲ Administer prophylactic heparin therapy as ordered. ▲ Maintain fluids and medications as needed *to keep BP from becoming hypotensive (which would result in graft occlusion) or hypertensive (which could result in hemorrhage/hematoma formation of the incisional areas and increased edema at the operative site).* • Avoid exposure to cold or excessive heat, *which could injure a poorly perfused area.* • Protect toes with lamb's wool or place cotton between the toes *to prevent areas of pressure.*

High Risk for Fluid Volume Deficit
 	
RISK FACTORS
Surgical procedure
Hemorrhage
	EXPECTED OUTCOMES
	Patient experiences adequate fluid volume as evidenced by urine output >30 ml/hr, normotensive BP, HR <100/min, and normal hematocrit.
	
	ONGOING ASSESSMENT
	• Check surgical site and donor site (if present) for signs/symptoms of hemorrhage:
	    Visualized bleeding from incision/graft.
	    Increased pain.
	    Change in color.
	    Decreased pulses.
	• Monitor vital signs. *Tachycardia may be the initial sign of developing fluid volume deficit.*
	• Assess patient's level of consciousness (LOC). Note nonverbal signs. *Early signs of cerebral hypoxia are restlessness and anxiety leading to agitation and confusion.*
	• Monitor I&O with Foley catheter. *Oliguria is a classic sign of inadequate renal perfusion.*
	▲ Monitor central venous pressure (CVP) *in order to closely monitor fluid balance and prevent iatrogenic fluid volume overload.*
	▲ Ensure that packed red blood cells (PRBCs) and fresh frozen plasma (FFP) are available for patient in blood bank.
	▲ Obtain hematocrit for suspected and/or active bleeding.
	• Obtain daily weights.
	▲ Monitor lab results as ordered: hemoglobin, hematocrit, PT, PTT, electrolytes.

NURSING DIAGNOSES	EXPECTED OUTCOMES AND NURSING INTERVENTIONS / *RATIONALE* (■ = INDEPENDENT; ▲ = COLLABORATIVE)

THERAPEUTIC INTERVENTIONS

- Ensure that surgical site is easily visualized; instruct patient/family to notify staff if bleeding is noted.
- ▲ Perform dressing changes per order. Document incision approximation, presence of sutures/staples, and overall appearance. Note presence, amount, and color of drainage.
- Keep adequate amounts of sterile gauze, Kerlix, gloves, and sutures in near proximity *in case of acute hemorrhage.*
- Protect the patient from trauma *to prevent injury to surgical area.*
- ▲ If bleeding is noted, administer IV fluids, colloids, and blood products as prescribed.

High Risk for Infection

RISK FACTORS

Surgery
Invasive procedures

EXPECTED OUTCOMES

Patient maintains reduced risk of infection as evidenced by afebrile state; no wound drainage, redness, or warmth; and negative cultures.

ONGOING ASSESSMENT

- Assess incisional sites for local symptoms of infection: redness, warmth, drainage.
- Monitor temperature. Notify MD if temperature >38.5° C or if patient shows other signs/symptoms of infection.
- ▲ Send cultures (wound, blood, etc.) as prescribed.

THERAPEUTIC INTERVENTIONS

- Wash hands before, after contact with patient *to prevent nosocomial infection.*
- Maintain aseptic technique during bedside procedures (e.g., catheter care, IV site care) *to prevent spread of disease.*
- ▲ Assist patient with selection of diet as prescribed *to promote healing.*
- Initiate measures for control of fever (i.e., tepid water bath for temperature >38.5° C). Avoid use of cooling mattress *(may decrease lower-extremity perfusion).*
- ▲ Administer medications as prescribed for infection or prevention of infection.

Pain

RELATED TO

Incision
Occlusion

DEFINING CHARACTERISTICS

Patient and/or significant others report pain
Guarding behavior, protective self-focusing, narrowed focus
Facial mask of pain
Alteration in muscle tone (rigid, tense)

EXPECTED OUTCOMES

Patient's pain is relieved as evidenced by verbalization of pain relief and relaxed facial expression.

ONGOING ASSESSMENT

- Solicit patient's description of pain.
- Assess pain characteristics. *The description of pain can help to decipher between incisional pain and occlusive pain.*
- Solicit techniques patient considers helpful in decreasing pain.
- Observe effectiveness of analgesic and/or therapies used to reduce pain.

THERAPEUTIC INTERVENTIONS

- ▲ Anticipate need for analgesics and respond immediately to complaint of pain.
- Use other comfort measures as appropriate (e.g., decrease the number of stressors in environment).
- Use distraction techniques. *Patient then focuses less on pain and more on television, newspaper, games, etc.*
- If pain is due to occlusion of graft, anticipate immediate evaluation by physician/surgeon.

Knowledge Deficit

RELATED TO

New surgical procedure

DEFINING CHARACTERISTICS

Multiple questions
Lack of questions
Misconceptions of health status
Request for information
Display of anxiety and/or fear
Noncompliance

EXPECTED OUTCOMES

Patient/significant others verbalize understanding of surgical procedure and related care.

ONGOING ASSESSMENT

- Assess knowledge regarding femoral popliteal bypass surgery and postoperative management.

THERAPEUTIC INTERVENTIONS

- Explain proper leg positioning and reasons for positioning. *Crossing legs may facilitate clot formation and graft closure.*
- Explain the need for frequent circulatory assessments. *This relieves patient's anxiety about the staff's need to be at the bedside often.*

Continued.

■ **Femoral-popliteal bypass—cont'd**

NURSING DIAGNOSES	EXPECTED OUTCOMES AND NURSING INTERVENTIONS / *RATIONALE* (■ = INDEPENDENT; ▲ = COLLABORATIVE)

DEFINING CHARACTERISTICS— cont'd
 	
 Inability to verbalize health maintenance regimen
 Development of complications
 	
 See also:
 Nutrition, altered: less than body requirements, p. 44
 Breathing pattern, ineffective, p. 10
 Skin integrity, imparied, high risk for, p. 59
	THERAPEUTIC INTERVENTIONS—cont'd
	 • Instruct patient to alert nurse of any change in sensation in lower extremities or any bleeding/swelling. *This prevents delay in detecting changes in circulation and allows prompt treatment.*
	 • Discuss patient's surgery and its relation to signs/symptoms patient is experiencing.
	 • Instruct on deep breathing exercises.
	 • Instruct in signs/symptoms to report after discharge:
	     Coolness in leg or foot.
	     Pain/discomfort/tingling/numbness.
	     Signs of incisional infection.

By: Sue Galanes, RN, MS, CCRN

Hypertension

HIGH BLOOD PRESSURE, INCREASED SYSTEMIC PRESSURE

Sustained elevation of arterial blood pressure above the normal upper limit of 140/90 or 20 points above that considered normal for one's age. This care plan focuses on patients with mild to moderate hypertension.

NURSING DIAGNOSES	EXPECTED OUTCOMES AND NURSING INTERVENTIONS / *RATIONALE* (■ = INDEPENDENT; ▲ = COLLABORATIVE)

Decreased Cardiopulmonary, Renal, Cerebral, or Peripheral Tissue Perfusion
 	
 RELATED TO
 Diminished blood flow caused by increased vascular resistance
 Hypervolemia
 	
 DEFINING CHARACTERISTICS
 Tachypnea
 Labored respiration
 Adventitious breath sounds
 Angina, palpitation
 Urine output less than 30 ml/hr
 Increasing BUN/creatinine
 Hematuria or proteinuria
 Mental status changes
 Restlessness/agitation/apathy
 Cool, clammy skin
 Pallor, cyanosis
 Mottled skin
 Decreased/absent peripheral pulse
	EXPECTED OUTCOMES
	 Patient maintains adequate tissue perfusion as evidenced by normal breathing pattern, urine output < 30 ml/hr, alert mentation, and warm, dry skin.
	
	 ONGOING ASSESSMENT
	 • Assess for evidence of decreased tissue perfusion as outlined in defining characteristics every 2-4 hr or more often as appropriate.
	 • Assess BP using proper equipment with cuff bladder that is two-thirds limb diameter *to ensure accurate measurements.*
	 • Assess breath sounds and heart sounds every 4 hr *to detect changes from baseline that indicate changes in cardiopulmonary status.*
	 • Assess and record I & O and daily weight.
	 ▲ Monitor for effectiveness and side effects of medications (e.g., hypokalemia, hypovolemia).
	
	 THERAPEUTIC INTERVENTIONS
	 ▲ Implement measures to reduce vascular resistance and improve tissue perfusion:
	     Maintain fluid and dietary sodium restrictions *to reduce fluid retention, which contributes to hypertension.*
	     Discourage intake of coffee, tea, colas, and chocolate, which are high in caffeine. *Caffeine stimulates sympathetic nervous system.*
	     Give antihypertensive drugs, diuretics as prescribed. *A wide range of medications is available for treatment: vasodilators, beta-blockers, calcium-channel blockers, and angiotensinogen-converting enzyme (ACE) inhibitors.*
	     Discourage smoking, *which causes vasoconstriction and contributes to decreased tissue oxygenation by reducing O_2 availability.*
	     Maintain physical and emotional rest. *Sedatives can be used to reduce stress and associated vasoconstriction.*
	 • Ensure adequate fluid intake unless contraindicated. *Volume depletion enhances potency of antihypertensive drugs and also reduces perfusion to kidneys.*

Hypertension

Knowledge Deficit: Nature of and Complications of Hypertension/Management Regimen

RELATED TO
Cognitive limitation
Lack of interest
Lack of information

DEFINING CHARACTERISTICS
Statement of misconceptions, knowledge gaps
Request for information

EXPECTED OUTCOMES
Patient verbalizes understanding of the disease and its long-term effects on target organs.
Patient describes self-help activities to be followed.

ONGOING ASSESSMENT
- Assess knowledge of disease and prescribed management.

THERAPEUTIC INTERVENTIONS
- Encourage questions about disease and prescribed treatments.
- Involve family or significant others *so they can effectively provide support upon discharge.*
- Plan teaching in stages, providing information in the following areas:
  Nature of disease and its effect on target organs (i.e., renal damage, visual impairment, heart failure, stroke).
  Risk factors (obesity, diet high in saturated fat and cholesterol, smoking, stress).
  Rationale for weight reduction (if overweight) and low-salt diet.
  Possible side effects of medications.
  Interaction with over-the-counter drugs such as cough and cold medicines and aspirin compounds, *which have vasoconstricting effect.*
  Avoidance of alcoholic drinks within 3 hr of medication *because of vasodilating effect, possible contribution to orthostatic hypotension.*
  Need for potassium-rich foods (e.g., fruit juices, bananas) as appropriate. *Most diuretics are potassium wasting.*
  Relaxation techniques to combat stress, *which can influence physiologic responses that aggravate hypertension.*
  Role of physical exercise in weight reduction
  Safety measures to observe:
    Avoid sudden changes in position *to reduce severity of orthostatic hypotension.*
    Avoid hot tubs and saunas, *which cause vasodilation and potential hypotension.*
    Avoid prolonged standing, *which can cause venous pooling.* Wear support stockings as needed.
  Signs and symptoms to report to physician: chest pain, shortness of breath, edema, weight gain greater than 2 lb/day or 5 lb/week, nose bleeds, changes in vision, and headaches and dizziness.
- Instruct patient to take own blood pressure, *to provide patient with sense of control and ability to seek prompt medical attention.*
- Assist in establishing medication routine considering his/her work and sleep habits. *This will minimize the chance of error and potentiate better compliance with therapy.*
- Instruct patient on use of sedatives and tranquilizers if prescribed *to assist patient in coping with situational stress.*
- Provide information about community resources and support groups (e.g., American Heart Association, weight loss programs, stop smoking programs) *that can assist and support patient in changing life-style.*

High Risk for Altered Nutrition: More Than Body Requirement

RISK FACTORS
Excessive intake in relation to metabolic needs resulting in overweight or obesity
High sodium intake which promotes fluid retention, weight gain, and hypertension

EXPECTED OUTCOMES
Patient maintains ideal body weight.
Patient demonstrates adherence to weight-reducing, salt-reducing diet.

ONGOING ASSESSMENT
- Assess attitudes toward food and salt.
- Assess need for psychological support in his/her effort to reduce weight and/or sodium intake.
- Instruct to weigh weekly and record.

THERAPEUTIC INTERVENTIONS
- ▲ Implement prescribed reducing, no-added-salt diet. *Excess caloric intake and sodium intake result in obesity and fluid retention, respectively; both predispose to hypertension and subsequent complications.*
- ▲ Communicate with dietitian regarding patient's likes and dislikes and cultural preferences.
- Support and reinforce patient's effort to adhere to prescribed diet.

Continued.

123

NURSING DIAGNOSES	EXPECTED OUTCOMES AND NURSING INTERVENTIONS / *RATIONALE* (■ = INDEPENDENT; ▲ = COLLABORATIVE)

High Risk for Discomfort: Headache and Dizziness

RISK FACTORS

Headache caused by increased arterial vascular pressure, which causes arterioles to dilate and exert pressure on surrounding tissues
Dizziness caused by hypotensive state related to drug therapy

EXPECTED OUTCOMES

Patient appears comfortable.
Patient verbalizes self-care measures to reduce/avoid discomfort.

ONGOING ASSESSMENT

- Assess for nonverbal signs of discomfort.
- Assess for complaints of occipital headache, usually upon waking.
- Assess precipitating and relieving factors.

THERAPEUTIC INTERVENTIONS

▲ Administer analgesics as prescribed. Anticipate need for sedative or tranquilizer as adjunct *to reduce stress and discomfort.*
- Minimize environmental stimuli. Restrict visitors if necessary. *Stress and anxiety can increase perception of pain and discomfort.*
- Encourage relaxation techniques (deep breathing exercise, imagery, etc.).
- Assist with ambulation if necessary *to prevent patient from falling if dizziness occurs. Dizziness is associated with both hypertension and hypotension secondary to drug therapy.*
- Elevate head of bed 30 degrees *to minimize changes in position that can trigger dizziness or lightheadedness.*
- Instruct to change position slowly. Sit before standing up from a lying position *to allow the body to adapt to redistribution of blood.*

High Risk for Ineffective Management of Therapeutic Regimen

RISK FACTORS

Complexity of therapeutic regimen
Social support deficits

EXPECTED OUTCOMES

Patient describes system for taking medications.
Patient describes positive efforts to lose weight, restrict sodium as appropriate.
Patient verbalizes intention to follow prescribed regimen.

ONGOING ASSESSMENT

- Assess previous patterns of compliant/noncompliant behavior.
- Assess for risk factors that may negatively affect compliance with regimen. *Knowledge of causative factors provides direction for subsequent interventions.*

THERAPEUTIC INTERVENTIONS

▲ Simplify the drug regimen. *The more often patients have to take medicines during the day, the greater the risk of noncompliance.*
- Include the patient in planning the treatment regimen. *Patients who become comanagers of their care have a greater stake in achieving a positive outcome.*
- Instruct in the importance of reordering medications 2 to 3 days before running out.
- Inform of the benefits of adherence to prescribed regimen. *Increased knowledge fosters compliance.*
- Instruct patient to take own blood pressure, *which will provide patient with immediate feedback and a sense of control.*
- Include significant others in explanations and teaching *to encourage their support and assistance in patient's compliance.*
- If negative side effects of prescribed treatment are a problem, explain that many side effects can be controlled or eliminated.
- If lack of adequate support in changing life-style exists, initiate referral to support group (e.g., American Heart Association, weight loss programs, stop smoking programs, stress management classes, social services). *Groups that come together for mutual support can be beneficial.*

By: Meg Gulanick, RN, PhD

Hypertensive crisis

ACCELERATED HYPERTENSION; MALIGNANT
HYPERTENSION; PHEOCHROMOCYTOMA

*A systolic blood pressure >200 mm Hg and/or a diastolic blood
pressure >120 mm Hg, associated with signs and symptoms of
end-organ damage such as renal failure, retinal hemorrhage, intracranial bleeding, and/or encephalopathy. Hypertensive crisis is
an immediate threat to life, and requires immediate treatment
and hospitalization.*

NURSING DIAGNOSES	EXPECTED OUTCOMES AND NURSING INTERVENTIONS / *RATIONALE* (■ = INDEPENDENT; ▲ = COLLABORATIVE)

High Risk for Injury

RISK FACTORS

Untreated/uncontrolled hypertension
Complications of nitroprusside
therapy
Hypotension secondary to
drug therapy

EXPECTED OUTCOMES

Patient maintains blood pressure within own normal range.
Patient maintains optimal cerebral perfusion, as evidenced by alert state, appropriate verbal responses.
Patient maintains optimal cardiac output, as evidenced by regular respiratory rate, no
shortness of breath, clear lungs, absence of edema.
Patient maintains optimal renal function as evidenced by normal BUN, creatinine, and
urine output >30 ml/hr.

ONGOING ASSESSMENT

- Assess vital signs closely. Continuously monitor blood pressure while administering antihypertensive medications. *Sudden drop in blood pressure will reduce perfusion, especially to brain, and may cause cerebral infarction.*
- Assess for signs of decreased cardiac output: tachypnea, dyspnea, cough, crackles, hypoxia noted on ABGs, tachycardia, edema, anxiety. *Elevated blood pressure increases left
ventricular afterload, which impairs emptying of left ventricle, leading to reduced cardiac
output.*
- Assess for signs of altered level of consciousness: change in alertness on verbal response, agitation, impaired thought processes. *Encephalopathy and cerebral vascular
accident are common complications of untreated hypertension.*
▲ Assess for signs of renal dysfunction: reduced urine output; increased serum BUN, K+,
creatinine.
▲ If nitroprusside is administered, monitor thiocyanate levels every 72 hr as appropriate.
Monitor for signs of thiocyanate accumulation: blurred vision, delirium, hypothyroidism,
convulsions, metabolic acidosis. *Nitroprusside is converted to thiocyanate when it is
metabolized.*

THERAPEUTIC INTERVENTIONS

▲ Administer "fast acting" antihypertensives as prescribed:
  Nitroprusside (Nipride): *A potent vasodilator that acts in seconds; has a short half life.
  Must be given by continuous IV infusion:*
    Dose: 0.5 to 10 μg/kg/min. Use infusion pump *for reliable dosing.*
    Change solution every 24 hr.
  Maintain separate IV line for nitroprusside *because of incompatibility with other
  medications.*
  Cover infusion container with opaque material *because nitroprusside is light-
  sensitive.*
  Maintain a constant infusion rate of main IV line while nitroprusside via piggyback
  is infusing *to prevent patient from receiving bolus of nitroprusside.*
  Titrate nitroprusside to maintain prescribed BP range. If hypotension occurs, stop
  nitroprusside immediately, notify physician, and lower head of bed to flat or Trendelenburg position *to increase venous return.*
  Discontinue medication if thiocyanate level is >10 mg/100 ml.
  Nifedipine (sublingual 10-20 mg): *Is a calcium-channel blocker agent with vasodilator
  effects. Sublingual administration has fast response.*
▲ Titrate medications to lower BP gradually (systolic to 160-180 mm Hg initially). *Sudden
drop in pressure reduces perfusion to vital organs.*
▲ Administer other antihypertensive medications as needed. *Other categories of drugs
such as diuretics, angiotensin-converting enzyme inhibitors, or adrenergic antagonists
may be indicated for continued oral therapy when blood pressure has stabilized.*
- Maintain head of bed at 30-degree elevation *to reduce intracranial pressure.*
- Maintain patient on complete bedrest; instruct patient to change positions gradually.
- Explain to patient the necessity of avoiding Valsalva maneuver *to prevent potential in-
creases in intracranial pressure:*
  Stress importance of exhaling when patient is being positioned.
  Provide stool softener as prescribed.
▲ Administer fluids as prescribed *to maintain adequate cardiac output and renal perfusion.*

Continued.

Hypertensive crisis—cont'd

NURSING DIAGNOSES	EXPECTED OUTCOMES AND NURSING INTERVENTIONS / *RATIONALE* (■ = INDEPENDENT; ▲ = COLLABORATIVE)

High Risk for Discomfort

RISK FACTORS

Increased intracranial pressure

EXPECTED OUTCOMES

Patient verbalizes comfort.

Patient appears calm and comfortable.

ONGOING ASSESSMENT

- Solicit patient's description of discomfort factors: headache, dizziness, nausea, vomiting, restlessness.

THERAPEUTIC INTERVENTIONS

- Provide rest periods *to facilitate comfort, sleep, relaxation.*
- Provide quiet environment. Keep lights low, noise minimal. Limit visitors.
- ▲ Give medications (e.g., acetaminophen [Tylenol], prochlorperazine [Compazine]) as prescribed, evaluating effectiveness and observing for any untoward effects.
- Use any additional comfort measures whenever appropriate: position of comfort, positive suggestion, and reassurance and contact.

Knowledge Deficit

RELATED FACTORS

Unfamiliarity with disease process, treatment, and procedures

DEFINING CHARACTERISTICS

Noncompliance with medications, diet, follow-up care, preventive measures

Patient verbalizes lack of knowledge, asks questions about hypertension

See also:

Ineffective management of therapeutic regimen, p. 39
Decreased cardiac output, p. 80
Altered level of consciousness, p. 252
Acute renal failure, p. 436

EXPECTED OUTCOMES

Patient verbalizes a basic understanding of the disease process, procedures, and treatment.

ONGOING ASSESSMENT

- Solicit patient's description and understanding of precipitating events, disease process, treatment, and procedures.

THERAPEUTIC INTERVENTIONS

- *To enhance compliance with therapy,* explain to patient/significant others:
  Disease process:
    Signs and symptoms of recurrence or progression (headache, diplopia, weakness, faintness, nausea).
    Possible complications.
  Treatment and procedures:
    Importance of decreasing or maintaining stable weight.
    Importance of low-fat, low-salt diet.
    Importance of maintaining proper fluid intake and observing limitations, such as caffeinated coffee, tea, and alcohol.
    Importance of knowing medications, dosages, and times.
    Importance of follow-up appointments.

By: Meg Gulanick, RN, PhD

Intra-aortic balloon pump (IABP)

COUNTERPULSATION DEVICE

The intra-aortic balloon pump (IABP) is a mechanical assist device for the failing heart aimed at increasing coronary perfusion and decreasing myocardial workload and O_2 consumption. It is indicated for unstable and postinfarction angina, refractory ventricular dysrhythmias, left ventricular pump failure (cardiogenic shock), acute myocardial infarction (MI), intraoperative MI, mechanical defects (ventricular septal defects, mitral regurgitation, papillary muscle dysfunction), septic shock, and perioperative support and stabilization for the patient with cardiovascular disease. It is contraindicated in patients with aortic valve incompetence, aortic aneurysm, severe peripheral vascular disease, and previous aortofemoral or aortoiliac bypass grafts.

NURSING DIAGNOSES	EXPECTED OUTCOMES AND NURSING INTERVENTIONS / *RATIONALE* (■ = INDEPENDENT; ▲ = COLLABORATIVE)

High Risk for Decreased Cardiac Output

RISK FACTORS

Balloon or pump malfunction, secondary to:
  Loss of or poor hemodynamic or ECG signals
  Arrhythmias/paced rhythms
  Inappropriate timing/ inadequate diastolic augmentation
  Kinked catheter
  Low helium
  Balloon catheter leak/ rupture/malposition/ migration
  System failure

EXPECTED OUTCOMES

Patient maintains adequate cardiac output, as evidenced by normal BP, HR between 60-100, urine output >30 ml/hr.
Integrity of balloon catheter is maintained.
Accurate pumping parameters are maintained.

ONGOING ASSESSMENT

▲ Assess hemodynamic status (BP, HR, PAP, PCWP) until patient stabilizes and thereafter as indicated. *If properly functioning, balloon inflation and deflation should improve cardiac output.*
■ Assess for adequate urine output (at least 30 ml/hr).
▲ Evaluate chest x-ray for correct position of catheter.
■ Assess and maintain clear ECG tracing with upright tall QRS segment to ensure proper balloon triggering. If paced rhythm, assess that "trigger select" of IABP is on "PACED MODE" to sense R-wave.
■ Assess and maintain clear arterial pressure waveform. *Balloon must inflate at dicrotic notch and deflate before systole.*
▲ Adjust "TIMING" of IABP for proper inflation and deflation.
■ Assess balloon patency *to rule out potential complications.*
■ Ensure that alarms are kept on at all times.
▲ Maintain "AUTO" mode for replenishment of helium/CO_2 and adequate balloon filling. *Helium is used most commonly because it is a lighter gas resulting in faster inflation/ deflation. However, in case of balloon rupture, CO_2 is more readily absorbed into the blood.*
▲ Initiate "IAB FILL" cycle to maintain adequate balloon filling.
▲ Verify correct "TRIGGER SELECT":
    ECG (skin): *preferred trigger mode; R-wave is trigger.*
    PACER AV: *only used with AV pacemaker and 100% paced rhythm.*
    PACER V: *only used with ventricular pacemaker and 100% paced rhythm.*
    PRESSURE: *trigger is the upslope of the arterial pressure waveform; not recommended as primary trigger mode, especially with irregular heart rates.*
    INTERVAL: *only used with cardiac arrest when the patient has no cardiac cycle or cardiac output.*
▲ Verify correct "IAB AUGMENTATION" for optimal perfusion during diastole.
■ Observe for cardiac dysrhythmias.
■ Monitor timing of inflation/deflation every hour *to ensure optimal afterload reduction and perfusion of coronary arteries.*
■ Assess for myocardial ischemia: chest pain, ST-T wave changes on ECG. *IABP may reverse myocardial ischemia through enhanced cardiac output and coronary blood flow.*
■ Document in chart arterial pressure tracing with balloon on and off:
    At insertion of balloon.
    Routinely q4h.
    For any change in tracing.
■ During weaning process, monitor for any changes in hemodynamics. *Pumping may have to be increased if patient is not tolerating weaning.*

Continued.

Cardiac and Vascular Care Plans

NURSING DIAGNOSES	EXPECTED OUTCOMES AND NURSING INTERVENTIONS / *RATIONALE* (■ = INDEPENDENT; ▲ = COLLABORATIVE)

THERAPEUTIC INTERVENTIONS

- Flush arterial lines after obtaining blood samples *to maintain patency. Wave forms are used to verify proper inflation/deflation.*
- Keep catheter system visible at all times. Keep tubing connection tight and catheter free of kinks.
▲ Administer medications for dysrhythmias *to regulate rhythm and optimize pumping effects.*
- If tachycardia (SVT, atrial fibrillation/flutter) results in inadequate pump augmentation, adjust pumping ratio to 1:2 as tolerated. Initiate "IAB FILL" cycle as needed to maintain adequate IAB filling.
▲ Wean from 1:1 to 1:2 to 1:3/1:4 slowly with 1 to 4 hr allowed for each new assist ratio as tolerated. *Caution must be used to ensure hemodynamic stability.*
▲ If technical problems resulting in hemodynamic compromise should occur:
  Institute IABP troubleshooting procedure per protocol.
  Notify physicians.
  Anticipate cardiovascular decompensation; titrate cardiotonic drugs to maintain pressure.
  Reassure patient *to prevent untoward cardiovascular response to anxiety.*

High Risk for Altered Peripheral Tissue Perfusion

RISK FACTORS

Presence of catheter, causing occlusion of femoral artery
Catheter malposition/migration
Thrombus from platelet aggregation on balloon catheter
Peripheral embolization
Arterial spasm
Traumatic insertion

EXPECTED OUTCOMES

Patient maintains adequate blood flow to affected extremity and general circulation, as evidenced by warm extremity, strong peripheral pulse, absence of pain, and good urine output.

ONGOING ASSESSMENT

- Assess and record quality of peripheral pulses, and color and temperature of extremity to be cannulated before insertion of catheter *to establish baseline. Suggested grading system: 0 = absent; 1+ = present; 2+ = strong.*
- Assess extremities for presence or development of any or all of the "6 Ps": Pain, Pallor, Pulselessness, Paresthesia (numbness, tingling), Poikilothermia (decreased temperature and coolness), Paralysis *to rule out peripheral ischemia/insufficiency. Limb ischemia is a common complication.*
▲ Observe for signs of obstruction of the subclavian, renal, or mesenteric artery due to catheter malposition. *Sites vary depending on positioning of balloon.*
  Subclavian:
    Change in level of consciousness (LOC), loss of radial pulse, catheter position too high on x-ray.
  Renal:
    Flank pain, decrease in absent urine output, catheter position too low on x-ray, lower extremity insufficiency.
  Mesentery:
    Abdominal pain/distention, GI bleeding, acidosis, catheter position too low on x-ray film, back pain (lumbar), lower extremity ischemia, sacral ischemia, change in elimination pattern.
▲ Monitor clotting time (PT/PTT, platelet count, Hgb, Hct) *to ensure adequate anticoagulation for duration of pumping.*

THERAPEUTIC INTERVENTIONS

- Apply TED hose to leg *to prevent peripheral thrombus.*
- Perform ROM exercise to arms and unaffected leg q2-4hr *to prevent venous stasis (may lead to thrombus formation).*
- Maintain safety measures *to prevent catheter displacement:*
  Keep cannulated leg straight. Log roll patient when turning *to prevent catheter displacement.*
  Do not raise head of bed more than 30 degrees.
  Weigh carefully on portable bed scale.
  Apply soft restraint to ankle when necessary *to prevent movement of extremity.*
▲ Administer anticoagulants (heparin, aspirin, rheomacrodex) as prescribed *to prevent peripheral embolization and/or thrombus from platelet aggregation on catheter.*
▲ Do not turn off balloon for more than 10-15 min, or wean at lower than 1:6 or 1:8 ratio. *Deflated balloon encourages thrombus formation*
▲ Should IAB pumping cease for longer than 30 min, manually inflate/deflate catheter using a syringe and stopcock once every 3-5 min. Use 20-50 cc helium, depending on size of catheter inserted. *Prevents thrombus formation on still balloon.*

NURSING DIAGNOSES	EXPECTED OUTCOMES AND NURSING INTERVENTIONS / *RATIONALE* (■ = INDEPENDENT; ▲ = COLLABORATIVE)

High Risk for Injury: Hematologic Disturbance

RISK FACTORS

Thrombocytopenia resulting from disruption of platelet integrity caused by trauma from balloon pumping
Bleeding from insertion site
Traumatic insertion
Aortic dissection
Overanticoagulation

EXPECTED OUTCOMES

Patient maintains adequate circulating blood volume.
Patient maintains PTT at 1.5-2 times control.

ONGOING ASSESSMENT

- ▲ Assess/monitor daily CBC, PTT, PT, platelets.
- ▪ Observe for swelling/hematoma at insertion site. *Percutaneous insertion usually results in less blood loss than arteriotomy.*
- ▪ Observe for other signs of bleeding: petechiae, hematuria, guaiac-positive stool/nasogastric drainage, and skin bruising.
- ▪ Monitor for side effects of anticoagulation therapy. *Bleeding/oozing from catheter site, bruising, and petechiae are common problems. NOTE: Visible signs of bleeding may be increased posteriorly (back, retroperitoneal) due to gravitational effects resulting from restricted activity and minimal patient movement.*
- ▪ Assess pain or discomfort in lower back, *to rule out aortofemoral dissection/injury or renal artery occlusion due to migration of catheter.*
- ▪ Assess abdominal pain or distention *to rule out mesenteric artery occlusion due to migration or rupture of catheter.*

THERAPEUTIC INTERVENTIONS

- ▲ Administer blood or platelets as necessary and as prescribed.
- ▲ Titrate heparin to maintain PTT as prescribed (1½-2 times control) *to prevent overanticoagulation.*
- ▲ If injury or aortic rupture occurs:
    Administer blood replacement as ordered.
    Anticipate cardiovascular decompensation:
        Prepare emergency medication.
        Anticipate emergency surgical repair of vessel.
    Provide emotional support to patient.

Impaired Physical Mobility

RELATED TO

Bed rest
Balloon insertion
Leg catheter
Critical physical condition
Restricted movement because of other invasive lines

DEFINING CHARACTERISTICS

Inability to move purposefully within physical environment (patient on bed rest)
Limited range of motion (ROM) (affected leg must be kept straight)

EXPECTED OUTCOMES

Patient does not experience complications of immobility, as evidenced by intact skin, normal muscle strength/motion, and clear breath sounds.

ONGOING ASSESSMENT

- ▪ Assess for signs and symptoms of complications of immobility: pulmonary complications, impaired skin integrity, decreased muscle strength, and foot drop.
- ▪ Assess respiratory rate, rhythm, and heart sounds.
- ▲ Monitor altered blood gases (ABGs) and chest x-ray films as appropriate.

THERAPEUTIC INTERVENTIONS

- ▪ Position patient q2h to either side or back. Use pillow support to maintain proper leg alignment.
- ▪ Perform ROM exercises to arms, unaffected leg, and ankle of affected leg q2-4h *to prevent joint stiffness and venous stasis.*
- ▪ Use footboard, boot, or shoe *to prevent foot drop.*
- ▪ Institute prophylactic antipressure devices *to help maintain skin integrity.*
- ▪ Encourage coughing, deep breathing exercises, and incentive spirometer q2h *to prevent atelectasis.*

Knowledge Deficit

RELATED TO

New procedure/equipment

Defining Characteristics

Questioning
Verbalized misconceptions
Lack of questions
Fearfulness

EXPECTED OUTCOMES

Patient/significant others verbalizes an understanding of the rationale behind insertion of balloon and use of pump, as well as activity restrictions.

ONGOING ASSESSMENT

- ▪ Assess level of understanding of balloon pump and activity restrictions.

THERAPEUTIC INTERVENTIONS

- ▪ Include significant others in teaching *to decrease feeling of helplessness and assist them in supporting patient.*
- ▪ Provide information about rationale for balloon use, insertion procedure, and ongoing care related to balloon.

Continued.

NURSING DIAGNOSES	EXPECTED OUTCOMES AND NURSING INTERVENTIONS / *RATIONALE* (■ = INDEPENDENT; ▲ = COLLABORATIVE)

THERAPEUTIC INTERVENTIONS— cont'd

- Prepare patient at times balloon is turned down: when listening to heart, recording baseline pressure, etc.
- Provide continuity of care by assigning staff members experienced in balloon functioning of pump *so patient and family feel confident about care rendered.*
- Avoid unnecessary conversations about pump function near patient *to increase patient's sense of security.*

By: Gail Smith-Jaros, RN, MSN

Mitral valve prolapse (MVP)

BARLOW'S DISEASE; FLOPPY VALVE

The mitral valve rests between the left atrium and ventricle. Prolapse of this valve refers to the upward movement of the mitral leaflets back into the left atrium during systole. Primary MVP usually results from abnormality in the connective tissue of the leaflets, annulus, or chordae tendinae and occurs in about 5% of the general population. Secondary causes of mitral valve prolapse include rheumatic fever, cardiomyopathy, and ischemic heart disease. Most persons with primary MVP are asymptomatic, though others may experience incapacitating symptoms: chest pain, palpitations, dizziness, fatigue, dyspnea, and anxiety. Diagnostic findings include midsystolic click, late systolic murmur, ECG and echocardiogram abnormalities, and angiographic findings.

NURSING DIAGNOSES	EXPECTED OUTCOMES AND NURSING INTERVENTIONS / *RATIONALE* (■ = INDEPENDENT; ▲ = COLLABORATIVE)

Knowledge Deficit

RELATED TO
New diagnosis

DEFINING CHARACTERISTICS
Asking multiple questions
Expressing fears
Being overly anxious
Asking no questions
Verbalizing misconceptions

EXPECTED OUTCOMES

Patient/significant others verbalizes understanding of occurrence of disease, causative factors, physiology of disease, diagnostic procedure, treatment, and complications.

ONGOING ASSESSMENT
- Assess knowledge of MVP: etiology, treatment, and prognosis.

THERAPEUTIC INTERVENTIONS
- Teach patient about occurrence of disease:
  Fairly common.
  Large number of undiagnosed, asymptomatic people in general population.
  Common in women but also diagnosed in men.
- Teach patient about causative factors *to increase understanding of disease process:*
  Etiology usually unknown.
  Can be primary or secondary to previous ischemic heart disease, rheumatic fever, cardiomyopathy, or ruptured chordae tendinae.
  Important to understand that serious heart disease is usually not present, that symptoms are more a nuisance than significant, and that prognosis for life is excellent.
- Teach patient the physiology of the disease: prolapse of one or both valve leaflets into the left atrium.
- Inform patient of usual diagnostic procedures:
  Cardiac auscultation for murmur or click.
  Echocardiogram to evaluate valve motion. *An echocardiogram is a particularly sensitive means of detecting minor degrees of mitral valve prolapse in apparently healthy adults. A negative echo does not exclude the diagnosis. A positive echo alone, without evidence of click/murmur, may result in overdiagnosis.*
- Teach patient about the treatment of the disease:
  Usually no treatment is indicated. *Patients need reassurance that this is not a severe cardiac condition.*
  Use of exercise *to reduce anxiety over condition and increase self-esteem.*
  β-blocker or calcium channel blocker medication *to reduce chest pain and control arrhythmias (if complication).*
  Self-limitation of activities, foods/drinks, and stresses that precipitate symptoms.

NURSING DIAGNOSES	EXPECTED OUTCOMES AND NURSING INTERVENTIONS / *RATIONALE* (■ = INDEPENDENT; ▲ = COLLABORATIVE)

THERAPEUTIC INTERVENTIONS— cont'd

- Teach patient about controversial use of prophylaxis for infective subacute bacterial endocarditis.
    It is believed that many common invasive procedures will leave a pathway in which bacteria can travel to the heart.
    Patient should contact physician for prophylactic antibiotics before any dental procedures (especially teeth cleaning), gynecologic procedures, or other invasive procedures.

High Risk for Body Image Disturbance

RISK FACTORS

Knowledge of "cardiac" condition

Fatigue secondary to beta blocker medication

Need for prophylactic antibiotics

EXPECTED OUTCOMES

Patient verbalizes positive feelings about altered heart function.

ONGOING ASSESSMENT

- Assess perception of change in body function and meaning of cardiac diagnosis. *A distinction should be made to patients between patients who present with no complaints and are "accidentally" diagnosed during routine examination versus patients who sought medical attention because of symptoms.*
- Note verbal references to heart and related discomfort and any change in life-style. *Symptoms are more common in patients who are told of the prolapse. Cardiac neurosis may develop when the condition is brought to the patient's attention.*

THERAPEUTIC INTERVENTIONS

- Provide accurate information about causes, prognosis, and treatment of condition. *Many patients have anxiety when diagnosed with a heart disease they and most people know little about.*
- Provide reassurance that it is possible to lead a "normal life" with MVP.
- For problems with fatigue:
    Encourage patient to allow several weeks for adjustment to β-blocker side effects.
    Encourage appropriate pacing of daily activities.
- Remind patient that though risk of bacterial endocarditis is small, appropriate prophylaxis may be warranted. *Knowledge of rationale for preventive therapy may reduce anxiety.*
- For female patients of childbearing years, instruct that pregnancy is usually not contraindicated. *Patients are encouraged to live normal lives.*
- See also Body Image disturbance, p. 7.

High Risk for Chest Pain

RISK FACTOR

The etiology of pain is uncertain but may be related to excessive stretch of chordae tendinae and papillary muscles

EXPECTED OUTCOMES

Patient verbalizes reduced or relieved pain.
Patient appears relaxed and comfortable.

ONGOING ASSESSMENT

- Assess whether complaints of chest pain are non-anginal in character:
    May last seconds to several hours.
    Typically left precordial, sharp, stabbing.
    May be substernal or diffuse.
    Usually not specifically related to exertion or stress.
    Usually not relieved by nitroglycerin (NTG).
    May present with inverted T waves and ST depression associated with exercise. *Patients with MPV can have a variety of types of chest pain, some of which can mimic angina. Primary MVP does not involve pathology of coronary arteries. However, some patients with MVP may also have unrelated but additional problem of coronary spasm causing angina.*
- Assess cardiac status during pain occurrence: HR, BP, skin changes.

THERAPEUTIC INTERVENTIONS

- Permit unrestricted activity if patient is asymptomatic.
- Encourage rest if pain is exertionally induced.
- Provide nonstressful environment.
- Provide psychological and emotional support *to allay fears of the seriousness of this benign disease.*

Continued.

Mitral valve prolapse—cont'd

NURSING DIAGNOSES	EXPECTED OUTCOMES AND NURSING INTERVENTIONS / *RATIONALE* (■ = INDEPENDENT; ▲ = COLLABORATIVE)
	THERAPEUTIC INTERVENTIONS— cont'd ▲ Administer medications as prescribed: β-blockers Calcium channel blockers *to provide relief of atypical* chest pain. ■ Instruct patient about positions that may reduce chest pain *by increasing venous return and lessening prolapse:* Lying down Squatting
High Risk for Decreased Cardiac Output **RISK FACTORS** Altered cardiac rate and rhythm, specifically paroxysmal tachycardia	**EXPECTED OUTCOMES** Patient maintains optimal cardiac output as evidenced by: Normal BP for patient. Regular cardiac rhythm. Strong peripheral pulses. No shortness of breath. **ONGOING ASSESSMENT** ■ Assess reports of palpitations, noting precipitating and relieving factors. *Stimulants such as caffeine, cigarettes, stress, and activity may increase occurrence of arrhythmias.* ■ Evaluate hemodynamic response to arrhythmias: BP, faintness, shortness of breath. **THERAPEUTIC INTERVENTIONS** ■ Provide reassurance that arrhythmias are usually benign in nature. ▲ Administer medications as prescribed. *β-blockers are usually the drug of choice.* ■ Instruct patient in avoidance of catecholamine stimulants. ■ Encourage exercise program as appropriate *to decrease sympathetic tone.*

By: Barbara Gallagher, RN, BSN

Myocardial infarction: acute phase (1 to 3 days)

CORONARY THROMBOSIS; "CORONARY" OR "HEART ATTACK;" MI

Acute myocardial infarction is a destructive process that produces irreversible tissue damage to regions of the heart muscle. It is caused by profound and sustained ischemia related to atherosclerotic narrowing of the coronary artery, spasm to the artery, thrombus formation, or any combination of these. This care plan focuses on the acute phase during hospitalization in the coronary care unit. Therapeutic goals are to establish reperfusion, to reduce infarct size, to prevent and treat complications, and to provide emotional support and education.

NURSING DIAGNOSES	EXPECTED OUTCOMES AND NURSING INTERVENTIONS / *RATIONALE* (■ = INDEPENDENT; ▲ = COLLABORATIVE)
Chest Pain **RELATED FACTORS** Myocardial ischemia/ myocardial infarction (MI) Reduced coronary blood flow Inadequate myocardial perfusion **DEFINING CHARACTERISTICS** Patient report and verbalizations of pain Restlessness, apprehension Facial mask of pain Diaphoresis	**EXPECTED OUTCOMES** Patient verbalizes relief of pain. Patient appears comfortable. **ONGOING ASSESSMENT** ■ Assess for characteristics of acute myocardial infarction pain: Occurs suddenly, usually when patient is at rest. Pain more intense than with angina; of longer duration (at least 30 min, usually several hours.) Quality varies: squeezing, aching, heaviness, "viselike," burning, pressure. Some patients experience *no pain,* rather discomfort or shortness of breath. Noted along anterior chest, usually substernal; may radiate to shoulder, arms, jaw, neck, and epigastrium. Not relieved with rest or nitrates. Usually requires narcotic analgesic for relief. Not affected by position change or breathing.

NURSING DIAGNOSES	EXPECTED OUTCOMES AND NURSING INTERVENTIONS / *RATIONALE* (■ = INDEPENDENT; ▲ = COLLABORATIVE)

DEFINING CHARACTERISTICS

Change in vital signs
Pallor, weakness
Nausea and vomiting

ONGOING ASSESSMENT—cont'd

May be associated with nausea and vomiting, dyspnea, anxiety, diaphoresis, fatigue. *Patients presenting with myocardial infarction can present with a variety of pain characteristics, making diagnosis difficult. Careful assessment facilitates early/appropriate treatment when time is critical for saving salvageable myocardium.*

- Note time since onset of first episode of chest pain. *If less than 6 hours patient may be a candidate for thrombolytic therapy.*
- Assess baseline EKG for diagnostic signs of MI and during each episode of pain. *Myocardial infarction occurs over several hours. The time course of ST-T wave changes and development of Q waves guides diagnosis and treatment.*
- Monitor serial myocardial enzymes (CK-MB). *Used to diagnose MI. Peak levels correlate with infarct size in absence of thrombolytic therapy.*
- Monitor heart rate and blood pressure during pain episodes and during medication administration. *Tachycardia and increased blood pressure are seen during pain and anxiety; hypotension is seen with nitrate and morphine administration; bradycardia is seen with morphine and beta blocker administration.*
- Monitor effectiveness of treatment.

THERAPEUTIC INTERVENTIONS

General
- Maintain bed rest, at least during periods of pain *to reduce workload of the heart.*
- Position patient comfortably, preferably in Fowler's position, *which allows for full lung expansion by lowering the diaphragm.*
- Maintain a quiet, relaxed atmosphere; display confident manner. *Physical and emotional rest is promoted in such a setting.*
- ▲ If patient complains of pain:
   Report immediately *for prompt treatment. Pain causes increased sympathetic stimulation, which increases O_2 demands on heart.*
   Administer O_2 at 3-5 L/min *to increase O_2 supply.*
   Institute medical therapy per order (see specific interventions that follow).

Specific
- ▲ Administer morphine sulfate per unit protocol. *Morphine sulfate is a narcotic analgesic that reduces the workload on the heart through vasodilation. It provides sedation and decreases patient's perception of pain. Side effects include: hypotension, bradycardia, decreased respirations, nausea.*
   Administer IV morphine at increments of 2-5 mg over 5 min.
   Repeat dose until pain is relieved or a total of 10 mg has been given if vital signs are stable.
   Have naloxone (Narcan) on standby *to reverse effect of morphine as needed.*
- ▲ Initiate IV nitrates per unit protocol. *Nitrates cause vasodilation and reduce workload of heart by decreasing venous return. Nitrates also dilate the coronary vessels, thus increasing the blood flow and O_2 supply to the myocardium.*
   Establish baseline BP and heart rate before beginning medication. *BP should be at least 100/70 mm Hg.*
   Prepare in a glass bottle with special tubing.
   Start at low dose, usually 5-10 μ/min through an infusion pump *to regulate delivery of the drug.*
   Titrate dose to relief of pain (usually <100 μ/min) as long as BP is stable. *Nitrates (Tridil) are both coronary dilators and peripheral vasodilators causing hypotension.*
   Expect reflex increased HR after initiating nitrates. Use cautiously in patients with possible/actual RV infarct and associated hypotension.
   Anticipate a fluid challenge *to correct hypotension.*
   If patient complains of headache (common side effect), treat with acetaminophen (Tylenol).
- ▲ Administer beta blocker agents per protocol. *Beta blockers reduce afterload and HR, thus decreasing myocardial O_2 demand.*
- ▲ Administer calcium channel blockers per protocol. *CCBs reduce afterload (BP), HR, and prevent vasospasm in acute MI.*
- Continually reassess patient's chest pain and response to medication. If no relief from optimal dose of medication, report to physician for evaluation for intra-aortic balloon pump, thrombolytic treatment, angioplasty, cardiac catheterization, or bypass surgery.
- Initiate SCP for Thrombolytic therapy (see p. 171) if applicable or appropriate *to reperfuse the infarct-related vessel.*

Continued.

Cardiac and Vascular Care Plans

NURSING DIAGNOSES	EXPECTED OUTCOMES AND NURSING INTERVENTIONS / *RATIONALE* (■ = INDEPENDENT; ▲ = COLLABORATIVE)

High Risk for Decreased Cardiac Output

RISK FACTORS

Electrical instability/irritability secondary to ischemia or necrosis, sympathetic nervous system stimulation, or electrolyte imbalance

EXPECTED OUTCOMES

Patient maintains normal cardiac rhythm with adequate cardiac output.

ONGOING ASSESSMENT

- Monitor patient's heart rate and rhythm continuously. *Eighty to 95% of patients experience some dysrhythmias.*
- Monitor appropriate lead *to facilitate prompt detection of conduction problem.*
  Monitor in lead II, observing for left anterior hemiblock (S-wave deep).
  If anterior MI with left anterior hemiblock is present, monitor in modified chest lead (MCL1) for right bundle branch block.
- Observe for/anticipate common dysrhthmias:
  With **anterior** MI: PVCs/ventricular tachycardia, second-degree heart block, complete heart block, right bundle branch block/left anterior hemiblock.
  With **inferior** MI: PVCs/ventricular tachycardia, sinus bradycardia/pause, and first- and second-degree heart block (Wenckebach phenomenon). *Areas of infarct correlate with expected dysrhythmias.*
- Assess for signs of decreased cardiac output that accompany dysrhythmias.
- Assess ventilation and oxygenation; note change in consciousness.
- Monitor PR, QRS, and QT intervals and note change *to reduce the potential for the occurrence of lethal arrhythmias. Many antiarrhythmic drugs also depress the conduction of normal impulses and can cause further arrhythmias.*
- Assess response to treatment and management.

THERAPEUTIC INTERVENTIONS

- Institute treatment as appropriate and as per protocol. See also Cardiac dysrhythmias, p. 114.
  Prophylactic lidocaine *(use is controversial). PVCs don't always predict V fibrillation; lidocaine does have side effects; prophylactic use should be avoided with older patients).*
  Lidocaine/procainamide (Pronestyl) for PVC, ventricular tachycardia.
  Atropine SO_4 for symptomatic bradycardia; external pacemaker on standby.
  Calcium channel blockers, beta blockers, adenosine, cardioversion for atrial arrhythmias.
  Isoproterenol/temporary pacemaker for complete heart block.
  Temporary pacemaker for Mobitz type II, new bifascicular bundle branch block, LBBB with anterior wall MI.
  Temporary pacemaker and overdrive pacing for recurrent ventricular tachycardia.
  Defibrillation for ventricular fibrillation.
  Precordial thump or CPR as appropriate.
  Potassium supplement as guided by serum electrolyte levels.

High Risk for Decreased Cardiac Output

RISK FACTORS

Acute MI (especially anterior site) affecting pumping ability of the heart
Right ventricular infarct with decreased ventricular filling
Papillary muscle rupture, mitral insufficiency
Ventricular aneurysm

EXPECTED OUTCOMES

Patient maintains adequate CO, as evidenced by: strong peripheral pulses, normal BP, clear breath sounds, good capillary refill, adequate urine output, and clear mentation.

ONGOING ASSESSMENT

- Assess for sinus tachycardia. *Early sign of heart failure.*
- Assess for changes in blood pressure.
- Auscultate lungs for crackles. *These abnormal breath sounds occur with left-sided failure, but are absent in right-sided failure.*
- Assess respiration for shortness of breath and tachypnea.
- Monitor for low urine output.
- If patient had inferior MI, assess for signs of RV infarct and failure. *RVI is seen in 30%-50% of patients presenting with inferior MI. Signs of ventricular dysfunction include increased CVP, increased JVD, absence of rales, decreased BP.*
- Assess for restlessness, fatigue, and change in mental status.
▲ Monitor ABGs/pulse oximeter.
- Auscultate for presence of S_3, S_4, or systolic murmur. *S_3 denotes LV dysfunction; S_4 is common finding with MI and is not significant; loud holosystolic murmur may be caused by papillary muscle rupture.*

NURSING DIAGNOSES	EXPECTED OUTCOMES AND NURSING INTERVENTIONS / *RATIONALE* (■ = INDEPENDENT; ▲ = COLLABORATIVE)

THERAPEUTIC INTERVENTIONS

▲ Anticipate insertion of hemodynamic monitoring catheters. *PAP/PCWP pressures are excellent guides of filling pressures in left ventricle; CVP/RAP monitoring guides management of RVI.*

▲ Administer IV fluids to keep PCWP at 16-18 mmHg *for optimal filling of ventricle. Too little fluid reduces preload/blood volume and BP; too much fluid can overtax heart and lead to pulmonary edema.*

▲ If signs of LVF occur:
   Administer diuretic and vasodilator medications as prescribed *to reduce filling pressures and reduce workload of infarcted heart.*
   Administer inotropic medications IV *to improve pumping of heart.*
   Initiate O₂ as needed *to increase arterial saturation.*

▲ If signs of RVF occur:
   Anticipate aggressive fluid resuscitation (3-6 L/24 hr) *to keep PCWP at 16-20 mm/Hg.*
   Carefully administer nitrates and morphine sulfate for pain *because they reduce preload.*

■ See also Decreased cardiac output, p. 12, and Cardiogenic shock, p. 159

Fear

RELATED FACTORS

Threat to or change in health status
Threat of death
Threat to self-concept
Change in environment
Unmet needs

DEFINING CHARACTERISTICS

Tense appearance, apprehension; feelings of impending doom
Frightened
Restless/unable to relax
Repeatedly seeking assurance
Increased alertness, wide-eyed
Expressed concern regarding changes in life-style

EXPECTED OUTCOMES

Patient verbalizes reduced fear.
Patient demonstrates positive coping mechanisms.

ONGOING ASSESSMENT

■ Assess level of fear. Note all signs and symptoms, especially nonverbal communication. *Controlling anxiety will help reduce sympathetic response that can aggravate condition.*

■ Assess patient's usual coping patterns.

THERAPEUTIC INTERVENTIONS

■ Explain in simple terms various aspects of MI, need for cardiac monitoring, etc.; identify and clarify misconceptions *to help patient adjust to emotional stress.*

■ Explain need for "high-tech" equipment. *Information can promote trust/confidence in medical management.*

■ Assure patient that close monitoring will ensure prompt treatment.

■ Foster patient's optimism that recovery is fully anticipated. Offer realistic assurances.

■ Assist patient to understand that emotions felt are normal, anticipated responses to acute MI.

■ Allow patient to verbalize fears of dying. Reassure patient that most deaths occur prior to reaching hospital.

■ Establish rest periods between care and procedures *to help patient relax and regain emotional balance.*

■ Provide diversional materials (e.g., newspapers, magazines, music, and television), *which can be relaxing and prevent feelings of isolation in private room.*

▲ Administer mild tranquilizers/sedatives as prescribed *to reduce stress.*

■ Involve family/significant other in visiting/care within limits.

High Risk for Activity Intolerance

RISK FACTORS

Generalized weakness
Imbalance between O₂ supply and demand

EXPECTED OUTCOMES

Patient tolerates progressive activity, as evidenced by heart rate/BP within expected range, no complaints of dyspnea or fatigue.
Patient verbalizes realistic expectations for progressive activity.

ONGOING ASSESSMENT

■ Assess patient's respiratory and cardiac status before initiating activity.

■ Observe and document response to activity. Signs of abnormal response include:
   Increased heart rate of >20 beats over resting rate during activity, or >120 bpm.
   Increased BP >20 mm Hg systolic during activity.
   Decreased BP of >10-15 mm Hg systolic during activity.
   Chest pain, dizziness.
   Skin color changes/diaphoresis.
   Dyspnea
   Increased dysrhythmias.
   Excessive fatigue.
   ST segment displacement on ECG.

Continued.

Myocardial infarction—cont'd

NURSING DIAGNOSES	EXPECTED OUTCOMES AND NURSING INTERVENTIONS / *RATIONALE* (■ = INDEPENDENT; ▲ = COLLABORATIVE)

THERAPEUTIC INTERVENTIONS

- Encourage adequate rest periods, especially before activities (e.g., ADL, visiting hours, meals).
- Instruct patient not to hold breath while exercising or moving about in bed and not to strain for bowel movement. *These activities stimulate Valsalva maneuver, which leads to bradycardia and resultant change in cardiac output.*
- Provide light meals (progress from liquids to regular diet as appropriate).
- ▲ Maintain progression of activity as ordered by physician and/or cardiac rehabilitation team by monitoring cardiac rehabilitation stages:
    Stage 1: Self-care activities (wash face, feed self, oral hygiene). Selected ROM exercises in bed. Dangle 15-30 min at bedside, tid. Use bedside commode with assistance. *Commode requires less energy expenditure than bedpan.*
    Stage 2: Up in chair for 30-60 min tid. Partial bath in chair. Continue ROM exercises in chair.
- Provide emotional support when increasing activity *to reduce possible anxiety about "overexertion" of heart.*
- Instruct patient that further cardiac rehabilitation/activity progression will occur after transfer from intensive care setting. (See Cardiac rehabilitation, p. 87.)

High Risk for Nausea/Vomiting

RISK FACTORS

Activation of a vagal reflex that occurs frequently with inferior site MIs and with severe pain

Common side effects of opiates

EXPECTED OUTCOMES

Patient verbalizes absence/relief of nausea/vomiting.

ONGOING ASSESSMENT

- Assess for signs and symptoms of epigastric distress.
- Assess color, consistency, and amount of emesis.
- Note any vasovagal responses from suppositories and straining. *Bradycardia, hypotension, dizziness, and lightheadedness are common side effects.*

THERAPEUTIC INTERVENTIONS

- Keep emesis basin at bedside.
- ▲ Administer antiemetics as ordered; prochlorperazine (Compazine) or trimethobenzamide (Tigan) suppositories prn.
- Offer ice chips as desired. *Ice is no longer prohibited for cardiac patients.*
- Offer general liquid to soft diet as tolerated.
- Provide mouth care/mouth wash as necessary.
- ▲ Anticipate atropine IV push if vasovagal bradycardia occurs. *Atropine blocks vagal responses, thereby increasing heart rate.*
- ▲ If vomiting persists, provide IV fluids as needed.

Chest Pain

RELATED FACTORS

Pericarditis secondary to acute MI

DEFINING CHARACTERISTICS

Complaint of pain

Pericardial friction rub (transient)

ST-segment elevation (concave) in most limb and precordial ECG leads without reciprocal ST-segment depression

Fever

EXPECTED OUTCOMES

Patient appears comfortable.

Patient verbalizes relief or reduction in "pericardial" discomfort.

ONGOING ASSESSMENT

- Assess characteristics of pericardial pain. It is similar to MI pain, except that pericardial pain:
    Increases with deep inspiration, turning of thorax, lying down.
    Is relieved by sitting up or leaning forward.
    Is sharp, stabbing, knifelike, "pleuritic."
    Occurs 2-3 days after MI.
    May be intermittent or continuous. *Accurate assessment facilitates appropriate treatment.*
- Auscultate chest for presence or change in pericardial rub. *Pericardial friction rub may be transient.*
- Monitor temperature. *Fever accompanies pericarditis.*

THERAPEUTIC INTERVENTIONS

- Position patient comfortably, preferably sitting up in bed at an angle of 90 degrees or leaning forward propped on a pillow on a side table *as these positions effectively relieve discomfort.*
- Offer assurance and emotional support through explanations of pericarditis. *Patients fear that this pain is another "heart attack" and need reassurance that pericarditis is an "inflammatory" response to some infarcts.*

THERAPEUTIC INTERVENTIONS—cont'd

▲ Give medications as prescribed, usually indomethacin (Indocin) or Motrin q8h *to reduce inflammation around the heart.* Give medications on full stomach *to prevent gastric irritation.*
▲ Administer antipyretics as indicated.

Knowledge Deficit

RELATED FACTORS

Unfamiliarity with disease process, treatment, recovery

DEFINING CHARACTERISTICS

Multiple or no questions
Confusion over events
Expressed need for information

EXPECTED OUTCOMES

Patient verbalizes understanding of condition, need for observation in CCU, diagnosis/ treatment of MI, and healing process of MI.

ONGOING ASSESSMENT

▪ Assess knowledge of acute MI: causes, treatment, early recovery process. *Many patients have been exposed to media information/family and friends experiencing an infarct. Misconceptions may exist.*

THERAPEUTIC INTERVENTIONS

▪ Encourage patients to ask questions and verbalize concerns.
▪ Provide information on the following (as appropriate), limiting each session to 10-15 min *so patient is not overwhelmed.*
　Positive aspects of the unit (CCU).
　Diagnosing of MI in CCU (e.g., with ECG, blood tests).
　Healing process *(takes 6 wk for necrotic tissue to be replaced by scar tissue; progressive activity required to optimize healing).*
　Cardiac anatomy.
　MI versus angina.
　Risk factors for MI.
　Recovery time in hospital (7-10 days).
　Expected return to prior life-style (2-3 months).
　Medications: anticoagulants (ASA/heparin) *to maintain patency of arteries;* antidysrhythmics; pain relievers (beta blockers, calcium channel blockers, nitrates.)
　Diagnostic procedures (echocardiogram, angiogram, stress test.)
▪ Inform patient that more extensive teaching sessions will be instituted after transfer to the medical floor and the next stage of cardiac rehabilitation will be initiated.

See also:
Cardiac rehabilitation, p. 87
Powerlessness, p. 52
Altered sexual patterns, p. 58
Health-seeking behavior,
　p. 33

By: Cynthia Antonio, RN, BSN
　　Meg Gulanick, RN, PhD

Myocardial Infarction: Acute Phase (1 to 3 Days)

Pacemaker external, (temporary/ noninvasive/invasive)

A device that delivers an artificial electrical stimulus to the heart for the acute management of: bradyarrhythmias (sinus node abnormalities, atrioventricular and intraventricular conduction abnormalities with hemodynamic compromise), certain types of tachyarrhythmias, and for use in provocative diagnostic cardiac procedures. Transcutaneous cardiac pacing (noninvasive, using antero-posterior patches to the chest wall) is an alternate method to transvenous pacing for the initial management of brady-asystolic arrest situation until definitive treatment can be instituted. It may also be used as standby prophylaxis for patients with acute myocardial infarction or those who are at high risk for conduction disturbances. Transvenous endocardial pacing stimulates the myocardial tissue directly with electrical current pulses via intravenous catheter electrodes. Epicardial pacing stimulates the myocardium via an epicardial catheter; it is most commonly used following open heart surgery for temporary relief of bradyarrhythmias.

NURSING DIAGNOSES

EXPECTED OUTCOMES AND NURSING INTERVENTIONS / *RATIONALE*
(■ = INDEPENDENT; ▲ = COLLABORATIVE)

High Risk for Decreased Cardiac Output

Risk Factors
External pacemaker malfunction caused by:
Pacemaker lead dislodgement
Improper placement of pacemaker lead(s) in the myocardium
Broken pacing lead wire
Poor electrical connections
Inadequate pacemaker parameter settings
External generator circuitry malfunction
Battery exhaustion
Improper technique in changing battery
Poor environmental and electrical safety measures
Pacemaker-induced dysrhythmia resulting from presence of competitive rhythm
Unstable pacing and sensing thresholds resulting from exit block (fibrosis) or lead position

Expected Outcomes
Patient maintains adequate cardiac output as evidenced by strong pulses, BP within normal limits for patient, skin warm and dry, lungs clear.

Ongoing Assessment
▲ Check that prescribed pacemaker parameters are maintained (rate, pacing output in mA, sensitivity). *Each patient has different pacing thresholds. Also, each type of pacemaker requires different settings (e.g., transvenous uses low mA (2-10) whereas transcutaneous may have 75-90 mA for capture.*
■ Observe/monitor ECG continuously for appropriate pacemaker function: sensing, capturing, and firing (pacing spikes).
■ Record rhythm strips:
　Routinely every_____hours.
　When changes in pacing parameters are made.
　For presence of spontaneous rhythm
■ If pacemaker is on standby, evaluate pacemaker capture daily and as needed. *Capture is represented by a pacing spike followed by ventricular depolarization (QRS).*
■ Assess for proper environmental and electrical safety measures, *because the pacemaker lead is directly in contact with the myocardium.*
■ If signs of pacemaker malfunction/dysrhythmia occur, assess hemodynamic status until stable.
■ Assess for pacemaker-induced dysrhythmias *which may be caused by competitive rhythm secondary to asynchronous pacing or tissue excitability.*

Therapeutic Interventions
■ Keep monitor alarm on at all times.
■ When transcutaneous pacemaker is used, ensure that a large R wave is obtained on the ECG monitor. *This pacing system reads/senses the signal from the surface ECG, not intracardiac as with the transvenous and epicardial pacemakers.*
If failure to sense is noted, *the pacemaker is not sensing spontaneous rhythm, which could lead to dysrhythmias. Pacing stimulus may excite a repolarized cell during relative refractory period (R on T phenomenon).*
■ Check that dial is *not* on "asynchronous" pacing (fixed rate).
■ Check for loose connections. *Pacemaker is not picking up cardiac signal when the line of communication is interrupted.*
■ Reposition limb of body if lead insertion is through brachial or femoral vein. *Malpositioning can dislodge pacemaker lead from wall of ventricle.*
▲ Notify physician of need to adjust sensitivity dial. *Increasing sensitivity will increase the gain of the spontaneous cardiac rhythm signal.*
▲ Check position of lead by chest x-ray examination. If problem is not corrected and patient has adequate rhythm, check with physician whether pacemaker should be on "standby." *Avoids risk of pacemaker-induced dysrhythmia from competitve rhythms.*

Continued.

NURSING DIAGNOSES	EXPECTED OUTCOMES AND NURSING INTERVENTIONS / *RATIONALE* (■ = INDEPENDENT; ▲ = COLLABORATIVE)

Therapeutic Interventions— cont'd

▲ If problem is not corrected, and patient is hemodynamically compromised, with transvenous lead, anticipate use of transcutaneous external pacemaker while awaiting electrode repositioning; with epicardial pacing, anticipate removal of lead and use of transcutaneous external pacemaker, or insertion of transvenous pacemaker, depending on patient's status.

If loss of capture is noted, *the pacemaker fails to depolarize the myocardium:*
- Check all possible connections.
- Turn patient on left side (endocardial catheter) *to facilitate optimal lead placement (right ventricular apex).*

▲ Increase pacing output (mA) and evaluate for good capture.

If loss of pacing spikes are noted, *the pacemaker fails to emit electrical stimulus:*
- Check that power switch is ON.
- Check whether needle gauge on pacemaker box is fluctuating.
- If needle gauge is not fluctuating, replace batteries in generator.
- Check all possible connections.
- Check for electromagnetic interference. *Interference from equipment such as radiation, cautery, or imaging resonance can inhibit pacing output by temporarily turning off pacemaker.*
- Replace generator as needed.

If pacemaker malfunction is noted and not easily corrected by the preceding steps:
- Evaluate adequate spontaneous rhythm. *(Unreliable escape rhythm will lead to hemodynamic collapse.)*
- Monitor vital signs every 15-30 min.

▲ Prepare atropine sulfate, isoproterenol, and epinephrine for standby. *Atropine is an anticholinergic drug that increases cardiac output and heart rate by blocking vagal stimulation in the heart. Isuprel and epinephrine are sympathetic drugs that increase heart rate and cardiac output by stimulating beta receptors in the heart.*

If pacemaker-induced arrhythmia is noted, treat patient according to unit protocol:
- Maintain proper environmental and electrical safety measures. *Stray electrical current may enter the heart through the external lead, which can cause dysrhythmia.*
- Ensure that all electrical equipment is properly grounded with 3-prong plugs.

▲ Ensure that a biomedical engineer has checked room to ensure a safe environment.
- Ensure that exposed pacing wire terminals and generator are insulated in rubber glove or enclosed in a plastic case.
- Ensure that bed linen/gown is kept dry.

Impaired Physical Mobility

Related to

Imposed activity restriction secondary to transvenous pacemaker lead insertion and need to guard against any tension

Defining Characteristics

Limited ROM
Reluctance to attempt movement
Verbalization of inability to perform activities

Expected Outcomes

Patient engages in activity within prescribed restrictions.
Patient avoids any complications of immobility.

Ongoing Assessment

- Assess specific activity restrictions for site of pacemaker insertion: femoral vein site necessitates complete bed rest; brachial or internal jugular approach is less restrictive. *Bending the leg with a femoral insertion site may dislodge the pacing lead. Patients with brachial or internal jugular leads may dangle, or sit in chair with assistance depending on their medical condition and institutional policy.*
- Assess for potential complications related to restricted movement:
  Assess for discomfort.
  Assess skin integrity. Check for redness or tissue ischemia.
  Observe for signs of pulmonary embolism.
  Assess for developing thrombophlebitis.

Therapeutic Interventions

▲ Ensure bed rest if pacemaker lead is inserted via femoral vein.
- Secure arm with an armboard and wrap with gauze if pacemaker lead is in the antecubital fossa and instruct not to raise arm over head *to prevent lead displacement.*
- Turn and position every 2 hours. Watch terminal pacing leads when turning. Avoid right-side positioning if transvenous catheter is inserted *to prevent pacing wire dislodgement.*
- Instruct patient to perform ROM to nonaffected extremities. Assist with modified ROM to extremity with lead insertion *(to reduce risks of immobility).*
- Encourage patient to dangle or sit up in chair if permitted.
- Institute prophylactic use of antipressure devices as needed.
- Encourage patient to cough and deep breathe every hour while awake *to prevent pulmonary stasis.*

Continued.

NURSING DIAGNOSES	EXPECTED OUTCOMES AND NURSING INTERVENTIONS / *RATIONALE* (■ = INDEPENDENT; ▲ = COLLABORATIVE)

Knowledge Deficit:

RELATED TO

Misinterpretation of information
New procedure and pacemaker equipment

DEFINING CHARACTERISTICS
Overwhelmed
Increased questioning
Verbalized misconceptions

EXPECTED OUTCOMES

Patient and family verbalize understanding of temporary pacemaker function and follow-up care.

ONGOING ASSESSMENT

- Assess understanding of condition, the electrical conduction system of the heart, and pacemaker function.

THERAPEUTIC INTERVENTIONS

- Provide instruction on: anatomy and physiology of the heart, function of the pacemaker, insertion procedure, and importance of activity restrictions.
- Refer more specific questions to clinical nurse specialist and physician.

Pain/Discomfort

RELATED TO

Insertion/application of temporary pacemaker
Imposed activity restrictions

DEFINING CHARACTERISTICS

Restlessness, patient reports discomfort
Hiccupping; intercostal or abdominal muscle twitching

EXPECTED OUTCOMES

Patient verbalizes relief or reduction in pain/discomfort.
Patient appears relaxed and comfortable.

ONGOING ASSESSMENT

- Assess level, location, and onset of discomfort.
- Assess for hiccups or muscle twitching *that may occur with lead displacement or very high pacing output (mA) in transvenous leads.*
- Assess for skin irritation or burns under skin patches if transcutaneous pacemaker is used at high mA.

THERAPEUTIC INTERVENTIONS

- Provide comfort measures (e.g., change in position, back rubs, pillows for immobilized limb, analgesics) as prescribed. *Analgesics or sedatives prn are usually needed to reduce painful skeletal muscle contractions with transcutaneous pacemaker.*
- Secure terminal portion of transvenous/epicardial pacing wires with 4 × 4 dressing *to prevent accidental pulling of leads.*
- ▲ If hiccups or muscle twitching are noted, call physician to evaluate lead placement. *Inaccurate position of leads can stimulate the diaphragm. Repositioning will relieve pain.*

High Risk for Infection

RISK FACTORS

Invasive procedure with possible introduction of bacteria (transvenous or epicardial)

EXPECTED OUTCOMES

The patient exhibits no signs of infection, as evidenced by normal temperature and WBC, negative cultures, skin incision well healed.

ONGOING ASSESSMENT

- Assess catheter site for signs of infection.
- Evaluate amount and characteristics of any drainage from catheter site.
- Monitor temperature every 4 hours and as needed.
- Monitor length of time pacemaker catheter is in place. *Temporary catheter in place for >72 hours increases risk of infection.*
- ▲ Follow up on WBC, blood and fluid cultures if infection is suspected.

THERAPEUTIC INTERVENTIONS

- Keep dressing dry and intact *to prevent contamination with bacteria.*
- ▲ Change dressing routinely or as needed per infection control policy. Use sterile technique *to reduce risk of infection to open wounds.*
- Avoid frequent and unnecessary contact with the catheter site.
- ▲ Administer antibiotics as prescribed.

See also:
Anxiety, p. 5
Fear, p. 23

By: Marilyn Samson-Hinton, RN, BSN

Pacemaker, implantable (permanent)

A battery-powered electronic device that delivers an electrical stimulus to the heart muscle when needed. Types of pacemakers currently available: (1) Bradycardia pacemaker—its mode of response is either inhibited, triggered, or asynchronous. Indicated for chronic symptomatic bradydysrhythmias including sinus arrest, sinoatrial block, and sinus bradycardia, or for chronic symptomatic second-degree or third-degree atrioventricular block. A dual-chamber pacemaker is indicated for bradycardia with competent sinus node to provide AV synchrony and rate variability. (2) Rate-modulated pacemaker—indicated for patients who can benefit from an increase in pacing rate, either atrial or ventricular, in response to their body's metabolic (physiologic) needs or to activity (nonphysiologic) for increased cardiac output. Contraindicated for patients who can tolerate only limited increases in heart rate as a result of concomitant disease states. (3) Antitachycardia pacemaker—indicated for pace-terminable conditions: recurrent SVT (e.g., A-V reciprocating tachydysrhythmias [as in WPW], atrial flutter, and other atrioventricular tachydysrhythmias).

NURSING DIAGNOSES	EXPECTED OUTCOMES AND NURSING INTERVENTIONS / *RATIONALE* (■ = INDEPENDENT; ▲ = COLLABORATIVE)

High Risk for Decreased Cardiac Output

RISK FACTORS

Permanent pacemaker malfunction caused by:
  Lead dislodgement
  Faulty connection between lead and pulse generator
  Faulty lead system (e.g., lead fracture, insulation break)
  Pulse generator circuitry failure
  Battery depletion
  Inadequate parameter settings
  Inappropriate type of pacemaker
Ventricular arrhythmias caused by irritation from pacing electrode, asynchronous pacing resulting from malsensing problem
Change in myocardial threshold
Competitive rhythms

EXPECTED OUTCOMES

Patient maintains adequate cardiac output, as evidenced by strong pulses, BP within normal limits for patient, skin warm and dry, lungs clear.

ONGOING ASSESSMENT

- Assess apical/radial pulses.
- Assess hemodynamic status.
- If ECG monitored:
    Assess for proper pacemaker function: capture, sensing, firing, and configuration of paced QRS (difficult to assess pace artifact on digital ECG).
    Assess for pacemaker-induced dysrhythmias.
▲ Immediately after pacemaker implantation:
    Check implant data for:
      Type of pacemaker (e.g., AV sequential, single-chamber, demand, programmable, rate response) and programmed parameters. *Certain types of pacemakers have variable functions, which can be difficult to interpret.*
    Monitor chest x-ray films and ECG studies after patient returns from OR and as prescribed *to verify correct placement of lead and pacemaker function. Ventricular lead placement is usually in the right ventricular apex; atrial lead placement is in the right atrial appendage*
    Keep monitor alarms on at all times.
    Record rhythm strips:
      Routinely every _____ hours.
      If pacemaker malfunction is suspected.
      When pacemaker parameter adjustments are made.
▲ If pacemaker malfunction is suspected.
    Assess hemodynamic stability with spontaneous/competitive rhythm.
    Obtain 12-lead ECG study *to verify function of pacemaker and lead placement. LBBB-paced QRS configuration suggests good right ventricular lead position.*

If failure to sense is noted:
▲ Monitor chest x-ray films *to check for placement and status of pacemaker electrode.*
- Observe for phrenic nerve stimulation (hiccups) and intercostal or abdominal muscle twitching. *Stimulation of chest wall and diaphragm indicates possible dislodged pacemaker.*
- Observe for induced ventricular dysrhythmias caused by pacemaker competition. *Pacing stimulus may excite a repolarized cell during the relative refractory period when the heart is at risk of fibrillation; represents an "R on T" phenonemon.*

If loss of capture is noted:
- Follow the three steps under "failure to sense," above.
- Assess for factors that increase myocardial threshold (i.e., ischemia, fibrosis around the tip of the electrode, acidosis, electrolyte imbalance, antidysrhythmic drugs). *Threshold is the minimum amount of electrical energy needed to pace and capture the heart.*

Continued.

Pacemaker, implantable (permanent)—cont'd

NURSING DIAGNOSES	EXPECTED OUTCOMES AND NURSING INTERVENTIONS / *RATIONALE* (■ = INDEPENDENT; ▲ = COLLABORATIVE)

ONGOING ASSESSMENT— cont'd
- If ventricular dysrhythmias occur, assess hemodynamic status.

THERAPEUTIC INTERVENTIONS
If pacemaker malfunction is suspected:
- Turn patient on left side (for endocardial pacemaker) *to facilitate good ventricular wall contact. Malpositioning is a common cause of malfunction.*
- Notify physician.
- ▲ Call the pacemaker specialist to evaluate further pacemaker function and to make changes in parameters if needed through the use of pacemaker programmer. *This is a noninvasive technique of pacemaker programming via radio frequency signal.*
- ▲ Prepare atropine sulfate, isoproterenol, epinephrine for standby. *Atropine is an anticholinergic drug that increases cardiac output and heart rate by blocking vagal stimulation in the heart. Isuprel and epinephrine are sympathetic drugs that increase heart rate and cardiac output by stimulating beta receptors in the heart.*
- ▲ Prepare for temporary pacemaker insertion. *Transcutaneous pacing is effective in providing adequate heart rate and rhythm to patients in an emergency situation.*
- Initiate basic life support measures as needed.
- Anticipate possible return to OR for repositioning.

Impaired Physical Mobility

RELATED TO
Imposed activity restriction
Reluctance to attempt movement because of pain at site of pulse generator/fear of lead dislodgement

DEFINING CHARACTERISTICS
Restlessness, irritability
Crying
Helplessness
Verbalization of inability to move about
Limited ROM
Muscle weakness
Complaints of shoulder joint stiffness/pain

EXPECTED OUTCOMES
Patient engages in activity within prescribed restrictions.
Patient avoids any complications of immobility.

ONGOING ASSESSMENT
- Assess whether patient is restricting activity because of physician order, discomfort, or fear of malfunction. *Many patients avoid moving for fear of dislodging pacemaker.*
- Assess for potential complications related to immobility/reduced activity:
  Assess respiratory status.
  Assess skin integrity. Check for redness or tissue ischemia.
  Assess for pulmonary embolism.
  Assess for signs of thrombophlebitis. *Though uncommon with pacemakers, thrombophlebitis can develop with prolonged bed rest/inactivity.*

THERAPEUTIC INTERVENTIONS
- Explain the importance of imposed activity restriction (24 to 48 hours after implant) *to prevent pacing electrode displacement.*
- Assist in turning every 2 hours. For endocardial pacemaker, avoid turning to the right side. *The pacing lead is positioned in the right ventricular apex. Turning to the right side can cause the lead to float/move away from the apex, thereby causing pacemaker malfunction.*
- Assist with active ROM exercises to nonaffected extremities tid.
- Assist patient in using affected extremity carefully.
- Provide passive ROM exercise to shoulder on operative side *to prevent "frozen" shoulder.*
- Advise to cough and deep breathe every hour while awake *to prevent atelectasis.*

Pain/Discomfort

RELATED TO
Insertion of permanent pacemaker
Self-imposed and imposed activity restriction
Lead displacement
High pacing energy output
"Frozen" shoulder

DEFINING CHARACTERISTICS
Restlessness, irritability
Verbalized discomfort
Splints wound with hands

EXPECTED OUTCOMES
Patient verbalizes relief or reduction in pain/discomfort.
Patient appears relaxed and comfortable.

ONGOING ASSESSMENT
- Assess level of discomfort, source, quality, location, onset, precipitating and relieving factors.
- Assess for hiccups or muscle twitching. *Hiccups occur with phrenic nerve stimulation; muscle twitching occurs with high energy output.*
- Palpate affected site for presence of pulse generator pocket stimulation. *High pacing output or lead detachment from generator can cause stimulation.*

THERAPEUTIC INTERVENTIONS
- Provide comfort measures (e.g., backrubs, change in position, gentle massage of shoulder on operative side).

NURSING DIAGNOSES	EXPECTED OUTCOMES AND NURSING INTERVENTIONS / *RATIONALE* (■ = INDEPENDENT; ▲ = COLLABORATIVE)

Pain Discomfort
 	
RELATED TO
Reluctance to move
Hiccuping (phrenic nerve stimulation); intercostal or pectoral muscle stimulation
	THERAPEUTIC INTERVENTIONS— cont'd
	▲ Administer pain medication as prescribed.
	■ Instruct patient to report pain and effectiveness of interventions.
	■ Explain reasons for activity restriction. Emphasize that most are temporary.
	▲ If hiccups/muscle twitching/pulse generator pocket stimulation are present:
	   Notify physician.
	   Obtain chest x-ray films *to check for lead status and placement and ECG studies to check for proper function of pacemaker.*
	   Anticipate return to OR for lead repositioning. *These discomforts will not be relieved until the lead is repositioned or the energy output is reduced.*

Knowledge Deficit:
 	
RELATED TO
Advanced age of patient
Inability to comprehend
New procedure/equipment
Misinterpretation of information
 	
DEFINING CHARACTERISTICS
Lack of questions
Verbalized misconceptions
Questioning
	EXPECTED OUTCOMES
	Patient and family verbalizes understanding about pacemaker and patient accepts activity limitation.
	
	ONGOING ASSESSMENT
	■ Assess level of understanding about the pacemaker and reasons for insertion.
	
	THERAPEUTIC INTERVENTIONS
	■ Preoperatively, explain:
	   Anatomy and physiology of the heart, pacemaker function and its advantages, and insertion procedure.
	■ Postoperatively (acute):
	   Stress the importance of complete bed rest 24-48 hours after implant *to prevent lead displacement.*
	   Instruct patient to avoid turning to the right side if endocardial pacemaker was inserted *to ensure good ventricular wall contact.*
	   Explain the importance of notifying the nurse of:
	      Any pain, or drainage from insertion site.
	      Complaints of headache, dizziness, confusion, chest pain, shortness of breath, hiccups, or muscle twitching *that may suggest pacemaker malfunction.*
	   Explain the need for chest x-ray evaluation and 12-lead ECG to assess pacemaker function.
	■ Before discharge, teach patient
	   The need for regular follow-up care.
	   Signs and symptoms of pacemaker malfunction.
	   Signs and symptoms of infection.
	   Wound care for insertion site.
	   To discuss with physician type of sports activities patient can participate in (avoid contact sports).
	   To avoid over-the-head arm motion or overstretching for 1 month *to prevent lead displacement, because it takes about 1 month for the scar tissue to form around the tip of the electrode.*
	   The need to carry pacemaker ID card.
	   Type of pacemaker, brand name, and model number.
	   Programmed pacing rate.
	   How to take and record pulse as needed.
	   To notify physician/pacemaker follow-up office if pulse rate is at least 5 beats slower than programmed rate or of any signs and symptoms of pacemaker malfunction.
	   Pacemaker longevity and the need for pacemaker battery replacement when elective replacement indication (ERI) time has been reached.
	   That the pulse generator replacement (battery) using the same electrode can be done on an outpatient basis.
	   To avoid strong magnetic field (magnetic resonance, electrocautery equipment, laser, diathermy, lithotripsy, direct radiation [should be shielded], current industrial machinery); *these may cause pulse generator circuitry failure, or certain pacemakers will go into backup mode.*
	   That it is safe to use newer-model microwave ovens. Should dizziness be felt while near the appliance being used, advise patient to step away from it; *pacemaker will assume normal function without permanent effects.*
	   To alert airport personnel, dentist, and others of presence of pacemaker

Continued.

NURSING DIAGNOSES	EXPECTED OUTCOMES AND NURSING INTERVENTIONS / *RATIONALE* (■ = INDEPENDENT; ▲ = COLLABORATIVE)
High Risk for Infection **RISK FACTORS** Insertion technique Presence of foreign object	**EXPECTED OUTCOMES** Patient exhibits no signs of infection, as evidenced by normal temperature and WBC, negative cultures, and well-healed skin incision. **ONGOING ASSESSMENT** ▪ Assess insertion site for signs of infection. ▪ Evaluate amount and characteristics of any drainage. ▪ Assess body temperature. ▲ Follow up on WBC, blood and fluid cultures if infection is suspected. **THERAPEUTIC INTERVENTIONS** ▪ Ensure sterile technique when changing dressing. *With a skin incision there is a great chance of pathogens, particularly staphylcoccus, to penetrate through the open wound if sterile technique is not maintained.* ▪ Keep dressing dry and intact *to reduce chance of migration of pathogens.* ▪ Avoid frequent and unnecessary contact with the incision site. ▪ Notify physician if infection is suspected and to report excessive drainage, if any. ▪ Encourage a high-protein, high-calorie diet *to facilitate wound healing.* ▲ Administer antibiotics as prescribed. ▪ Before discharge, teach: Avoidance of shower or full bath for a week after implant. Proper technique on dressing change if needed. Signs and symptoms of infection. To avoid frequent contact with the incision site.

See also:
Anxiety, p. 5
Fear, p. 23
Body Image Disturbance, p. 7
Coping, imparied individual,
  p. 18

By: Marilyn Sampson-Hinton, RN, BSN

Percutaneous balloon valvuloplasty

BALLOON DILATION

Percutaneous balloon valvuloplasty is a nonsurgical procedure that involves the transluminal dilation of stenotic valvular (mitral valve, aortic valve) lesions by using balloon catheters. It is indicated for symptomatic patients who no longer respond to medical therapy and who are not candidates for valve replacement surgery. A percutaneous retrograde approach via the femoral artery is most commonly used for aortic valves. The femoral vein is used in the antegrade approach across the intraatrial septum for the mitral valve, and at times the aortic valve. The procedure is performed under fluoroscopy in the cardiac catheterization laboratory.

NURSING DIAGNOSES	EXPECTED OUTCOMES AND NURSING INTERVENTIONS / *RATIONALE* (■ = INDEPENDENT; ▲ = COLLABORATIVE)
Knowledge Deficit **RELATED TO** New procedure **DEFINING CHARACTERISTICS** Expressed need for more information Multiple questions or lack of questions Anxiousness Restlessness Verbalized misconceptions	**EXPECTED OUTCOMES** The patient/significant others verbalize basic understanding of valvuloplasty and the care associated with it. **ONGOING ASSESSMENT** ▪ Note baseline level of knowledge of heart anatomy, disease, valvuloplasty procedure, and possible risks/complications. **THERAPEUTIC INTERVENTIONS** ▪ Provide information about: Heart anatomy and physiology. Patient's heart problem (mitral or aortic stenosis). *Mitral stenosis is associated with fibrous valve leaflets that reduce the valve orifice. Aortic stenosis is associated with thickened and fibrous cusps and valve calcification.* Prevalvuloplasty preparations.

NURSING DIAGNOSES	EXPECTED OUTCOMES AND NURSING INTERVENTIONS / *RATIONALE* (■ = INDEPENDENT; ▲ = COLLABORATIVE)

THERAPEUTIC INTERVENTIONS— cont'd

    Procedure.
        Insertion of catheter.
        Balloon inflation at 3-5 atmospheres for seconds.
        Monitoring of pressure gradients across valve to verify results.
    Postvalvuloplasty care.
    Discharge instructions:
        May resume normal activities in 1 wk.
        Notify physician of weight gain, dyspnea, edema *[signs of valve dysfunction]*.
- Be in room when physicians discuss risk/complications of procedure *so that patient's subsequent questions can be answered accurately.*

High Risk for Decreased Cardiac Output

RISK FACTORS

Fluid volume deficit related to radiographic dye and restricted oral intake before procedure (NPO)
Valve tear or rupture, leading to valvular insufficiency
Dysrhythmia
↑ Pulmonary artery pressures and pulmonary vascular resistance secondary to left to right shunt with transseptal approach

EXPECTED OUTCOMES

Patient maintains adequate cardiac output as evidenced by warm, dry skin, normal BP, HR 60-100/min, absence of rales, and normal PAP, PCWP.

ONGOING ASSESSMENT

- Assess patient's hemodynamic status closely: obtain vital signs q15min until stable. *The first few hours are crucial to recovery.* Note and report changes.
- ▲ Assess the following parameters as available: pulmonary artery pressure (PAP), pulmonary capillary wedge pressure (PCWP), central venous pressure (CVP), cardiac output (CO), oxygen saturation. *PAP and PCWP pressures are elevated with new mitral regurgitation. Venous O_2 saturation will be more than 70% with L → R shunt.*
- Assess 12-lead ECG on arrival in ICU and monitor each morning. *ECG is necessary to assess changes and to monitor potential arrhythmias.*
- Assess heart sounds for change in murmur. *A blowing high-pitched murmur denotes valvular insufficiency.*
- Auscultate lungs. Observe for changes in respiratory pattern and report.
- Assess fluid balance closely (strict I & O).
- Monitor voiding/urine output closely. Report if there is no voiding for 8 hr or if urine output is less than 20 ml/hr.
- Assess for increased restlessness, fatigue, confusion, and disorientation.
- ▲ Monitor ABGs as necessary.

THERAPEUTIC INTERVENTIONS

- If signs of hemodynamic compromise are observed, institute treatment for Cardiac output, decreased, p. 12.
- ▲ Administer O_2 therapy *to increase oxygen availability to tissues.*
- ▲ If cardiac output is decreased secondary to fluid volume deficit, anticipate fluid resuscitation.
- ▲ If cardiac output is decreased secondary to valve rupture or tear:
    Administer afterload reducers (nitroprusside).
    Anticipate emergency open heart surgery for valve replacement.
- ▲ If cardiac output is decreased secondary to pulmonary hypertension, anticipate use of vasodilators (nitrates, hydralizine) *to reduce pulmonary vascular resistance.*

High Risk for Altered Peripheral Tissue Perfusion

RISK FACTORS

Mechanical obstruction from arterial and venous sheaths
Arterial vasospasm
Thrombus formation
Embolization of calcium debris
Bleeding/hematoma

EXPECTED OUTCOMES

Patient maintains peripheral tissue perfusion in affected extremity, as evidenced by strong pulse, and warm extremity.

ONGOING ASSESSMENT

Pre-procedure:
- Assess and document presence or absence and quality of all distal pulses.
- Obtain Doppler ultrasonic reading for faint, nonpalpable pulses. Indicate if pulse check is with Doppler. Mark location of faint pulses with *X for easier location during post-procedure monitoring.*
- Assess and document skin color and temperature, presence or absence of pain, numbness, tingling, movement, and sensation of all extremities. *Knowledge of baseline circulatory status of extremities will assist in monitoring for post-procedure changes.*
Post-procedure:
- Assess presence and quality of pulses distal to arterial cannulation site 15 min×4, q30min×4, q1h×2, then q2h until stable.
- Check cannulation site for swelling and hematoma *(may hinder peripheral circulation by constricting vessels).*

Continued.

Cardiac and Vascular Care Plans

NURSING DIAGNOSES	EXPECTED OUTCOMES AND NURSING INTERVENTIONS / *RATIONALE* (■ = INDEPENDENT; ▲ = COLLABORATIVE)
	THERAPEUTIC INTERVENTIONS Post-procedure: • Ensure safety measures to prevent displacement of sheaths *(may compromise circulation or traumatize artery)*: 　Maintain complete bed rest in supine position. 　Keep cannulated extremity straight at all times. Apply knee immobilizer or soft restraint *to remind patient not to bend it.* 　Do not elevate HOB more than 30 degrees. Assist with meals, use of bedpan, and position changes appropriate to activity limitations. ▲ Continue prescribed dose of heparin infusion *to ensure proper anticoagulation.* Check PTT 4h after start of infusion and after change in dose. *PTT is usually kept at 1½ times control.* • Do passive ROM exercises to unaffected extremities q2-4h as tolerated *to prevent venous stasis and joint stiffness.* • Instruct patient to report presence of pain, numbness, tingling, decrease or loss of sensation and movement immediately. *Important for quick assessment, diagnosis, and treatment.* • Immediately report to physician decrease or loss of pulse, change in skin color and temperature, presence of pain, numbness, tingling, delayed capillary refill, decrease or loss of sensation and motion *(may signify ischemia).* • Anticipate removal of catheter sheath *(presence may obstruct blood flow).* ▲ Prepare for possible embolectomy *to remove blood clot obstructing or compromising circulation.*
High Risk for Bleeding **RISK FACTORS** Presence of large catheter sheaths Overheparinization Arterial trauma	**EXPECTED OUTCOMES** Patient does not experience abnormal bleeding at insertion site. Risk of injury from bleeding is reduced through early assessment and intervention. **ONGOING ASSESSMENT** • Assess cannulation site for evidence of bleeding. *Fresh blood on dressing, oozing, pain/tenderness, swelling, hematoma are all signs of bleeding.* • Assess for signs of retroperitoneal bleeding. *These may include flank or thigh pain, loss of lower extremity pulse.* • Post procedure, monitor vital signs q15min×4, q30min×4, q1h×2, then q2h until stable. *Increased HR and decreased BP are commonly noted with bleeding.* ▲ Monitor PT, PTT, and platelets. *Provides information on coagulation status. Usually PTT is kept at 1½ times control.* • If significant bleeding occurs: 　Monitor vital signs at least q15min until bleeding controlled. 　Observe for circulatory compromise in affected extremity. • Note amount of drainage if fresh blood noted on dressing. Circle or outline size of hematoma if noted *to help assess further bleeding.* **THERAPEUTIC INTERVENTIONS** Before removal of catheter sheaths: • Maintain bedrest in supine position with affected extremity straight *to minimize risk of bleeding from cannulation site.* • Do not elevate head of bed more than 30 degrees. Observe appropriate positioning for meals, bowel and bladder elimination, and position changes. *Significant changes in position cause catheter to bend or move, which interferes with clot formation and can facilitate bleeding.* • Avoid sudden movement of affected extremity *to prevent displacement of catheter sheaths (may cause bleeding).* • Instruct patient to apply light pressure on dressing when coughing, sneezing, or raising head off pillow *to facilitate clot formation.* • Instruct patient to notify nurse immediately of signs of bleeding from cannulation site (e.g., feeling of wetness, warmth, "pop" at catheter sheath site, and feeling of faintness). ▲ Administer heparin drip via infusion pump *to ensure prescribed dose, depending on PTT result.*

THERAPEUTIC INTERVENTIONS

▲ If significant bleeding occurs:
  Turn off heparin drip.
  Notify physician immediately.
  Remove dressing and apply manual pressure directly to bleeding site *to provide temporary hemostasis.*
  Anticipate fluid challenge to treat hypotension.
  Administer protamine sulfate as ordered *to reverse effect of heparin.*
  Anticipate removal of catheter sheaths *to facilitate better control of bleeding.*
After removal of catheter sheaths:
▲ Maintain bed rest in supine position with affected extremity straight for 6 hr *to promote clot formation.*
▪ Avoid sudden movement of affected extremity *to facilitate clot formation and wound closure at insertion site.*
▲ Maintain occlusive pressure dressing on cannulation site.
▲ Apply 5-lb sandbag over dressing on cannulation site for 4 hr.
▲ For 6 hr after removal, do not elevate head of bed more than 30 degrees.
▲ Allow patient to dangle at bedside, then ambulate 6 hr after sheath removal if no evidence of bleeding. *Protocols may vary according to institutional policy.*

See also:
Pain, p. 49
Anxiety, p. 5
Fear, p. 23
Fluid volume deficit, p. 25

By: Cynthia Antonio, RN, BSN

Percutaneous Balloon Valvuloplasty

Percutaneous coronary intervention: PTCA, atherectomy, lasers, stents

These interventions provide a means to nonsurgically improve coronary blood flow and revascularize the myocardium. A variety of techniques have been developed. Though PTCA remains the mainstay, clinical trials are under way to determine the effectiveness of other, newer procedures. To date, restenosis remains a critical problem with all techniques.

Percutaneous Transluminal Coronary Angioplasty (PTCA): Utilizes a balloon-tipped catheter that is positioned at the site of the lesion. Multiple balloon inflations are performed until the artery is satisfactorily dilated.

Coronary atherectomy: Refers to removal of plaque material by excision or ablation. It may be performed in conjunction with PTCA. Several types of devices are being evaluated:

a) Directional: has rotating cutter blade that shaves the plaque; the tissue obtained is collected in a cone for removal.

b) Rotational: uses a burr at the tip of the catheter, which rotates at high speeds (150,000-200,000 rpms) to abrade hard plaque. The removed microparticles are released into the distal circulation rather than collected as in directional atherectomy.

c) Transluminal extraction: has low-speed rotator that excises the atheroma, then removes fragments by vacuum suction.

Lasers: Devices that use high energy to "pulverize" lesions and improve blood flow. They have been used successfully in peripheral arteries and in total coronary occlusions.

Stents: Are metallic coils that are inserted following dilation to provide structural support ("internal scaffolding") to the vessel.

NURSING DIAGNOSES	EXPECTED OUTCOMES AND NURSING INTERVENTIONS / *RATIONALE* (■ = INDEPENDENT; ▲ = COLLABORATIVE)

Knowledge Deficit

RELATED TO

Unfamiliarity with procedure
Information misinterpretation
Cognitive limitation

DEFINING CHARACTERISTICS

Request for more information
Statement of misconception
Increase in anxiety level
Lack of questions

EXPECTED OUTCOMES

Patient demonstrates basic understanding of heart anatomy and physiology, coronary artery disease, and anticipated procedure.

ONGOING ASSESSMENT

▪ Assess patient's knowledge of cardiac anatomy and physiology, coronary artery disease, and anticipated procedure.

THERAPEUTIC INTERVENTIONS

▪ Provide information about:
  Heart anatomy and physiology.
  Coronary artery disease.
  Type of procedure: *PTCA vs atherectomy, laser, use of stents.*
  Indications for interventional procedure: *significant obstruction (70%-100%) in areas reachable by catheterization.*
  Vessels requiring intervention: *may be single lesion/single vessel to multilesion/ multivessel.*
  Success rate: *above 90% in most cardiac centers.*
  Procedure room/environment.
  Expected length of procedure: *depends on number of vessels attempted, number of catheters required.*
  Expected discomfort: *Local anesthetic used at insertion site; however, patient is awake and may be uncomfortable when PTCA balloon is inflated, and because of prolonged lying in the same position.*
  Immediate postprocedure care:
    Activity restrictions: *usually bedrest until next day when femoral sheath is removed.*
    Routine vital signs.
    Pushing of oral fluids.
    Monitoring for complications: *bleeding at site, restenosis of vessel.*

NURSING DIAGNOSES	EXPECTED OUTCOMES AND NURSING INTERVENTIONS / *RATIONALE* (■ = INDEPENDENT; ▲ = COLLABORATIVE)

THERAPEUTIC INTERVENTIONS— cont'd

Recovery:
Discharge 1-3 days after procedure.
Avoidance of lifting heavy objects for 1 wk.
Possible return to work within 1 wk.
When to notify physician (e.g., chest pain).
Medications: *ASA for antiplatelet effect; calcium channel blockers for antispasm effect.*
Follow-up tests: *Exercise stress test may be performed early (1-2 wk) to provide new baseline for followup. Later testing (3-6 wks) may be done to assess for restenosis.*

- Stay with patient when physician explains procedure and evaluates patient. Clarify and reinforce physician's explanation of potential need for CABG surgery. *Dissection of the coronary artery during procedure may require emergency surgery.*
- Encourage patient to verbalize questions and concerns *to correct misunderstanding and misconceptions.*
- Include cardiac clinical nurse specialist, cath lab nurse, coronary care nurses as resource persons.

Chest Pain

RELATED TO

Myocardial ischemia caused by reocclusion of affected coronary artery, coronary artery spasm, possible myocardial infarction

Residual pain from manipulation/dilation of coronary artery

DEFINING CHARACTERISTICS

Patient complains of pain
Restlessness, apprehension
Facial mask of pain
Diaphoresis
↑↓ BP, ↑ heart rate

EXPECTED OUTCOMES

Patient is free of pain post procedure.
Patient appears comfortable.

ONGOING ASSESSMENT

- Assess for characteristics of myocardial ischemia. *Restenosis usually presents with a symptom pattern similar to before the interventional procedure.*
- Assess HR and BP during episode of pain.
- Monitor effectiveness of treatment.

THERAPEUTIC INTERVENTIONS

- Instruct patient to report pain immediately *so that relief measures can be initiated before additional myocardium is jeopardized. Early restenosis results from elastic recoil of vessel and/or thrombosis.*
- Notify physician of chest pain immediately. *Necessary to differentiate expected residual pain from coronary dilation and manipulation from pain related to restenosis.*
- ▲ Obtain 12-lead ECG stat. *Necessary to document new ST-T wave changes subsequent to procedure.*
- ▲ Administer medications as ordered:
  Nitroglycerin: *useful for spasm.*
  Calcium channel blockers: *for spasm.*
  Tylenol: *for residual pain from dilation of coronary artery.*
  Morphine sulfate: *needed for myocardial ischemia/infarct.*
- Anticipate need for possible emergency cardiac catheterization and repeat procedure. *Restenosis occurs in 25%-50% of cases, with the greatest occurrence in first 24 hr.*
- Prepare patient for possibility of CABG surgery.
- Stay with patient during pain *to provide emotional support and reassurance.*

High Risk for Bleeding

RISK FACTORS

Presence of large catheter sheaths
Overheparinization
Arterial trauma

EXPECTED OUTCOMES

Patient does not experience abnormal bleeding at insertion site.
Risk of injury from bleeding is reduced through early assessment and intervention.

ONGOING ASSESSMENT

- Assess cannulation site for evidence of bleeding. *Fresh blood on dressing, oozing, pain/tenderness, swelling, hematoma are all signs of bleeding.*
- Assess for signs of retroperitoneal bleeding (*these may include flank or thigh pain, loss of lower extremity pulses*).
- Post procedure, monitor vital signs q15min×4, q30min×4, q1h×2, then q2h until stable. *Increased HR and decreased BP are commonly noted with bleeding.*
- ▲ Monitor PT, PTT, and platelets. *Provides information on coagulation status. Usually PTT is kept at 1.5-2 × control.*
- If significant bleeding occurs:
  Monitor vital signs at least q15min until bleeding controlled.
  Observe for circulatory compromise in affected extremity.
- Note amount of drainage if fresh blood noted on dressing. Circle or outline size of hematoma if noted *to help assess further bleeding.*

Continued.

NURSING DIAGNOSES	EXPECTED OUTCOMES AND NURSING INTERVENTIONS / *RATIONALE* (■ = INDEPENDENT; ▲ = COLLABORATIVE)

THERAPEUTIC INTERVENTIONS

Before removal of catheter sheaths:
- ▲ Maintain bedrest in supine position with affected extremity straight *to minimize risk of bleeding from cannulation site.*
- ■ Do not elevate head of bed more than 30 degrees. Observe appropriate positioning for meals, bowel and bladder elimination, and position changes. *Significant changes in position cause catheter to bend or move which interferes with clot formation and can facilitate bleeding.*
- ■ Avoid sudden movement of affected extremity *to prevent displacement of catheter sheaths (may cause bleeding).*
- ■ Instruct patient to apply light pressure on dressing when coughing, sneezing, or raising head off pillow *to facilitate clot formation.*
- ■ Instruct patient to notify nurse immediately of signs of bleeding from cannulation site (e.g., feeling of wetness, warmth, "pop" at catheter sheath site, and feeling of faintness).
- ▲ Administer heparin drip via infusion pump *to ensure prescribed dose, depending on PTT result.*
- ▲ If significant bleeding occurs:
    Turn off heparin drip.
    Notify physician immediately.
    Remove dressing and apply manual pressure directly to bleeding site, observing aseptic technique.
    Anticipate fluid challenge to treat hypotension.
    Administer protamine sulfate as ordered *to reverse effect of heparin.*
    Anticipate removal of catheter sheaths *to facilitate better control of bleeding.*

After removal of catheter sheaths:
- ▲ Maintain bed rest in supine position with affected extremity straight for 6 hr.
- ■ Avoid sudden movement of affected extremity *to facilitate clot formation and wound closure at insertion site.*
- ▲ Maintain occlusive pressure dressing on cannulation site.
- ▲ Apply 5-lb sandbag over dressing on cannulation site for 4 hr.
- ▲ For 6 hr after removal, do not elevate head of bed more than 30 degrees.
- ▲ Allow patient to dangle at bedside, then ambulate 6 hr after sheath removal if no evidence of bleeding. *Protocols may vary according to institutional policy.*

Altered Peripheral Tissue Perfusion

RELATED TO

Mechanical obstruction from arterial and venous sheaths
Arterial vasospasm
Thrombus formation
Embolization
Immobility
Swelling of tissues
Bleeding/hematoma

DEFINING CHARACTERISTICS

Decrease or loss of peripheral pulses
Decrease in skin temperature of extremity
Presence of mottling, pallor, cyanosis, rubor in skin of distal extremity
Delayed capillary refill in affected extremity
Decrease or loss of sensation and motion

EXPECTED OUTCOMES

Patient maintains peripheral tissue perfusion in affected extremity, as evidenced by strong pulse, and warm extremity.

ONGOING ASSESSMENT

Pre-procedure:
- ■ Assess and document presence or absence and quality of all distal pulses.
- ■ Obtain Doppler ultrasonic reading for faint, nonpalpable pulses. Indicate if pulse check is with Doppler. Mark location of faint pulses with X *for easier location during postprocedure monitoring.*
- ■ Assess and document skin color and temperature, presence or absence of pain, numbness, tingling, movement, and sensation of all extremities. *Knowledge of baseline circulatory status of extremities will assist in monitoring for post-procedure changes.*

Post-procedure:
- ■ Assess presence and quality of pulses distal to arterial cannulation site (radial for brachial artery; dorsalis pedis and/or posterior tibialis pulses for femoral artery) q15min×4, q30min×4, q1h×2, then q2h until stable.
- ■ Check cannulation site for swelling and hematoma *(may hinder peripheral circulation by constricting vessels).*

THERAPEUTIC INTERVENTIONS

Post-procedure:
- ■ Ensure safety measures to prevent displacement of arterial and venous sheaths *(may compromise circulation or traumatize artery):*
    Maintain patient at complete bedrest in supine position.
    Keep cannulated extremity straight at all times. Apply knee immobilizer or soft restraint *to remind patient not to bend it.*
    Do not elevate HOB more than 30 degrees. Assist with meals, use of bedpan, and position changes appropriate to activity limitations.

| NURSING DIAGNOSES | EXPECTED OUTCOMES AND NURSING INTERVENTIONS / *RATIONALE*
(■ = INDEPENDENT; ▲ = COLLABORATIVE) |

THERAPEUTIC INTERVENTIONS— cont'd

▲ Continue prescribed dose of heparin infusion *to ensure proper anticoagulation.* Check PTT 4h after start of infusion and after change in dose. *PTT is usually kept at 1½-2 times control.*

▲ Administer aspirin as prescribed *to prevent platelet aggregation and systemic clot formation.*

▪ Do passive ROM exercises to unaffected extremities q2-4h as tolerated *to prevent venous stasis and joint stiffness.*

▪ Instruct patient to report presence of pain, numbness, tingling, decrease or loss of sensation and movement immediately. *Important for quick assessment, diagnosis, and treatment.*

▪ Immediately report to physician decrease or loss of pulse, change in skin color and temperature, presence of pain, numbness, tingling, delayed capillary refill, decrease or loss of sensation and motion *(may signify ischemia).*

▪ If altered tissue perfusion is noted, anticipate removal of catheter sheath *(presence may obstruct blood flow).*

▪ Prepare for possible embolectomy *to remove blood clot obstructing or compromising circulation.*

See also:
Incisional pain, p. 49
Cardiac Dysrhythmias, p. 114
Physical mobility, impaired, p. 47
Anxiety, p. 25
Fear, p. 23

By: Maureen Kangleon, RN
    Meg Gulanick, RN, PhD

Peripheral chronic arterial occlusive disease

INTERMITTENT CLAUDICATION; ARTERIAL INSUFFICIENCY

Reduced arterial blood flow to peripheral tissues causing decreased nutrition and oxygenation at cellular level. Management is directed at removing vasoconstricting factors, improving peripheral blood flow, and reducing metabolic demands on the body.

| NURSING DIAGNOSES | EXPECTED OUTCOMES AND NURSING INTERVENTIONS / *RATIONALE*
(■ = INDEPENDENT; ▲ = COLLABORATIVE) |

Altered Peripheral Tissue Perfusion

RELATED FACTORS

Atherosclerosis
Vasoconstriction secondary to medications, tobacco, etc.
Arterial spasm

DEFINING CHARACTERISTICS

Pain, cramping, ache in extremity
Intermittent claudication (pain or weakness in one or both legs relieved by rest)
Numbness of toes on walking, relieved by rest
Foot pain at rest
Tenderness, especially at toes
Cool extremities
Pallor of toes/foot when leg is elevated for 30 sec
Dependent rubor (20 sec to 2 min after leg is lowered)
Decreased capillary refill
Diminished or absent arterial pulses

EXPECTED OUTCOMES

Patient maintains optimal tissue perfusion, as evidenced by warm extremities, palpable pulses, reduction in pain, and prevention of ulceration.

ONGOING ASSESSMENT

▪ Assess extremities for color, temperature, and texture. *This disease occurs primarily in the legs.* See Defining characteristics for changes.

▪ Assess quality of peripheral pulses, noting capillary refill. *Routine examination should include palpation of femoral, popliteal, posterior tibial, and dorsalis pedis pulses. In approximately 10% of normal people the dorsalis pedis pulse is absent without disease.*

▪ If no pulses are noted, assess arterial blood flow using Doppler ultrasonic instrumentation (if available).

▪ Assess for dependent changes. *In advanced disease the lower extremities become pale when the leg is elevated, and become red (rubor) when placed in a dependent position.*

▪ Assess for ulcerated areas on the skin. *They are commonly seen over bony prominences and on the toes and feet. Ulcers develop from chronic ischemia. If not treated they can lead to gangrene.*

▪ Assess pain/numbness/tingling as to causative factors, time of onset, quality, severity, relieving factors. *Intermittent claudication is the most common symptom of peripheral vascular disease. It is muscle pain that is precipitated by exercise/activity and is relieved with rest. It commonly occurs in the calf muscles or buttocks. Pain that occurs at rest signifies more extensive disease requiring immediate attention. Tingling or numbness represent impaired perfusion to nerve tissue cells.*

▲ Monitor results of diagnostic tests: Doppler ultrasound, arteriography. *Used to identify location and severity of disease.*

Continued.

NURSING DIAGNOSES	EXPECTED OUTCOMES AND NURSING INTERVENTIONS / *RATIONALE* (■ = INDEPENDENT; ▲ = COLLABORATIVE)

DEFINING CHARACTERISTICS—cont'd

Shiny skin
Loss of hair
Thickened, discolored nails
Ulcerated areas/gangrene
Edema
Change in skin texture
See Skin integrity, impaired, high risk for, p. 59.

THERAPEUTIC INTERVENTIONS

- Maintain affected extremity in a *dependent* position *to increase peripheral blood flow.* Do not elevate bed at the knee gatch.
- Keep extremity warm (socks/blankets) *to prevent vasoconstriction and promote comfort.*
- ▲ Administer analgesics as ordered.
- Bathe patient in warm bath water—never hot. *Cleanliness is important to prevent infection. However, heat increases tissue metabolism at already compromised site and can lead to further tissue impairment.*
- Assist with progressive activity program, noting claudication. *During exercise, tissues do not receive adequate oxygenation from obstructed arteries and convert to anerobic metabolism of which lactic acid is a byproduct. Accumulation of lactic acid causes muscle spasm and discomfort. However, gradual progressive exercise helps promote collateral circulation.*
- If ulcerated area exists, keep clean with dressing *to provide protection from infection.*

Knowledge Deficit

RELATED FACTORS

New condition
Lack of resources

DEFINING CHARACTERISTICS

Many questions
Lack of questions
Misconceptions

EXPECTED OUTCOMES

Patient verbalizes self-care measures required to treat disease and prevent complications.

ONGOING ASSESSMENT

- Assess knowledge of physiology of disease, and treatment/preventive techniques prescribed.

THERAPEUTIC INTERVENTIONS

- Instruct on the physiology of blood supply to the tissues.
- Instruct patient on appropriate diagnostic tests: Doppler studies, arteriography.
- Instruct patient on how to prevent progression of disease. *The three major risk factors for atherosclerosis are smoking, hyperlipidemia, and hypertension. Atherosclerosis is not confined just to the lower extremities, but may occur in the coronary, cerebral, and renal vessels.*
  Smoking:
    Avoid all tobacco, *which further decreases an already compromised circulation. Nicotine is a vasoconstrictor; ↑s blood viscosity.*
    Consider referral to stop smoking clinics as needed.
  Diet:
    If atherosclerotic problem exists, provide diet counseling on need for reduction in fats.
    If overweight, provide diet counseling regarding attainment of ideal body weight.
- Instruct on prevention of complications:
  Effects of temperature:
    Keep extremities warm. Wear stockings to bed.
    Keep house/apartment as warm as possible.
    Wear enough clothes during winter.
    Never apply hot water bottles or electric pads to feet/legs. *Burns may occur secondary to impaired nerve function.*
    Avoid local cold applications.
    Avoid cold temperatures.
  Foot care *to prevent ulceration and infection:*
    Inspect daily. *Patients with concomitant diabetes are at increased risk.*
    Wash feet daily with warm soap/water. Dry thoroughly by gentle patting.
    Never rub dry.
    Trim toenails carefully and only after soaking in warm water. Trim straight across. See podiatrist as needed.
    Lubricate skin *to prevent cracking.*
    Wear clean stockings.
    Do not walk barefoot. *Ulceration or gangrene of the toe/foot may follow mild trauma.*
    Wear correctly fitting shoes.
    Inspect feet frequently for signs of ingrown toenails, sores, blisters, etc.
- Provide information on ways to improve collateral circulation.
  Begin a daily exercise program *to promote collateral circulation.*
    Walk on flat surface.
    Walk about half a block after intermittent claudication is experienced, unless otherwise ordered by the physician.
    Stop and rest until all discomfort subsides. *Once the lactic acid clears from the local blood system, pain should subside.*
    Repeat same procedure for total of 30 min, 2 to 3 times/day.

Continued.

NURSING DIAGNOSES	EXPECTED OUTCOMES AND NURSING INTERVENTIONS / *RATIONALE* (■ = INDEPENDENT; ▲ = COLLABORATIVE)

THERAPEUTIC INTERVENTIONS— cont'd

- Discuss available drug treatment:
    Pentoxifylline (Trentyl) *Decreases blood viscosity, increases blood flow by increasing flexibility of RBCs. Also reduces platelet aggregation. Therapeutic response may take 4-6 wk.*
    Antiplatelets *To improve circulation through narrowed vessel.*
- Explain that these medicines do not replace other preventive/treatment measures.
- Provide information on other available medical-surgical therapies:
    Nonsurgical:
    Percutaneous transluminal angioplasty: *uses special balloon catheter to dilate obstructed artery.*
    Laser.
    Atherectomy—*uses special catheter to "shave" plaque away.*
    Surgical:
    Bypass surgery.
    Endarterectomy.
    Sympathectomy.
    Amputation: *Required if gangrene is present.*

See also:
Pain, p. 23
Skin integrity, impaired, high risk for, p. 59
Activity Intolerance, p. 3
Coping, impaired individual, p. 18

By: Meg Gulanick, RN, PhD

Pulmonary edema, acute

PULMONARY CONGESTION

Pulmonary edema is a pathologic state in which there is an abnormal accumulation of fluid in the alveoli and interstitial spaces of the lung. This fluid causes impaired gas exchange by interfering with diffusion between the pulmonary capillaries and the alveoli. It is commonly caused by left ventricular failure, altered capillary permeability of the lungs, ARDS, neoplasms, overhydration, and hypoalbumenemia. Acute pulmonary edema is considered a medical emergency.

NURSING DIAGNOSES	EXPECTED OUTCOMES AND NURSING INTERVENTIONS / *RATIONALE* (■ = INDEPENDENT, ▲ = COLLABORATIVE)

Impaired Gas Exchange

RELATED TO:

Pulmonary-venous congestion
Alveolar-capillary membrane changes

DEFINING CHARACTERISTICS

Restlessness
Irritability
Pink, frothy sputum
Hypercapnia
Hypoxia
Cough
Crackles
Dyspnea
Cyanosis

EXPECTED OUTCOMES

Patient exhibits signs and symptoms of improved ventilation and oxygenation, as evidenced by:
    Normal ABGs.
    O_2 saturation >90%.
    Decreased crackles, rales; clear breath sounds.
    RR 12-16/min.
    Relaxed, comfortable appearance.

ONGOING ASSESSMENT

- Assess respiratory rate, depth; presence of shortness of breath; use of accessory muscles. *In the early stages there is mild increase in respiratory rate. As it progresses, severe dyspnea, gurgling respirations, use of accessory muscles, and extreme breathlessness, as if "drowning in own secretions," are noted.*
- Assess breath sounds in all lung fields, noting aerations, presence of rales, wheezes. *Bubbling rales, wheezes, and rhonchi are easily heard over the entire chest reflecting fluid-filled airways.*
- Assess secretions. *Frothy, blood-tinged sputum is characteristic of pulmonary edema.*
- ▲ Obtain and monitor serial ABGs: *In early stages there is a decrease in both pO_2 and pCO_2, secondary to hypoxemia and respiratory alkalosis from tachypnea. In later stages the pO_2 continues to drop while the pCO_2 may increase, reflecting metabolic acidosis.*
- ▲ Monitor O_2 saturation with pulse oximeter.
- Monitor mental status. *Hypoxia is reflected in restlessness and irritability.*
- ▲ Monitor chest x-ray films. *As interstitial edema accumulates, the x-rays show cloudy white lung fields. Eventually Kerley B lines appear.*

Continued.

Cardiac and Vascular Care Plans

NURSING DIAGNOSES	EXPECTED OUTCOMES AND NURSING INTERVENTIONS / *RATIONALE* (■ = INDEPENDENT; ▲ = COLLABORATIVE)

	THERAPEUTIC INTERVENTIONS
	
	· Position patient for optimal breathing patterns (high Fowler's position; feet dangling at bedside). *Upright position reduces venous filling.*
	· Encourage slow, deep breaths as appropriate.
	· Assist with coughing or suctioning prn.
	▲ Provide O_2 as needed to maintain Po_2 at acceptable level. Anticipate endotracheal intubation and use of mechanical ventilation. See Mechanical ventilation, p. 202.
	▲ If ABGs are expected to be drawn more frequently than at four 1-hr intervals, suggest appropriateness of an arterial line *for patient comfort and ease in obtaining necessary ABGs.*
	▲ Administer prescribed medication carefully:
	  Morphine sulfate: *Reduces preload by vasodilation, decreases respiratory rate and reduces anxiety. Side effects include respiratory depression, bradycardia, and nausea.*
	  Keep naloxone (Narcan) available in the event of morphine overdose. *Narcan reverses effects of morphine.*
	  Nitrates: *Reduce preload.*
	  Diuretics: *Reduce intravascular fluid volume.*
	  Aminophylline: *Dilates bronchioles, dilates venous vessels. However, it is also a cardiac stimulant. Patients must be observed for cardiac dysrhythmias.*

Decreased Cardiac Output **RELATED TO:** Increased preload Increased afterload Decreased contractility Combined etiologies **DEFINING CHARACTERISTICS** Variations in hemodynamic parameters Arrhythmias/ECG changes Weight gain, edema, ascites Abnormal heart sounds Anxiety, restlessness Dizziness, weakness, fatigue	**EXPECTED OUTCOMES** Patient maintains cardiac output as evidenced by warm, dry skin, heart rate 60-100/min, clear breath sounds, good capillary refill, adequate urine output, and normal mentation. **ONGOING ASSESSMENT** · Assess mentation. *Restlessness is noted in early stages; severe anxiety, confusion seen in later stages.* · Assess heart rate and blood pressure. *Sinus tachycardia and increased arterial blood pressure are seen in early stages; BP drops as condition deteriorates.* · Assess skin color, temperature. *Cold, clammy skin is secondary to compensatory increase in sympathetic nervous system stimulation and low cardiac output and desaturation.* · Assess fluid balance and weight gain. *Compromised regulatory mechanisms may result in fluid and sodium retention.* · Assess heart sounds, noting murmurs, gallops, S_3, and S_4. ▲ Monitor O_2 saturation with pulse oximeter. ▲ Assess hemodynamic parameters. Monitor pulmonary artery (PA), pulmonary capillary wedge (PCWP) waveforms closely. *Usually PA diastolic and PCWP pressures are greater than 30 mm Hg. If PCWP correlates within 10% of pulmonary artery diastolic pressure, monitor PA diastolics instead of PCWP to prevent pulmonary infarction or balloon rupture from repeated readings.* **THERAPEUTIC INTERVENTIONS** ▲ Anticipate need for hemodynamic monitoring. See also: Hemodynamic monitoring, p. 167. *Swan-Ganz catheter guides treatment.* · Position patient for optimal reduction of preload (high Fowler's position, dangling feet at bedside). · Anticipate use of vasodilators: *they reduce preload and afterload.* **If nitrates are used:** ▲ Prepare IV nitrate in glass bottle using special tubing *because IV nitroglycerin is absorbed into the plastic.* ▲ Evaluate need to prepare as a multiple concentration *to decrease total amount of IV fluids administered.* ▲ Titrate dose to desired effect. *Usually used to reduce PCWP below 20-25 mm Hg.* **If nitroprusside (Nipride) is used:** · Make certain patient has a clear, audible BP by cuff. If not, evaluate need for arterial line *for continuous BP monitoring.* · Administer via infusion pump *for reliable dosing.* ▲ Titrate dose 0.5-10 µg/kg/min. ▲ Do not infuse with any other medicines. ▲ Protect from sunlight *because nitroprusside is light-sensitive.* · Anticipate potential side effects: hypotension, sweating, nausea, confusion. ▲ Monitor thiocyanate levels prn. *Nitroprusside is converted to cyanide when it is metabolized.*

NURSING DIAGNOSES	EXPECTED OUTCOMES AND NURSING INTERVENTIONS / *RATIONALE* (■ = INDEPENDENT; ▲ = COLLABORATIVE)

THERAPEUTIC INTERVENTIONS—cont'd

If hypotension or decreased ventricular contraction is a related problem:
- Evaluate need for hemodynamic monitoring/arterial line *for continuous BP monitoring.*
- Anticipate use of pressor agents.

If dopamine or dobutamine (Dobutrex) is prescribed *(increases contractility; causes vaso-constriction in blood vessels):*
- ▲ Titrate dose: 0.5-20 µg/kg/min for dopamine.
- ▲ Titrate dose: 0.5-10 µg/kg/min for dobutamine.
- ▲ Keep phentolamine (Regitine) on standby *in the event of extravasation of dopamine.*
- Anticipate potential side effects: tachycardia, decreased urine output (with high doses of dopamine).
- If necessary, dopamine and dobutamine may be infused through the same central line.

Anxiety/Fear

RELATED TO

Dyspnea
Excessive monitoring equipment
Increased staff attention
Impact of illness
Threat of death

DEFINING CHARACTERISTICS

Sympathetic stimulation
Restlessness
Increased awareness
Increased questioning
Avoidance of looking at equipment
Constant demands, complaints
Uncooperative behavior

EXPECTED OUTCOMES

Patient appears relaxed and comfortable.
Patient verbalizes reduced fear.

ONGOING ASSESSMENT

- Assess patient's level of anxiety and normal coping pattern. *Controlling fear/anxiety will help decrease physiologic reactions that can aggravate the condition.*

THERAPEUTIC INTERVENTIONS

- Remain with patient during periods of acute respiratory distress. *During acute episodes, patients become extremely anxious, gasping for breath and thrashing around. They fear they might "drown to death" in their secretions.*
- Promote an environment of confidence and reassurance.
- Anticipate need and use of morphine sulfate *to reduce anxiety and fear associated with shortness of breath.*
- Avoid unnecessary conversations between team members in front of patient. *This will reduce patient's misconceptions and fear/anxiety.*
- Briefly explain the need for/function of high-tech equipment. *Information can promote trust/confidence in medical management.*
- Institute treatment for Fear, p. 23.

Discomfort

RELATED TO

Dyspnea
Prolonged bed rest
Fatigue
Uncomfortable therapeutic interventions

DEFINING CHARACTERISTICS

Complaints of discomfort
Diaphoresis
Pain; dyspnea
Restlessness
Uncomfortable feeling from mask or Foley catheter

See also:

Breathing pattern, ineffective, p. 10
Infection, high risk for, p. 40
Knowledge deficit, p. 41
Tissue perfusion, altered, p. 69
Fluid volume excess, p. 26
Swan-Ganz catheterization, p. 167
Intra-aortic balloon pump, p. 127
Cardiac dysrhythmias, p. 114
Sleep pattern disturbance, p. 61

EXPECTED OUTCOMES

Patient appears comfortable.
Patient verbalizes comfort.

ONGOING ASSESSMENT

- Assess patient's level of comfort, noting both verbal and nonverbal communication.
- ▲ Monitor ABGs closely, *so that most comfortable mode of O_2 delivery (cannula vs. mask) is used without compromising oxygenation.*

THERAPEUTIC INTERVENTIONS

- Position patient in preferred position. *Sitting upright, dangling at bedside provide changes in position as well as therapeutic benefit.*
- Offer frequent back rubs and massages.
- Turn patient from side to side q2h as tolerated by respiratory status.
- Obtain egg crate mattress/flotation pad as needed.
- Keep patient's linens dry. *Diaphoresis occurs secondary to peripheral vasoconstriction.*
- Provide frequent oral hygiene. *Usually patients breathe through their mouth, have increased respiratory rate, and may even have an ET tube in place.*
- Provide ice chips *to lessen complaints of thirst and dry mouth.* Maintain accurate I & O records.
- Ensure that tubes have enough slack so pulling is avoided.

By: Meg Gulanick, RN, PhD
Nancy J. Cooney, RN, BSN, MBA

Shock, anaphylactic

ALLERGIC REACTION

An exaggerated form of hypersensitivity (antigen-antibody interaction) that occurs within 1-2 min after contact with an antigenic substance and progresses rapidly to respiratory distress, vascular collapse, systemic shock, and possibly death, if emergency treatment is not initiated.

NURSING DIAGNOSES	EXPECTED OUTCOMES AND NURSING INTERVENTIONS / *RATIONALE* (■ = INDEPENDENT; ▲ = COLLABORATIVE)

Decreased Cardiac Output

RELATED TO
Severe reactions to drugs, insect bites, diagnostic agents, or food

DEFINING CHARACTERISTICS
Hypotension
Tachycardia
Decreased CVP
Decreased pulmonary pressures
Decreased cardiac output
Oliguria
Decreased peripheral pulses

EXPECTED OUTCOMES
Patient achieves adequate cardiac output as evidenced by: strong peripheral pulses, normal vital signs, urine output >30 ml/hr, warm dry skin, and alert, responsive mentation.

ONGOING ASSESSMENT
- Assess skin warmth and peripheral pulses. *Peripheral vasoconstriction causes cool, pale, diaphoretic skin.*
- Assess level of consciousness. *Early signs of cerebral hypoxia are restlessness and anxiety leading to agitation and confusion.*
- Monitor vital signs with frequent monitoring of BP. *Direct intra-arterial monitoring of pressure should be anticipated for a continuing shock state. Auscultatory BP may be unreliable secondary to vasoconstriction.*
- Monitor for dysrhythmias. *Cardiac dysrhythmias may occur from the low perfusion state, acidosis, or hypoxia.*
- ▲ If hemodynamic monitoring is in place, assess CVP, PAP, PCWP, and CO. *CVP provides information on filling pressures of right side of the heart; PAP and PCWP reflect left-side fluid volumes.*
- Monitor urine output with Foley catheter. *Oliguria is a classic sign of inadequate renal perfusion.*
- ▲ Monitor ABG results.

THERAPEUTIC INTERVENTIONS
- If ingested drugs or foods are the cause of the reaction, assist with forced emesis to delay absorption of the drug.
- If injected agents or insect bites are the cause of the reaction, apply a tourniquet above injection site or insect bite followed by infiltration of the site with epinephrine as ordered. Inspect the site for a stinger following an insect sting, and remove if present. Remove tourniquet every 15 min and then reapply, *to ensure perfusion to the distal extremity.*
- ▲ Administer medications as prescribed, noting responses:
  Epinephrine: *An endogenous catecholamine with both α- and β-receptor stimulating actions that provides rapid relief of hypersensitivity reactions. It is unknown whether epinephrine prevents mediator release or whether it reverses the action of mediators on target tissues, but its early administration is critical. For prolonged reactions, it may be necessary to repeat the dose.*
  Benadryl: *An antihistamine with anticholinergic and sedative side effects that is a useful therapeutic adjunct to epinephrine after the acute episode is controlled.*
  Vasopressors: *Useful to reverse vasodilation in the acute state. Vasopressors may be necessary to raise the BP in acute situations. However, infusion rate must be monitored closely and vital signs monitored frequently with titration of the drip, as necessary, to maintain hemodynamic parameters at prescribed levels.*
  Corticosteroids: *May be used to suppress immune and inflammatory response.*
- Place patient in the physiologic position for shock: head of bed flat with the trunk horizontal and lower extremities elevated 20-30 degrees with knees straight. *This will promote venous return.* Do not use Trendelenburg's (head down) position *because it causes pressure against the diaphragm.*

Continued.

NURSING DIAGNOSES	EXPECTED OUTCOMES AND NURSING INTERVENTIONS / *RATIONALE* (■ = INDEPENDENT; ▲ — COLLABORATIVE)

Ineffective Breathing Pattern

RELATED TO

Facial angioedema
Bronchospasm
Laryngeal edema

DEFINING CHARACTERISTICS

Dyspnea
Wheezing
Tachypnea
Stridor
Tightness of chest
Cyanosis

EXPECTED OUTCOMES

Patient's breathing pattern is restored as evidenced by eupnea, regular respiratory rate/rhythm, and improved breath sounds.

ONGOING ASSESSMENT

- Monitor respiratory status and observe for changes (e.g., increased shortness of breath, tachypnea, dyspnea, wheezing, stridor, hoarseness, coughing).
▲ Monitor ABGs and note changes.
- Auscultate breath sounds and report changes.
- Assess patient for the sensation of a narrowed airway.
- Assess presence of facial/angioedema.

THERAPEUTIC INTERVENTIONS

- Position patient *for optimal lung expansion and ease of breathing.*
▲ Administer O_2 as prescribed.
- Instruct patient to breathe deeply and slow down respiratory rate. *Focusing on breathing may help to calm patient and facilitate improved gas exchange.*
- Provide reassurance and allay anxiety by staying with the patient during acute distress. *Air hunger can produce an extremely anxious state.*
▲ If patient is wheezing, administer aminophylline, *which is a bronchodilator, pulmonary vasodilator, and smooth muscle relaxant that inhibits bronchospasm.*
▲ Give medications (e.g., steroids, antihistamines, aminophylline, 1 : 1000 aqueous epinephrine) as prescribed *to reverse bronchospasm and record effects.*
▲ Administer epinephrine by inhaler or nebulizer if laryngeal edema is present.
- Maintain patent airway. Anticipate emergency intubation or tracheostomy. *Respiratory distress may progress rapidly.*

Fluid Volume Deficit

RELATED TO

Loss of intravascular fluid into the interstitial spaces

DEFINING CHARACTERISTICS

Decreased urine output
Concentrated urine
Decreased venous filling
Hypotension
Thirst
Tachycardia

EXPECTED OUTCOMES

Patient experiences adequate fluid volume as evidenced by urine output >30 ml/hr, normotensive BP, and HR <100/min.

ONGOING ASSESSMENT

- Closely monitor I & O, assessing urine for concentration.
- Obtain daily weights.
- Assess for edema.
- Assess for presence of tachycardia and hypotension. *Stimulation of sympathetic nervous system occurs to compensate for the fluid shift.*

THERAPEUTIC INTERVENTIONS

▲ Maintain optimal fluid balance.
▲ Administer parenteral fluid *to reverse hypovolemia,* as ordered.
▲ Give fluid challenges as ordered and closely monitor and record effects.
▲ Anticipate the administration of volume expanders (e.g., plasma, dextran) *to correct the hypovolemia. Unless the shock state is treated early, the body will not be able to compensate and death will occur.*
▲ Administer vasopressors as necessary *to raise the BP [e.g., dopamine (Intropin), levarterenol bitartrate (Levophed)].*

High Risk for Altered Cerebral Tissue Perfusion

RISK FACTORS

Anaphylactic reaction
Shock
Hypovolemia

EXPECTED OUTCOMES

Patient experiences improved cerebral perfusion as evidenced by absence of headache/dizziness, improved neurological state, and absence of seizure activity.

ONGOING ASSESSMENT

- Assess patient for complaints of headache or dizziness.
- Assess for presence of parasthesia. *Headache, dizziness, and parasthesia occur during an anaphylactic reaction.*
- Monitor with complete neurologic checks.
- Observe for seizure activity.

THERAPEUTIC INTERVENTIONS

- Protect patient from possible injuries (seizures, decreased gag reflex).
- Maintain BP in prescribed range *to increase cerebral perfusion.*
▲ Give fluids as ordered *to maintain BP.*

Continued.

NURSING DIAGNOSES	EXPECTED OUTCOMES AND NURSING INTERVENTIONS / *RATIONALE* (■ = INDEPENDENT; ▲ = COLLABORATIVE)

High Risk for Impaired Skin Integrity

RISK FACTORS

Manifestations of allergic reaction

EXPECTED OUTCOMES

Patient experiences decrease in urticaria, and skin condition returns to normal.

ONGOING ASSESSMENT

- Observe for signs of flushing (localized or generalized).
- Watch for development of rashes; note character: macules, papules, pustules, petechia, uticaria. *Rashes occur as a manifestation of the allergic reaction.*
- Assess for swelling/edema.

THERAPEUTIC INTERVENTIONS

▲ Give medications (e.g., Benadryl) as prescribed.
- Instruct patient not to scratch. *Scratching can cause further skin damage.*
- Clip nails if patient is scratching in sleep.
- Mitten hands if necessary *to prevent excessive scratching.*

High Risk for Anxiety/Fear

RISK FACTORS

Alteration in breathing
Shock state
Another allergic reaction
Other possible allergens
Threat of death

EXPECTED OUTCOMES

Patient experiences reduced anxiety/fear as evidenced by calm and trusting appearance. Patient verbalizes fears and concerns.

ONGOING ASSESSMENT

- Recognize patient's level of anxiety/fear and note signs and symptoms.
- Assess patient's coping mechanisms. *Shock is an acute life-threatening illness that will produce high levels of anxiety in the patient as well as in significant others.*

THERAPEUTIC INTERVENTIONS

- Reduce patient's/significant others' anxiety by explaining all procedures/treatment.
- Maintain confident, assured manner. *Staff's anxiety may be easily perceived by patient.*
- Assure patient and significant others of close, continuous monitoring that will ensure prompt interventions.
- Reduce unnecessary external stimuli (e.g., clear unnecessary personnel from room; decrease volume of cardiac monitor).
- Reassure patient/significant others as appropriate; allow them to express their fears.
▲ Refer to other support systems, (e.g., clergy, social workers, other family/friends) as appropriate.

Knowledge Deficit: Allergens

RELATED TO

No previous experience

DEFINING CHARACTERISTICS

Recurrent allergic reactions
Inability to identify allergens

EXPECTED OUTCOMES

Patient/significant others verbalize understanding of allergic reaction, prevention, and treatment.

ONGOING ASSESSMENT

- Assess knowledge of patient's condition and exposure to allergens.

THERAPEUTIC INTERVENTIONS

- Explain symptoms and interventions to help prevent anaphylactic shock.
- Instruct patient/significant others about factors that can precipitate a recurrence of shock and ways to prevent or avoid these precipitating factors. *The patient is at high risk for developing anaphylactic shock in the future if exposed to the same antigenic substance.*
- Explain environmental factors that may increase risk of anaphylaxis (i.e., certain drugs, bee stings, food).
- Instruct patient on use of insect sting kits (containing a chewable antihistamine, epinephrine in prefilled syringe, and instructions for use), as appropriate, and how they are to be obtained.
- Discuss the possibility of undergoing desensitization therapy, as appropriate, *to lessen the risk of a life-threatening allergic reaction.*
- Instruct patient with known allergies to wear Medic-Alert tags. *In case of emergency, persons providing care will then be aware of this significant history.*
- Ensure that patient/significant others are made aware that when giving past medical history they should include all allergies.

See also:
Nutrition, altered: less than body requirements, p. 44

By: Sue Galanes RN, MS, CCRN

Shock, Cardiogenic

PUMP FAILURE; CONGESTIVE HEART FAILURE

An acute state of decreased cardiac output tissue perfusion usually associated with myocardial infarction, massive pulmonary embolism, cardiac surgery or cardiac tamponade. It is a self-perpetuating condition because coronary blood flow to the myocardium is compromised, causing further ischemia and ventricular dysfunction. This care plan focuses on the care of an unstable patient in a shock state.

NURSING DIAGNOSES	EXPECTED OUTCOMES AND NURSING INTERVENTIONS / *RATIONALE* (■ = INDEPENDENT; ▲ = COLLABORATIVE)

Decreased Cardiac Output

RELATED TO

Mechanical:
  Impaired left ventricular
    contractility
Dysrhythmias
Structural:
  Valvular dysfunction
  Septal defects

DEFINING CHARACTERISTICS

Mental status changes
Variations in hemodynamic
  parameters
Pale, cool, clammy skin
Cyanosis, mottling of extremities
Oliguria, anuria
Sustained hypotension with
  narrowing of pulse pressure
Pulmonary congestion
Respiratory alkalosis or metabolic acidosis

EXPECTED OUTCOMES

Patient achieves adequate CO, as evidenced by: strong peripheral pulses, normal vital signs, urine output >30 ml/hr, warm, dry skin, and alert, responsive mentation.

ONGOING ASSESSMENT

- Assess skin color, temperature, moisture *Peripheral vasoconstriction causes cool, pale, and diaphoretic skin.*
- Assess mental status. *Early signs of cerebral hypoxia are restlessness and anxiety.*
- Assess BP and pulse pressure. *Auscultatory BP may be unreliable secondary to vasoconstriction; direct intra-arterial monitoring of pressure should be initiated. Pulse pressure (systolic minus diastolic) falls in shock.*
- Assess central and peripheral pulses. *Provides information about stroke volume and peripheral perfusion.*
- Assess urine output with Foley catheter. *Oliguria is a classic sign of inadequate renal perfusion.*
- Assess respiratory rate, rhythm, and breath sounds. *Rapid shallow respirations and presence of crackles and wheezes are characteristic of shock.*
- ▲ Assess ABGs.
- ▲ If hemodynamic monitoring in place, assess CVP, PAP, PCWP, and CO. *CVP provides information on filling pressures of right side of heart; PAP and PCWP reflect left-sided fluid volumes.*

THERAPEUTIC INTERVENTIONS

- Place patient in optimal position, usually supine with head of bed slightly elevated *to promote venous return and facilitate ventilation.*
- ▲ Administer IV fluids to maintain optimal filling pressure. *Too little fluid reduces circulating blood volume and ventricular filling pressures; too much fluid can cause pulmonary edema in a failing heart.*
- ▲ Initiate and titrate drug therapy as ordered. *Therapy is more effective when initiated early. Goal is to maintain systolic BP >90-100 mm/Hg.*
  Inotropic agents
    Dopamine: *Positive inotropic and chronotropic effect on the heart that improves stroke volume and cardiac output. High dose, however, can cause peripheral vasoconstriction and can be arrhythmiogenic.*
    Dobutamine: *Positive inotropic effect increases cardiac output. Reduces afterload by decreasing peripheral vasoconstriction, also resulting in higher cardiac output.*
    Inocor: *Increased contractility and vasodilation.*
  Vasodilators
    Nipride: *Increases cardiac output by decreasing afterload. Produces peripheral and systemic vasodilation by direct action to smooth muscles of blood vessels.*
    Nitroglycerin IV: *May be used to reduce excess preload, if contributing to pump failure, and to reduce afterload.*
  Diuretics: *Used when volume overload is contributing to pump failure.*
  Antiarrhythmics: *Used when cardiac arrhythmias are further compromising a low-output state.*
  Vasopressors: *Augment the vasoconstriction that occurs with shock to increase perfusion pressure.*
- ▲ If mechanical assistance by counterpulsation is indicated, institute intra-aortic balloon pump, p. 127. *IABP increases coronary perfusion while decreasing myocardial O_2 demands.*
- If ventricular assist device is indicated, see VAD, p. 177.

Continued.

Cardiac and Vascular Care Plans

NURSING DIAGNOSES	EXPECTED OUTCOMES AND NURSING INTERVENTIONS / *RATIONALE* (■ = INDEPENDENT; ▲ = COLLABORATIVE)

Impaired gas exchange

RELATED TO

Altered blood flow
Alveolar capillary membrane changes

DEFINING CHARACTERISTICS

Fast, labored breathing
May have Cheyne-Stokes respirations
Crackles
Tachycardia
Hypoxia
Restlessness
Confusion

EXPECTED OUTCOMES

Patient achieves adequate oxygenation, as evidenced by respiratory rate <20/min, pO_2 >80 mm, and baseline heart rate for patient.

ONGOING ASSESSMENT

- Assess rate, rhythm, and depth of respiration.
- Assess for abnormal breath sounds.
- Assess for tachycardia *[occurs with tissue hypoxia]*.
- Assess skin, nailbeds, and mucous membranes for pallor or cyanosis.
- ▲ Assess ABGs with changes in respiratory status and 15-20 min after each adjustment in O_2 therapy *to evaluate effectiveness of O_2 therapy.*

THERAPEUTIC INTERVENTIONS

- Place patient in optimal position for ventilation. *Slightly elevated head of bed (HOB) facilitates diaphragmatic movement.*
- ▲ Initiate O_2 therapy as prescribed *to maintain pO_2 at acceptable level. The patient in shock has great need for O_2 to offset the hypoperfusion and metabolic state.*
- ▲ Prepare patient for mechanical ventilation if noninvasive O_2 therapy is ineffective:
    Explain need for mechanical ventilation *to allay anxiety and gain compliance.*
    Assist in intubation procedure.
    Institute Mechanical ventilation, p. 202.
- Suction as needed.

Fear/Anxiety

RELATED TO

Guarded prognosis; mortality rate 80%
Unfamiliar environment
Dyspnea
Dependence on IABP or mechanical ventilation
Fear of death

DEFINING CHARACTERISTICS

Sympathetic stimulation
Restlessness
Increased awareness
Increased questioning
Uncooperative behavior
Avoids looking at equipment or keeps vigilant watch over equipment

See also:
Spiritual distress, p. 62
Hopelessness, p. 36
Nutrition, altered: less than body requirements, p. 44
Knowledge deficit, p. 41

EXPECTED OUTCOMES

Patient appears calm and trusting of medical care.
Patient verbalizes fears and concerns.

ONGOING ASSESSMENT

- Assess patient's level of anxiety. *Controlling anxiety will help decrease physiologic reactions that can aggravate condition.*

THERAPEUTIC INTERVENTIONS

- Assure patient and significant others of close, continuous monitoring that will ensure prompt interventions. *Promotes a feeling of security.*
- Avoid unnecessary conversations between team members in front of patient. *This will reduce patient's misconceptions and fear/anxiety.*
- Contact religious representative/counselor *to provide spiritual care and support, if appropriate.*
- Briefly explain the need for/function of high-tech equipment. *Information can promote trust/confidence in medical management.*
- Encourage visiting by patient's support system.
- Allow patient to express fears of dying.
- See Anxiety, p. 4, 5.

By: Meg Gulanick, RN, PhD

Shock, hypovolemic

Hypovolemic shock occurs from an actual loss of intravascular fluid volume. This loss can be whole blood, plasma, or water and electrolytes. Common causes include: hemorrhage (external or internal); vomiting; and diarrhea. Hemorrhagic shock frequently occurs after trauma, GI bleeding, or rupture of organs/aneurysms.

NURSING DIAGNOSES	EXPECTED OUTCOMES AND NURSING INTERVENTIONS / *RATIONALE* (■ = INDEPENDENT; ▲ = COLLABORATIVE)

Fluid Volume Deficit

RELATED TO
Estimated blood volume loss up to 30%

DEFINING CHARACTERISTICS
Tachycardia
Hypotension
Capillary refill normal or >2 sec
Tachypnea
Urine output may be normal (>30 ml/hr) or as low as 20 ml/hr
Cool, clammy skin
Thirst
Dry mouth
Lightheadedness/dizziness
Mild to moderate anxiety

EXPECTED OUTCOMES
Patient experiences adequate fluid volume as evidenced by: urine output >30 ml/hr, normotensive BP, HR <100/min, and warm & dry skin.

ONGOING ASSESSMENT
- Obtain baseline vital signs and continue frequent monitoring of BP. *Direct intra-arterial monitoring of pressure should be anticipated for a continuing shock state. Ausculatory BP may be unreliable secondary to vasoconstriction.*
- Evaluate, document extent of patient's injuries; use Primary Survey (or another consistent survey method) or ABCs: airway with cervical spine control, breathing, circulation. *Primary Survey helps identify imminent/potentially life-threatening injuries. This is a quick, initial assessment.*
- Perform secondary survey after all life-threatening injuries are ruled out/treated. *Secondary survey uses methodical head to toe inspection.* Anticipate potential causes of shock state from ongoing assessment.
- Assess for early warning signs of hypovolemia. *Mild to moderate-anxiety may be first sign of impending hypovolemic shock; unfortunately it may also bee asily overlooked, attributed to pain, psychological trauma, and fear. (BP is not good indicator of early hypovolemic shock).*
- Monitor possible sources of fluid loss: chest tube drainage, diarrhea, vomiting, increasing abdominal girth, increasing extremity girth.
- If the only visible injury is obvious head injury, look for other causes of hypovolemia (i.e., long bone fractures, internal bleeding, external bleeding).
- ▲ Assess CVP to distinguish hypotension caused by hypovolemia (low CVP reading of <6cm H_2O) versus hypotension caused by pericardial tamponade/tension pneumothorax (high CVP reading of >10cm H_2O).
- Record and evaluate I & O.
- Monitor for signs and symptoms of continued blood loss.
- ▲ Obtain spun Hct, reevaluate q30min-4h, depending on stability. *Hct decreases as fluids are administered because of dilution. Rule of thumb: Hct decreases 1%/1L lactated Ringer's or NS used. Any other Hct drop must be evaluated as indication of continued blood loss.*
- ▲ Monitor coagulation studies including PT, PTT, fibrinogen, fibrin split products, and platelet counts, as appropriate.
- Monitor for arrhythmias. *Mild tachycardia (<120 beats/min) can be expected as sign of anxiety/mild hypovolemia.*

THERAPEUTIC INTERVENTIONS
- Prevent blood volume loss by trying to control source of bleeding. If external, apply direct pressure.
- ▲ If bleeding source is internal (e.g., pelvic fracture), military antishock trousers (MAST)/pneumatic antishock garment (PASG) may be used *to tamponade bleeding. Hypovolemia from long bone fractures (e.g., femur fractures) may be controlled by splinting with air splints, Hare traction splints, or MAST/PASG trousers, may be used to reduce tissue and vessel damage from manipulation of unstable fractures.*
- ▲ Initiate IV therapy. Start two large-bore, shorter-length peripheral IVs *(amount of volume that can be infused inversely affected by length of IV catheter; best to use shorter-length, large-bore catheter).*
    Replacement therapy: infuse 3 cc IV fluid/1 cc estimated blood loss.
    Initiate IV therapy with lactated Ringer's solution or colloidal expanders.
- ▲ If patient is hypotensive, prepare to bolus with 1-2 L IV fluids as ordered (normal adult dosage). *Patient's response to treatment depends on extent of blood loss. If blood loss is mild (<20%), expected response is rapid return to normal blood pressure. If IV fluids are slowed, patient remains normotensive. If patient has lost 20%-40% of circulating blood volume or has continued uncontrolled bleeding, fluid bolus may produce normotension, but if fluids are slowed after bolus, BP will deteriorate.*
- ▲ Administer blood products (packed red blood cells, fresh frozen plasma, platelets) as prescribed.

Continued.

NURSING DIAGNOSES	EXPECTED OUTCOMES AND NURSING INTERVENTIONS / *RATIONALE* (■ = INDEPENDENT; ▲ = COLLABORATIVE)

Decreased Cardiac Output

RELATED TO
Volume loss ≥30%
Late uncompensated hypovolemic shock

DEFINING CHARACTERISTICS
Pulse rate >120 beats/min
Hypotension
Capillary refill >2 sec
Decreased pulse pressure
Decreased peripheral pulses
Cold and clammy skin
Agitation/confusion
Decreased urinary output <30 ml/hr
Abnormal ABGs:
　Acidosis
　Hypoxemia

EXPECTED OUTCOMES
Patient achieves adequate cardiac output as evidenced by strong peripheral pulses, normal vital signs, urine output >30 ml/hr, warm dry skin, and alert responsive mentation.

ONGOING ASSESSMENT
- Assess skin warmth and peripheral pulses. *Peripheral vasoconstriction causes cool, pale, diaphoretic skin.*
- Assess level of consciousness. *Early signs of cerebral hypoxia are restlessness and anxiety leading to agitation and confusion.*
- Monitor vital signs with frequent monitoring of BP. *Direct intra-arterial monitoring of pressure should be anticipated for a continuing shock state. Auscultory BP may be unreliable secondary to vasoconstriction.*
- Monitor for dysrhythmias. *Cardiac dysrhythmias may occur from low perfusion, acidosis, or hypoxia.*
- ▲ If hemodynamic monitoring is in place, assess CVP, PAP, PCWP, and CO. *CVP provides information on filling pressures of right side of the heart; PAP and PCWP reflect left-sided fluid volumes.*
- Monitor urine output with Foley catheter. *Oliguria is a classic sign of inadequate renal perfusion.*
- ▲ Monitor ABG results.

THERAPEUTIC INTERVENTIONS
- Place the patient in the physiologic position for shock: head of bed flat with the trunk horizontal and lower extremities elevated 20-30 degrees with knees straight. *This will promote venous return.*
- ▲ Maintain lactated Ringer's IV infusion wide open until BP >90 mm Hg systolic.
- ▲ In addition to two established peripheral lines, prepare for additional peripheral lines, cutdowns.
- ▲ Transfuse patient with whole blood-packed RBCs. *Preparing fully cross-matched blood may take up to 1 hr in some labs. Consider using uncrossmatched or type-specific blood until crossmatched blood is available. If type-specific blood is unavailable, type O blood may be used for exsanguinating patients. If available, Rh(−) blood preferred, especially for females of childbearing age.*
- ▲ Apply MAST/PASG trousers when systolic BP is below 90 mm Hg. Deflate *slowly* when systolic BP is >100 mm Hg.
- ▲ If possible, use fluid warmer/rapid fluid infuser *to keep core temperature warm, facilitate rapid IV fluids, blood infusion. Infusion of cold blood is associated with myocardial arrhythmias, paradoxical hypotension. Macropore filtering IV devices should also be used to remove small clots and debris.*
- Prepare patient for possible surgical procedure *to stabilize condition.* Advise patient/significant others of possible surgery.
- ▲ If patient's condition progressively deteriorates, initiate CPR, other lifesaving measures according to advanced cardiac life support (ACLS) guidelines, as indicated.

Anxiety/Fear

RELATED TO
Acute injury
Threat of death
Unfamiliar environment

DEFINING CHARACTERISTICS
Restlessness, agitation
Crying
Increased pulse, BP
Increased respirations
Irrational thought processes
Admitted anxiety
Questioning of patient's condition by patient/significant others

EXPECTED OUTCOMES
Patient appears calm and trusting.
Patient verbalizes reduction in fears and expresses concerns.

ONGOING ASSESSMENT
- Assess level of anxiety/fear. *Hypovolemic shock is an acute life-threatening illness that will produce high levels of anxiety in the patient as well as in the significant others.*

THERAPEUTIC INTERVENTIONS
- Maintain confident, assured manner. *Staff's anxiety may be easily perceived by patient.*
- Explain all procedures/treatment. Keep explanations basic.
- Assure patient and significant others of close, continuous monitoring that *will ensure prompt interventions.*
- Reduce unnecessary external stimuli (e.g., clear unnecessary personnel from room; decrease volume of cardiac monitor).
- Reassure patient/significant others as appropriate; allow them to express their fears.
- Provide quiet, private place for significant others to wait.
- ▲ Refer to other support systems, (e.g., clergy, social workers, other family/friends) as appropriate.

NURSING DIAGNOSES	EXPECTED OUTCOMES AND NURSING INTERVENTIONS / *RATIONALE* (■ = INDEPENDENT; ▲ = COLLABORATIVE)

Ineffective Breathing Pattern

RELATED TO

Acidosis
Shock state

DEFINING CHARACTERISTICS

Tachypnea
Change in depth of breathing
Complaint of shortness of breath
Use of accessory muscles

See also:
Tissue perfusion, altered, p. 69
Nutrition, altered: less than body requirements, p. 44
Gas exchange, impaired, p. 27
ARDS, p. 183

EXPECTED OUTCOMES

Patient's breathing pattern is maintained as evidenced by eupnea, regular respiratory rate/pattern, and verbalization of comfort with breathing.

ONGOING ASSESSMENT

- Assess respiratory rate, rhythm, and depth. *Rapid shallow respirations may occur from hypoxia or from the acidosis with the shock state. Development of hypoventilation indicates immediate ventilator support is needed.*
- Assess for any increase in work of breathing:
    Shortness of breath.
    Use of accessory muscles.
- Assess breath sounds.
▲ Monitor ABGs and note changes.

THERAPEUTIC INTERVENTIONS

- Position patient with proper body alignment *for optimal lung expansion.*
- Change position q2hr *to facilitate movement and drainage of secretions.*
- Suction as needed *to clear secretions.*
- Provide reassurance and allay anxiety by staying with patient during acute episodes of respiratory distress. *Air hunger can produce an extremely anxious state.*
▲ Maintain O$_2$ delivery system *so that the appropriate amount of O$_2$ is applied continuously and the patient does not desaturate.*
- Anticipate the need for intubation and mechanical ventilation. See Mechanical ventilation, p. 202.

By: Sue Galanes RN, MS, CCRN

Shock, septic

SEPSIS; BACTEREMIA; WARM SHOCK; COLD SHOCK

Septic shock occurs after bacteremia of gram-negative bacilli (most common) or gram-positive cocci that results in a systolic BP <90 mm Hg (or a drop >25%), urine output <30 ml/hr, and metabolic acidosis. The circulatory insufficiency is initiated by endotoxin, which causes an increase in capillary permeability and a decrease in systemic vascular resistance (SVR). Hyperdynamic, warm shock is present in 30% to 50% of patients in early septic shock and is characterized by strong beta-adrenergic stimulation of the heart, with tachycardia and increased cardiac output if adequate blood volume is available. Hypodynamic, cold septic shock tends to occur relatively late in septic shock as a result of hypovolemia and release of myocardial depressant factors, causing a fall in cardiac output.

NURSING DIAGNOSES	EXPECTED OUTCOMES AND NURSING INTERVENTIONS / *RATIONALE* (■ = INDEPENDENT; ▲ = COLLABORATIVE)

Actual Infection

RELATED TO

An infectious process of either gram-negative or gram-positive bacteria
The most common causative organisms and their related factors are:
Escherichia coli: commonly occurs in GU tract, biliary tract, IV catheter, colon or intra-abdominal abscesses

EXPECTED OUTCOMES

Cause of infection is determined and appropriate treatment initiated.

ONGOING ASSESSMENT

- Assess level of consciousness/mentation. Utilize neurologic checklist, using Glasgow Coma Scale.
- Assess skin turgor, color, temperature, and peripheral pulses.
- Assess for presence of chills. *Chills often precede temperature spikes.*
- Monitor temperature.

Continued.

Cardiac and Vascular Care Plans

NURSING DIAGNOSES	EXPECTED OUTCOMES AND NURSING INTERVENTIONS / *RATIONALE* (■ = INDEPENDENT; ▲ = COLLABORATIVE)

Actual Infection

RELATED TO—cont'd

Klebsiella: from the lungs, GI tract, intravenous catheter, urinary tract, or surgical wounds

Proteus: GU tract, respiratory tract, abscesses, or biliary tract

Bacteroides fragilis: female genital tract, colon, liver abscesses, decubitus ulcers

Pseudomonas aeruginosa: lungs, urinary tract, skin, and IV catheter

Candida albicans: line-related infection, especially hyperalimentation infusion, pulmonary and urinary abscesses

DEFINING CHARACTERISTICS

Changes in LOC: lethargy, confusion

Fever/chills may or may not be present

Ruddy appearance with warm, dry skin

Leucocytosis

ONGOING ASSESSMENT—cont'd

■ Assess related factors thoroughly *to identify a source for the sepsis:*
   Lungs: Assess breath sounds; assess presence of sputum, including color, odor, and amount.
   GU: monitor UA reports; assess color and opacity of urine; assess for presence of drainage/pus around Foley catheter.
   GI: check for abdominal distention; assess for bowel sounds and abdominal tenderness.
   IV catheters: assess all insertion sites for redness, swelling, and drainage.
   Surgical wounds: assess all wounds for signs of infection: redness, swelling, and drainage.
   Pain: obtain patient's subjective statement of location and description of pain or discomfort. *This may help to localize a site.*

▲ Obtain culture and sensitivity (C & S) samples as ordered. *C & S reports show which antibiotic will be effective against the invading organism.*

▲ Draw peak and trough antibiotic titers as needed. *This will help to ensure an appropriate level of antibiotic for the patient.*

▲ Monitor for toxicity from antibiotic therapy, especially with hepatic and/or renal insufficiency/failure patients:
   Aminoglycocides should be followed with urinalysis and serum creatinine levels at least three times/week.
   Chloramphenicol should be restricted from patients with liver disease.

THERAPEUTIC INTERVENTIONS

▲ Initiate early administration of antibiotics as prescribed. *Antibiotic therapy is begun with broad-spectrum antibiotics after obtaining the C & S but prior to receiving the C & S report. After the C & S report is received, the physician should be notified if the organism is not sensitive to the present antibiotic coverage. The antibiotic may then be changed or supplemented.*

■ Remove any possible source of infection, e.g., urinary catheter, IV catheter.

▲ Manage the cause of infection and anticipate surgical consult as necessary *to drain pus/ abscess, to resolve obstruction, or to repair perforated organ.*

▲ Assist with the incision and drainage of wounds, irrigation, and sterile application of saline soaked 4 × 4's as indicated.

▲ Maintain temperature in adequate range *to prevent stress on the cardiovascular system:*
   Administer antipyretics as prescribed.
   Apply cooling mattress.
   Administer tepid sponge baths.
   Limit number of blankets/linens used to cover patients.

▲ Initiate appropriate isolation measures *to prevent the spread of infection.*

Fluid Volume Deficit

RELATED TO

Early septic shock (warm shock)

Decrease in systemic vascular resistance (SVR)

Increased capillary permeability

DEFINING CHARACTERISTICS

Hypotension

Tachycardia

Decreased urine output <30 ml/hr

Concentrated urine

EXPECTED OUTCOMES

Patient experiences adequate fluid volume as evidenced by urine output >30 ml/hr, normotensive BP, and HR <100/min.

ONGOING ASSESSMENT

■ Assess for presence of hypotension and tachycardia.

■ Closely monitor I & O, assessing urine for concentration.

■ Obtain daily weights and record.

■ When initiating fluid challenges, closely monitor patient *to prevent iatrogenic volume overload.* Monitor CVP.

THERAPEUTIC INTERVENTIONS

▲ Perform fluid resuscitation aggressively, starting with 300 to 500 cc of crystalloid, followed by an additional 500 cc over 15-20 min. Continue with further fluid resuscitation as ordered. *The fluid needs in septic patients may exceed 8-20 L in the first 24 hr.*

■ Use caution in fluid replacement in the elderly patient, *who may be more prone to congestive heart failure. In these patients monitor closely for signs of iatrogenic fluid volume overload.*

▲ Adjust fluid as ordered *to obtain an optimal PCWP of 12 mm Hg in absence of MI and PCWP of 14-18 mm Hg if MI has occurred.*

NURSING DIAGNOSES	EXPECTED OUTCOMES AND NURSING INTERVENTIONS / *RATIONALE* (■ = INDEPENDENT; ▲ = COLLABORATIVE)

Shock, Septic

THERAPEUTIC INTERVENTIONS— cont'd
- Notify physician of response to fluid challenge.
- ▲ Administer vasoactive substances, such as dopamine, phenylephrine HCl (neo-synephrine), or norepinephrine bitartrate (Levophed) as prescribed, if poor or no response to fluid resuscitation. *In early septic shock the cardiac output is high or normal. At this point, the vasoactive agents are administered for their alpha effect.*

Decreased Cardiac Output

RELATED TO

Late septic shock: a decrease in tissue perfusion leads to increased lactic acid production and systemic acidosis, which causes a decrease in myocardial contractility
Gram-negative infections may cause a direct myocardial toxic effect.

DEFINING CHARACTERISTICS

Decreased peripheral pulses
Cold and clammy skin
Hypotension
Agitation/confusion
Decreased urinary output <30 ml/hr
Abnormal ABGs:
  Acidosis
  Hypoxemia

EXPECTED OUTCOMES

Patient achieves adequate cardiac output as evidenced by strong peripheral pulses, normal vital signs, urine output >30 ml/hr, warm dry skin, and alert responsive mentation.

ONGOING ASSESSMENT
- Assess skin warmth and peripheral pulses. *Peripheral vasoconstriction causes cool, pale, diaphoretic skin.*
- Assess level of consciousness. *Early signs of cerebral hypoxia are restlessness and anxiety leading to agitation and confusion.*
- Monitor vital signs with frequent monitoring of BP. *Direct intra-arterial monitoring of pressure should be anticipated for a continuing shock state. Auscultory BP may be unreliable secondary to vasoconstriction.*
- Monitor for dysrhythmias. *Cardiac dysrhythmias may occur from the low perfusion state, acidosis or from hypoxia.*
- ▲ If hemodynamic monitoring is in place, assess CVP, PAP, PCWP, and CO. *CVP provides information on filling pressures of right side of the heart; PAP and PCWP reflect left sided fluid volumes.*
- Monitor urine output with Foley catheter. *Oliguria is a classic sign of inadequate renal perfusion.*
- ▲ Monitor ABG results.
- ▲ Monitor blood lactate levels.

THERAPEUTIC INTERVENTIONS
- Place patient in the physiologic position for shock: head of bed flat with the trunk horizontal and lower extremities elevated 20-30 degrees with knees straight. *This will promote venous return.* Do not use Trendelenburg's (head down) position *because it causes pressure against the diaphragm.*
- ▲ Administer inotropic agents (Dobutrex) dobutamine HCl dopamine, digoxin, or amrinone (Inocor) *to improve myocardial contractility.* Continuously monitor their effectiveness.
- ▲ Administer sodium bicarbonate *to treat acidosis.*

Ineffective Breathing Pattern

RELATED TO

Lactic acidosis

DEFINING CHARACTERISTICS

Tachypnea
Change in depth of breathing
Complaint of shortness of breath
Use of accessory muscles

EXPECTED OUTCOMES

Patient's breathing pattern is maintained as evidenced by eupnea, regular respiratory rate/pattern, and verbalization of comfort with breathing.

ONGOING ASSESSMENT
- Assess respiratory rate, rhythm, and depth every hour. *Rapid shallow respirations may occur from hypoxia or from the acidosis with sepsis. Development of hypoventilation indicates that immediate ventilator support is needed.*
- Assess for any increase in work of breathing: shortness of breath and use of accessory muscles.
- Assess breath sounds.
- ▲ Monitor ABGs and note pattern of change.

THERAPEUTIC INTERVENTIONS
- Position patient with proper body alignment *for optimal lung expansion.*
- Change position q2hr *to facilitate movement and drainage of secretions.*
- Suction as needed *to clear secretions.*
- Provide reassurance and allay anxiety by staying with patient during acute episodes of respiratory distress. *Air hunger can produce an extremely anxious state.*
- ▲ Maintain O$_2$ delivery system *so that the appropriate amount of O$_2$ is applied continuously and the patient does not desaturate.*
- Anticipate the need for intubation and mechanical ventilation. See Mechanical ventilation, p. 202.

See also:
ARDS, p. 183
Pneumonia, p. 211
Gas exchange, impaired, p. 27.

Continued.

NURSING DIAGNOSES	EXPECTED OUTCOMES AND NURSING INTERVENTIONS / *RATIONALE* (■ = INDEPENDENT; ▲ = COLLABORATIVE)

Altered Renal Perfusion

RELATED TO

Hypotension
Nephrotoxic drugs (antibiotics)

DEFINING CHARACTERISTICS

Urine output <30 ml/hr
Elevated BUN and creatinine
Hematuria, proteinuria
Tubular casts in urine
Fixed specific gravity

See also:
Acute renal failure, p. 436

EXPECTED OUTCOMES

Patient's renal perfusion is maintained as evidenced by urine output >30 ml/hr, normal urinalysis, BUN, and creatinine within normal limits.

ONGOING ASSESSMENT

- Monitor and record I & O.
- Assess for patency of Foley catheter.
▲ Monitor blood and urine: BUN, creatinine, electrolytes, urinalysis.
- Monitor urine specific gravity and check for blood and protein every 4 hr.

THERAPEUTIC INTERVENTIONS

▲ Maintain IV fluids and inotropic agents at prescribed rates *to maintain BP, cardiac output, and, ultimately, renal perfusion.*

High Risk for Injury: Bleeding

RISK FACTORS

Sepsis:
Deficiency in clotting factors
DIC

EXPECTED OUTCOMES

Potential for injury from bleeding is reduced through early assessment and appropriate intervention.

ONGOING ASSESSMENT

- Assess for signs of bleeding:
Petechiae, purpura, hematomas.
Blood oozing from IV sites, drains, or wounds.
Bleeding from mucous membranes:
Hemoptysis.
Blood obtained during suctioning.
Bleeding from GI/GU tract.
- Determine blood loss and report to physician.
▲ Monitor PT, PTT, FSP, bleeding time, and hemoglobin/hematocrit.

THERAPEUTIC INTERVENTIONS

▲ Administer colloids and blood products as prescribed.
- Avoid injury to mucous membranes, e.g., rectal temperatures, aggressive suctioning.
- If bleeding is present, refer to Disseminated intravascular coagulation, p. 410.

Knowledge Deficit

RELATED TO

New condition

DEFINING CHARACTERISTICS

Increased frequency of questions posed by patient and significant others
Inability to respond correctly to questions asked
Family's/significant others' avoidance of patient's condition

See also:
Gas exchange, impaired, p. 27
Nutrition, altered: less than body requirements, p. 44
Anxiety, p. 5
Fear, p. 23

EXPECTED OUTCOMES

Patient/significant others demonstrate understanding of disease process and treatment utilized.

ONGOING ASSESSMENT

- Evaluate understanding of septic shock and patient's overall condition.

THERAPEUTIC INTERVENTIONS

- Explain all procedures before performing them. *This will help to decrease patient's fear of the unknown.*
- Orient patient and significant others to ICU surroundings, routines, equipment alarms, and noises. *The ICU is a busy and noisy environment, which can be very upsetting to both patient and significant others.*
- Keep patient/significant others informed of disease process and present status of patient. *Septic shock results in a critically ill patient with a tenuous baseline for recovery.*

By: Sue Galanes, RN, MS, CCRN

Swan-Ganz catheterization (hemodynamic monitoring)

PULMONARY ARTERY PRESSURES; WEDGE PRESSURES; THERMODILUTION; OXYGEN SATURATION

A multilumen, balloon-tipped, flow-guided catheter inserted into the pulmonary artery for monitoring of pulmonary artery pressure (PAP) and pulmonary capillary wedge pressure (PCWP). It also has the capability of monitoring right atrial pressure (RAP), measuring cardiac output by thermodilution techniques, and monitoring mixed venous saturation via oximetry. The proximal lumen of this catheter can be used solely for intravenous infusion. These catheters are routinely used in intensive care settings.

NURSING DIAGNOSES	EXPECTED OUTCOMES AND NURSING INTERVENTIONS / *RATIONALE* (▪ = INDEPENDENT; ▲ = COLLABORATIVE)

Knowledge Deficit

RELATED TO
Newness, complexity, and urgency of procedure

DEFINING CHARACTERISTICS
Extensive questioning
Excessive anxiety
Inability to talk about procedure
Lack of questioning

EXPECTED OUTCOMES
Patient/significant other verbalizes understanding of rationale for use, procedures involved, follow-up care.

ONGOING ASSESSMENT
- Assess knowledge regarding S/G catheter.
- Assess learning capabilities of patient/significant other.

THERAPEUTIC INTERVENTIONS
- Provide information about Swan-Ganz catheter:
  Purpose: *to provide information on left ventricular function. Some catheters also monitor right ventricular parameters.*
  Insertion procedure: *through jugular, subclavian, antecubital vein into right side of heart.*
  Complications: *embolus, dysrhythmias, pulmonary infarction.*
  Ongoing care: *balloon inflation; dressing changes.*
  Activity restrictions: *necessary for arm or leg insertion sites to prevent malpositioning of catheter.*
- Reinforce previous learning. *The critical care environment can cause sensory overload, sleep deprivation, and anxiety; all affect retention of information.*

High Risk for Cardiac Dysrhythmias (PVCs)

RISK FACTORS
Irritation of ventricular endocardium by catheter during insertion/repositioning
Migration of catheter from pulmonary artery to right ventricle
Excessive looping of catheter in right ventricle

EXPECTED OUTCOMES
Patient maintains baseline cardiac rhythm.

ONGOING ASSESSMENT
- Document precatheterization baseline arrhythmias, noting frequency and type.
- Observe cardiac monitor continuously for arrhythmias during and after catheter positioning. *Transient ventricular arrhythmias are commonly observed while catheter is passed through the right ventricle.*
- ▲ Monitor catheter position on chest x-ray daily and when arrhythmias occur. *Catheter may have moved back to right ventricle.*
- Assess insertion site; note length of inserted catheter (check markings). *Change in markings alerts staff of catheter movement.*
- Monitor pulmonary artery waveform closely. *Change in waveform to right ventricle tracing signals malpositioned catheter.*
- Assess and document amount of air needed to wedge catheter. *Amount increases as catheter migrates to right ventricle, or catheter does not wedge.*
- If arrhythmias occur:
  Assess patient for complaints of dizziness, palpitations, lightheadedness, shortness of breath.
  Document rhythm strip and notify physician.
  Observe contributing factors that may have potentiated arrhythmias (e.g., patient/catheter position; other medical problems). *Correct assessment guides appropriate treatment.*

THERAPEUTIC INTERVENTIONS
- Maintain appropriate positioning of extremity if femoral or brachial site is used *to prevent malposition of catheter.*
- ▲ Have lidocaine bolus available. *Most dysrhythmias are ventricular in origin.*
- If catheter slips back to right ventricle, anticipate repositioning (if sterile sleeve in place) or removal and reinsertion of catheter.
- See Cardiac dysrhythmias, p. 114.

Continued.

Swan-Ganz catheterization—cont'd

NURSING DIAGNOSES	EXPECTED OUTCOMES AND NURSING INTERVENTIONS / *RATIONALE* (■ = INDEPENDENT; ▲ = COLLABORATIVE)

High Risk for Injury: Pulmonary Artery Infarction or Hemorrhage

RISK FACTORS

Continuous or prolonged wedging of catheter
Overinflation of balloon
Migration of catheter to pulmonary capillary seen on x-ray film

EXPECTED OUTCOMES

Patient does not exhibit signs of pulmonary infarction, as noted by absence of hypotension and shortness of breath.

ONGOING ASSESSMENT

▲ Monitor pulmonary artery position of catheter on x-ray *to verify correct placement.*
■ Monitor pulmonary arterial pressure waveform continuously. *PCWP is only measured intermittently.*
■ Monitor pulmonary artery diastolic pressure instead of PCWP pressure when both values are correlated. *This reduces risk of permanent "wedging" of catheter. Values are not correlated if mitral valve incompetence exists.*
■ Assess for signs of pulmonary artery infarction or hemorrhage: c/ shortness of breath, hemoptysis.

THERAPEUTIC INTERVENTIONS

■ Inject only enough air to obtain pulmonary capillary artery wedge pressure. *Waveform will change from PAP to PCWP tracing.*
■ Do not inflate balloon past recommended volume *to prevent rupture.* Document amount used. *Changes in the amount of air needed to float the catheter into pulmonary arteriole provide information on migration of catheter.*
■ Leave balloon deflated when not directly measuring *to prevent pulmonary infarction.*
■ Never forcefully flush catheter; *may rupture balloon or cause infarction.*
■ Do not infuse anything through distal port except standardized continuous flush solution.
■ If catheter appears permanently wedged:
  Verify that cause is not false wedge pressure waveform, as with dampening or other technical problems.
  Have patient take deep breaths, raise arm, turn on left side, cough *to attempt to unwedge.*
  Notify physician immediately *to pull back catheter to pulmonary artery.*
  Determine catheter/balloon position on chest x-ray.

High Risk for Injury: Pneumothorax

RISK FACTORS

Use of subclavian insertion site
Patient movement during insertion

EXPECTED OUTCOMES

Patient has normal respirations and breathing pattern

ONGOING ASSESSMENT

■ Assess breath sounds, respiratory pattern, and chest movement before and immediately after insertion. *Shortness of breath, decreased breath sounds on affected side, and unequal thoracic wall movement are seen with pneumothorax.*
▲ When checking for catheter placement on x-ray, note lung expansion. *A shift of trachea toward affected side can be noted with pneumothorax.*

THERAPEUTIC INTERVENTIONS

▲ Keep patient still during procedure. *Sudden movements increase risks of pneumothorax.* Provide sedatives, local anesthesia, and reassurance as needed.
■ Provide optimal positioning of insertion area (back/shoulder/subclavian region).
■ If symptoms of pneumothorax are noted, refer to physician and anticipate chest tube insertion.

See also:
Pneumothorax with chest tube, p. 214
Pain, p. 49
Infection, high risk for, p. 40

By: Meg Gulanick, RN, PhD

Tamponade

CHEST TRAUMA; CARDIAC SURGERY; PERICARDIAL
EFFUSION

Cardiac tamponade is a life-threatening condition caused by fluid accumulation in the mediastinum or pericardium. As fluid collects, it causes compression of the cardiovascular structures. This impairs cardiac filling and greatly reduces cardiac output. Rapidly accumulating fluid is most often blood and is usually caused by chest trauma or surgery. Chronic effusions are often serous fluid that accumulates gradually secondary to infection (viral, bacterial), inflammation (rheumatoid, uremia, radiation, etc.), or neoplastic conditions (primary, metastatic). Rapid recognition and intervention are essential. Treatment modalities include pericardiocentesis, pericardiocentesis with pigtail catheter placement for drainage, open chest drainage, pericardiectomy, and pleuropericardial window.

NURSING DIAGNOSES

EXPECTED OUTCOMES AND NURSING INTERVENTIONS / *RATIONALE*
(■ = INDEPENDENT; ▲ = COLLABORATIVE)

Decreased Cardiac Output

RELATED TO

External compression of cardiovascular structures causing reduced diastolic filling

DEFINING CHARACTERISTICS

Decreased BP
Narrow pulse pressure
Pulsus paradoxus (systolic pressure falls 15 mm Hg or more during inspiration)
Tachycardia
Electrical alternans (decreased QRS voltage during inspiration)
Equalization of pressures (CVP, PAP, PCWP)
Jugular venous distention
Chest tubes (if present) suddenly stop draining (suspect clot)
Distant or muffled heart tones
Restlessness, confusion, anxiety
Fall in Hgb and Hct
Cool, clammy skin
Diminished peripheral pulses
Decreased urine output
Decreased arterial and venous O$_2$ saturation
Acidosis

EXPECTED OUTCOMES

Patient maintains adequate cardiac output as evidenced by:
  Blood pressure within normal limits for patient.
  Strong regular pulses.
  Absence of JVD.
  Absence of pulsus paradoxus.
  Skin warm and dry.
  Clear mentation.

ONGOING ASSESSMENT

- Assess for classic signs associated with acute cardiac tamponade:
  Low arterial blood pressure.
  Tachypnea.
  Pulsus paradoxus *(accentuation of normal drop in arterial blood pressure with inspiration).*
  Distant/muffled heart sounds *(due to distention in pericardial sac).*
  Sinus tachycardia related to compensatory catecholamine release.
  Jugular venous distention. *(The venous pulse may rise to 15-20 cm water due to reduced circulating volume).*
  Cardiac tamponade is a life-threatening condition. Early assessment of reduced cardiac output facilitates early emergency treatment.
- Assess mental status. *Symptoms may range from anxiety to altered level of consciousness in shock.*
- Monitor chest tube drainage. *Sudden cessation of drainage suggests clot.*
▲ Assist with performance of echocardiogram if time permits. *Provides most helpful diagnostic information. Effusions seen with acute tamponade are usually smaller than with chronic. However, in light of circulatory collapse, treatment may be indicated before the echocardiogram can be performed.*
▲ If patient is in an ICU setting, assess hemodynamic profile using pulmonary artery catheter; assess for equalization of pressures. *The RAP, RVDP, PADP, and PCWP pressures are all elevated in tamponade, and within 2-3 mm Hg of each other. These pressures confirm diagnosis.*

THERAPEUTIC INTERVENTIONS

If cardiac tamponade is secondary to a slowly developing effusion and the patient's compensatory mechanisms are maintaining temporary cardiovascular stability:
- Anticipate transfer to ICU.
▲ Initiate O$_2$ therapy *to maximize O$_2$ saturation.*
▲ Administer parenteral fluids as ordered. *Optimal state of hydration will increase venous return and therefore cardiac output.*
▲ Type and cross match as ordered. Anticipate blood product replacement *to correct any existing alterations in hematology or coagulation factors.*
- Place patient in Fowler's position (unless condition requires supine).

Continued.

Cardiac and Vascular Care Plans

NURSING DIAGNOSES	EXPECTED OUTCOMES AND NURSING INTERVENTIONS / *RATIONALE* (■ = INDEPENDENT; ▲ = COLLABORATIVE)

THERAPEUTIC INTERVENTIONS— cont'd

In ICU:

▲ Maintain IV access. *Aggressive fluid resuscitation may be required to raise venous pressure above pericardial pressure.*

▲ Assemble equipment for pericardiocentesis. *Indicated when systolic BP is reduced more than 30 mm from baseline. However, if patient can be stabilized, drainage of fluid should be delayed until surgical or open resection/drainage can be performed. Pericardiocentesis should be performed under sterile conditions.*

▲ Have emergency resuscitative equipment and medications readily available. *Bedside pericardiocentesis can be a high-risk, though life-saving procedure. Complications include pneumothorax, and myocardial or coronary artery lacerations.*

If cardiac tamponade is rapidly developing (as in trauma or as a complication of cardiac surgery) with cardiovascular decompensation and collapse:

▲ Maintain aggressive fluid resuscitation.

▲ Administer vasopressor agents (dopamine hydrochloride, norepinephrine bitartrate [Levophed bitartrate]) as ordered *to maximize systemic perfusion pressure to vital organs.*

▲ Assemble open chest tray for bedside intervention; prepare patient for transport to surgery. *Acute tamponade is a life-threatening complication, but immediate prognosis is good with fast, effective treatment. Open resection and drainage should be performed in a sterile environment.*

If acute tamponade reoccurs and repeated pericardiocentesis fails to prevent such, anticipate surgical pericardiotomy or resection of a portion of the pericardium.

Impaired Gas Exchange

RELATED TO

Decreased blood flow to lungs
Decreased respiratory drive secondary to cerebral hypoxia
Decreased vital capacity secondary to fluid in mediastinum
Chest trauma

DEFINING CHARACTERISTICS

Tachypnea early; decreased respiratory rate or respiratory arrest later
Hypoxia
Hypercapnia
Restlessness
Somnolence
Dusky nailbeds
Pneumothorax or hemothorax may also be associated with chest trauma

EXPECTED OUTCOMES

Patient manifests normal ABGs.
Patient breathes easily without dyspnea.

ONGOING ASSESSMENT

· Assess airway and efficacy of breathing.

▲ Assess arterial blood gases. *Reduced pO_2 and O_2 saturation are early signs of impaired gas exchange. Increased pCO_2 follows later.*

· Assess changes in level of consciousness (LOC). *Restlessness and anxiety can be early signs of cerebral hypoxia.*

If chest trauma is present:

▲ Assess and evaluate x-ray stability of bony structures of thorax.

· Assess for subcutaneous emphysema, *which is a sign of pneumothorax.*

THERAPEUTIC INTERVENTIONS

· Have airway and intubation equipment at bedside.

· Have suction equipment available.

· Avoid sedation. *Although patient may appear agitated and anxious, sedation would further compromise cardiopulmonary status.*

▲ Anticipate use of supplemental O_2 to maximize O_2 saturation of circulating blood volume. *Positive-pressure O_2 must not be used because it will increase intrapericardial pressure and aggravate the tamponade.*

▲ Notify anesthesiologist and respiratory therapy of potential need for intubation and mechanical ventilation.

· If indicated, institute Mechanical ventilation, p. 202.

▲ Anticipate chest tube insertion if pneumothorax or hemothorax are present.

▲ In the event of cardiopulmonary arrest, open chest massage is indicated if sternum or ribs are unstable *to prevent further trauma to heart, lungs, and vasculature.*

Anxiety/Fear

RELATED TO

Unfamiliar environment
Chest pain
Dyspnea
Invasive procedures

EXPECTED OUTCOMES

Patient appears as relaxed as situation warrants.
Patient verbalizes trust in health care providers.

ONGOING ASSESSMENT

· Assess patient's level of anxiety. *Acute tamponade is a life-threatening condition. The patient may also sense anxiety on the part of staff.*

| NURSING DIAGNOSES | EXPECTED OUTCOMES AND NURSING INTERVENTIONS / *RATIONALE* (■ = INDEPENDENT; ▲ = COLLABORATIVE) |

DEFINING CHARACTERISTICS

Sympathetic stimulation
Restlessness
Increased questioning
Uncooperative behavior
Avoids looking at equipment
  or keeps vigilant watch over
  equipment

THERAPEUTIC INTERVENTIONS

- Maintain a calm, supportive environment during evaluation and acute intervention.
- Remain with patient as much as possible. *Presence provides support.*
- Prepare patient for transfer to ICU if appropriate. *Fear of unknown increases catecholamine release, which can aggravate condition.*
- Explain procedure and equipment (pericardiocentesis, Swan-Ganz catheter placement).
- Institute treatment, see Anxiety, p. 5.

Knowledge Deficit

RELATED TO

New procedures/equipment
Unfamiliarity with disease process

DEFINING CHARACTERISTICS

Questioning
Verbalized misconceptions
Lack of questions

See also:
Infection, high risk for, p. 40
Chest Pain, p. 49

EXPECTED OUTCOMES

Patient/significant others verbalize a basic understanding of disease process and therapy.

ONGOING ASSESSMENT

- Assess knowledge of cardiac anatomy and physiology.
- Assess patient's/significant others' physical/emotional readiness to learn. *During the acute stages family or significant others may require the most teaching. This will minimize their feelings of helplessness and assist them in providing support to patient.*

THERAPEUTIC INTERVENTIONS

- When appropriate, provide information about:
    Disease process and rationale for prescribed therapy. *This will help allay anxiety.*
    Follow-up care.

By: Donna McDonald, RN, BS, CCRN
    Carol Ruback, RN, MSN, CCRN
    Meg Gulanick, RN, PhD

Thrombolytic therapy in myocardial infarction

t-PA; STREPTOKINASE; UROKINASE, EMINASE; ANISOYLATED PLASMIN STREPTOKINASE ACTIVATOR COMPLEX (APSAC)

Thrombolytic agents are drugs that activate the fibrinolytic system to dissolve fibrin clots. Thrombolytic therapy is used in the management of acute myocardial infarction secondary to coronary artery thrombus formation. Eighty to 90% of acute MIs are secondary to thrombus formation. Treatment with thrombolytic agents in the early hours of MI restores perfusion to jeopardized myocardium, thereby reducing the progressive ischemia, salvaging myocardium and reducing mortality. Several thrombolytic agents are available: streptokinase, urokinase, tissue plasminogen activator (tPA), and anisoylated plasmin streptokinase activator complex (APSAC).

| NURSING DIAGNOSES | EXPECTED OUTCOMES AND NURSING INTERVENTIONS / *RATIONALE* (■ = INDEPENDENT; ▲ = COLLABORATIVE) |

Chest Pain

RELATED TO

Myocardial infarction

DEFINING CHARACTERISTICS

Patient reports pain
Restlessness, apprehension
Moaning, crying
Facial mask of pain
Diaphoresis
↑ HR, ↑ B/P

EXPECTED OUTCOMES

Patient verbalizes relief of pain.
Patient appears relaxed and comfortable.

ONGOING ASSESSMENT

- Assess for characteristics of myocardial pain: (see Myocardial infarction, p. 132).
- Assess whether chest pain is less than 6 hr in duration. *Necrosis begins in the endocardium after 20 min of ischemia; transmural necrosis is complete between 4 to 6 hr; thus early intervention may limit infarct size, preserve left ventricular function, and ultimately prolong life.*
- Verify if ECG changes are consistent with acute myocardial infarction: ST-segment elevations in at least two contiguous ECG leads.

Continued.

Cardiac and Vascular Care Plans

NURSING DIAGNOSES	EXPECTED OUTCOMES AND NURSING INTERVENTIONS / *RATIONALE* (▪ = INDEPENDENT; ▲ = COLLABORATIVE)

ONGOING ASSESSMENT—cont'd

- Assess for contraindications to thrombolytic agents. *Thrombolytic agents will not distinguish a pathologic occlusive coronary thrombus from a protective hemostatic clot, therefore patient selection is critical.* Patients with absolute contraindications include those with:
  - History of cerebrovascular accident (CVA).
  - Severe uncontrolled hypertension (SBP >200 mm Hg; DBP >115 mm Hg).
  - Active internal bleeding.
  - Known bleeding disorder.
  - Recent (within 2 mo) intracranial or intraspinal surgery.
  - Recent major surgery or trauma.
  - Recent prolonged CPR (>10 minutes), organ biopsy or puncture involving noncompressible vessel.
- Assess for other relative contraindications. *With the following conditions, the risks of thrombolytic agents must be weighed against the anticipated benefits.*
  - Unknown or suspected pregnancy.
  - High likelihood of heart thrombus (seen in dilated cardiomyopathy, left ventricular aneurysm, mitral stenosis with atrial fibrillation).
  - Oral anticoagulant use.
  - Hemorrhagic opthalmic condition.
  - Hemostatic defects secondary to severe hepatic/renal dysfunction.
- If streptokinase type agent is to be used:
  - Assess for previous strep infection or previous administration of streptokinase. *Streptokinase and APSAC (Eminase) are derived from β-hemolytic streptococci; previous exposure will have activated the patient's immune system; thus streptokinase administration may trigger allergic reaction.*
  - Assess for allergic reaction during infusion.
  - Monitor BP closely during infusion. *Hypotension is a side effect of all thrombolytics.*
- After thrombolytic medication is injected/infused, assess for evidence of reperfusion. *Successful reperfusion manifests as relief of chest pain, normalization of ST segments, reperfusion dysrhythmias (primarily ventricular), and early peaking of CPK (wash out secondary to rapid reinfusion into the circulation of enzymes released by damaged myocardial cells following restoration of blood flow).*

THERAPEUTIC INTERVENTIONS

▲ Administer test dose of sublingual nitroglycerin (NTG) tablet *to rule out angina. Stable angina does not involve thrombus formation; therefore, thrombolytic therapy is contraindicated.*

▲ Institute measures to relieve pain. See Myocardial infarction: acute phase (1-3 days), p. 132.

▲ Before streptokinase/eminase administration, give hydrocortisone, 100 mg IVP, and Bendadryl, 50 mg IVP, as prescribed *as prophylaxis for allergic reaction.*

▲ Administer thrombolytic agent (t-PA, streptokinase, or urokinase) per unit protocol. *May be intracoronary, IV push and/or continuous drip. IV therapy is preferred because it is fastest.*

▲ For IV infusion, ensure complete dosage administration by adding 10-20 cc of 0.9 NS to empty IV bag or bottle and infuse at current rate to "flush" tubing.

▲ If signs of reperfusion are not evident and the patient continues to infarct, prepare for possible cardiac catheterization, PTCA, or coronary artery bypass grafting.

High Risk for Injury: Bleeding

RISK FACTORS

Dissolution of protective hemostatic clots
Heparin therapy

EXPECTED OUTCOMES

Risk for bleeding is reduced through preventive measures, early assessment, and intervention.

ONGOING ASSESSMENT

- Monitor for signs of bleeding: puncture sites, gingiva, prior cuts. *All agents except tPA have systemic effects.*
- Observe for presence of occult or frank blood in urine, stool, emesis, and sputum.
- Monitor for signs of internal bleeding: ↑ HR, ↓ B/P, restlessness, ↓ UO.
- Postcatheterization, assess patient for retroperitoneal bleeding. *Low back pain, numbness of lower extremities, and diminishing pedal pulses are signs of retroperitoneal bleeding.*
- Assess for intracranial bleeding by frequent monitoring of neurologic status. *Confusion, visual disturbances, and headaches are frequent signs of intracranial bleeding.*
▲ Assess Hgb/Hct, fibrinogen, and PTT levels. *Need to monitor coagulation studies to determine expected changes with thrombolytics vs. bleeding.*

Thrombolytic Therapy in Myocardial Infarction

THERAPEUTIC INTERVENTIONS

To prevent bleeding:
▲ Establish all IVs before therapy: *2-3 lines are started in case of later need.*
- Avoid noncompressible IV access sites (subclavian, internal jugular). *Any interruption of vascular integrity may cause bleeding secondary to patient's temporary inability to form a hemostatic clot.*
▲ Insert a heparin lock device with a stopcock *to obtain venous blood samples without additional venipuncture.*
- Avoid unnecessary arterial or venous punctures or IM injections.
▲ Avoid discontinuing any arterial/venous lines during thrombolytic infusion and 24 hr after therapy. *The catheters will occlude the puncture sites until coagulation proteins are restored.*
- If arterial/venous puncture is unavoidable, use small-gauge (i.e., 25-gauge) needle and apply direct pressure to all arterial/venous puncture sites for 30 min. Apply pressure dressing to all arterial/venous puncture sites.
▲ Administer prophylactic antiulcer therapy (Mylanta, Tagamet, Zantac, Sucralfate) as ordered *to reduce risk of bleeding from gastritis or stress ulcer (may develop in response to acute MI event).*
▲ Obtain type and cross match before therapy as prescribed.
Management of *minor* bleeding (superficial):
- Apply direct pressure *to control bleeding. Minor bleeding is to be expected.*
- Gingival bleeding: assist patient with rinsing mouth using ice water *to provide comfort and cause vasoconstriction.*
▲ Continue medication, infusions; monitor patient.
Management of *major* bleeding (frank, GI, intracranial, retroperitoneal):
▲ Discontinue thrombolytic agent infusion.
▲ Discontinue heparin infusion. Administer protamine sulfate *to reverse anticoagulant effect of heparin.*
▲ Administer IV fluids as ordered.
▲ Anticipate blood product replacement.

High Risk for Decreased Cardiac Output

RISK FACTORS
Reperfusion dysrhythmias

EXPECTED OUTCOMES
Patient maintains adequate cardiac output, as evidenced by strong pulses, baseline blood pressure, warm dry skin, and alert mentation.

ONGOING ASSESSMENT
- Monitor ECG for reperfusion dysrhythmias. *These frequently but not always occur when the artery is reopened. Common reperfusion dysrhythmias include: accelerated idioventricular rhythm (most common), ventricular tachycardia, premature ventricular contractions, sinus bradycardia, and AV block.*
- Assess for signs of reduced cardiac output that may accompany dysrhythmia: ↓ B/P, dizziness, change in mental status, cool skin, shortness of breath, and ↑ JVD.

THERAPEUTIC INTERVENTIONS
▲ Administer prophylactic lidocaine before initiation of thrombolytic therapy *to prevent ventricular ectopy:*
 Lidocaine bolus, 1 mg/kg, as ordered; may repeat *Dose adjusted for advanced age/ liver disease.*
 Lidocaine continuous infusion, 2-4 mg/min, as ordered.
▲ Keep atropine sulfate at bedside *for treatment of bradyarrhythmias commonly associated with reperfusion of right coronary artery (inferior wall MI).*
▲ Have emergency resusitative equipment and medications readily available. *Any arrhythmia can decompensate into an unstable rhythm such as ventricular tachycardia or ventricular fibrillation with an accompanying compromise in cardiac output.*
- Initiate treatment for Cardiac output, decreased, p. 12; Cardiac dysrhythmias, p. 114.

High Risk for Chest Pain

RISK FACTORS
Reocculsion of coronary artery (rethrombosis of infarct-related artery) after successful thrombolysis

EXPECTED OUTCOMES
Patient remains pain free.
If chest pain recurs, it will be treated promptly.

ONGOING ASSESSMENT
- Assess for complaints of myocardial pain. *Reocclusion occurs in about 12%-15% of cases.*
- Assess ECG for ST-segment elevation.
▲ Assess PT/PTT every day and 4-6 hr after any change in heparin dose.

Continued.

Cardiac and Vascular Care Plans

NURSING DIAGNOSES	EXPECTED OUTCOMES AND NURSING INTERVENTIONS / *RATIONALE* (■ = INDEPENDENT; ▲ = COLLABORATIVE)

	THERAPEUTIC INTERVENTIONS
	Prevention:
	▲ Maintain infusion of thrombolytic agent at appropriate dose and rate.
	▲ Administer heparin therapy as ordered. *Concomitant use of heparin reduces risk of re-occlusion and thrombosis of infarct-related artery (may develop in response to re-exposure of vessel injury after thrombolysis). Length of administration varies among protocols from 1 vs. 3 vs. 5 days.*
	▲ Titrate heparin to maintain PTT at 1.5-2 times control value.
	▲ Administer antiplatelet agents (aspirin, Persantine) as ordered *to prevent platelet aggregation and subsequent clot formation.*
	Recurrence of ischemia:
	· Notify physician of return of any signs and symptoms of myocardial ischemia.
	▲ Obtain 12-lead ECG.
	▲ Administer appropriate pharmacologic therapy for treatment of pain (nitrates, morphine sulfate, etc). See Myocardial infarction: acute phase (1-3 days), p. 132.
	▲ Prepare patient for possible emergency procedures:
	    Repeat administration of thrombolytic agent: *to lyse newly formed occlusive thrombus. For Eminase/streptokinase, if readministered more than 5 days after prior Eminase/streptokinase therapy, may not be as effective due to development of antistreptokinase antibody.*
	    Cardiac catheterization: *to evaluate and diagnose underlying pathology responsible for recurrent myocardial ischemia.*
	    PTCA: *to reduce residual stenosis and improve blood flow.*
	    CABG: *to bypass occluded artery.*

Knowledge Deficit **RELATED TO** New treatment of acute MI Unfamiliarity with disease process, treatment, recovery **DEFINING CHARACTERISTICS** Multiple questions or lack of questions Confusion about events Expressed need for more information	**EXPECTED OUTCOMES** Patient/significant others verbalizes understanding of patient's condition, healing process of MI, need for observation in CCU, diagnosis of MI, and treatment with thrombolytic agents. **ONGOING ASSESSMENT** · Assess knowledge of thrombolytic therapy. **THERAPEUTIC INTERVENTIONS** · Explain indications for and benefits and risks of thrombolytic therapy. · Inform patient of possible surface bleeding and bruising as minor side effects. · Instruct patient to report recurrence of chest pain. · Inform patient of need for frequent inspection for bleeding, VS, and cardiac monitoring. · Provide information on recovery from MI. See Myocardial infarction: acute phase (1-3 days), p. 132. *The patient has experienced an MI and will have the same educational needs as one experiencing an MI managed without thrombolytic therapy.*

By: Anne Paglinawan, RN, BSN

Thrombophlebitis

DEEP VEIN THROMBOSIS (DVT); PHLEBITIS;
PHLEBOTHROMBOSIS

Thrombophlebitis is the inflammation of the wall of a vein, usually resulting in the formation of a blood clot (thrombosis) that may partially or completely block the flow of blood through the vessel. Venous thrombophlebitis usually occurs in the lower extremities. It may occur in superficial veins, which, though painful, are not life-threatening and do not require hospitalization, or it may occur in a deep vein that can be life-threatening because clots may break free (embolize) and cause a pulmonary embolism.

NURSING DIAGNOSES	EXPECTED OUTCOMES AND NURSING INTERVENTIONS / *RATIONALE* (■ = INDEPENDENT; ▲ = COLLABORATIVE)

Altered Peripheral Tissue Perfusion

RELATED FACTORS
Venous stasis
Injury to vessel wall
Hypercoagulability of blood

DEFINING CHARACTERISTICS
Deep vein thrombosis (DVT):
　Usually involves femoral, popliteal, or small calf veins
　Pain
　Edema
　Swelling
　Tenderness
　+ Homan's sign (not always reliable)
　May be asymptomatic
Superficial thrombophlebitis:
　Usually involves saphenous vein
　Aching and swelling, usually localized into a "knot" or "bump"
　A firm mass may be palpable along vein
　Redness
　Warmth
　Tenderness
　May be asymptomatic

EXPECTED OUTCOMES
Patient has adequate blood flow to extremity, as evidenced by warm skin and absence of edema and pain.
Patient does not experience pulmonary embolism as evidenced by normal breathing, normal heart rate, and absence of chest pain.

ONGOING ASSESSMENT
- Assess for signs and symptoms of superficial versus deep vein thrombosis (see Defining characteristics). *Differentiation is important because treatment goals are different.*
- Assess for contributing factors: immobility, leg trauma, varicose veins, pregnancy, obesity, surgery, malignancy, and use of oral contraceptives. *Many patients are asymptomatic. Knowledge of high-risk situations aids in early detection.*
- With deep vein thrombosis, measure circumference of affected leg with a tape measure. *This is to document progression or resolution of swelling.*
- ▲ Monitor results of blood flow studies *to document location of clot and status of affected vein.*
　Doppler ultrasound—*uses Doppler probe to document reduced flow, especially in popliteal and iliofemoral veins.*
　Impedance plethysmography—*uses blood pressure cuffs to record changes in venous flow.*
　Radionuclide scan—*uses radioactive injection (e.g., fibrinogen) followed by scanning to localize areas of obstructed blood flow.*
　Venography—*uses radiopaque contrast media injected through foot vein to localize thrombi in deep venous system.*
- ▲ Monitor coagulation profile (PT/PTT). *Hospitalized patient are treated with anticoagulants.*
- Observe for side effects of anticoagulant therapy (see next diagnosis).

THERAPEUTIC INTERVENTIONS
For deep vein thrombosis: *goal is prevention of emboli and relief of discomfort.*
- Encourage and maintain bedrest with affected leg elevated. *Elevation of leg will reduce venous pooling and edema and prevent further clot formation.*
- Provide warm moist heat. *Heat will relieve pain and inflammation.*
- ▲ Apply elastic stockings as prescribed *to promote venous blood flow and decrease venous stagnation.* Ensure that stockings are of correct size and are applied correctly. *Inaccurately applied stockings can serve as a tourniquet and can facilitate clot formation.*
- ▲ Administer analgesics as indicated. *Analgesics will relieve pain and promote comfort.*
- ▲ Administer and monitor anticoagulant therapy as ordered (heparin/warfarin [Coumadin]). *Therapy will prevent further clot formation by decreasing normal activity of clotting mechanism.*
- Use mechanical infusion device *to ensure accurate dosing and prevention of adverse effects of anticoagulant medications.*
- ▲ Anticipate thrombolytic therapy *to dissolve the clot if diagnosed within 3 days of acute occlusion. Lysis carries a higher risk of bleeding than anticoagulation. Therefore, the use is restricted to patients with severe embolism that significantly compromises blood flow to tissues.*

Continued.

Cardiac and Vascular Care Plans

NURSING DIAGNOSES	EXPECTED OUTCOMES AND NURSING INTERVENTIONS / *RATIONALE* (■ = INDEPENDENT; ▲ = COLLABORATIVE)

THERAPEUTIC INTERVENTIONS— cont'd

▲ Maintain adequate hydration. *Hydration prevents increased viscosity of blood.*

▲ If patient shows no response to conventional therapy, or if patient is not a candidate for anticoagulation, anticipate surgical treatment: (a) thrombectomy to excise the clot if a major vein is occluded, or (b) placement of a vena cava filter *to trap any migrating clots and prevent pulmonary embolism.*

For superficial veins: *goal is symptomatic relief.*

· Explain that hospitalization is not usually required.

· Instruct patient on need for bedrest at home with legs elevated. *(May require 2-3 days.)*

· Instruct patient to apply warm moist heat and/or take warm baths. *Warm moist heat will relieve pain.*

· Explain schedule for nonsteroidal anti-inflammatory medications as ordered. *Medications will reduce swelling and promote comfort.*

▲ Provide analgesics are prescribed.

· Instruct patient on use of support stockings. *Stockings will promote venous return and provide comfort.*

· Explain that surgical ligation of the veins may be indicated if therapy attempted is ineffective.

High Risk for Injury

RISK FACTORS

Heparin therapy

EXPECTED OUTCOMES

Patient maintains therapeutic blood level of anticoagulant, as evidenced by PTT within desired range.

ONGOING ASSESSMENT

▲ Monitor for adverse effects of "too much heparin" *to reduce risk of bleeding.*

    Increase in bleeding from sites (e.g., GI and GU tracts, IV sites, respiratory tract, wounds).

    Development of new purpura, petechiae, or hematomas.

    Bone and joint pain.

    Mental status changes *indicating an intracranial bleed.*

    PTT >2-$2\frac{1}{2}$ times normal.

▲ Monitor for adverse effects of "too little heparin" *to prevent clot formation.*

    Continued evidence of further clot formation (newly developed signs of pulmonary embolus or peripheral thromboemboli).

    PTT below desired level.

THERAPEUTIC INTERVENTIONS

· Ensure that infusion is not interrupted (e.g., infiltrated IV, malfunctioning infusion device. *This will maintain therapeutic blood level of anticoagulant.*

▲ Re-evaluate heparin dose and administer it as prescribed.

▲ If bleeding occurs, stop heparin infusion as prescribed.

Knowledge Deficit

RELATED TO

Unfamiliarity with pathology, treatment, and prevention

DEFINING CHARACTERISTICS

Multiple questions
Lack of questions
Misconceptions

EXPECTED OUTCOMES

Patient and/or significant others verbalize understanding of disease, management, and prevention.

ONGOING ASSESSMENT

· Assess understanding of causes, treatment, and prevention plan. *Patients with superficial thromboses will be treated at home and must understand treatment plan. Both types of thrombophlebitis may recur.*

THERAPEUTIC INTERVENTIONS

· Explain conditions that place people at risk for blood clots:

    Persons with varicose veins.

    Pregnancy.

    Obesity.

    Surgery (especially pelvic or abdominal).

    Immobility.

    Advanced age.

· Explain the rationale for treatment differences between superficial and deep vein thrombosis:

    Superficial thrombosis treated at home with supportive care, symptom relief.

    Deep vein thromboses may be life-threatening and require additional treatment with anticoagulation.

NURSING DIAGNOSES	EXPECTED OUTCOMES AND NURSING INTERVENTIONS / *RATIONALE* (■ = INDEPENDENT; ▲ = COLLABORATIVE)

THERAPEUTIC INTERVENTIONS— cont'd

- Explain need for bedrest and elevation of leg. *Bedrest and elevation of leg prevents embolization with deep vein thrombosis.*
- Instruct patient on correct application of support stockings. *Stockings applied incorrectly can act as a tourniquet and "facilitate" clot formation.*
- Instruct patient to avoid rubbing or massaging calf. *Avoidance will prevent breaking off clot, which may circulate as embolus.*
- For patients with deep vein thrombosis, instruct on signs of pulmonary embolus:
    Sudden chest pain.
    Tachypnea.
    Tachycardia.
    Shortness of breath.
    Restlessness. *Can be caused by a clot that breaks off from original clot in leg and travels to lungs.*
- Discuss preventive measures to prevent recurrence:
    Avoiding staying in one position for long periods. *Avoidance will prevent venous stasis (at home, on train or plane, at desk).*
    Not sitting with legs crossed.
    Maintaining ideal body weight. *This will reduce pressure on legs and venous system.*
    Wearing properly sized, correctly applied elastic stockings as prescribed.
    Quitting smoking. *Nicotine is a vasoconstrictor that promotes clotting.*
    Participating in an exercise program. *Exercise promotes circulation.*
    Avoiding constricting garters or socks with tight bands.

See also:
Diversional activity deficit,
  p. 21
Pulmonary embolus, p. 216.

By: Meg Gulanick, RN, PhD
  Gloria Young, RN, BS

Ventricular assist device

LVAD; RVAD; HEARTMATE

Ventricular assist devices (VADs) are flow assistance devices that provide temporary circulatory support for the failing ventricle. The VAD can be inserted in either the right ventricle (RVAD) or left ventricle (LVAD), depending on the site of ventricular failure. They can be used for patients with deteriorating heart failure who are on the waiting list for heart transplant, for acute MI patients with severe left ventricular dysfunction not responsive to traditional therapies, or for cardiac surgery patients who cannot be weaned from cardiopulmonary bypass with an intra-aortic balloon pump and pharmacological therapy. Optimal postoperative nursing management involves awareness of patient's preoperative history, operative course, and potential problems related to both surgical recovery and insertion of the VAD. Some patients have the device in place for only a few days. Others awaiting transplant may have a portable device such as a "Heartmate" that allows patients to ambulate.

NURSING DIAGNOSES	EXPECTED OUTCOMES AND NURSING INTERVENTIONS / *RATIONALE* (■ = INDEPENDENT; ▲ = COLLABORATIVE)

Decreased Cardiac Output

RELATED TO
Myocardial dysfunction
Technical problems with VAD
Dysrhythmias

EXPECTED OUTCOMES
Patient maintains hemodynamic stability as evidenced by adequate CO and BP, strong peripheral pulses, urine output >30 ml/hr, alert, responsive mentation, and warm and dry skin.

Continued.

Ventricular assist device—cont'd

NURSING DIAGNOSES	EXPECTED OUTCOMES AND NURSING INTERVENTIONS / *RATIONALE* (■ = INDEPENDENT; ▲ = COLLABORATIVE)

DEFINING CHARACTERISTICS

Left ventricular failure:
Increased LAP
Increased PAD/PCWP
Tachycardia
Decreased BP
Decreased CO
Sluggish capillary refill
Diminished peripheral
  pulses
Changes in chest x-ray; en-
  larged heart
Crackles
Decreased arterial and ve-
  nous oxygenation
Acidosis
Decreased urine output
Change in mental status

Right ventricular failure:
Increased RAP
Increased CVP
Jugular vein distention
Decreased BP
Decreased CO

ONGOING ASSESSMENT

▲ Monitor hemodynamics for signs of left and/or right ventricular failure (see Defining characteristics).

▲ If only LVAD is in place, monitor for signs of right ventricular dysfunction.

▲ Monitor assist device flows and cardiac output.

· Assess skin color, temperature, and quality and presence of peripheral pulses.

· Monitor strict I & O, daily weights.

· Monitor and document cardiac rhythm for signs of dysrhythmias.

▲ Monitor drug infusion rates as prescribed.

· Monitor VAD tubing for kinks and tension *so perfusion is not compromised.*

· Assess for accurate triggering.

THERAPEUTIC INTERVENTIONS

▲ Maintain hemodynamic parameters as prescribed. *Hemodynamic parameters may be maintained by titration of vasoactive drugs and administration of volume such as crystalloids and/or colloids.*

▲ Administer vasopressors as prescribed:
  Use infusion pump *to ensure accuracy.*
  Administer through central line.
  Keep drug cards at bedside with patient's name, weight, amount of drug, and rate of infusion.
Drugs:
  Dopamine: *increases contractility; increases renal blood flow in low doses.*
  Dobutamine: *increases contractility; may slightly vasodilate.*
  Inocor: *increases contractility and vasodilation.*
  Isoproterenol: *increases HR, contractility; decreases pulmonary resistance for RV failure.*
  Epinephrine: *Strengthens myocardial contractility.* Monitor glucose every q4h while on epinephrine. *Epinephrine raises blood glucose by promoting conversion of glycogen reserves in liver to glucose and inhibiting insulin release in pancreas.*
  Neosynephrine: *Vasoconstricts and increases SVR.*

· Administer vasodilators as prescribed.
  Nitroglycerin: *Dilates coronary vasculature, dilates venous system, prevents coronary spasm.*
  Nitroprusside: *Lowers BP, lowers systemic vascular resistance (SVR). Elevated pressure on new grafts may cause bleeding.*
  Prostaglandin E. *Vasodilates pulmonary vascular bed to reduce pulmonary hypertension and protect right ventricle.*

▲ Maintain assist device flows as prescribed. If left atrial pressure (LAP) is elevated (e.g., >20 mm Hg) may need to increase flow of LVAD *to assist failing left ventricle and maintain LAP within prescribed range.* If RVAD is present, may need to increase flow of RVAD *to maintain RA at prescribed range.*

· Keep VAD tubing in full view. Avoid kinking and pulling tubing. Keep patient's hands in safety restraints or mittened as needed *to prevent disconnection of tubing.*

▲ If dysrhythmias occur, treat according to etiology and protocol. See SCP: Cardiac dysrhythmias, p. 114.

▲ If ventricular tachycardia or fibrillation occurs, defibrillate or cardiovert as indicated. *Countershock can be performed safely with VAD.*

▲ Keep temporary pacemaker at bedside at all times; attach temporary epicardial wires to pacemaker as indicated. *Ectopy usually results from irritability caused by ischemia, electrolytic imbalance, or mechanical irritation.*

▲ If cardiac arrest occurs, anticipate/prepare to open chest for cardiac massage. *Cardiac compressions are always contraindicated because dislodgment of cannula results in rapid exsanguination.*

High Risk for Impaired Gas Exchange

RISK FACTORS

Surgery
Secretions
Pulmonary vascular conges-
  tion

EXPECTED OUTCOMES

Patient maintains optimal gas exchange as evidenced by clear breath sounds, normal respiratory pattern, absence of secretions, and ABGs within normal limits.

ONGOING ASSESSMENT

· Monitor respiratory rate/pattern. *Note: Device noises may make this difficult.*

· Auscultate lung fields.

· Assess for restlessness or changes in mental status. *Hypoxemia results in cerebral hypoxia.*

NURSING DIAGNOSES	EXPECTED OUTCOMES AND NURSING INTERVENTIONS / *RATIONALE* (■ = INDEPENDENT; ▲ = COLLABORATIVE)

ONGOING ASSESSMENT—cont'd

▲ Monitor serial ABGs and O_2 saturation *for hypoxemia.*

▲ Monitor serial x-rays.

▲ Verify that ventilator settings are maintained as prescribed:
   TV 10-15 cc/kg.
   Rate 10-14/min.
   FiO_2 to maintain pO_2 >80 mm.
   PEEP + 5 cm.

▲ Adjust ventilator settings as ordered *to maintain ABGs within accepted limits. PEEP may be increased in increments of 2.5 cm to maintain adequate oxygenation on FiO_2 of 50%. Patients can usually tolerate up to 20 cm H_2O of PEEP if not hypovolemic or hypotensive.*

▪ Suction prn. Hyperventilate and hyperoxygenate patients *to prevent desaturation.*

▲ Administer sedation as needed:
   Morphine sulfate.
   Versed: short-acting central nervous system depressant.
   Pavulon: skeletal muscle relaxant.
   Sedation helps to decrease anxiety (in turn helping decrease myocardial O_2 consumption).

▲ Wean patient from ventilator and extubate as soon as possible.

▪ After extubation, encourage coughing and deep breathing. *Assists in mobilizing secretions.*

▲ Provide supplemental O_2 as indicated.

▪ Encourage dangling/progressive activity as tolerated. *Increases lung volume and ventilation.*

High Risk for Fluid Volume Deficit

RISK FACTORS

Fluid leaks into extravascular spaces

Bleeding caused by coagulopathies from prolonged time on extracorporeal circulation (ECC)

Need for anticoagulation

Diuretics

EXPECTED OUTCOMES

Patient maintains fluid volume sufficient to meet metabolic demands, as evidenced by balanced I and O, normal urine specific gravity, and BP within normal limits.

ONGOING ASSESSMENT

▲ Assess hemodynamics for signs of decreased filling pressure: decreased LAP, CVP, RA, PAD, PCWP, BP, and tachycardia.

▪ Monitor I & O and daily weights. *Total fluid volume may be normal or increased, but because of changes in membrane integrity from extracorporeal circulation during insertion, fluid leaks into extravascular spaces, causing deficit.*

▪ Check for ↑ urine specific gravity.

▪ Assess chest tube drainage and report excess.

▲ Check CBC, PT, PTT, and active clotting time for signs of overcoagulation.

▲ Repeat CBC or spin Hct if bleeding persists.

▲ Monitor electrolytes, BUN, and creatinine.

▪ Assess for obvious postoperative blood loss from sternum or chest tube (if present), and line sites.

THERAPEUTIC INTERVENTIONS

▲ Administer IV fluids as prescribed *to maintain positive fluid balance.*

▲ Maintain patient at prescribed anticoagulation parameter. Notify physician of deviations. *Depending on the type of assist device in use, patients may receive heparin or Dextran initially. In the long term they may require only ASA and/or Persantine.*

▲ Administer coagulation factors/drugs (FFP, platelets, vitamin K, cryoprecipitate, vasopressin) as ordered *to correct deficiencies.*

▲ Use autotransfusion when possible *to minimize use of bank blood.*

▪ Milk chest tubes *to maintain patency. Clotted tubes may precipitate cardiac tamponade.*

High Risk for Infection

RISK FACTORS

Invasive lines, catheters, assist device cannulas

Open chest (sternum is not closed with some devices)

EXPECTED OUTCOMES

Patient shows no signs of infection, as evidenced by absence of fever, no purulent drainage, and no adventitious breath sounds.

ONGOING ASSESSMENT

▪ Assess incisions and central and peripheral line sites for signs and symptoms of infection. *Early identification of infection can facilitate early treatment.*

▪ Monitor temperature.

▲ Assess CBC daily for increased WBC.

Continued.

Ventricular assist device—cont'd

NURSING DIAGNOSES	EXPECTED OUTCOMES AND NURSING INTERVENTIONS / *RATIONALE* (■ = INDEPENDENT; ▲ = COLLABORATIVE)

ONGOING ASSESSMENT— cont'd
- Assess lungs; monitor sputum for signs of infection.
- Monitor urine. *Cloudy, foul-smelling urine indicates infection.*
- ▲ Obtain relevant cultures as indicated.

THERAPEUTIC INTERVENTIONS
- Maintain aseptic technique *to prevent risk of infection.*
- Maintain sterile barrier to chest. Change dressing per unit policy.
- Maintain occlusive dressings to central and peripheral line sites. Change dressing per unit policy.
- Cap open stopcocks; change if contaminated.
- Ensure that central line sites are changed q72h. Rotate peripheral IVs.
- Change IV bags and tubing per unit protocol.
- ▲ Draw blood cultures postoperative day 2, as ordered. If temperature >38.5° C, obtain urine and sputum cultures as indicated.
- ▲ Administer prophylactic antibiotics.
- ▲ Provide respiratory treatments PRN.
- ▲ Discontinue lines and catheters as prescribed as soon as possible. *The are potential sources of infection.*
- Increase activity of patients as tolerated (sitting, ambulating). *Activity serves to mobilize secretions and reduce risk of pneumonia.*

Anxiety/Fear

RELATED TO

Insertion of VAD
Dependence on proper functioning of VAD
Inability to control environment
Uncertain prognosis
Gravity of illness
ICU environment

DEFINING CHARACTERISTICS

Many questions from family
Vigilant watch over equipment
Restlessness
Fear of sleep (if not sedated)
Tearfulness, restlessness
Wide-eyed appearance
Tense appearance

EXPECTED OUTCOMES

Patient appears relaxed and comfortable.
Patient verbalizes ability to cope with situation.
Patient verbalizes concerns/fears.

ONGOING ASSESSMENT
- Assess level of anxiety.
- Assess patient's/family's coping style.

THERAPEUTIC INTERVENTIONS
- Explain purpose/functioning of device as appropriate. Include significant others *to decrease their feelings of helplessness.*
- Display calm, confident manner *to increase feeling of security.*
- Provide continuity of care by assigning staff members experienced in function of assist device *so patient/family feel confident of care rendered.*
- Prevent unnecessary conversations about assist device near patient/family *to increase patient's sense of security.*
- ▲ Keep patient sedated as appropriate.
- Encourage visiting by family or significant others *so patient does not feel alone.*
- Keep family honestly informed of patient's condition.
- ▲ Refer family to crisis intervention if necessary.
- Provide diversional activities if possible.
- Implement stress reduction management techniques.
- ▲ Refer to pastoral care as requested.
- See Anxiety, p. 5.
- If extubated, encourage patient to verbalize feelings.
- Encourage family to bring personal items from home.

High Risk for Decreased Level of Consciousness

RISK FACTORS

Anesthesia effects
Embolization
Inadequate anticoagulation

EXPECTED OUTCOMES

Risk for altered level of consciousness is reduced through early assessment and intervention.

ONGOING ASSESSMENT
- Perform neurologic assessment, noting focal deficit upon awakening, unequal pupils, and abnormal reflexes.
- Check ability to follow commands.
- Observe for signs of seizure activity.
- ▲ Monitor ACT, PT, and PTT.
- ▲ Monitor flow function of assist device. *Reduced perfusion facilitates clot formation.*

NURSING DIAGNOSES	EXPECTED OUTCOMES AND NURSING INTERVENTIONS / *RATIONALE* (■ = INDEPENDENT; ▲ = COLLABORATIVE)

THERAPEUTIC INTERVENTIONS

- Reorient patient to surroundings as needed.
- Regulate anticoagulant as prescribed. *Depending on the type of device in use, patients may require heparin or Dextran initially.*
- Notify surgeon immediately of any changes seen in neurologic assessment.
- See Consciousness, alteration in level of, p. 252.

Knowledge Deficit

RELATED FACTORS

Inexperience with device
Lack of resources

DEFINING CHARACTERISTICS

Many questions
Lack of questions
Verbalized misconceptions

See also:

Nutrition, altered: less than
  body requirements, p. 44
Physical mobility, impaired,
  high risk for, p. 47
Skin integrity, altered, p. 59
Sleep pattern disturbance,
  p. 61
Pain, p. 49

EXPECTED OUTCOMES

Patient verbalizes "working" knowledge of VAD.
Patient verbalizes rationale for ongoing monitoring.
If ambulatory, patient verbalizes troubleshooting/safety procedures required for safe operation.

ONGOING ASSESSMENT

- Assess patient/family's knowledge about device.

THERAPEUTIC INTERVENTIONS

- Provide information on purpose, insertion techniques, and ongoing monitoring.
- Encourage patient to express questions and concerns. *Providing information may reduce anxiety and foster compliance with treatment plan.*
- Prepare patient for the many alarms and machines which he/she will be exposed to in the critical care setting.
- If device is a "bridge to transplant," also provide information on cardiac transplantation as appropriate. *It is important to assess patient readiness for learning about such complex, high-tech, life-threatening treatments.*

By: Linda Kamenjarin, RN, BSN, CCRN
    Meg Gulanick, RN, PhD
    Kathleen L. Grady, RN, PhD

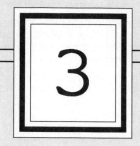

Pulmonary Care Plans

Adult respiratory distress syndrome

(ARDS; SHOCK LUNG; NONCARDIOGENIC PULMONARY EDEMA; ADULT HYALINE MEMBRANE DISEASE; OXYGEN PNEUMONITIS; POST-TRAUMATIC PULMONARY INSUFFICIENCY)

ARDS is a form of respiratory failure that was not recognized as a syndrome until the 1960s, when advances in medical care allowed for prolonged survival of trauma victims who previously would have died. Many causal factors have been related to ARDS (aspiration, trauma, O_2 toxicity, shock, sepsis, disseminated intravascular coagulation (DIC), pancreatitis, etc.), but the exact causative event is unknown. Nursing care must focus upon maintenance of pulmonary function as well as treatment of the causal factor, and even then mortality remains at 50 to 60%.

NURSING DIAGNOSES	EXPECTED OUTCOMES AND NURSING INTERVENTIONS / *RATIONALE* (■ = INDEPENDENT; ▲ = COLLABORATIVE)

Ineffective Breathing Pattern

RELATED FACTORS

Decreased lung compliance:
 Low amounts of surfactant
 Fluid transudation
Fatigue and decreased energy:
 Increased work of breathing
 Primary medical problem

DEFINING CHARACTERISTICS

Dyspnea
Shortness of breath
Tachypnea
Abnormal ABGs
Cyanosis
Cough
Use of accessory muscles

EXPECTED OUTCOMES

Patient maintains optimal breathing pattern, with assistance as appropriate, as evidenced by decreased work of breathing and normal ABGs.

ONGOING ASSESSMENT

- Assess respiratory rate and depth.
- Assess for dyspnea, shortness of breath, cough, and use of accessory muscles. *Initially, respiratory rate increases with the decreasing lung compliance. Work of breathing increases greatly as compliance decreases.*
▲ Assess for cyanosis and monitor ABGs. *As the patient becomes fatigued from the increased work of breathing, he/she may no longer be capable of adequately maintaining his/her own ventilation: CO_2 begins to elevate on ABGs.*

THERAPEUTIC INTERVENTIONS

▲ Maintain the O_2 delivery system applied to the patient *so that the patient does not desaturate.*
- Provide reassurance and allay anxiety:
 Have an agreed-upon method for calling for assistance (e.g., call light or bell).
 Stay with the patient during episodes of respiratory distress. *Air hunger can cause a patient to be extremely anxious.*
▲ Keep physician informed of respiratory status.
▲ Anticipate the need for intubation and mechanical ventilation. *Being prepared for intubation prevents full decompensation of the patient to cardiopulmonary arrest. Early intubation and mechanical ventilation are recommended.*
- See also Mechanical ventilation, p. 202, as appropriate.

Impaired Gas Exchange

RELATED FACTORS

Diffusion defect:
 Hyaline membrane formation
Increased shunting:
 Collapsed alveoli
 Fluid-filled alveoli
Increased dead space:
 Microembolization in the pulmonary vasculature

DEFINING CHARACTERISTICS

Confusion
Somnolence
Restlessness
Irritability
Inability to move secretions
Hypercapnia
Hypoxia

EXPECTED OUTCOMES

Patient maintains optimal gas exchange as evidenced by normal ABGs and alert responsive mentation/or no further reduction in mental status.

ONGOING ASSESSMENT

- Assess respirations, noting quality, rate, pattern, depth, and breathing effort.
- Assess breath sounds and note changes.
▲ Monitor chest radiograph reports. *Keep in mind that radiographic studies of lung water lag behind clinical presentation by 24 hr.*
- Assess for changes in orientation and behavior.
▲ Closely monitor ABGs and note changes.
▲ Use pulse oximetry *to monitor O_2 saturation and pulse rate continuously. Keep alarms on at all times. Pulse oximetry has been found to be a useful tool in the clinical setting to detect changes in oxygenation.*

THERAPEUTIC INTERVENTIONS

▲ Use a team approach in planning care with the physician and respiratory therapist. *Timely and accurate communication of assessments is a must to keep pace with the needed ventilator setting changes: F_iO_2 and PEEP.*
▲ Administer sedation, as prescribed, *to decrease patient's energy expenditure during mechanical ventilation and to deliver adequate positive pressure.*
- Combine nursing actions (i.e., bath, bed, and dressing changes) and intersperse with rest periods *to minimize energy expended by patient and to prevent a decreased O_2 saturation. Temporarily discontinue activity if saturation drops, to decrease O_2 consumption,* and make any necessary F_iO_2, PEEP, or sedation changes *to improve saturation.*
- Change patient's position q2h *to facilitate movement and drainage of secretions.*
- Suction as needed *to clear secretions.*

Continued.

Adult respiratory distress syndrome cont'd

NURSING DIAGNOSES	EXPECTED OUTCOMES AND NURSING INTERVENTIONS / *RATIONALE* (■ = INDEPENDENT; ▲ = COLLABORATIVE)

High Risk for Decreased Cardiac Output

RISK FACTOR

Positive pressure ventilation

EXPECTED OUTCOMES

Patient achieves adequate cardiac output as evidenced by strong peripheral pulses, normal vital signs, urine output > 30 ml/hr, and warm dry skin.

ONGOING ASSESSMENT

▲ Assess vital signs and hemodynamic pressures (CVP, pulmonary artery pressures) q1h; with changes in positive pressure ventilation; and with changes in inotrope administration.

▲ Obtain cardiac output measurement, after positive pressure ventilation changes and with inotrope administration change. *Mechanical ventilation decreases venous return to the heart (preload), which decreases cardiac output. As positive pressure ventilation is increased, the changes in pressure will further impede venous return. There is no absolute value for maximum PEEP. This must be individualized for each patient to maintain cardiac output at optimal PEEP levels. In addition, ABGs must be closely monitored.*

· Monitor urine output with Foley catheter. *Oliguria is a classic sign of inadequate renal perfusion.*

· Assess skin warmth and quality of peripheral pulses.

THERAPEUTIC INTERVENTIONS

▲ Administer inotropic agents as prescribed, noting response and observing for side effects.

▲ Administer IV fluids, as prescribed, *to maintain optimal fluid balance.*

· Anticipate need to decrease level of PEEP *to range that allows improved cardiac output,* if fluid administration and inotropes are not successful.

· See also Decreased cardiac output, p. 12. as necessary.

High Risk for Injury: Barotrauma

RISK FACTORS

Positive-pressure ventilation
Decreased pulmonary compliance

EXPECTED OUTCOMES

Potential for injury from barotrauma is reduced as a result of ongoing assessment and early intervention.

ONGOING ASSESSMENT

· Assess for signs of barotrauma q1h: crepitus, subcutaneous emphysema, altered chest excursion, asymmetrical chest, abnormal ABGs, shift in trachea, restlessness, evidence of pneumothorax on chest radiograph. *Frequent assessments are needed since barotrauma can occur at any time and the patient will not show signs of dyspnea, shortness of breath, or tachypnea if heavily sedated to maintain ventilation.*

▲ Monitor chest radiograph reports daily and obtain a stat portable chest radiograph if barotrauma suspected.

THERAPEUTIC INTERVENTIONS

▲ Notify physician of signs of barotrauma immediately.

▲ Anticipate need for chest tube placement, and prepare as needed. *If barotrauma is suspected, intervention must follow immediately to prevent tension pneumothorax.*

Impaired Physical Mobility

RELATED FACTORS

Acute respiratory failure
Monitoring devices
Mechanical ventilation

DEFINING CHARACTERISTICS

Imposed restrictions of movement
Decreased muscle strength
Limited range of motion (ROM)

EXPECTED OUTCOMES

Patient's optimal physical mobility is maintained.

ONGOING ASSESSMENT

· Assess for imposed restrictions of movement. *Patients with ARDS initially are bedridden and may have multiple IV sites, which, depending on their location, may limit movement. In addition, the patient who is intubated and ventilated is restricted by the ventilator tubing and may need bilateral wrist restraints, as well, to prevent dislodgment or self-extubation.*

· Assess muscle strength.

· Assess range of motion of extremities.

THERAPEUTIC INTERVENTIONS

· Turn and reposition patient q2h.

· Maintain limbs in functional alignment (with pillows). Support feet in dorsiflexed position *to prevent footdrop.*

· Perform/assist with passive ROM exercises to extremities *to prevent contractures.*

NURSING DIAGNOSES	EXPECTED OUTCOMES AND NURSING INTERVENTIONS / *RATIONALE* (■ = INDEPENDENT; ▲ = COLLABORATIVE)

THERAPEUTIC INTERVENTIONS—cont'd

▲ Initiate activity increases (dangling, sitting in chair, ambulation) as condition allows. *The pulmonary changes with ARDS may result in activity intolerance, so oxygen saturation via pulse oximetry should be monitored closely with any increase in activity.*

High Risk for Impaired Skin Integrity

RISK FACTORS

Prolonged bed rest
Immobility
Sensory deficit
Altered vasomotor tone
Altered nutritional state
Prolonged intubation

EXPECTED OUTCOMES

Patient's skin integrity is maintained as a result of ongoing assessment and early intervention.

ONGOING ASSESSMENT

- Assess bony prominences for signs of threatened or actual breakdown of skin.
- Assess around endotracheal (ET) tube for crusting of secretions, redness, or irritation.
- Assess for signs of skin breakdown beneath ET-securing tape.

THERAPEUTIC INTERVENTIONS

- Turn and reposition patient q2h.
- Institute prophylactic use of pressure-relieving devices.
- Maintain skin integrity:
     If patient is nasally intubated, notify physician if skin is red or irritated or breakdown is noted.
     If patient is orally intubated, the tube should be repositioned from side to side q24-48h *(this will help prevent pressure necrosis on the lower lip).*
- Provide mouth care q2h.
- Keep ET tube free of crusting of secretions.
- See also Skin integrity, impaired, p. 59 (as needed)

Knowledge Deficit

RELATED FACTORS

New equipment
New environment
New condition

DEFINING CHARACTERISTICS

Increased frequency of questions posed by patient and significant others
Inability to respond correctly to questions

EXPECTED OUTCOMES

Patient/significant others demonstrate understanding of serious nature of disease and treatment regimen.

ONGOING ASSESSMENT

- Evaluate understanding of ARDS.

THERAPEUTIC INTERVENTIONS

- Explain all procedures to patient before performing them. *This will help decrease patient's anxiety. Fear of unknown can make patient extremely anxious, uncooperative.*
- Orient patient and significant others to ICU surroundings, routines, equipment alarms, and noises. *The ICU is a busy environment that can be very upsetting to patient/significant others.*
- Keep the patient/significant others informed of current patient status. *ARDS is a very serious syndrome with high mortality rates. Significant others must be informed of changes that occur.*

See also:
Nutrition: less than body requirements, p. 44.
Activity Intolerance, p. 2.
Anxiety, p. 5.
Pain/Discomfort, p. 49.

By: Susan Galanes, RN, MS, CCRN

Bronchial asthma (status asthmaticus)

A clinical syndrome characterized by an increased responsiveness of the tracheobronchial tree to a variety of stimuli. This results in paroxysmal dyspnea accompanied by adventitious sounds (wheezing) caused by swelling and spasm of bronchial tubes. This reversible condition is commonly precipitated by antigen-antibody reactions, respiratory infection, cold weather, physical exertion, emotions, and some drugs.

NURSING DIAGNOSES	EXPECTED OUTCOMES AND NURSING INTERVENTIONS / *RATIONALE* (■ = INDEPENDENT; ▲ = COLLABORATIVE)

Ineffective Breathing Pattern

RELATED FACTORS

Swelling and spasm of the bronchial tubes in response to allergies, drugs, stress, infection, inhaled irritants

DEFINING CHARACTERISTICS

Dyspnea
Tachypnea
Cyanosis
Cough
Nasal flaring
Wheezing
Respiratory depth changes
Use of accessory muscles
Prolonged expiratory phase

EXPECTED OUTCOMES

Patient maintains optimal breathing pattern as evidenced by regular respiratory rate/pattern and eupnea.

ONGOING ASSESSMENT

- Assess respiratory rate and depth; monitor breathing pattern. *Respiratory rate and rhythm changes can be an early warning sign to impending respiratory difficulties.*
- Assess for dyspnea, use of accessory muscles, retractions, and flaring of nostrils.
- Assess relationship of inspiration to expiration.
▲ Monitor peak expiratory flow rates and forced expiratory volumes as obtained per the respiratory therapist. *The severity of the exacerbation can be measured objectively by monitoring these values.*
- Assess vital signs q1hr and prn while in distress.

THERAPEUTIC INTERVENTIONS

- Keep head of bed elevated *to allow for adequate lung excursion and chest expansion.*
- Encourage slow deep breathing. Instruct patient to utilize pursed lip breathing for exhalation. *Pursed lip breathing during exhalation produces a positive distending pressure within the bronchioles, which facilitates expiratory airflow by helping to keep the bronchioles open.* Instruct to time breathing so that exhalation takes 2-3 times as long as inspiration. *Prolonged expiration prevents air trapping.*
▲ Utilize β_2-adrenergic agonist drugs by metered-dose inhaler (MDI) or nebulizer (per respiratory therapist) as prescribed. *β_2-adrenergic agonist drugs are the treatment of choice for acute exacerbations of asthma. Their action occurs within minutes.*
▲ Administer other medications as ordered. *IV aminophylline may be ordered for severe attacks; corticosteroids are indicated in severe attacks or when the patient has previously been receiving steroid therapy.*

Ineffective Airway Clearance

RELATED FACTORS

Bronchospasm
Excessive mucus production
Ineffective cough and fatigue

DEFINING CHARACTERISTICS

Abnormal breath sounds (rhonchi, wheezes)
Changes in respiratory rate or depth
Cough
Cyanosis
Dyspnea
Abnormal ABGs
Verbalized chest tightness

EXPECTED OUTCOMES

Patient's airway is maintained free of secretions as evidenced by normal/improved breath sounds and normal ABGs.

ONGOING ASSESSMENT

- Auscultate lungs with each routine vital sign check *to allow for early detection and correction of abnormalities.*
- Assess for changes in respiratory rate or depth.
- Assess cough for effectiveness and productivity. *Consider possible causes of an ineffective cough: respiratory muscle fatigue, severe bronchospasm, thick tenacious secretions.*
- Note color changes (lips, buccal mucosa, nail beds).
▲ Monitor laboratory work as ordered:
  Theophylline level.
  ABGs. *CO_2 retention occurs as the patient becomes fatigued from the increased work of breathing caused by the bronchoconstriction.*
  CBC.

THERAPEUTIC INTERVENTIONS

- Keep the patient as calm as possible. *Anxiety during an asthma attack can further potentiate the exacerbation.*
- Pace activities *to prevent fatigue.*
▲ Ensure that respiratory treatments are given as prescribed; notify the respiratory therapists as the need arises.
- Encourage the patient to cough, especially after treatments. Teach effective coughing techniques, e.g., huff.
▲ Maintain humidified O_2 as prescribed *to decrease viscosity of secretions.*
▲ Administer medications and IV fluids as prescribed. *Mucolytic agents may be used in conjunction with a bronchodilator.*
- Anticipate the need for intubation and mechanical ventilation if ABGs begin to deteriorate.

NURSING DIAGNOSES	EXPECTED OUTCOMES AND NURSING INTERVENTIONS / *RATIONALE* (■ = INDEPENDENT; ▲ = COLLABORATIVE)

High Risk for Fluid Volume Deficit

RISK FACTORS

Fatigue resulting in decreased fluid intake

Tachypnea or diaphoresis resulting in fluid loss

EXPECTED OUTCOMES

Patient's hydration is maximized as evidenced by moist mucous membranes and urine output > 30 ml/hr.

ONGOING ASSESSMENT

- Monitor vital signs.
- Assess turgor and mucous membranes for signs of dehydration.
- Assess color and amount of urine. Report urine output <30 ml/hr for 2 consecutive hours. *Concentrated urine denotes fluid deficit.*
- Assess specific gravity.
- Weigh daily with same scale, preferably at the same time of day, *to evaluate true fluid status and to monitor trends.*
- Assess sputum for color, tenacity, viscosity, amount.

THERAPEUTIC INTERVENTIONS

- Encourage oral fluid intake by providing water and preferred liquids at bedside.
- Provide oral hygiene *to promote interest in drinking.*
- ▲ Maintain IV infusion at proper rate. *Adequate intake will enhance liquification of bronchial secretions. Thinner, liquid secretions are more easily expectorated.*
- Provide assistance with bedpan/commode at frequent intervals. *Some patients decrease intake to decrease frequent need for urination.*

Anxiety

RELATED FACTORS

Respiratory distress
Change in health status
Change in environment

DEFINING CHARACTERISTICS

Complaints of inability to breathe
Uncooperative behavior
Restlessness
Apprehensiveness
Insomnia
Increased heart rate
Frequent requests for someone to be in room
Diaphoresis

EXPECTED OUTCOMES

Patient's anxiety is reduced as evidenced by cooperative behavior and calm appearance.

ONGOING ASSESSMENT

- Assess anxiety level, including vital signs, respiratory status, irritability, apprehension, and orientation. *Anxiety increases as breathing becomes more difficult. Also, anxiety can affect respiratory rate and rhythm, causing rapid shallow breathing.*

THERAPEUTIC INTERVENTIONS

- Stay with patient and encourage slow deep breathing.
- Explain all procedures to patient before starting; be simple and concise. *An informed patient who understands the treatment plan will be more cooperative.*
- Make patient as comfortable as possible:
  Be available. Place in room near nurses station if possible.
  Be reassuring.
- Provide quiet diversional activities.
- Explain importance of remaining as calm as possible. *Maintaining calm will decrease O_2 consumption and work of breathing.*
- Explain that nurses will be available if needed *to promptly treat any exacerbations.*
- Teach relaxation techniques as appropriate.

Pain/Discomfort

RELATED FACTORS

Excessive exertion of accessory respiratory musculature as result of acute asthma attack

DEFINING CHARACTERISTICS

Complaints of pain when breathing
Complaints of inability to get comfortable
Restlessness
Insomnia
Increased respiratory distress

EXPECTED OUTCOMES

Patient's pain/discomfort is relieved as evidenced by verbalization of pain relief and comfortable appearance.

ONGOING ASSESSMENT

- Monitor respiratory function.
- Assess ability to relax.
- Assess complaints of pain (degree, location) and intervention effectiveness.
- Assess for changes in physical tolerance. *Fatigue may indicate increasing distress leading to status asthmaticus and respiratory failure.*

THERAPEUTIC INTERVENTIONS

- Make patient as comfortable as possible:
  Raise head of bed.
  Position with pillows.
  Maintain in upright position.
- ▲ Provide medications as prescribed.
- Explain need to remain as calm as possible.
- Explain need to inform nurses of any discomfort. *Relief of respiratory distress will relieve source of pain.*
- Keep significant other informed of patient's progress *to relieve apprehension. Anxiety may be readily transferred to the patient.*

Continued

Pulmonary Care Plans

NURSING DIAGNOSES	EXPECTED OUTCOMES AND NURSING INTERVENTIONS / *RATIONALE* (■ = INDEPENDENT; ▲ = COLLABORATIVE)
Knowledge Deficit **RELATED FACTORS** Chronicity of disease Long-term medical management **DEFINING CHARACTERISTICS** Absence of questions Anxiety Inability to answer questions properly Ineffective self-care	**EXPECTED OUTCOMES** Patient/significant others verbalize knowledge of disease and its management. **ONGOING ASSESSMENT** · Assess knowledge of asthma. · Assess knowledge of medications. · Evaluate self-care activities: preventive care and home management of acute attack. · Assess knowledge of care for status asthmaticus, as appropriate. **THERAPEUTIC INTERVENTIONS** · Explain disease to patient/significant others. · Reinforce need for taking prescribed medications as prescribed *to reduce incidence of full-blown attacks.* · Identify precipitating factors for the patient and instruct patient how to avoid them (e.g., cigarette smoke, aspirin, air pollution, allergens). · Teach warning signs and symptoms of asthma attack and importance of early treatment of impending attack. · Reinforce what to do in an asthma attack: Home management When to go to emergency room Prevention · Instruct to keep emergency phone numbers by telephone. · Teach how to administer metered-dose inhalers (MDIs). · Instruct in use of peak flow meters, as appropriate, and develop an individualized plan on how to adjust medications and when to seek medical advice. · Reinforce need of keeping follow-up appointments. ▲ Refer to social services, as needed. · Refer to support groups, as appropriate. · Address long-term management issues: environmental controls, avoidance of precipitators, good health habits.

By: Susan Galanes, RN, MS, CCRN

Chest trauma

(PNEUMOTHORAX; TENSION PNEUMOTHORAX; FLAIL CHEST; FRACTURED RIBS; PULMONARY CONTUSION; HEMOTHORAX; MYOCARDIAL CONTUSION; CARDIAC TAMPONADE)

A blunt or penetrating injury of the thoracic cavity that can result in a potentially life-threatening situation secondary to hemothorax, pneumothorax, tension pneumothorax, flail chest, pulmonary contusion, myocardial contusion, and/or cardiac tamponade.

NURSING DIAGNOSES	EXPECTED OUTCOMES AND NURSING INTERVENTIONS / *RATIONALE* (■ = INDEPENDENT; ▲ = COLLABORATIVE)
Ineffective Breathing Pattern **RELATED FACTORS** Simple pneumothorax Tension pneumothorax Pain Flail chest Simple hemothorax (<400 cc blood) Massive hemothorax (>1500 cc blood) Pulmonary contusion	**EXPECTED OUTCOMES** Patient experiences effective breathing pattern as evidenced by eupnea, normal skin color, and regular respiratory rate/pattern. **ONGOING ASSESSMENT** · Assess airway for patency. *Maintaining airway is always first priority.* · Assess for respiratory distress signs/symptoms: breathing patterns, breath sounds (presence/absence), use of accessory muscles, changes in orientation, restlessness, skin color, change in ABGs. · Assess chest excursion. *Paradoxical movement is a sign of flail chest. Decreased chest expansion on affected side is a sign of pneumothorax/hemothorax.* · Assess for pain, increase with inspiration (*sign of rib fracture*), decrease with inspiration (*sign of flail chest*). · Assess trachea position. *Deviation from midline is a sign of tension pneumothorax.*

NURSING DIAGNOSES	EXPECTED OUTCOMES AND NURSING INTERVENTIONS / *RATIONALE* (■ = INDEPENDENT; ▲ = COLLABORATIVE)

DEFINING CHARACTERISTICS

Shortness of breath
Dyspnea
Tachypnea
Chest pain
Decreased breath sounds on affected side
Hyperresonance on affected side to percussion (pneumothorax)
Dullness on affected side to percussion (hemothorax)
Unequal chest expansion
Abnormal ABGs
Anxiety, restlessness
Cyanosis
Jugular venous distension
Tracheal deviation toward unaffected side
Subcutaneous emphysema
Paradoxical chest movements (flail chest)

ONGOING ASSESSMENT—cont'd

- Assess, inspect chest wall for obvious injuries that allow air to enter pleural cavity.
- Assess for presence of contusions, abrasions, and bruising on chest. *Further injuries may have occurred beneath these integumentary manifestations of trauma (e.g., fractured ribs, pulmonary contusion, myocardial contusion).*
- ▲ Monitor chest radiographs *to confirm correct placement of chest tubes, signs of improvement of pneumothorax or hemothorax.*
- Assess for subcutaneous emphysema/crepitus (*a sign of air escaping into the subcutaneous tissues*).

THERAPEUTIC INTERVENTIONS

- Suction *to clear secretions, optimize gas exchange.*
- Insert oral/nasal airway as condition warrants *to maintain airway.*
- Place in sitting position, if not contraindicated, *to assist lung expansion.*
- ▲ Provide oxygen therapy *to meet specific need.*
- If flail chest is present, tape flail segment or place manual pressure over the flail segment *to stabilize. Patients with increasing respiratory distress may require external pressure until more definitive treatment (intubation, surgical stabilization) initiated. This will prevent the outward motion of flail chest. The flail segment will still move inward with respirations, but stopping the outward motion will help to decrease the pendulluft motion to the mediastinum and great vessels.*
- If open pneumothorax:
  Cover chest wall defect with sterile vaseline and 4 by 4 dressing.
  Tape on three sides with waterproof tape. *Untaped side allows air escape from pleural cavity (flutter-valve effect) so tension does not continue to increase.*
- ▲ If patient *not* in severe respiratory distress, prepare for chest radiograph *to determine pneumothorax/hemothorax size and/or confirm suspected diagnosis. Patients with small pneumothoraces, hemothoraces, and minimal symptoms may not require chest tube. However, if the patient's condition deteriorates with the need to be intubated/mechanically ventilated, a chest tube will be required even with small pneumothoraces because of the high risk of developing a tension pneumothorax in that circumstance.*
- ▲ If tension pneumothorax is suspected, anticipate/prepare for emergency thoracentesis *to relieve air tension in pleural space on affected side.*
- ▲ If severe respiratory distress/respiratory status is steadily deteriorating, prepare for chest tube placement. *Larger chest tubes are inserted for hemothorax than for pneumothorax to help alleviate chest tube clotting. Chest tube then connected to underwater seal; closed drainage suction device applied to reinflate lung, remove secretions from the pleural space.* See also p. 225, Thoracotomy, as appropriate.
- ▲ Prepare for intubation if patient's condition warrants. *Note: Patients with flail chest may be stable initially because of compensatory mechanisms (e.g., splinting of flail segment and shallow respirations). As these compensatory mechanisms fail, increasing respiratory distress develops. Intubation and positive-pressure ventilation are means of stabilizing flail segment by preventing patient from breathing independently.*
- Refer to Acute respiratory failure care plan, p. 223, as appropriate.

Fluid Volume Deficit

RELATED FACTORS

Trauma
Hemothorax
Chest tube drainage

DEFINING CHARACTERISTICS

Tachycardia
Hypotension
Cool, clammy skin
Pallor
Restlessness
Anxiety
Mental status changes
Decreased urine output

EXPECTED OUTCOMES

Patient experiences adequate fluid volume as evidenced by urine output > 30 ml/hr, normotensive BP, and HR < 100/min.

ONGOING ASSESSMENT

- Assess vital signs until stable. Note heart rate; *tachycardia is an early indication of fluid volume deficit. Blood pressure is not a good indicator of early shock.*
- ▲ Assess CVP to distinguish hypotension caused by hypovolemia (low CVP reading < 6 cm H_2O) versus hypotension caused by pericardial tamponade/tension pneumothorax (high CVP reading > 10 cm H_2O).
- Assess for jugular venous distension, *which may occur with cardiac tamponade as a result of the increased heart pressures, or with tension pneumothorax from the mediastinum's shifting toward the unaffected side.*
- Assess anxiety level. *Mild to moderate anxiety may be first early warning sign before vital sign changes. Anxiety may also indicate pain, psychological traumas, etc.*
- Monitor I & O, document. *Decreased urine output indicates progressive shock.*
- ▲ Obtain specimens; evaluate lab tests for CBC, electrolytes, BUN, creatinine levels, type, and crossmatch.
- Assess, measure, document amount of blood in chest tube collection chamber. Estimate blood lost to sterile towels, etc.
- Monitor chest tube drainage q10-15 min until blood loss slows to <25 cc/hr.
- ▲ Establish baseline Hct/Hb; monitor and continue to assess.

Chest trauma cont'd

NURSING DIAGNOSES	EXPECTED OUTCOMES AND NURSING INTERVENTIONS / *RATIONALE* (■ = INDEPENDENT; ▲ = COLLABORATIVE)

THERAPEUTIC INTERVENTIONS

- Attempt to control bleeding source by using direct pressure with sterile 4 by 4 bandage.
- ▲ Insert one to two large-bore peripheral IVs. Administer crystalloid/colloid fluids as prescribed. *Rule for fluid replacement: Infuse 3 cc IV fluid per 1 cc blood volume lost.*
- ▲ Prepare patient for transfusions, if prescribed, with typed and crossmatched blood if it is available and time permits. *Type-specific blood may be used if unable to obtain type and crossmatch. O negative blood may be used as last resort.*
- ▲ Prepare patient for autotransfusion; *may be used in cases of blunt/penetrating injuries of chest only.*
- Prepare for transfer to OR as condition warrants.
- If patient is hypotensive, see also Hypovolemic shock, p. 161, as appropriate.

Decreased Cardiac Output

RELATED FACTORS

Acute pericardial tamponade
Tension pneumothorax
Severe volume loss

DEFINING CHARACTERISTICS

Decreased BP
Narrow pulse pressure
Pulsus paradoxus (systolic pressure falls >15 mm Hg during inspiration)
Tachycardia
Electrical alterans (decreased QRS voltage during inspiration)
Equalization of pressures (CVP, PAP, PCWP)
Jugular venous distention
Widened mediastinum/ enlarged heart on chest radiograph
Chest tubes (if present) suddenly stop draining (suspect clot)
Distant/muffled heart tones
Restlessness, confusion, anxiety
Fall in Hb, Hct
Cool, clammy skin
Diminished peripheral pulses
Decreased urine output
Decreased arterial venous O_2 saturation
Acidosis

EXPECTED OUTCOMES

Patient maintains adequate cardiac output as evidenced by blood pressure within normal limits for patient, strong regular pulses, absence of JVD, absence of pulsus paradoxus, warm and dry skin, and clear mentation.

ONGOING ASSESSMENT

- Assess for classic signs associated with acute cardiac tamponade:
  Low arterial blood pressure
  Tachypnea
  Pulsus paradoxus *(accentuation of normal drop in arterial blood pressure with inspiration)*
  Distant/muffled heart sounds *(caused by distention in pericardial sac)*
  Sinus tachycardia *related to compensatory catecholamine release*
  Jugular venous distention *(The venous pulse may rise to 15-20 cm water as a result of reduced circulating volume).*
  Pericardial tamponade can decrease cardiac output as the pericardial sac fills with blood to the point that it compresses the myocardium, causing decreased ability of the heart to pump blood out and accept blood in.
- Assess mental status. *Symptoms may range from anxiety to altered level of consciousness in shock.*
- Monitor chest tube drainage. *Sudden cessation of drainage suggests clot.*
- ▲ Assist with performance of echocardiogram if time permits. *Provides most helpful diagnostic information. Effusions seen with acute tamponade are usually smaller than with chronic. However, in light of circulatory collapse, treatment may be indicated before the echocardiogram can be performed.*
- ▲ If patient is in ICU setting, assess hemodynamic profile using pulmonary artery catheter; assess for equalization of pressures. *The RAP, RVDP, PADP, and PCWP pressures are all elevated in tamponade, and within 2-3 mm Hg of each other. These pressures confirm diagnosis.*
- ▲ Monitor serial chest radiographs; evaluate for widened mediastinum/increased heart size.
- Assess for midline shift of trachea. *Tension pneumothorax will cause a midline shift of the trachea and mediastinum to the opposite side with compression of the great vessels, decreasing cardiac output.*

THERAPEUTIC INTERVENTIONS

- ▲ Initiate O_2 therapy *to maximize O_2 saturation.*
- ▲ Establish large-bore IV access.
- ▲ Administer parenteral fluids as prescribed. *Optimal hydration state increases venous return.*
- ▲ Type and crossmatch as prescribed. Anticipate blood product replacement *to correct existing hematologic or coagulation factor alterations.*
- Place patient in optimal position *to increase venous return.*
- Have emergency resuscitative equipment, medications readily available. *Bedside pericardiocentesis can be a high-risk lifesaving procedure. Complications include pneumothorax and myocardial or coronary artery lacerations.*

NURSING DIAGNOSES	EXPECTED OUTCOMES AND NURSING INTERVENTIONS / *RATIONALE* (■ = INDEPENDENT; ▲ = COLLABORATIVE)

Therapeutic Interventions—cont'd

▲ Assemble pericardiocentesis tray/open chest tray for bedside intervention/prepare patient for transport to surgery. *Tamponade must be relieved to improve cardiac output. Indicated when systolic BP is reduced more than 30 mm Hg from baseline. However, if patient's condition can be stabilized, drainage of fluid should be delayed until surgical or open resection/drainage can be performed. Pericardiocentesis should be performed under sterile conditions. Acute tamponade is a life-threatening complication, but immediate prognosis is good with fast, effective treatment.*

▲ Maintain aggressive fluid resuscitation (*may be required to raise venous pressure above pericardial pressure*).

▲ Administer vasopressor agents (dopmaine, levophed) as ordered *to maximize systemic perfusion pressure to vital organs.*

▲ If repeated pericardiocentesis fails to prevent recurrence of acute tamponade, anticipate surgical correction.

Pain

Related Factors

Rib fractures
Chest tube incision
Contusions/abrasions

Defining Characteristics

Anxiety
Wincing, grimacing
Shallow respiration to minimize pain
Tachycardia
Agitation
Verbalization of pain

Expected Outcomes

Patient's pain is reduced or relieved as evidenced by verbalization of pain relief, normotension, and HR < 100/min.

Ongoing Assessment

- Assess pain level and characteristics. *It is important to determine the type of pain the patient is experiencing to aid in the diagnosis.*
- Evaluate effectiveness of all pain medication. *Unlike all other body fractures, rib fractures cannot be casted to reduce pain. The rib cage is in continuous motion; therefore, more difficult to manage.*

Therapeutic Interventions

▲ Anticipate need for analgesics and respond immediately to complaint of pain.
- Use other comfort measures as appropriate (e.g., decrease the number of stressors in environment).
- Use distraction techniques. *Patient then focuses less on pain and more on television, newspaper, games, etc.*
- Assist patient in splinting chest with pillow to minimize discomfort *and to assist with effective cough and deep breathing.*
▲ Assist with insertion/maintenance of intrapleural catheter, epidural catheter, or intercostal nerve block as appropriate.

Anxiety/Fear

Related Factors

Acute injury
Threat of death
Unfamiliar environment

Defining Characteristics

Apprehension
Restlessness
Look of fear
Crying
Agitation

See also:
Knowledge Deficit, p. 41.
Impaired Gas Exchange, p. 27.
High Risk for Infection, p. 40.

Expected Outcomes

Patient appears calm and trusting.
Patient verbalizes fears and concerns.

Ongoing Assessment

- Assess anxiety level (mild, severe). Note signs/symptoms, especially nonverbal communication. *Chest trauma can result in an acute life-threatening injury that will produce high levels of anxiety in the patient as well as the significant others.*

Therapeutic Interventions

- Reduce patient's/significant others' anxiety by explaining all procedures/treatment. Keep explanations basic.
- Maintain confident, assured manner. *Staff's anxiety may be easily perceived by patient.*
- Assure patient and significant others of close, continuous monitoring that will ensure prompt interventions.
- Reduce unnecessary external stimuli (e.g., clear unnecessary personnel from room; decrease volume of cardiac monitor).
- Reassure patient/significant other as appropriate; allow them to express their fears.
- Provide quiet, private place for significant others to wait.
- When appropriate, provide information about disease process and reasoning for prescribed therapy *to help allay anxiety.*
▲ Refer to other support systems (e.g., clergy, social workers, other family/friends) as appropriate.

By: Susan Galanes, RN, MS, CCRN

Chronic obstructive pulmonary disease (COPD)

(CHRONIC BRONCHITIS; EMPHYSEMA)

Chronic obstructive pulmonary disease (COPD) refers to a group of diseases, including chronic bronchitis, asthma, and emphysema, that cause a reduction in expiratory outflow. It is usually a slow, progressive debilitating disease, affecting those with a history of heavy tobacco abuse and prolonged exposure to respiratory system irritants such as air pollution, noxious gases, and repeated upper respiratory tract infections. It is also regarded as the most common cause of alveolar hypoventilation with associated hypoxemia, chronic hypercapnia, and compensated acidosis.

NURSING DIAGNOSES

EXPECTED OUTCOMES AND NURSING INTERVENTIONS / *RATIONALE*
(■ = INDEPENDENT; ▲ = COLLABORATIVE)

Ineffective Airway Clearance

RELATED FACTORS

Hyperplasia and hypertrophy of mucus-secreting glands
Increased mucus production in bronchial tubes
Decreased ciliary function
Thick secretions
Decreased energy and fatigue
Bronchospasm

DEFINING CHARACTERISTICS

"Smoker's cough"
Coarse rales over larger airways
Persistent cough for months
Copious amount of secretions
Wheezing
Loud, prolonged exploratory phase
Dyspnea (air hunger)

EXPECTED OUTCOMES

Patient's airway is free of secretions.
Patient has clear breath sounds after suctioning.

ONGOING ASSESSMENT

- Auscultate lungs as needed *to note and document significant change in breath sounds:*
  Decreased or absent breath sounds *may indicate presence of mucus plug or other major airway obstruction.*
  Presence of fine rales *may indicate cardiac involvement.*
  Wheezing *may indicate increasing airway resistance.*
  Coarse rales *indicate presence of fluid along larger airways.*
- Assess characteristics of secretions: consistency, quantity, color, odor.
- Assess hydration status: skin turgor, mucous membranes, tongue.
- Monitor accurate I & O. Include accurate approximation of secretions and insensible loss from increased work of breathing.
- Obtain daily weights.
- Assess patient's physical strength including ability to expectorate sputum and ability to use incentive spirometer.

THERAPEUTIC INTERVENTIONS

- Encourage patient to cough out secretions; suction as needed.
- Assist with effective coughing techniques:
  Splint chest for comfort.
  Have patient use abdominal muscles for more forceful cough.
  Utilize cough techniques as appropriate (e.g., quad, huff).
- ▲ Assist in mobilizing secretions *to facilitate airway clearance by:*
  Increasing room humidification *to liquify secretions.*
  Administering mucolytic agents in conjunction with respiratory therapist.
  Performing chest physiotherapy: postural drainage, percussion, and vibration.
  Encouraging 2-3 L fluid intake unless contraindicated *to prevent dehydration from increased insensible loss and to keep secretions thin.*
- ▲ Anticipate administration of bronchodilators (IV or inhalation) *to relieve bronchoconstriction.*
- ▲ Anticipate intubation and mechanical ventilation if needed. See also Mechanical ventilation, p. 202.
- Demonstrate effective technique in use of incentive spirometer *to conserve energy with positive result.* Emphasize not to overexert self (15-20 times maximum) *to prevent respiratory muscle fatigue.*
- Perform nasotracheal suctioning as indicated. Use a well-lubricated soft catheter, preferably rubber, *to minimize irritations.*

Impaired Gas Exchange

RELATED FACTORS

Increase in dead space caused by:
  Loss of lung tissue elasticity
  Atelectasis
  Increased residual volume

EXPECTED OUTCOMES

Patient maintains optimal gas exchange as evidenced by ABGs within baseline for the patient and alert responsive mentation or no further reduction in mental status.

ONGOING ASSESSMENT

- Assess for altered breathing patterns:
  Increased work of breathing
  Abnormal rate, rhythm, and depth of respiration
  Abnormal chest excursions

NURSING DIAGNOSES	EXPECTED OUTCOMES AND NURSING INTERVENTIONS / *RATIONALE* (■ = INDEPENDENT; ▲ = COLLABORATIVE)

RELATED FACTORS—cont'd

Increased upper and lower airway resistance caused by:
Overproduction of secretions along bronchial tubes
Bronchoconstriction

DEFINING CHARACTERISTICS

Altered I:E ratio (prolonged expiratory phase)
Active expiratory phase: use of accessory muscles of breathing
Decreased vital capacity (VC)
Increased residual volume (RV)
Hypoxemia/hypercapnia
$Paco_2 > 55$ mm Hg
$Pao_2 < 55$ mm Hg
Tachycardia
Restlessness
Diaphoresis
Headache
Lethargy
Confusion
Cyanosis
Increase in rate and depth of respiration
Increase in BP

ONGOING ASSESSMENT—cont'd

- Assess for signs and symptoms of hypoxemia/hypercapnia: restlessness, diaphoresis, headache, lethargy, confusion, cyanosis, tachypnea.
- Monitor vital signs with frequent monitoring of BP. *Hypoxia/hypercarbia may cause initial hypertension with restlessness and progress to hypotension and somnolence.*
- ▲ Monitor ABGs. *Increasing $Paco_2$ and decreasing Pao_2 are signs of respiratory failure. As the patient begins to fail, respiratory rate will decrease and $Paco_2$ will begin to rise. The COPD patient has a significant decrease in pulmonary reserves, and any physiologic stress may result in acute respiratory failure.*

THERAPEUTIC INTERVENTIONS

- ▲ Promote more effective breathing pattern for better gas exchange:
  Position properly for optimal breathing. *Upright and high Fowler's position will favor better lung expansion; diaphragm is pushed downward. If patient is bedridden, turning from side to side at least q2hr will promote better aeration of all lung lobes, thus minimizing atelectasis.*
  Teach patient pursed-lip breathing *for more complete exhalation.*
  Teach patient to use abdominal and other accessory muscles to exhale *for more forceful exhalation.*
  Administer bronchodilators as prescribed *to decrease work of breathing:*
  Monitor for therapeutic and side effects.
  Monitor blood levels.
- ▲ Administer low-flow O_2 therapy as indicated (e.g., 2 L/min nasal cannula). If insufficient, switch to high-flow O_2 apparatus (e.g., Venturi mask) for more accurate O_2 delivery. *COPD patients who chronically retain CO_2 depend upon "hypoxic drive" as their stimulus to breathe. When applying O_2, close monitoring is imperative to prevent unsafe increases in the patient's Pao_2, which would result in apnea.*
- ▲ If Pao_2 level is significantly lower or if $Paco_2$ level is higher than patient's usual baseline (varies from patient to patient), anticipate:
  Vigorous pulmonary toilet and suctioning
  Increase in Fio_2 with use of controlled high flow system
  Use of diuretics
  Possible need for intubation and mechanical ventilation
- Assist in performing related procedures and tests (bronchoscopy, pulmonary function tests).

Altered Nutrition: Less than Body Requirements

RELATED FACTORS

Increased metabolic need caused by increased work of breathing
Poor appetite resulting from fever, dyspnea, and fatigue

DEFINING CHARACTERISTICS

Body weight 20% or more below ideal for height and frame
Indifference to food
Caloric intake inadequate for metabolic demands of disease state
Muscle wasting
Abnormal lab values (e.g., low serum albumin level)

EXPECTED OUTCOMES

Patient's optimal nutritional status is maintained as evidenced by maintenance of body weight and adequate caloric intake.

ONGOING ASSESSMENT

- Assess caloric requirements and caloric intake record.
- Assess for possible cause of poor appetite (see Related Factors).
- Compile diet history, including preferred foods and dietary habits.
- ▲ Consult and work with the dietician to estimate caloric requirements.

THERAPEUTIC INTERVENTIONS

- Offer small feedings of nutritious soft foods/liquids frequently. *They are easier to digest and require less chewing.*
- Assist patient with meals.
- Give frequent oral care *to promote comfort and appetite.*
- Instruct patient to avoid very hot/cold foods, gas-producing foods, carbonated beverages *to prevent possible abdominal distention.*
- Plan activities to allow rest before eating.
- Substitute nasal prongs for O_2 mask during mealtime *to maintain patient's oxygenation.*

High Risk for Infection

RISK FACTORS

Retained secretions (good medium for bacterial growth)
Poor nutrition
Impaired pulmonary defense system secondary to COPD

EXPECTED OUTCOMES

Risk for infection is reduced through early assessment and intervention.

ONGOING ASSESSMENT

- Auscultate lungs *to monitor significant changes in breath sounds. Bronchial breath sounds and rales may indicate pneumonia.*
- Assess for significant change in sputum *that may indicate presence of infection:*
  Sudden increase in production

Continued.

Chronic obstructive pulmonary disease (COPD) cont'd

NURSING DIAGNOSES	EXPECTED OUTCOMES AND NURSING INTERVENTIONS / *RATIONALE* (■ = INDEPENDENT; ▲ = COLLABORATIVE)

RISK FACTORS—cont'd

Use of respiratory equipment

ONGOING ASSESSMENT—cont'd

Change in color (rusty, yellow, greenish)
Change in consistency (thick)
- Assess for other signs and symptoms of infection: fever, chills, increase in cough, elevated WBC, shortness of breath, nausea, vomiting, diarrhea, anorexia.

THERAPEUTIC INTERVENTIONS

- Encourage an increase in fluid intake, unless contraindicated, *to maintain good hydration. Insensible loss is markedly increased during infection because of fever and increase in respiratory rate.*
- Ensure that O_2 humidifier is properly maintained. Never add new water to old water. *Stagnant old water is medium for bacterial growth.*
- Minimize retained secretions by encouraging patient to cough and expectorate secretions frequently. If patient is unable to cough and expectorate, perform nasotracheal or oropharyngeal suctioning. *Retained secretions provide bacterial growth medium*

Knowledge Deficit

RELATED FACTORS

Recent diagnosis
Ineffective past teaching/
learning

DEFINING CHARACTERISTICS

Display of anxiety/fear
Noncompliance
Inability to verbalize health
maintenance regime
Repeated acute exacerbations
Development of complications
Misconceptions about health
status
Multiple questions or none

EXPECTED OUTCOMES

Patient verbalizes understanding of disease process and treatment.

ONGOING ASSESSMENT

- Assess knowledge base of COPD.
- Assess environmental, social, cultural, and educational factors that may influence teaching plan.

THERAPEUTIC INTERVENTIONS

- Establish common goals with the patient.
- Instruct patient in basic anatomy and physiology of respiratory system, with attention to structure and airflow.
- Discuss relation of disease process to signs and symptoms patient experiences; introduce the following words: *mucus, spasm, narrowing, obstruction, elasticity, trapping, inflammation.*
- Discuss purpose and method of administration for each medication.
- Instruct patient to avoid CNS depressants.
- Discuss appropriate nutritional habits.
- Discuss concept of energy conservation. Encourage: resting as needed during activities, avoiding overexertion/fatigue, sitting as much as possible, alternating heavy and light tasks, carrying articles close to body, organizing all equipment at beginning of activity, and working slowly.
- Discuss signs/symptoms of infection.
- Discuss common factors that lead to exacerbations of lung problems: smoking, environmental temperature, and humidity.
- Refer patient/significant other to smoking cessation support groups as appropriate.
- Discuss importance of specific therapeutic measures as listed:
  Breathing exercises
    Exercise 1: Purpose: to strengthen muscles of respiration.
      Technique: Lie supine, with one hand on chest and one on abdomen. Inhale slowly through mouth, raising abdomen against hand. Exhale slowly through pursed lips while contracting abdominal muscles and moving abdomen inward.
    Exercise 2: Purpose: to develop slowed, controlled breathing
      Technique: Walk, stop to take deep breath, exhale slowly while walking.
    Exercise 3: Purpose: to decrease air trapping and airway collapse.
      Technique: For pursed-lip breathing, inhale slowly through nose. Exhale twice as slowly as usual through pursed lips.

THERAPEUTIC INTERVENTIONS—cont'd

Cough: Lean forward; take several deep breaths with pursed-lip method. Take last deep breath, cough with open mouth during expiration, and simultaneously contract abdominal muscles.

Chest physiotherapy/pulmonary postural drainage: *Purpose: to facilitate expectoration of secretions and prevent waste of energy.* Demonstrate correct methods for postural drainage: positioning, percussion, vibration.

Hydration: Discuss importance of maintaining good fluid *intake to decrease viscosity of secretions.* Recommend 1½-2 L/d.

Humidity: Discuss various forms of humidification *to prevent drying of secretions.*

- Discuss home oxygen therapy:

Use of equipment:

Demonstrate how to open oxygen cylinder, regulate flowmeter, and use humidifier. *Patient or others who will be primarily responsible for O₂ therapy at home should be able to demonstrate process perfectly at least 3 times before discharge.*

Safety precautions: *Oxygen is not combustible itself, but it will feed a fire if one occurs.*

Do not use around a stove or gas space heater.

Do not smoke or light matches around cylinder when O₂ is in use.

Post "No Smoking" sign and call to visitors' attention.

Care of humidifier:

Change water in humidifier once a day *to decrease risk of infection.*

▲ Discuss available resources:

Arrange for visiting nurse to check patient as appropriate.

Refer to local Lung Association if available for support.

See also:
Activity Intolerance, p. 2.
Self Care Deficit, p. 53.
Sleep Pattern Disturbance, p. 61.

By: Lumie L. Perez, RN, BSN, CCRN
Susan Galanes, RN, MS, CCRN

High-frequency jet ventilation

(HFJV)

HFJV is a type of mechanical ventilation that uses high-frequency rates (40 to 150 cycles/min is approved by FDA for adults, as nonexperimental) with very low tidal volumes (3-5 ml/kg) to achieve ventilation (30-35 L/min ventilation). It is useful for patients with bronchopleural fistulas and large pulmonary air leaks and is indicated for patients who have failed on conventional ventilation.

NURSING DIAGNOSES	EXPECTED OUTCOMES AND NURSING INTERVENTIONS / *RATIONALE* (■ = INDEPENDENT; ▲ = COLLABORATIVE)

Impaired Gas Exchange (Requiring HFJV)

RELATED FACTORS

Adult respiratory distress syndrome
Barotrauma
Aspiration pneumonitis
Bronchopleural fistula
Interstitial air leak syndromes

EXPECTED OUTCOMES

Patient maintains optimal gas exchange as evidenced by normal ABGs, peak inspiratory pressures less than 50 cm H₂O, normal intrathoracic pressures, and regular respiratory rate/rhythm.

ONGOING ASSESSMENT

- Assess respiratory rate, rhythm, and character.
- Auscultate lungs to check for aeration both before and after jet ventilation begins. *Patients exhibiting low pulmonary compliance are at a higher risk for development of barotrauma.*

Continued.

High-frequency jet ventilation—cont'd

NURSING DIAGNOSES	EXPECTED OUTCOMES AND NURSING INTERVENTIONS / *RATIONALE* (■ = INDEPENDENT; ▲ = COLLABORATIVE)

DEFINING CHARACTERISTICS

Hypercapnia
Hypoxia
Abnormal ABGs
Low pulmonary compliance exhibited by high peak pressures ($\geq$ 55 cm H_2O)
Presence of increased intrathoracic pressures
Abnormal breathing pattern
Decreased LOC/increasing anxiety

ONGOING ASSESSMENT—cont'd

- Observe for abnormal breathing patterns: bradypnea, tachypnea, Kussmaul or Cheyne-Stokes respirations, apneustic, Biot's, and ataxic patterns.
- Assess level of consciousness and level of anxiety, *both of which may be affected in the presence of hypercapnea and hypoxia.*
- Assess skin color (presence/absence of cyanosis), temperature, capillary refill, and peripheral perfusion.
- ▲ Monitor vital signs, watching for increased central venous pressure, increased pulmonary capillary wedge pressure (PCWP), decreased BP, and decreased cardiac output.
- ▲ Monitor cardiac output as indicated, especially after ventilator changes or changes in patient's condition.
- Monitor for complaints of pain, *which may increase respirations, making patient ventilation more difficult.* Assess location and duration.
- ▲ Monitor ABGs as indicated (i.e., after changes in Fio_2, rate, drive pressure, or continuous positive airway pressure).

THERAPEUTIC INTERVENTIONS

- ▲ Administer O_2 as prescribed and indicated.
- ▲ Obtain informed consent for jet therapy if possible. *Although jet ventilation is approved by FDA, it is still not generally a first-line treatment mode.*
- ▲ Prepare patient for intubation with Hi-Lo Jet Tracheal Tube (National Catheter Co.). *This endotracheal tube has two additional ports: for jet driveline and for continuous intratracheal pressure monitoring. Note: Hi-Lo Jet Tracheal Tube outer diameter is half-size larger than conventional ET tubes (e.g., 7.5 Hi-Lo single-lumen cuffed ET tube = 7.0 Hi-Lo Jet Tracheal Tube).*
  Administer sedation (e.g., diazepam [Valium]) and neuromuscular blocking agent (e.g., pancuronium [Pavulon] or succinylcholine) as prescribed.
  Provide comfort measures/reassurance (verbal and nonverbal contact).
  Obtain baseline status before instituting therapy (PCWP, cardiac output, and ABGs) as prescribed.
- ▲ Maintain adequate blood volume, treating any sources of hemorrhage or changes in vascular compartments with appropriate fluids (i.e., blood, crystalloid, colloid) as prescribed. *Hemoglobin is the primary vehicle of oxygen delivery.*
- Combine nursing actions (i.e., bath, bed, and dressing changes) *to minimize energy expended by patient and allow frequent periods of rest.*
- Provide frequent attendance *since there are few alarms on present jet system to detect patient disconnect or low volumes.* Be prepared to use Ambu bag *in case of emergency failure of machinery or acute change in condition. Ambu bag ventilation may be difficult because of the decreased compliance and elasticity of the patient's lungs.*
- ▲ Administer medications (e.g., antibiotics) as prescribed. *The primary cause of the patient's respiratory failure many times is infection (e.g., aspiration pneumonia, some cases of ARDS).*
- ▲ Administer sedation and/or pain relievers as prescribed, and provide other comfort measures as needed. Be aware that sedation to maintain ventilation control will decrease with jet ventilation. *Most patients on HFJV have cessation of their ventilatory effort at supraphysiologic ventilatory rates. However, when weaning back to conventional ventilation, the need for sedation may recur.*

Ineffective Airway Clearance

RELATED FACTORS

Presence/irritation by ET tube
Secretions
Drying of mucosa
Decreased energy and fatigue

EXPECTED OUTCOMES

Patient maintains patent clear airway as evidenced by clear breath sounds, regular respiratory rate, and eupnea.

NURSING DIAGNOSES	EXPECTED OUTCOMES AND NURSING INTERVENTIONS / *RATIONALE* (■ = INDEPENDENT; ▲ = COLLABORATIVE)

DEFINING CHARACTERISTICS

Abnormal breath sounds
Change in rate, depth, and character of respirations
Tachypnea
Cough
Cyanosis
Dyspnea or shortness of breath

ONGOING ASSESSMENT

- Assess for alteration in airway clearance.
▲ Assess ET tube placement and the adequacy of the cuff to prevent air leakage. *Underinflation may cause aspiration of oral secretions. Overinflation of the cuff may obliterate perfusion to left or right bronchus resulting in deterioration of ABGs.*
   Notify respiratory therapist to check cuff pressure.
   Notify physician of problems with ET tube maintenance (e.g., placement, suctioning, cuff).

THERAPEUTIC INTERVENTIONS

- Institute aseptic suctioning of airway as needed *to prevent airway obstruction. Potential for mucous plug is present because of drying of mucosa from high-frequency ventilation* (respiratory therapist will maintain humidification).
▲ Turn off jet ventilator or disconnect during suctioning; *otherwise increased airway resistance may increase potential for pneumothorax.*
▲ Be aware that respiratory therapist will use Ambu bag or "sigh" q1h, with jet off, *to prevent atelectasis or atrophy of respiratory muscles as result of low tidal volume.*

High Risk for Injury: Barotrauma

RISK FACTORS

Pressure-cycled ventilation
High-peak airway pressures

EXPECTED OUTCOMES

Potential for injury from barotrauma is reduced due to ongoing assessment and early intervention.

ONGOING ASSESSMENT

- Assess for signs of barotrauma q1h: crepitus, subcutaneous emphysema, altered chest excursion, asymmetrical chest, abnormal ABGs, shift in trachea, restlessness. *Frequent assessments are needed since barotrauma can occur at any time and the patient may not show signs of dyspnea, shortness of breath, or tachypnea while on HFJV.*
▲ Monitor chest radiograph reports daily; obtain stat portable chest radiograph if barotrauma suspected.

THERAPEUTIC INTERVENTIONS

- Notify physician immediately of any signs of barotrauma.
▲ Anticipate the need for chest tube placement; prepare as needed. *If barotrauma is suspected, intervention must be immediate to prevent a tension pneumothorax.*

High Risk for Impaired Skin Integrity

RISK FACTORS

Prolonged bedrest
Immobility
Sensory deficit
Altered vasomotor tone and/or altered nutritional state
Prolonged intubation

EXPECTED OUTCOMES

Patient maintains intact skin around ET tube.
Patient is free of skin breakdown as evidenced by pink intact skin and absence of redness or blisters.

ONGOING ASSESSMENT

- Assess around ET tube for crusting of secretions, redness, or irritation.
- Assess for signs of skin breakdown beneath ET-securing tape.
- Assess bony prominences for signs of threatened or actual skin breakdown.

THERAPEUTIC INTERVENTIONS

- Change tape securing ET tube when loosened or soiled, taking care to maintain tube position.
   If patient is nasally intubated, notify physician if skin is red or irritated or breakdown is noted.
   If patient is orally intubated, the tube should be repositioned from side to side q24-48hr. *This will help prevent pressure necrosis on the lower lip.*
- Provide mouth care q2hr *to decrease oral bacteria.*
- Keep ET tube free of crusting of secretions.
- Institute changes in position carefully *because of limitations in length of ventilator tubing, which is designed to minimize compressible volume, increasing efficiency. Changes in position may change ability to ventilate patient but should be made q2hr.*
- Institute prophylactic use of pressure-relieving devices.
- See Impaired skin integrity, p. 59 (as needed).

Continued.

NURSING DIAGNOSES	EXPECTED OUTCOMES AND NURSING INTERVENTIONS / *RATIONALE* (■ = INDEPENDENT; ▲ = COLLABORATIVE)

Knowledge Deficit

RELATED FACTORS

New equipment
New environment

DEFINING CHARACTERISTICS

Increased frequency of questions posed by patient and/or significant others
Inability to ask or correctly respond to questions asked by medical personnel

EXPECTED OUTCOMES

Patient/significant others demonstrate understanding of, rationale for, safety of, and routines associated with jet ventilation.

ONGOING ASSESSMENT

- Evaluate understanding of patient's overall condition and need for jet ventilation.

THERAPEUTIC INTERVENTIONS

- Explain all procedures to patient before performing them, especially during period of intubation and initial use of jet ventilation. *This will help to decrease patient's anxiety. Fear of the unknown could otherwise produce an extremely anxious uncooperative patient.*
- Provide reassurance of safety of jet ventilatory system.
- Orient and reorient patient to ICU surroundings, routines, equipment alarms, and noises. *The ICU is a busy and noisy environment that can be very upsetting to the patient who doesn't know what the noises and alarms mean.*
- Include significant others in explanations of jet therapy.
- Allow patient to ventilate feelings through alternative methods of communication (picture boards, sign language, written messages, alphabet board).
- Explain methods/procedures of "weaning off" HFJV. Be aware that sedation, which may have been used before jet therapy, may have to be reinstituted during weaning process. Reassure that sedation is not meant as a means of punishment but may provide an easier transition to conventional ventilation and eventual extubation.

See also:
Anxiety/Fear, p. 53.
Impaired Verbal Communication, p. 14.
Decreased Cardiac Output, p. 12.
Impaired Physical Mobility, p. 47.
Sleep Pattern Disturbance, p. 61.
Altered Nutrition: Less than Body Requirements, p. 44.

By: Susan Galanes, RN, MS, CCRN

Lung cancer

Lung cancer is the most common and lethal cancer in the United States. Epidermoid (squamous) carcinomas of the lung are the most frequently identified cell type and account for about 35% of lung cancers. Adenocarcinoma accounts for about 25% of cases. Small cell undifferentiated carcinoma is biologically and clinically distinct from the other major histologic types and accounts for about 25% of cases. Large cell undifferentiated lung cancer is the least common cell type. Mixed tumors comprise all combinations of major lung cancer types and may represent 10% of all cases. The diagnosis and stage of lung cancer subtype are critical to the determination of appropriate treatment. Non—small cell cancer can be surgically resected in early stages and treated with chemotherapy if symptomatic disease develops. Small cell cancer is always treated with chemotherapy and radiation therapy.

NURSING DIAGNOSES	EXPECTED OUTCOMES AND NURSING INTERVENTIONS / *RATIONALE* (■ = INDEPENDENT; ▲ = COLLABORATIVE)

Knowledge Deficit

RELATED FACTORS

Unfamiliarity with causes, diagnostic evaluation, and treatment

DEFINING CHARACTERISTICS

Many questions
Lack of questions
Verbalized misconceptions

EXPECTED OUTCOMES

Patient describes probable cause of his/her cancer.
Patient describes the diagnostic evaluation for lung cancer.
Patient explains the treatment regimen for own type of lung cancer.

ONGOING ASSESSMENT

• Elicit patient's understanding of causes, diagnostic evaluation, and treatment interventions for lung cancer.

THERAPEUTIC INTERVENTIONS

• Explain possible causes of lung cancer: tobacco, passive exposure to smoke, radon, asbestos, air pollution containing benzypyrenes and hydrocarbons, and exposure to occupational agents such as petroleum, chromates, and arsenic.
• If patient is a smoker, discuss strategies for stopping smoking, such as use of nicotine patch, nicotine gum, behavior modification, and stop smoking support groups. *Continued smoking in the face of a diagnosis of treatable lung cancer may hasten the patient's death. However, the perceived pressure to stop smoking is an added stressor to patient with newly diagnosed lung cancer.*
• Communicate information on risk to children and nonsmokers caused by environmental tobacco smoke. *Passive smoke is a known carcinogen in individuals with long-term exposure. Children exposed to smoke also have an increased incidence of respiratory complications/disease.*
• Discuss evaluation of home for detection of radon and inexpensive removal, if necessary.
• Discuss the diagnostic evaluation:
  Chest radiograph. *Films are repeated at frequent intervals and may be the initial test performed when new symptoms are reported.*
  Collection of sputum for cytologic evaluation.
  Bronchoscopy. *Brush biopsies and multiple bronchial washings are performed to obtain a tissue diagnosis. Bronchoscopy is mandatory for small cell cancer.*
  Percutaneous transthoracic needle aspiration/biopsy under fluoroscopy, and/or computed tomography (CT). *Indicated for non—small cell cancer; done if bronchoscopy has not yielded an adequate tissue diagnosis or if lesion is not central and accessible by bronchoscope.*
  Mediastinoscopy. *Performed if previous two procedures have not yielded a tissue diagnosis. Used to sample lymph nodes; is mandatory for staging non—small cell cancer if surgery is contemplated.*
  Pulmonary function tests. *Predict whether lung function is sufficient to tolerate a surgical resection. Most patients with lung cancer are chronic smokers with poor lung function.*
• Describe the following tests for patients with small cell cancer:
  Brain/head CT and MRI scans *to look for brain metastases*
  Liver and abdominal CT scans *to evaluate the liver and adrenals*
  Bone scan *if patient has bone pain*
  Bone marrow aspiration and biopsy

Continued.

NURSING DIAGNOSES	EXPECTED OUTCOMES AND NURSING INTERVENTIONS / *RATIONALE* (■ = INDEPENDENT; ▲ = COLLABORATIVE)

THERAPEUTIC INTERVENTIONS—cont'd

- Discuss staging classifications:

    For small cell cancer:

    "Limited stage" *Includes lesions confined to a hemithorax that can be encompassed in a single radiation therapy port. "Port" refers to the anatomic location designated to receive radiation therapy.*

    "Extensive stage" *Includes all other disease.*

    For non–small cell cancer:

    Revised tumor, node, metastasis (TNM) staging classification. *The clinical diagnostic stage is based on pretreatment scans, radiographs, biopsies, and mediastinoscopy and is used to determine resectability. The postsurgical pathologic stage is based on analysis of tissue obtained at thoracotomy and is used to determine prognosis as well as the need for additional treatment.*

- Explain "Performance Status Assessment." *This is probably is the most important prognostic factor for nonresectable cases.*

    Fully ambulatory patients tolerate therapy better and live longer.

    Patients with restricted activities, out of bed > 50% of day, survive longer than more restricted patients.

    Totally bedridden patients tolerate all forms of therapy poorly and have short survival.

- Explain treatments for **non–small cell cancer.** *The cure rate for all newly diagnosed lung cancer patients remains below 15%, primarily because the disease has spread beyond the scope of surgical therapy before a diagnosis is made.*

    Chemotherapy: systemic treatment with platinum based combination therapy. *Offers palliation of symptoms. See also: Chemotherapy, p. 403.*

    Radiation therapy for regional inoperable tumor. *Relieves symptoms in a significant percentage of patients, especially those with superior vena cava syndrome, dyspnea, cough, hemoptysis, and pneumonia secondary to obstruction.*

    Describe radiation therapy protocol:

    Radiation ports must be carefully marked before initiating therapy.

    Don't remove skin markings. *They serve as "landmarks" for therapy doses.*

    Use gentle soap and water cleansing on skin within ports; avoid perfumed lotions and known skin irritants.

    Treatment schedule: can be 5 days/wk × 6 weeks.

    Complications to report:

    Shortness of breath, sore throat, or altered sensation associated with spinal cord damage.

    In patients with central lesions, esophagitis may occur. Medicated oral suspensions may be prescribed.

    Surgery for Resectable Disease (Stages I-IIIA): *Surgical resection offers the best chance for long-term survival. Selection of the type of operation is determined by tumor location and size.*

    Pneumonectomy. *Reserved for extensive disease that is technically resectable. See also Thoracotomy, p. 225.*

    Lobectomy: *Performed when the tumor is contained within a lobe and adequate margins can be obtained or when lymph node extension is limited to lobar nodes totally encompassed in the enbloc dissection.*

    Wedge resection. *Performed for small (<2 cm) peripheral nodules without lymph node or other extensive involvement. See also Thoracotomy, p. 225.*

- Explain treatments for **small cell cancer:**

    Chemotherapy: *Because SCLC more frequently spreads from the primary site and because of its increased sensitivity to chemotherapy, combination chemotherapy is the major treatment and has improved survival fivefold. See also Chemotherapy, p. 403.*

    Prophylactic cranial radiation: *Utilized in patients who have limited disease and those who go for 6 months without relapse.*

NURSING DIAGNOSES	EXPECTED OUTCOMES AND NURSING INTERVENTIONS / *RATIONALE* (■ = INDEPENDENT; ▲ = COLLABORATIVE)

High Risk for Injury

RISK FACTORS

Paraneoplastic syndromes
Oncologic emergencies

EXPECTED OUTCOMES

Risk for injury is reduced by early assessment of complications and appropriate treatment.

ONGOING ASSESSMENT

- Assess for common paraneoplastic syndromes. *These are extrapulmonary clinical manifestations of lung cancer that affect multiple body systems.*
    Endocrine (caused by secretion of a hormonelike substance by the tumor).
    Hypercalcemia: Most often with squamous cell cancer.
        Lethargy, polyuria, nausea, vomiting, abdominal pain, and constipation
        Inappropriate ADH and hyponatremia
        Ectopic ACTH and Cushing's syndrome
    Neurologic: Most common extrathoracic manifestations of lung cancer characterized by:
        Weakness of muscles, especially of pelvis and thighs
        Eaton-Lambert syndrome, myasthenic syndrome
        Peripheral neuropathy
        Cerebellar degeneration
        Polymyositis
    Hematologic
        Migratory thrombophlebitis
        Nonbacterial thrombotic endocarditis
        Disseminated intravascular coagulation: *DIC results from liberation of clot-promoting agents by tumor cells into circulating plasma. Patient may hemorrhage into vital organs.*
- Assess for common oncologic emergencies. These can be life-threatening and lead to permanent damage.
    Neurologic:
        Headache, vomiting, papilledema *caused by increased intracranial pressure*
        Stroke and seizures *caused by CNS metastases, infection, metabolic consequences*
    Cardiovascular:
        Cardiac tamponade *caused by accumulation of fluid containing tumor cells in the pericardial sac and by encasement of the heart by tumor.* Signs include chest pain, apprehension, dyspnea.
        Superior vena caval syndrome *caused by partial or complete obstruction of blood flow per SVC to right atrium.* Signs: facial and upper extremity edema, tracheal edema, cough, shortness of breath, dizziness, visual changes, hoarseness.

THERAPEUTIC INTERVENTIONS

▲ Anticipate appropriate treatment for each type of paraneoplastic syndrome:
    For hypercalcemia: hydration and bisphosphanates.
    For neuromyopathies: first concern is treatment of the primary tumor, then steroids and physical therapy may be added.
    For DIC: heparin, cryoprecipitates, platelets, and packed RBCs.
▲ Anticipate treatment for neurologic oncologic emergencies.
    Glucocorticoids. *Improve neurologic deficits in 70% of patients with increased ICP.*
    Brain irradiation
    For seizures: maintenance of airway, anticonvulsant drug therapy
▲ Anticipate the following treatment for cardiovascular oncologic emergencies:
    For cardiac tamponade: Decompression of the heart either surgically or by pericardiocentesis.
    For prevention of reaccumulation of effusions:
        Catheter drainage with instillation of tetracycline
        Radiation therapy
        Surgical intervention with creation of pericardial window
    For superior vena caval syndrome: radiation therapy, chemotherapy, surgery, anticoagulation, corticosteroids, diuretics

Continued.

Lung cancer cont'd

NURSING DIAGNOSES	EXPECTED OUTCOMES AND NURSING INTERVENTIONS / *RATIONALE* (■ = INDEPENDENT; ▲ = COLLABORATIVE)

Pain

RELATED FACTORS

Original tumor and metastatic
disease

DEFINING CHARACTERISTICS

Complaints of pain
Moaning/crying
Grimacing
Restlessness
Irritability

EXPECTED OUTCOMES

Patient verbalizes relief of/ability to tolerate pain.
Patient appears relaxed and comfortable.

ONGOING ASSESSMENT

- Assess for pain characteristics. *Bone pain is common at site of metastasis.*
- Monitor effectiveness of pain relief therapies.

THERAPEUTIC INTERVENTIONS

▲ Administer prescribed medications:
  Nonsteroidal antiinflammatory agents. *Used to treat muscle spasm associated with progressive tumor spread.*
  Short- and long-acting narcotics. *Most often used with bone metastasis. It is essential to work for pain relief and patient comfort and not fear escalating doses as narcotic tolerance develops or patients manifest symptoms of disease progression.*
  Long-acting with short-acting. *Prevents breakthrough pain.*
  Transdermal.
  Morphine and oxygen. *Are palliative therapies for end stage disease.*

By: Mary T. McCarthy, RN, MSN, CS

Mechanical ventilation

The patient who requires mechanical ventilation must have an artificial airway (endotracheal [ET] tube or tracheostomy). A mechanical ventilator will facilitate movement of gases into and out of the pulmonary system (ventilation), but it cannot ensure gas exchange at the pulmonary and tissue levels (respiration). It provides either partial or total ventilatory support for patients with respiratory failure.

NURSING DIAGNOSES	EXPECTED OUTCOMES AND NURSING INTERVENTIONS / *RATIONALES* (■ = INDEPENDENT; ▲ = COLLABORATIVE)

Inability to Sustain Spontaneous Ventilation

RELATED FACTORS

Metabolic factors
Respiratory muscle fatigue
Acute respiratory failure:
  Pneumonia
  Chronic obstructive pulmonary disease (COPD)
  Acute respiratory distress syndrome (ARDS)
  Tuberculosis
  Pulmonary embolus
  Pulmonary edema
  Airway obstruction
  Copious amounts of secretions
  Drug overdosage
  Diabetic coma
  Uremia
  Various CNS disorders
  Smoke inhalation
  Aspiration
  Chest trauma
  Status asthmaticus
  Guillian-Barré
  Myasthenia gravis

EXPECTED OUTCOMES

Patient's ventilatory demand is decreased as evidenced by eupnea, no use of accessory muscles, and ABGs normal for patient.

ONGOING ASSESSMENT

- Assess vital signs. *Hypotension, tachycardia, and tachypnea may result from hypoxia and/or hypocarbia.*
- Assess lung sounds *(allows early detection of deterioration or improvement)*. Listen closely for rhonchi, rales (crackles), wheezing, and diminished breath sounds in each lobe, assessing right to left, *to compare lung sounds.* Reassess lung sounds after coughing/suctioning *to determine whether they have improved or cleared.*
- Assess breathing rate, pattern, depth; note position assumed for breathing.
▲ Observe ABGs for abrupt changes or deteriorations. Normal ranges: pH 7.35-7.45, Po_2 80-90 torr, Pco_2 35-45 torr, O_2 saturation 85%-98%, O_2 content 16-23 vol%, HCO_3 23-29 mEq/L, Base excess 0 ± 2 mEq/L. *Oxygenation must be closely monitored to prevent hypoxia or hyperoxia, both of which could cause additional injury.*
- Assess for changes in mental status and LOC. *Signs of hypoxia include anxiety, restlessness, disorientation, somnolence, lethargy, and/or coma.*
- Assess skin color, checking nail beds and lips for cyanosis. *Cyanosis is a late sign of hypoxia because 5 g of hemoglobin must be desaturated for cyanosis to occur.*
▲ Use pulse oximetry, as available, *to continuously monitor O_2 saturation, rapidly assess changes, and prevent acute hypoxia.*
▲ Observe laboratory data, especially noting changes in Hb, electrolyte, and blood glucose levels.

DEFINING CHARACTERISTICS

pH < 7.35
P_{O_2} < 50-60
P_{CO_2} ≥ 50-60
Decrease in available Hb resulting in decreased O_2 content
Changes in mental status (e.g., apprehension, increased restlessness)
Increased or decreased respiratory rate
Apnea
Inability to maintain airway (i.e., depressed gag, depressed cough, emesis)
Forced vital capacity <10 cc/kg)
Rales (crackles), rhonchi, wheezing
Diminished breath sounds

ONGOING ASSESSMENT—cont'd

▲ After intubation, assess for ET tube position:
Inflate cuff until no audible leaks are heard. *Cuff pressure should not exceed 30 mm Hg. Cuff overinflation increases incidence of tracheal erosions.*
Auscultate for bilateral breath sounds while patient is being manually ventilated by Ambu bag *to assure good ET tube position. If diminished breath sounds are present over left lung field, the ET tube is most likely below the carina, in the right main stem bronchus, and must be pulled back.*
Observe for abdominal distention *(may indicate gastric intubation and can also occur after CPR when air is inadvertently blown/bagged into the esophagus as well as the trachea).*
Ensure that chest radiograph evaluation is obtained *to determine ET tube placement.*

THERAPEUTIC INTERVENTIONS

Before intubation:
▪ Maintain patient's airway:
Encourage patient to cough and breathe deeply.
If coughing and deep breathing not effective, use nasotracheal suction as needed *to clear airway.*
Use oral or nasal airway as needed *to prevent tongue from occluding oropharynx.*
Provide O_2 therapy as prescribed and indicated. *Increasing O_2 tension in the alveoli may result in more O_2 diffusion into the capillaries.*
Coordinate respiratory therapy treatments.
▪ Place patient in high Fowler's position, if tolerated, *to promote lung expansion. Check position frequently so that patient does not slide down, causing the abdomen to compress the diaphragm, which would cause respiratory embarrassment.*
▪ Notify physician:
If vital signs are out of prescribed range or trending from baseline
Immediately for signs of impending respiratory failure
Prepare for endotracheal intubation:
▲ Notify respiratory therapist to bring mechanical ventilator.
▪ If possible, before intubation, explain to patient need for intubation, steps involved, and temporary inability to speak.
▪ Prepare equipment:
ET tubes of various sizes, noting size used.
Benzoin and waterproof tape or other methods *for securing ET tube*
A syringe for inflating balloon after ET tube is in position
Local anesthetic agent (e.g., Cetacaine spray, cocaine, lidocaine [Xylocaine] spray or jelly, and cotton tip applicators) *for comfort and suppression of gag reflex*
Sedation as prescribed by physician *to decrease combative resistance to intubation*
Stylet *to make ET tube firmer and give additional support to direction*
Magill forceps
Laryngoscope and blades
Ambu bag and mask connected to oxygen *to provide assisted ventilation with 100% O_2*
Suction equipment *to maintain clear airway*
Oral airway if patient is being orally intubated *to prevent occlusion or biting of ET tube*
Bilateral soft wrist restraints *to prevent self-extubation of ET tube*
Assist with intubation:
▪ Place patient in supine position, hyperextending neck (if not contraindicated) and aligning patient's oropharynx, posterior nasopharynx, and trachea.
▲ Oxygenate and ventilate patient as needed before and after each intubation attempt. If intubation is difficult, physician will stop periodically so that oxygenation will be maintained with artificial ventilation by Ambu bag and mask.
After intubation:
▪ Continue with manual ventilation until ET tube is stabilized.
▪ Insert oral airway for orally intubated patient *to prevent patient from biting down on ET tube.*
▪ Assist in securing ET tube (if in proper placement per examination).
▪ Document ET tube position, noting the centimeter reference marking on ET tube *to monitor for possible displacement.*
▪ Institute aseptic suctioning of airway.
▲ Institute mechanical ventilation with settings as prescribed.

Continued.

Mechanical ventilation—cont'd

NURSING DIAGNOSES	EXPECTED OUTCOMES AND NURSING INTERVENTIONS / *RATIONALES* (■ = INDEPENDENT; ▲ = COLLABORATIVE)

THERAPEUTIC INTERVENTIONS—cont'd

- Apply bilateral soft wrist restraints as needed, explaining reason for use. *Although all patients do not require restraints to prevent extubation, many do.*
▲ Administer muscle paralyzing agents, sedatives, and narcotic analgesics as indicated *to decrease the patient's work of breathing and to decrease myocardial work.*
- Anticipate need for nasogastric (NG) suction *to prevent abdominal distention.*

High Risk for Injury

RISK FACTORS

Improper ventilator settings
Improper alarm settings
Disconnection of ventilator

EXPECTED OUTCOMES

Patient remains free of injury as evidenced by ABGs within normal limits for patient and appropriate ventilator settings.

ONGOING ASSESSMENT

▲ Check ventilator settings q1h *to see that patient is receiving correct:*
    Mode:
        Synchronized intermittent mandatory ventilation (*SIMV: preset TV; preset rate in synchronization with patient's own spontaneous breathing*).
        Controlled mandatory ventilation (*CMV: preset TV; preset rate with no sensitivity to patient's respiratory effort. Patient cannot initiate breaths or alter pattern*).
        Assist control (*AC: Preset TV; preset rate that is sensitive to patient's inspiratory effort. Delivers a preset TV for each patient-initiated breath*)
    Rate of mechanical breaths
    Tidal volume
    Fio_2
    Continuous positive airway pressure
    Pressure support (*PS*): *Positive airway pressure during the inspiratory cycle of a spontaneous inspiratory effort.*
▲ Monitor ABGs.
- Assess rate/rhythm of respiratory pattern, including work of breathing. *It is important to maintain the patient in synchrony with the ventilator; not "fighting" it.*

THERAPEUTIC INTERVENTIONS

▲ Notify respiratory therapist of discrepancy in ventilator settings immediately.
- Ensure that ventilator alarms are on.
▲ Listen for alarms; know range in which ventilator will alarm and respond to alarms: *The ventilator is a life-sustaining treatment that requires prompt intervention to alarms.*
    High peak pressure alarm *may indicate bronchospasm, retained secretions, obstruction of ET tube, atelectasis, ARDS, pneumothorax, etc.*
        If patient is agitated, give sedation as prescribed.
        Empty water from water traps as appropriate.
        Auscultate breath sounds; institute suctioning as needed. Notify respiratory therapist and physician if high pressure alarm persists.
    Low-pressure alarm *indicates possible disconnection or mechanical ventilatory malfunction.*
        If disconnected, reconnect patient to mechanical ventilator.
        If malfunctioning, remove patient from mechanical ventilator and use Ambu bag. Notify respiratory therapist to correct malfunction.
    Low exhale volume *indicates patient is not returning delivered tidal volume (i.e., leak or disconnection).*
        Reconnect patient to ventilator if disconnected, or reconnect exhale tubing to the ventilator. If problem is not resolved, notify physician and respiratory therapist.
        Check cuff volume by assessing whether patient can talk or make sounds around tube or whether exhaled volumes are significantly less than volumes delivered. To correct, slowly reinflate cuff with air until no leak is detected. Notify respiratory therapist to check cuff pressure: *Cuff pressure should be maintained at <30 mm Hg.*
        Maintenance of low-pressure cuffs prevents many tracheal complications formerly associated with ET tubes. Notify physician if leak persists. *ET tube cuff may be defective, requiring physician to change tube.*
    Apnea alarm *is indicative of disconnection or absence of spontaneous respirations.*
        If disconnected, reconnect patient to ventilator.
        If apnea persists, use Ambu bag to ventilate; notify physician.

NURSING DIAGNOSES	EXPECTED OUTCOMES AND NURSING INTERVENTIONS / *RATIONALES* (■ = INDEPENDENT; ▲ = COLLABORATIVE)

Ineffective Airway Clearance

RELATED FACTORS
Endotracheal intubation

DEFINING CHARACTERISTICS
Copious secretions
Abnormal breath sounds
Dyspnea

EXPECTED OUTCOMES
Patient's secretions are mobilized and airway remains patent as evidenced by eupnea and clear breath sounds after suctioning.

ONGOING ASSESSMENT
- Assess breath sounds as needed.
- Note quantity, color, consistency, and odor of sputum.

THERAPEUTIC INTERVENTIONS
- Institute suctioning of airway as needed on the basis of presence of adventitious breath sounds and/or increased ventilatory pressures.
▲ Administer pain medications, as appropriate, before suctioning.
- Silence ventilator alarms during suctioning *to decrease the frequency of false alarms and reduce stressful noise to the patient.*
- Use sterile saline instillations during suctioning as needed *to help facilitate removal of tenacious sputum.*
- Turn patient q2hr *to mobilize secretions.*
▲ Administer adequate fluid intake (IV and NG, as appropriate) *to promote patient's hydration and to keep secretions liquid.*

Impaired Verbal Communication

RELATED FACTORS
Endotracheal intubation

DEFINING CHARACTERISTICS
Patient inability to communicate verbally because of intubation
Difficulty in being understood with nonverbal methods
Increasing frustration and/or anxiety at inability to verbalize

EXPECTED OUTCOMES
Patient attains a nonverbal means to express needs and concerns.

ONGOING ASSESSMENT
- Assess patient's ability to use nonverbal communication. *An endotracheal tube passes through the vocal cords and, when the cuff is effectively inflated, prevents airflow across the vocal cords. Therefore, phonation is not possible with an ET tube.*

THERAPEUTIC INTERVENTIONS
- Provide nonverbal means of communication: writing equipment, communication board, or generalized list of questions/answers.
▲ Refer to speech therapy for alternate forms of speech (e.g., electrolarynx), as appropriate.
- Reassure patient that inability to speak is temporary effect of ET tube's passing vocal cords.
- Enlist significant other's assistance in understanding needs/communication.
- See also Impaired communication, p. 14.
- When long-term ventilation is anticipated and tracheostomy is performed, see also Tracheostomy, p. 229.

Fear/Anxiety

RELATED FACTORS
Inability to breathe adequately without support
Inability to maintain adequate gas exchange
Fear of unknown outcome

DEFINING CHARACTERISTICS
Restlessness
Fear of sleeping at night
Uncooperative behavior
Withdrawal
Indifference
Vigilant watch on equipment
Facial tension
Focus on self

EXPECTED OUTCOMES
Patient demonstrates reduced fear/anxiety as evidenced by calm manner and cooperative behavior.

ONGOING ASSESSMENT
- Assess for signs of fear/anxiety. *Anxiety can affect respiratory rate and rhythm, resulting in rapid shallow breathing.*

THERAPEUTIC INTERVENTIONS
- Display confident, calm manner and understanding attitude.
- Inform patient of alarms in ventilatory system and reassure patient of close proximity of health care personnel *to respond to alarms. An informed patient who understands the treatment plan will be more cooperative.*
- Be available to patient/significant other and offer support as well as explanations of patient's care and progress.
- Reduce distracting stimuli *to provide quiet environment.* Schedule care to provide frequent rest periods.
- Encourage visiting by family/friends.
- Encourage sedentary diversional activities *to enhance patient's quality of life and to help pass time (e.g., television, reading, being read to, writing, occupational therapy).*
- Provide calendar and clock at bedside.
- Provide relaxation techniques *to promote relaxation (tapes, imagery, progressive muscle relaxation, etc).*
▲ Refer to psychiatric liaison clinical nurse specialist, psychiatrist, or hospital chaplain as appropriate.

Continued.

NURSING DIAGNOSES	EXPECTED OUTCOMES AND NURSING INTERVENTIONS / *RATIONALES* (■ = INDEPENDENT; ▲ = COLLABORATIVE)

Decreased Cardiac Output

RELATED FACTORS
Mechanical ventilation
Positive-pressure ventilation

DEFINING CHARACTERISTICS
Hypotension
Tachycardia
Dysrhythmias
Anxiety, restlessness
Decreased peripheral pulses
Weight gain
Edema

EXPECTED OUTCOMES
Patient achieves adequate cardiac output as evidenced by strong peripheral pulses, normal vital signs, warm dry skin, and alert responsive mentation.

ONGOING ASSESSMENT
▲ Assess vital signs and hemodynamic parameters (CVP, pulmonary artery pressures, cardiac output). *Mechanical ventilation can cause decreased venous return to the heart, resulting in decreased cardiac output (this may occur abruptly with ventilator changes: rate, tidal volume, or positive-pressure ventilation). Close monitoring during ventilator changes is imperative.*
▪ Assess skin color, temperature; note quality of peripheral pulses.
▪ Assess fluid balance through:
  Daily weights
  I & O: *After the initial decrease in venous return to the heart, volume receptors in the right atrium signal a decrease in volume, which triggers an increase in the release of antidiuretic hormone from the posterior pituitary and a retention of H_2O by the kidneys.*
▪ Assess mentation. *Early signs of cerebral hypoxia are restlessness and anxiety, leading on to agitation and confusion.*
▪ Monitor for dysrhythmias. *Cardiac dysrhythmias may result from the low perfusion state, acidosis, or hypoxia.*

THERAPEUTIC INTERVENTIONS
▲ Maintain optimal fluid balance. *Fluid challenges may initially be used to add volume. However, if pulmonary artery pressures rise and cardiac output remains low, fluid restriction may be necessary.*
▲ Notify physician immediately of signs of decrease in cardiac output and anticipate possible ventilator setting changes.
▲ Administer medications (diuretics, inotropic agents, bronchodilators) as ordered.
▪ See also Decreased cardiac output, p. 12.

High Risk for Impaired Skin Integrity

RISK FACTORS
Prolonged intubation

EXPECTED OUTCOMES
Patient's skin integrity is maintained as evidenced by clean dry skin around ET tube and intact skin.

ONGOING ASSESSMENT
▪ Observe skin for buildup of secretions, crusting around ET tube, redness, or breakdown.

THERAPEUTIC INTERVENTIONS
▪ Support ventilator tubing *to prevent pressure on nose or lips.*
▪ Change tape when loosened or soiled *to ensure adequate stabilization of ET tube.*
▪ Provide mouth care q2hr (e.g., may use $1:1$ H_2O_2 and H_2O and mouthwash afterward). *This will help decrease oral bacteria and prevent crusting of secretions.* Apply lip lubrication after mouth care *to prevent drying/cracking of lips.*
▪ If patient is nasally intubated, notify physician of red or irritated skin or breakdown.
▪ If patient orally intubated, reposition tube from side to side q24-48hr. *to prevent pressure breakdown on lip beneath ET tube.*

High Risk for Injury: Barotrauma

RISK FACTORS
Positive-pressure ventilation
Decreased pulmonary compliance

EXPECTED OUTCOMES
Potential for injury from barotrauma is reduced by ongoing assessment and early intervention.

ONGOING ASSESSMENT
▲ Assess for signs of barotrauma q1h: crepitus, subcutaneous emphysema, altered chest excursion, asymmetrical chest, abnormal ABGs, shift in trachea, restlessness, evidence of pneumothorax on chest radiograph. *Frequent assessments are needed since barotrauma can occur at any time and the patient will not show signs of dyspnea, shortness of breath, or tachypnea if heavily sedated to maintain ventilation.*
▲ Monitor chest radiograph reports daily and obtain a stat portable chest radiograph if barotrauma suspected.

NURSING DIAGNOSES	EXPECTED OUTCOMES AND NURSING INTERVENTIONS / *RATIONALES* (■ = INDEPENDENT; ▲ = COLLABORATIVE)

THERAPEUTIC INTERVENTIONS

- Notify physician of signs of barotrauma immediately.
▲ Anticipate need for chest tube placement, and prepare as needed. *If barotrauma is suspected, intervention must follow immediately to prevent tension pneumothorax.*

High Risk for Infection

RISK FACTORS

ET intubation
Suctioning of airway

EXPECTED OUTCOMES

Risk of infection is reduced through proper techniques, continued assessment, and early intervention.

ONGOING ASSESSMENT

- Monitor temperature; notify physician of temperature >38.5° C.
▲ Monitor WBC.
▲ Monitor sputum culture and sensitivity reports.
- Observe for changes in tracheal secretions: color, consistency, amount, and odor.
▲ Monitor radiograph results *for signs of infiltration or atelectasis.*

THERAPEUTIC INTERVENTIONS

- Maintain aseptic suctioning techniques *to lessen probability of infection acquisition.*
- Administer antibiotics as ordered.
▲ Limit the number of visitors as appropriate and screen all visitors for communicable disease.
- Administer mouth care *to limit bacterial growth and to promote patient comfort.*
- Maintain patient's personal hygiene, nutrition, and rest *to increase natural defenses.*

Knowledge Deficit

RELATED FACTORS

New treatment
New environment

DEFINING CHARACTERISTICS

Multiple questions
Lack of concern
Anxiety

EXPECTED OUTCOMES

Patient/significant other state basic understanding of mechanical ventilation and care involved.

ONGOING ASSESSMENT

- Assess perception and understanding of mechanical ventilation.

THERAPEUTIC INTERVENTIONS

- Allow patient/significant other to express feelings and ask questions.
- Explain that patient will not be able to eat or drink while intubated but assure him/her that alternative measures (i.e., gastric feedings or hyperalimentation) will be taken to provide nourishment. *Risk of aspiration is high if patient eats or drinks while intubated.*
- Explain necessity for procedures (e.g., obtaining ABGs).
- Explain to patient inability to talk while intubated: *ET tube passes through vocal cords and attempts to talk can cause more trauma to cords.*
- Explain that alarms may periodically sound off, which may be normal, and that the staff will be in close proximity.
- Explain the need for frequent assessments (i.e., vital signs, auscultation of breath sounds).
- Explain probable need for restraints *to gain cooperation in preventing an accidental extubation.*
- Explain the need for suctioning as needed.
- Explain the weaning process and explain that extubation will be attempted after the patient has demonstrated adequate respiratory function and a decrease in pulmonary secretions.

See also:
Altered nutrition: less than
body requirements, p. 44.
Sleep pattern disturbance,
p. 61.
Impaired physical mobility,
p. 47.
Dysfunctional ventilatory
weaning response, p. 21.
Caregiver role strain, p. 13.
Dependence/Powerlessness,
p. 52.

By: Susan Galanes, RN, MS, CCRN

Near-drowning

Survival at least 24 hours after submersion in a fluid medium. Aspiration of salt water causes plasma to be drawn into the lungs, resulting in hypoxemia and hypovolemia. Freshwater aspiration causes hypervolemia resulting from absorption of water through alveoli into the vascular system. These fluids are further absorbed into the interstitial space. Hypoxemia results from the decrease in pulmonary surfactant caused by the absorbed water and leading to damage of the pulmonary capillary membrane. Severe hypoxia can also result from asphyxia related to submersion without aspiration of fluid. Of drowning victims 10%-20% are "dry" drowning victims who experience severe laryngospasm without aspiration of fluid.

NURSING DIAGNOSES	EXPECTED OUTCOMES AND NURSING INTERVENTIONS / *RATIONALES* (■ = INDEPENDENT; ▲ = COLLABORATIVE)

Impaired Gas Exchange

RELATED FACTORS

Surfactant elimination
Bronchospasm
Aspiration
Pulmonary edema

DEFINING CHARACTERISTICS

Cyanosis
Retractions
Tachypnea
Stridor
Hypoxemia
Frothy, pink-tinged expectorant (saltwater-induced pulmonary edema)

EXPECTED OUTCOMES

Patient maintains optimal gas exchange as evidenced by ABGs within baseline for the patient, decrease in work of breathing (eupnea, absence of retractions).

ONGOING ASSESSMENT

- Assess breath sounds.
▲ Monitor ABGs.
- Assess for signs of respiratory distress: retractions, stridor, nasal flaring, use of accessory muscles.
▲ Assess for signs of hypoxemia: altered LOC, tachycardia, deteriorating serial ABG results, tachypnea, cyanosis, increasing respiratory distress.
▲ Assess serial chest radiographic examination reports.
- Monitor for evidence of increasing pulmonary edema *(may indicate need for mechanical ventilation).*

THERAPEUTIC INTERVENTIONS

- Maintain the airway and assist ventilations as needed while protecting the C-spine. *C-spine injuries should always be considered in victims of near-drowning, especially after a dive.*
- Place patient in position to allow maximum lung inflation. *Head and chest down position is indicated in seawater near-drowning patients to drain the lungs. This position is of no use in fresh water near-drowning, as the water is rapidly absorbed into the circulation, no longer remaining in the lungs.*
▲ Maintain O$_2$ delivery system as needed.
- Suction only as needed; *hypoxia and Valsalva maneuver with suctioning may increase ICP, metabolic acidosis.*
▲ Anticipate the need for intubation and mechanical ventilation. See also Mechanical ventilation, p. 202.
- See also ARDS, p. 183. *The results of pulmonary injury are a clinical picture of ARDS: pulmonary edema, atelectasis, hyaline membrane formation, and pulmonary capillary injury.*

Altered Cerebral Perfusion

RELATED FACTORS

Impaired gas exchange
Increased intracranial pressure (ICP) caused by fluid shifts with freshwater aspiration/hypoxia
Prolonged hypoxemia

DEFINING CHARACTERISTICS

Deficit in cranial nerve responses
Altered LOC
Inappropriate behavior
Altered pupillary response

EXPECTED OUTCOMES

Patient's cerebral perfusion is maximized as evidenced by alert responsive mentation or no further reduction in mental status.

ONGOING ASSESSMENT

- Assess LOC, using Glasgow Coma Scale.
- Determine cranial nerve response, especially vagus (breathing, gag, cough). *Absence indicates need for artificial airway maintenance.*
▲ Monitor for increasing intracranial pressure:
   Increased ICP monitor readings
   Narrowed pulse pressure and decreased heart and respiratory rates
   Alteration of pupil response
   Alteration of LOC (from admission level)
- Assess for seizure activity.
- Assess environment for degree of stimulation.

NURSING DIAGNOSES	EXPECTED OUTCOMES AND NURSING INTERVENTIONS / *RATIONALES* (■ = INDEPENDENT; ▲ = COLLABORATIVE)

THERAPEUTIC INTERVENTIONS

- Elevate head of bed (HOB) 30 degrees; maintain midline head, body alignment.
- ▲ Administer anticonvulsants as prescribed *to prevent seizure activity.*
- Maintain seizure precautions *to prevent patient from injuring self in event of seizure.*
- Minimize frequency of suctioning. *Hypoxia and Valsalva maneuver associated with suctioning may elevate ICP.*
- ▲ Sedate patient before beginning procedures (i.e., blood drawing, invasive procedures) *to prevent ICP elevation.*
- ▲ Administer medication as prescribed to maintain patient in barbiturate coma (*protects brain from athetoid movements, grunting, and straining, which may increase ICP*).
- ▲ Administer hyperventilation, as prescribed in collaboration with respiratory therapist, *to blow off CO_2 to control cerebral blood flow and in turn control increases in ICP.*
- ▲ Maintain oxygenation levels *to prevent further hypoxemic damage.*
- ▲ Control decerebrate activity with muscle paralyzing agents as prescribed (e.g., d-tubocurarine or pancuronium) *to control rises in ICP.*
- ▲ Administer corticosteroids, furosemide, and mannitol infusions as prescribed *to treat an increased ICP.*
- Minimize exposure to unnecessary stimuli.
- ▲ Maintain body temperature at *30° C with cooling or warming blankets (as appropriate) to reduce total O_2 requirements and prevent additional damage.*

Fluid Volume Excess/Deficit

RELATED FACTORS
EXCESS:

Aspiration of fresh water
Fluid shift from interstitial to intravascular space

DEFICIT:

Aspiration of salt water
Fluid shift from intravascular to interstitial space

DEFINING CHARACTERISTICS
EXCESS:

Decreased Hb, Hct levels
Increased CVP
Increased BP
Jugular venous distention

DEFICIT:

Hypotension
Tachycardia
Decreased urine output <30 ml/hr
Concentrated urine

EXPECTED OUTCOMES

Patient experiences adequate fluid volume as evidenced by urine output > 30 ml/hr, normotensive BP, and HR < 100/min.

ONGOING ASSESSMENT

- Assess vital signs. *Fresh water aspiration entering the circulation will expand the blood volume and increase BP. Salt water aspiration pulls water from the circulation into the alveoli, decreasing blood volume, and causing hypotension.*
- Monitor heart rate/rhythm.
- ▲ Assess serial electrolytes and assess pH results for acidosis/alkalosis.
- ▲ Assess Hct *to determine level of hemodilution/concentration.*
- Assess urine output q1hr; maintain accurate I & O.
- Assess specific gravity.
- Monitor CVP. *Severe hypovolemia will cause decreasing CVP, indicating the need for volume expanders. Note: Presence of crackles on auscultation or pulmonary congestion on radiograph may not indicate fluid overload if patient has had salt water aspiration, which pulls water from the circulation into the alveoli.*

THERAPEUTIC INTERVENTIONS

- Assist the physician with insertion of a central venous line and arterial line as indicated *for more effective fluid administration and monitoring.*
- ▲ Administer IV fluids as prescribed *to correct fluid imbalance.*
- ▲ Administer fluid volume expanders as prescribed.
- ▲ Administer sodium bicarbonate as prescribed *to correct metabolic acidosis.*

High Risk for Decreased Cardiac Output

RISK FACTORS

Hypothermia induced dysrhythmias
Hypoxic damage

EXPECTED OUTCOMES

Patient achieves adequate cardiac output as evidenced by strong peripheral pulses, normal vital signs, urine output > 30 ml/hr, warm, dry skin, and no further reduction in mental status.

ONGOING ASSESSMENT

- Assess temperature with routine vital sign checks. *Severe acute submersion hypothermia may be present. Myocardial contractility and vasomotor tone are decreased by hypothermia.*
- Monitor BP frequently. *Vasodilatation occurs during rewarming and hypotension may result unless closely monitored with intervention as necessary. Direct intra-arterial monitoring of pressure should be anticipated for a continuing shock state.*

Continued.

NURSING DIAGNOSES	EXPECTED OUTCOMES AND NURSING INTERVENTIONS / *RATIONALES* (■ = INDEPENDENT; ▲ = COLLABORATIVE)
	ONGOING ASSESSMENT—cont'd • Assess skin warmth and peripheral pulses every hour. *Peripheral vasoconstriction causes cool, pale, diaphoretic skin.* • Assess level of consciousness every hour. *Early signs of cerebral hypoxia are restlessness and anxiety, leading on to agitation and confusion.* • Monitor for dysrhythmias. *Cardiac dysrhythmias may result from the low perfusion state, acidosis, or hypoxia.* ▲ If hemodynamic monitoring is in place, assess CVP, PAP, PCWP, and CO. *CVP provides information on filling pressures of right side of the heart; PAP and PCWP reflect left-sided fluid volumes.* • Monitor urine output every hour with Foley catheter. *Oliguria is a classic sign of inadequate renal perfusion.* **THERAPEUTIC INTERVENTIONS** ▲ Rewarm patient as appropriate (e.g., blankets, head wrap, warmed O_2, rewarming blankets). *Note: Warming should be limited to a maximum of 30° C.* ▲ Administer inotropic agents dobutamine HCl (Dobutrex), dopamine, digoxin, or amrinone (Inocor) *to improve myocardial contractility.* Continuously monitor their effectiveness. ▲ *Treat acidosis* with sodium bicarbonate.
High Risk for Infection **RISK FACTORS** Aspiration of contaminated water	**EXPECTED OUTCOMES** Risk for infection is decreased through ongoing assessment and early intervention. **ONGOING ASSESSMENT** • Monitor temperature. ▲ Monitor results of cultures and serial white blood cell counts, which *may indicate infection.* • Assess for increased respiratory distress and notify physician if present. ▲ Monitor chest radiograph reports; *aspiration of contaminated water during near-drowning puts patient at risk for pneumonia.* See also Pneumonia, p. 211, as indicated. • Assess color, odor, and amount of sputum. **THERAPEUTIC INTERVENTIONS** • Suction secretions as needed; send secretion sample for culture and sensitivity testing. ▲ Administer antibiotics is ordered. • Position *for ease in lung expansion.* • Reposition *to promote drainage (postural drainage);* perform chest physical therapy as needed. • Encourage use of incentive spirometer when patient is neurologically stable.

See also:
Impaired Skin Integrity, p. 59.
Knowledge Deficit, p. 41.

By: Susan Galanes, RN, MS, CCRN

Pneumonia

(PNEUMONITIS)

Pneumonia is caused by a bacterial or viral infection that results in an inflammatory process in the lungs. It is an infectious process that is spread by droplets or by contact. Predisposing factors to the development of pneumonia include upper respiratory infection, excessive alcohol ingestion, central nervous system depression, cardiac failure, any debilitating illness, chronic obstructive pulmonary disease, endotracheal intubation, postoperative effects of general anesthesia; at risk are patients who are bedridden, patients with lowered resistance, and hospitalized patients in whom a superinfection may develop.

NURSING DIAGNOSES	EXPECTED OUTCOMES AND NURSING INTERVENTIONS / *RATIONALE* (■ = INDEPENDENT; ▲ = COLLABORATIVE)

Ineffective Airway Clearance

RELATED FACTORS

Increased sputum production in response to respiratory infection
Decreased energy and increased fatigue with predisposing factors present
Aspiration

DEFINING CHARACTERISTICS

Abnormal breath sounds (e.g., rhonchi, bronchial breath sounds)
Decreased breath sounds over affected areas
Cough
Dyspnea
Change in respiratory status
Infiltrates on chest radiograph film

EXPECTED OUTCOMES

Patient's airway is free of secretions as evidenced by eupnea and clear breath sounds after coughing/suctioning.

ONGOING ASSESSMENT

- Assess vital signs and auscultate breath sounds, noting areas of decreased ventilation and presence of adventitious sounds.
- Assess respiratory movements and use of accessory muscles. *Use of accessory muscles to breathe indicates an abnormal increase in work of breathing.*
- ▲ Monitor chest radiograph reports *to determine progression of disease process (e.g., clearing of infiltrates)*
- Observe sputum color, amount, and odor and report significant changes.
- ▲ Monitor sputum Gram's stain and culture and sensitivity reports.
- Assess for presence of cough and monitor its effectiveness.

THERAPEUTIC INTERVENTIONS

- Assist patient with coughing and deep breathing, splinting, as necessary *to improve coughing.*
- Encourage patient to cough unless cough is frequent and nonproductive. *Frequent nonproductive coughing can result in hypoxemia.*
- Use positioning *to facilitate clearing secretions.*
- ▲ Consult respiratory therapist for chest physiotherapy and nebulizer treatments, as appropriate.
- Use humidity *to loosen secretions (humidified O₂ or humidifier at bedside).*
- Maintain adequate hydration *(fluids are lost by diaphoresis, fever, and tachypnea and are needed to aid in the mobilization of secretions).*
- ▲ Administer medication (e.g., antibiotics, expectorants *[for productive coughs]*, cough suppressants *[for hacking nonproductive coughs]*) as prescribed/indicated, noting effectiveness.
- Institute suctioning of airway as needed *to remove sputum and mucous plugs.*
- ▲ Assist with bronchoscopy and thoracentesis as needed.
- Use nasopharyngeal/oropharyngeal airway as needed.
- ▲ Anticipate possible need for intubation if patient's condition deteriorates.

Impaired Gas Exchange

RELATED FACTORS

Collection of mucus in airways

DEFINING CHARACTERISTICS

Dyspnea
Decreased Pao₂
Increased Paco₂
Cyanosis
Tachypnea
Air hunger
Tachycardia
Decreased activity tolerance
Restlessness
Disorientation/confusion

EXPECTED OUTCOMES

Patient maintains optimal gas exchange as evidenced by eupnea, normal ABGs, and alert responsive mentation or no further reduction in mental status.

ONGOING ASSESSMENT

- Assess respirations: note quality, rate, pattern, depth, dyspnea on exertion, use of accessory muscles, position assumed for easy breathing.
- Assess skin color for development of cyanosis.
- Assess for changes in orientation and note increasing restlessness. *These can be early signs of hypoxia and/or hypercarbia.*
- Assess for activity intolerance.
- Monitor for changes in vital signs. *With initial hypoxia and hypercapnia, BP, heart rate, and respiratory rate all rise. As the hypoxia and/or hypercapnia becomes more severe, BP may drop, heart rate tends to continue to be rapid with arrhythmias, and respiratory failure may ensue, with the patient unable to maintain the rapid respiratory rate.*
- ▲ Monitor ABGs; note differences.

Continued.

NURSING DIAGNOSES	EXPECTED OUTCOMES AND NURSING INTERVENTIONS / *RATIONALES* (■ = INDEPENDENT; ▲ = COLLABORATIVE)

THERAPEUTIC INTERVENTIONS

- Pace activities to patient's tolerance. *Activities will increase O$_2$ consumption and should be planned so patient does not become hypoxic.*
▲ Maintain O$_2$ administration device as ordered. Avoid high concentrations of O$_2$ in patients with COPD. *Hypoxia stimulates the drive to breathe in the chronic CO$_2$ retainer patient.*
- Anticipate need for intubation, and, possibly, mechanical ventilation if condition worsens. See also Mechanical ventilation, p. 202 (as needed).

Infection

RELATED FACTORS
Invading bacterial/viral organisms

DEFINING CHARACTERISTICS
Elevated temperature
Elevated WBC
Tachycardia
Chills
Positive sputum culture report
Changing character of sputum

EXPECTED OUTCOMES

Patient experiences improvement in infection as evidenced by normothermia, normal WBC count, and negative sputum culture report on repeat culture.

ONGOING ASSESSMENT

- Elicit patient's description of illness, including onset, chills, chest pain.
- Assess for predisposing factors: medications *(patients receiving high dosages of corticosteroids have reduced resistance to infections.)*; recent exposure to illness; alcohol, tobacco, or drug abuse; chronic illness.
- Assess vital signs, closely monitoring temperature fluctuations. *Continued fever may be caused by drug allergy, drug-resistant bacteria, superinfection, or inadequate lung drainage.*
▲ Monitor Gram's stain, sputum, culture, and sensitivity reports.
▲ Obtain fresh sputum for Gram's stain/culture and sensitivity, as prescribed:
    Instruct patient to expectorate into sterile container. Be sure the specimen is coughed up and is not saliva.
    If patient is unable to cough up specimen effectively, use sterile nasotracheal suctioning with a Luken's tube.
▲ Monitor WBC.
- Continue to monitor the effectiveness of the prescribed antimicrobial agents. *Parenteral IV antibiotics are usually given for the first few days of acute cases, and then changed to oral antibiotics (which may be adequate for milder cases from day one). To prevent a relapse of pneumonia the patient needs to complete the course of antibiotics as prescribed. Antiviral drugs (e.g., amantadine, rimantadine) are available for parenteral administration in viral respiratory infections. Antibiotics are not effective against viral pneumonia but may be utilized when concurrent viral and bacterial pneumonias are present.*

THERAPEUTIC INTERVENTIONS

▲ Use appropriate therapy for elevated temperatures: antipyretics, cold therapy.
▲ Administer prescribed antimicrobial agent(s) on schedule *so that a blood level is maintained to fight the organism adequately in order to prevent a relapse or the development of a resistant strain of the organism.*
- Provide tissues and waste bags for disposal of sputum.
- Isolate patient as necessary after review of culture and sensitivity results.
- Keep patient away from other patients who are at high risk of developing pneumonia.

Pain/Discomfort

RELATED FACTORS
Respiratory distress
Coughing

DEFINING CHARACTERISTICS
Complaints of discomfort
Guarding
Withdrawal
Moaning
Facial grimace
Irritability
Anxiety
Tachycardia
Increased BP

EXPECTED OUTCOMES
Patient verbalizes relief/reduction in pain.
Patient appears relaxed and comfortable.

ONGOING ASSESSMENT

- Assess complaints of discomfort: pain or discomfort with breathing, shortness of breath, muscle pains, pain with coughing, etc.
- Monitor for nonverbal signs of discomfort (e.g., grimacing, irritability, tachycardia, increased BP).

THERAPEUTIC INTERVENTIONS

▲ Administer appropriate medications to treat the cough:
    Do not suppress a productive cough; use moderate amounts of analgesics to relieve pleuritic pain.
    Use cough suppressants and humidity for dry, hacking cough. *An unproductive hacking cough irritates airways and should be suppressed.*

NURSING DIAGNOSES	EXPECTED OUTCOMES AND NURSING INTERVENTIONS / *RATIONALES* (■ = INDEPENDENT; ▲ = COLLABORATIVE)

THERAPEUTIC INTERVENTIONS—cont'd

▲ Administer analgesics as prescribed and as needed. Encourage patient to take analgesics before discomfort becomes severe *to prevent peak periods of pain.*

■ Evaluate medication effectiveness. Use additional measures to relieve discomfort, including positioning and relaxation techniques *to facilitate effective respiratory excursion.*

High Risk for Altered Nutrition: Less than Body Requirements

RISK FACTORS

Pneumonia, resulting in increased metabolic needs, lack of appetite, decreased intake

EXPECTED OUTCOMES

Patient's optimal nutritional status is maintained as evidenced by stabilized weight and adequate caloric intake.

ONGOING ASSESSMENT

■ Document patient's actual weight.
■ Obtain nutritional history and monitor present caloric intake.

THERAPEUTIC INTERVENTIONS

■ Maintain bed rest *to decrease metabolic needs.*
■ Increase activity gradually as patient tolerates.
■ Provide high-protein/high-carbohydrate diet, and assist with meals as needed.
■ Provide small, frequent feedings.
■ Provide a pleasing environment for meals by decreasing negative stimuli.
▲ Maintain O_2 delivery system (e.g., nasal cannula if appropriate) while patient eats. *This will help prevent desaturation and shortness of breath, with resultant loss of appetite.*
▲ Administer vitamin supplements, as prescribed.
▲ Administer enteral supplements and parenteral nutrition, as prescribed.

Knowledge Deficit

RELATED FACTORS

New condition and procedures
Unfamiliarity with disease process and transmission of disease

DEFINING CHARACTERISTICS

Questions
Confusion about treatment
Inability to comply with treatment regimen, including appropriate isolation procedures
Lack of questions

EXPECTED OUTCOMES

Patient and significant others demonstrate understanding of disease process and compliance with treatment regimen and isolation procedures.

ONGOING ASSESSMENT

■ Determine understanding of pneumonia complications and treatment.
■ Observe for compliance with treatment regimen.

THERAPEUTIC INTERVENTIONS

■ Teach patient to continue deep breathing exercises and techniques to cough effectively.
■ Provide information about need to:
　Maintain natural resistance to infection through adequate nutrition, rest, and exercise.
　Avoid contact with people with upper respiratory infections.
　Obtain immunizations against influenza for the elderly and chronically ill.
　Use pneumococcal vaccine for those at greatest risk: elderly patients with chronic systemic disease, patients with COPD, patients with sickle cell anemia, patients who have had splenectomy, patients who have had pneumonectomy and are immunosuppressed.
■ Instruct patient and significant other on isolation procedure used, *so they understand importance of protecting the patient and themselves for the time isolation is needed.*

See also:
Diversional activity deficit, p. 21.
Anxiety/fear, p. 5, 23.
Altered LOC, p. 252.
Activity intolerance, p. 2.

By: Susan Galanes, RN, MS, CCRN

Pneumothorax with chest tube

The presence of air in the intrapleural space, causing partial or complete collapse of the lung. Pneumothorax can be iatrogenic, spontaneous, or the result of injury. A chest tube drainage system is utilized to reestablish negative pressure in the intrapleural space to facilitate lung reexpansion.

RELATED FACTORS	EXPECTED OUTCOMES AND NURSING INTERVENTIONS / *RATIONALES* (■ = INDEPENDENT; ▲ = COLLABORATIVE)

Ineffective Breathing Pattern

RELATED FACTORS

Partially or completely collapsed lung
Pain
Anxiety

DEFINING CHARACTERISTICS

Shallow respirations
Rapid respirations
Diminished breath sounds on affected side
Dyspnea, shortness of breath
Asymmetrical chest expansion
Use of accessory muscles

EXPECTED OUTCOMES

Patient maintains effective breathing pattern, as evidenced by respiratory rate 12-20/min, clear breath sounds, and equal breath sounds bilaterally.

ONGOING ASSESSMENT

- Assess respiratory rate and effort, and use of accessory muscles.
- Auscultate lungs for areas of diminished or absent breath sounds.
- Assess patient's pain level.
- Assess chest tube drainage system for:
  Secure connections. *A loose connection can allow air entry and positive pressure in the intrapleural space, resulting in further lung collapse.*
  Intact water seal *to prevent air entry into intrapleural space.*
  Presence of fluctuation or tidaling fluid *caused by pressure changes in the intrapleural space during inspiration and expiration. Cessation of fluctuating/tidaling of fluid can indicate lung reexpansion or, if abrupt, can indicate clogged or kinked tube.*
  Presence of air leak or bubbling in the water seal. *Bubbling indicates air removal from the intrapleural space, especially during expiration or coughing. Cessation of bubbling can indicate lung reexpansion. Continuous bubbling can indicate air leak within patient's chest or within system.*
- ▲ Monitor serial chest radiographs to document lung reexpansion.

THERAPEUTIC INTERVENTIONS

- Explain the procedure for chest tube insertion *to prepare patient and decrease fear.*
- Assist physician during chest tube insertion.
- Maintain chest tube drainage system:
  Secure connections.
  Maintain proper H_2O levels in water seal and suction control chamber. *The amount of the suction is determined by the depth of the tubing in the suction control chamber. As water evaporates, additional water will need to be added to each chamber.*
- Encourage deep breathing while awake *to decrease atelectasis and enhance gas exchange.* Encourage coughing after deep breathing as needed.
- ▲ Administer pain medication as prescribed before activity: deep breathing, coughing, and physical mobility.
- Offer reassurance to decrease fear/anxiety. *Anxiety can result in rapid shallow respirations.*

Pain

RELATED FACTORS

Chest tube placement
Collapse of lung
Reexpansion of lung

DEFINING CHARACTERISTICS

Complaint of pain
Reluctance to participate in activities
Shallow respirations
Facial mask of pain

EXPECTED OUTCOMES

The patient experiences decrease in pain as evidenced by verbalization of comfort, relaxed facial expression, increase in activity tolerance, and normal respirations.

ONGOING ASSESSMENT

- Assess intensity and characteristics of pain. Determine whether pain is related to the respiratory cycle or is continuous.
- Evaluate effectiveness of pain relief medications.

THERAPEUTIC INTERVENTIONS

- ▲ Administer pain medication as prescribed/needed.
- Instruct patient is splinting chest tube site with pillow during coughing and with movement *to support area.*
- Assist patient in repositioning q2-3hr for comfort.
- Assist patient in relaxation techniques *to decrease need for medication.*
- Instruct patient that pain medication may not completely relieve pain, but should decrease it.
- Instruct patient to notify nurse of pain before it gets too severe *so that medication will be more effective.*

RELATED FACTORS	EXPECTED OUTCOMES AND NURSING INTERVENTIONS / *RATIONALES* (■ = INDEPENDENT; ▲ = COLLABORATIVE)

High Risk for Impaired Gas Exchange

RISK FACTORS

Collapsed lung
Shallow breathing
Malfunctioning chest tube
  drainage system

EXPECTED OUTCOMES

The patient maintains adequate gas exchange as evidenced by normal ABGs for patient, normal skin color, and clear mentation.

ONGOING ASSESSMENT

▲ Assess ABG results for abnormalities and report.
▲ Assess pulse oximetry levels and report if <90% or as prescribed.
▪ Assess color of skin, mucous membranes, and nailbeds.
▪ Assess mentation for signs of hypoxia and hypercapnia: *restlessness, inappropriateness, lethargy, confusion.*

THERAPEUTIC INTERVENTIONS

▲ Administer supplemental oxygen as prescribed.
▪ Elevate HOB *to enhance lung expansion.*
▪ Utilize incentive spirometry as needed to *enhance deep breathing, thereby decreasing potential for atelectasis.*
▪ Maintain chest tube drainage system; troubleshoot as necessary *to assure patency.*

Knowledge Deficit

RELATED FACTORS

Change in health status

DEFINING CHARACTERISTICS

Multiple questions
Lack of questions

EXPECTED OUTCOMES

The patient verbalizes understanding of physical condition, reason for chest tube, importance of deep breathing, follow-up care, and signs and symptoms to report.

ONGOING ASSESSMENT

▪ Assess knowledge of pneumothorax and its treatment.

THERAPEUTIC INTERVENTIONS

▪ Encourage questions to facilitate open communication.
▪ Instruct patient and significant other regarding:
  Physical condition.
  Purpose of chest tube in lung reexpansion.
  Importance of keeping chest drainage unit below level of chest *to prevent backup of drainage or air into intrapleural space.*
  Importance of deep breathing, coughing, and gradually increasing physical activity *to enhance lung expansion.*
  Medication actions and side effects.
  Chest tube insertion site care *to decrease incidence of infection.*
  Signs and symptoms to report: *fever, purulent drainage from insertion site, reddened wound edges, and signs of lung collapse, chest pain, dyspnea, shortness of breath.*
▲ Collaborate with physician *to determine likelihood for recurrence of pneumothorax and instruct patient as appropriate.*

See also:
Fear, p. 23.
High risk for infection, p. 40.
Impaired physical mobility,
  p. 47.

By: Robin R. Young, RN, MS, CCRN

Pulmonary thromboembolism

(PULMONARY EMBOLUS [PE])

Pulmonary thromboembolism occurs when there is an obstruction in the pulmonary vascular bed (pulmonary artery or one of the branches) caused by blood clots (thrombi). It is one of the most common causes of death in hospitalized patients, resulting from a variety of factors that predispose to intravascular clotting. These include postoperative states, trauma to vessel walls, obesity, diabetes mellitus, infection, venous stasis caused by immobility, postpartum state, and other circulatory disorders. The clinical picture varies according to size and location of the embolus. The primary objective when pulmonary embolism occurs is to prevent recurrence.

NURSING DIAGNOSES	EXPECTED OUTCOMES AND NURSING INTERVENTIONS / *RATIONALES* (■ = INDEPENDENT; ▲ = COLLABORATIVE)

Ineffective Breathing Pattern

RELATED FACTORS

Hypoxia (from the V/Q disorder caused by the pulmonary embolus)
Pain
Anxiety

DEFINING CHARACTERISTICS

Dyspnea
Tachypnea
Cyanosis
Cough
Use of accessory muscles

EXPECTED OUTCOMES

Patient's breathing pattern is maintained as evidenced by eupnea, normal skin color, and regular respiratory rate/pattern.

ONGOING ASSESSMENT

- Assess respiratory rate and depth by listening to breath sounds. *Respiratory rate and rhythm changes are early warning signs of impending respiratory difficulties. Tachypnea is a typical finding of pulmonary embolus. The rapid shallow respirations result from hypoxia. Development of hypoventilation (a slowing of respiratory rate) without improvement in patient condition indicates respiratory failure.*
- Assess for any increase in work of breathing: shortness of breath, use of accessory muscles.
- Assess breath sounds.
- ▲ Monitor ABGs and note changes. *ABGs of the pulmonary embolus patient typically exhibit respiratory alkalosis from a blowing off of CO_2 and hypoxemia. Development of respiratory acidosis in this patient indicates respiratory failure, and immediate ventilator support is indicated.*
- Assess characteristics of pain, especially in association with the respiratory cycle.

THERAPEUTIC INTERVENTIONS

- Position patient with proper body alignment for optimal breathing pattern. *If not contraindicated, a sitting position allows good lung excursion and chest expansion.*
- ▲ Assure that O_2 delivery system is applied to the patient *so that the appropriate amount of oxygen is continuously delivered and the patient does not become desaturated.*
- Provide reassurance and allay anxiety by staying with patient during acute episodes of respiratory distress. *Air hunger can produce extreme anxiety.*
- Change position q2hr *to facilitate movement and drainage of secretions.*
- Assist patient with coughing and deep breathing to help keep airways open. Suction as needed *to clear secretions.*
- Anticipate the need for intubation and mechanical ventilation. See also Mechanical ventilation, p. 202.

Impaired Gas Exchange

RELATED FACTORS

Decreased perfusion to lung tissues caused by obstruction in pulmonary vascular bed by embolus
Increased alveolar dead space
Increased physiologic shunting caused by collapse of alveoli produced by loss of surfactant

EXPECTED OUTCOMES

Patient maintains optimal gas exchange as evidenced by normal ABGs, alert responsive mentation or no further reduction in mental status.

ONGOING ASSESSMENT

- Auscultate breath sounds every shift, noting areas of decreased ventilation and presence of adventitious sounds. *Common clinical findings include rales, tachypnea, and tachycardia.*
- Monitor vital signs, noting any changes. *In initial hypoxia and hypercapnia, BP, heart rate, and respiratory rate all rise. As the hypoxia and/or hypercapnia becomes more severe, BP may drop, heart rate tends to continue to be rapid and include dysrhythmias, and respiratory failure may ensue, with the patient unable to maintain the rapid respiratory rate.*

NURSING DIAGNOSES	EXPECTED OUTCOMES AND NURSING INTERVENTIONS / *RATIONALES* (■ = INDEPENDENT; ▲ = COLLABORATIVE)

DEFINING CHARACTERISTICS

Confusion
Somnolence
Restlessness
Irritability
Hypoxemia
Hypercapnea

ONGOING ASSESSMENT—cont'd

- Assess for changes in orientation and behavior.
- Assess for signs/symptoms of hypoxemia: tachycardia, restlessness, diaphoresis, headache, lethargy/confusion, skin color changes.
- Assess for presence of signs/symptoms of atelectasis: diminished chest expansion, limited diaphragm excursion, bronchial/tubular breath sounds, rales, tracheal shift to affected side.
- Assess for presence of signs/symptoms of infarction: cough, hemoptysis (*hemoptysis occurs as a result of tissue destruction associated with pulmonary infarction*), pleuritic pain, consolidation, pleural effusion, bronchial breathing, pleural friction rub, fever.
- ▲ Monitor arterial blood gases (ABGs) and note changes, *to monitor for signs of respiratory failure (e.g., low Pao_2, elevated $Paco_2$).*
- Assess for calf tenderness, swelling, redness, and/or hardened area. Assess for presence of Homan's sign (pain when foot is forcefully dorsiflexed). *PE frequently arises from a deep vein thrombosis and may have been previously overlooked.*

THERAPEUTIC INTERVENTIONS

- ▲ Administer O_2 as needed *to prevent severe hypoxemia.*
- ▲ Utilize pulse oximetry, as available, *to continuously monitor O_2 saturation and pulse rate.* Keep alarms on at all times. Pulse oximetry has been found to be a useful tool in the clinical setting to detect changes in oxygenation.
- Position patient properly *to promote optimal lung perfusion. When patient is positioned on side, affected area should not be dependent. Upright and sitting positions optimize diaphragmatic excursions.*
- Pace and schedule activities *to conserve energy.*
- Use nursing measures to maintain normal body temperature. *Fever causes tachycardia, which increases O_2 demand.*

High Risk for Decreased Cardiac Output

RISK FACTORS

Failure of right side of heart resulting from pulmonary hypertension
Failure of left side of heart secondary to failure of right side

EXPECTED OUTCOMES

Patient achieves adequate cardiac output as evidenced by strong peripheral pulses; normal vital signs; warm, dry skin; and alert, responsive mentation.

ONGOING ASSESSMENT

- Assess vital signs, skin warmth, and peripheral pulses. *Peripheral vasoconstriction causes cool, pale, diaphoretic skin.*
- Monitor for dysrhythmias: *atrial dysrhythmias caused by right side strain and ventricular dysrhythmias caused by hypoxemia.*
- ▲ If hemodynamic monitoring is in place, assess CVP, PAP, PCWP, and CO. *CVP provides information on filling pressures of right side of the heart; PAP and PCWP reflect left sided fluid volumes.*
- Assess level of consciousness. *Early signs of cerebral hypoxia are restlessness and anxiety, which lead on to agitation and confusion.*
- Monitor weight daily. *Gain of 2-3 lb/day is significant for heart failure.*
- Observe and document clinical findings that indicate impending or present failure of right side of heart: accentuated pulmonic component of second heart sound (S_2); splitting of S_2; engorged neck veins, positive hepatojugular reflex; increased CVP readings; palpable liver and spleen; altered coagulation values; ECG change associated with right atrial hypertrophy; atrial dysrhythmias; pedal edema; weight gain.
  Note: *Embolus causes decreased cross-sectional area of pulmonary vascular bed that results in increased pulmonary resistance. This increases the workload of the right side of the heart.*
- Auscultate lung and heart sounds q2-4hr *to identify abnormalities indicating impending or present failure of left side of heart:* fine rales (bases of the lungs); increased pulmonary artery wedge pressure; presence of S_3; gallop rhythms; frothy secretions; dyspnea; tachycardia; cough; wheezing; orthopnea; hypoxemia; respiratory acidosis; ECG changes associated with left atrial hypertrophy.
  Note: *Decreased right ventricular contractility decreases left side blood volume. This decreases left ventricular pumping power if not treated promptly.*

THERAPEUTIC INTERVENTIONS

- Elevate legs/feet and apply/maintain TED hose *to promote peripheral blood flow and decrease venous stasis.*

Continued.

Pulmonary thromboembolism—cont'd

NURSING DIAGNOSES	EXPECTED OUTCOMES AND NURSING INTERVENTIONS / *RATIONALES* (■ = INDEPENDENT; ▲ = COLLABORATIVE)

THERAPEUTIC INTERVENTIONS—cont'd

▲ For massive pulmonary thromboembolism, anticipate the following:
  Mechanical ventilation (see also Mechanical ventilation, p. 202).
  Insertion of invasive monitoring lines: arterial line *(auscultory BP may be unreliable secondary to vasoconstriction associated with the decreased cardiac output)*; Swan-Ganz catheter (see also Swan-Ganz catheter, p. 167).
  Inotropic agents
  Anticoagulant therapy
  Thrombolytic therapy
  Vena caval interruption
  Pulmonary embolectomy (rarely done)
▪ If cardiac output is a problem, see also treatment for Decreased cardiac output, p. 12.

High Risk for Bleeding

RISK FACTORS

Anticoagulant/thrombolytic therapy

EXPECTED OUTCOMES

Patient's risk for bleeding is reduced through ongoing assessment and early intervention.

ONGOING ASSESSMENT

▪ Assess for high-risk bleeding condition: liver disease, kidney disease, severe hypertension, cavitary tuberculosis, bacterial endocarditis.
▲ Monitor IV dosage and delivery system (tubing/pump) *to minimize risk of overcoagulation/undercoagulation.*
▲ Monitor partial thromboplastin time (PTT) level. *Goal is PTT level at least twice control level to maintain anticoagulated state.* Notify physician immediately if higher or lower than designated range. *Higher level could result in bleeding; lower level could result in further thrombus formation.*
▪ Assess for signs and symptoms of bleeding: petechiae, purpura, hematoma; bleeding from catheter insertion sites; GI, GU bleeding; bleeding from respiratory tract; bleeding from mucous membranes; decreasing Hb and Hct.

THERAPEUTIC INTERVENTIONS

▲ Administer anticoagulant therapy as prescribed (continuous IV heparin infusion). *Heparin is given to prevent further thrombus formation.*
▲ If bleeding occurs, anticipate the following:
  Stop the infusion.
  Recheck PTT level stat.
  Administer protamine sulfate *(heparin antagonist)* as ordered.
  Take vital signs frequently *to assess status.*
  Reevaluate dose of heparin on basis of PTT result.
  Notify blood bank to ensure blood availability if needed.
▲ Discontinue anticoagulant infusion cautiously:
  Taper dose on basis of PTT result, as prescribed.
  Administer oral anticoagulant, usually warfarin (Coumadin), while heparin dose is tapered. *Heparin dosage is gradually tapered during the addition of an oral anticoagulant for long-term therapy.*
  Monitor both prothrombin time (PT) and PTT levels.
  Continue to observe closely for signs of bleeding.
  Instruct conscious and reliable patients to report signs of bleeding immediately.
▲ Administer thrombolytic therapy as prescribed. *Lytic agents are indicated for patients with massive pulmonary embolus that results in hemodynamic compromise.* Be aware of contraindications for thrombolytic therapy in order to minimize complications: recent surgery, recent organ biopsy, paracentesis/thoracentesis, pregnancy, recent stroke, recent or active internal bleeding.
▲ Institute precautionary measures:
  Use only compressible vessels for IV sites.
  Compress IV sites for at least 10 min and arterial sites for 30 min.
  Discontinue anticoagulants and antiplatelet aggregates before thrombolytic therapy.
  Limit physical manipulation of patients *to prevent disruption of formed blood clots.*
  Pad side rails *to prevent further bleeding injury.*
  Provide gentle oral care.
  Avoid IM injections: *any needle stick is potential bleeding site.*
  Draw all laboratory specimens through existing line: arterial line or venous hep-lock line.
  Send specimen for type and crossmatch as prescribed.

NURSING DIAGNOSES	EXPECTED OUTCOMES AND NURSING INTERVENTIONS / *RATIONALES* (■ = INDEPENDENT; ▲ = COLLABORATIVE)

THERAPEUTIC INTERVENTIONS—cont'd
- Discuss and provide patient with a list of what to avoid when taking anticoagulants:
  Do not use blade razor (electric razors preferred).
  Do not take new medications without consulting physician, pharmacist, or nurses.
  Do not eat foods high in vitamin K (e.g., dark green vegetables, cauliflower, cabbage, bananas, tomatoes).
  Do not ingest aspirin or other salicylates.
- Discuss and give patient list of measures *to minimize recurrence of emboli:*
  Take medicines as prescribed.
  Keep medical checkup and blood test appointments.
  Perform leg exercises as advised, especially during long automobile and airplane trips, *to prevent venous stasis.*
  Do not cross legs *(pressure alters circulation and may lead to clotting).*
  Use TED stockings as prescribed *to prevent venous stasis.*
  Maintain adequate hydration *to prevent increased blood viscosity.*

Anxiety

RELATED FACTORS

Threat of death
Change in health status
Overall feeling of intense sickness
Multiple laboratory tests
Increased attention of medical personnel
Increasing respiratory difficulty

DEFINING CHARACTERISTICS

Verbalization of anxiety
Restlessness, inability to relax
Multiple questions
Tremors, shakiness
Tense/anxious appearance
Crying
Withdrawal

EXPECTED OUTCOMES

Patient experiences reduced anxiety/fear as evidenced by calm and trusting appearance, and verbalized fears and concerns.

ONGOING ASSESSMENT

- Assess level of anxiety. *A patient with a pulmonary embolus experiencing increasing respiratory difficulty and shortness of breath may have a high level of anxiety.*

THERAPEUTIC INTERVENTIONS

- Reduce patient's/significance others' anxiety by explaining all procedures/treatment. Keep explanations basic.
- Maintain confident, assured manner. *Staff's anxiety may be easily perceived by patient.*
- Encourage patient to ventilate feelings of anxiety. *Understanding patient's feelings of anxiety will guide staff in planning and implementing care plan to allay individualized anxiety.*
- Provide adequate rest:
  Organize activities (e.g., morning care, meals, hospital staff rounds, treatments).
  Decrease sensory stimulations:
  Dim lights when appropriate.
  Remove unnecessary equipment from room *to maintain more relaxed environment.*
  Limit visitors and phone calls *(to prevent tiring). Patients feel obligated to entertain (may be physically and emotionally taxing).*
- ▲ Administer pain medicines or sedatives as indicated *to assist in allaying anxiety. Anxiety may increase oxygen consumption.*
- ▲ Refer to other support systems (e.g., clergy, social workers, other family/friends) as appropriate.

Knowledge Deficit

RELATED FACTORS

New medical condition

DEFINING CHARACTERISTICS

Expresses inaccurate perception of health status
Verbalizes deficiency in knowledge
Multiple questions or none

EXPECTED OUTCOMES

Patient understands importance of medications, signs of excessive anticoagulation, and means to reduce risk of bleeding and recurrence of emboli.

ONGOING ASSESSMENT

- Assess present knowledge of pulmonary embolus: severity, prognosis, risk factors, therapy

THERAPEUTIC INTERVENTIONS

- Provide information on cause of the problem; effects of pulmonary embolus on body functioning; common risk factors: immobilization; trauma: hip fracture, major burns; certain heart conditions; oral contraceptives.
- Instruct about medications, their actions, dosages, and side effects.
- Discuss and give patient list of signs and symptoms of excessive anticoagulation: easy bruising, severe nosebleed, black stools, blood in urine or stools, joint swelling and pain, coughing up of blood, severe headache.
- Inform of the need for routine laboratory testing of PT while on oral anticoagulant.
- Discuss safety/precautionary measures to use while on anticoagulant therapy to prevent bleeding: need to inform dentist or other care givers before treatment, use of electric razor, use of soft toothbrush.

By: Lumie Perez, RN, BSN, CCRN
Susan Galanes RN, MS, CCRN

Radical neck surgery

(LARYNGECTOMY; HEAD AND NECK CANCER)

Radical neck surgery is a surgical procedure for cancer of the larynx. This procedure involves laryngectomy and removal of cervical lymph nodes and lymphatics. Dissection includes fascia, muscle, nerves, salivary glands, and veins in an attempt to eradicate metastatic cancer.

RELATED FACTORS	EXPECTED OUTCOMES AND NURSING INTERVENTIONS / *RATIONALE* (■ = INDEPENDENT; ▲ = COLLABORATIVE)

Ineffective Airway Clearance

RELATED FACTORS

Thick, copious secretions
Tracheostomy tube
Pain
Edema
Fatigue
Refusal to cough

DEFINING CHARACTERISTICS

Diminished breath sounds
Coarse breath sounds
Cough
Dyspnea
Tachypnea

EXPECTED OUTCOMES

Patient maintains effective airway clearance as evidenced by normal breath sounds, eupnea, and an airway free of secretions with effective cough.

ONGOING ASSESSMENT

- Auscultate lungs for normal and abnormal breath sounds.
- Assess respiratory rate, rhythm, and effort.
- Assess effectiveness of cough.
- Assess color, consistency, and quantity of secretions.
- ▲ Monitor ABGs for abnormalities and compare to preoperative values.
- ▲ Assess pulse oximetry and report O_2 saturation <90%.
- Assess color of skin, nailbeds, and mucous membranes.
- Assess level of consciousness for lethargy, change in behavior, or disorientation, *which may be indicative of poor air exchange.*
- Assess for pain. *Postoperative pain can result in shallow breathing and an ineffective cough.*

THERAPEUTIC INTERVENTIONS

- ▲ Maintain humidified oxygen per tracheostomy collar *to thin secretions.*
- Encourage patient deep breathing q1-2hr while awake *to prevent atelectasis and enhance gas exchange.*
- Encourage effective coughing after taking deep breaths.
- Suction tracheostomy with sterile technique if patient is unable to clear own secretions.
- Position with head of bed elevated *to decrease edema and increase lung expansion.*
- Encourage and assist patient to change position q2-3hr and increase activity as tolerated *to facilitate mobilization of secretions.*
- Change tracheostomy inner cannula q8hr if disposable inner cannula is used, or cleanse inner cannula q8hr if nondisposable inner cannula used. *Retained secretions can obstruct airway.*
- Maintain secure tracheostomy ties *to prevent tracheostomy tube dislodgment.*
- Keep same size sterile tracheostomy tube at bedside *for insertion if dislodgment should occur.*
- ▲ Consult respiratory therapy staff as needs arise.

Impaired Verbal Communication

RELATED FACTORS

Laryngectomy (results in permanent loss of voice)

DEFINING CHARACTERISTICS

Inability to speak
Frustration
Withdrawal

EXPECTED OUTCOMES

The patient effectively communicates needs.

ONGOING ASSESSMENT

- Assess patient's presurgical communication ability *to help determine best nonverbal method to use.*
- Frequently assess patient's need to communicate *to decrease anxiety and enhance communication.*
- Assess effectiveness of nonverbal communication methods and alter as necessary.
- Assess for additional obstacles to communication (i.e., patient is hard of hearing, is mentally retarded, or has arthritis of the hands).

THERAPEUTIC INTERVENTIONS

- Keep call light within reach at all times. Answer call light promptly *to decrease anxiety and feelings of helplessness.*
- Instruct patient and significant others in alternative methods of communication: hand gestures, writing tablet with pen, picture board, word board, electronic communication system, electronic voice box.
- ▲ Consult speech therapy staff regarding alternate forms of speech. *Voice prosthesis, electrolarynx, and esophageal speech may be used for patient.*
- Anticipate needs *to decrease frustrations:*
- Allow patient time to communicate needs.
- Provide emotional support to patient and significant others.
- Encourage patient to obtain before discharge an audiotape for home use that can be played in an emergency when 911 is called. *Promotes security in home environment.*

RELATED FACTORS	

High Risk for Altered Tissue Perfusion

RISK FACTORS

Tissue edema
Malfunction of wound drainage tubes
Preoperative radiation to surgical area
Extensive surgical dissection of blood vessels
Infection of surgical area

EXPECTED OUTCOMES

Patient maintains adequate tissue perfusion, as evidenced by normal incisional healing, gradual decrease in edema, gradual decrease in wound drainage, and no signs and symptoms of infection.

ONGOING ASSESSMENT

- Assess surgical wound drainage system for amount and color of drainage. *An abrupt cessation of drainage can indicate a clogged tube. Excessive drainage can indicate a leaking vessel in the area. Purulent drainage can indicate infection.*
- Assess edema at surgical wound. *Excessive edema can impede blood flow to or from the area and result in necrosis or infection.*
- Monitor body temperature.
- Assess color of wound and surrounding skin for signs of decreased circulation: pale, blue, or dark in color.
- Assess wound edges. *Wound edges should be proximate (next to each other). Wound edges separate with excessive edema, necrosis, and infection.*

THERAPEUTIC INTERVENTIONS

- ▲ Gently milk drainage tubes as needed *to maintain patency and prevent buildup of fluid at surgical site, causing excessive edema and possible infection or necrosis.* Maintain suction as prescribed (e.g., Jackson-Pratt drain).
- Keep head of bed elevated *to decrease edema.*
- Perform tracheostomy tube and site cleaning as needed *to keep respiratory secretions away from surgical wound.*
- Promptly change tracheostomy or wound dressings when wet *to prevent maceration of skin.*

Alteration in Nutrition: Less than Body Requirements

RELATED FACTORS

NPO status
Decreased appetite
Dysphagia
Radiation therapy
Chemotherapy
Edema

DEFINING CHARACTERISTICS

Weight loss
Decreased caloric intake

EXPECTED OUTCOMES

The patient has adequate caloric intake as evidenced by body weight greater than or equal to admission weight.

ONGOING ASSESSMENT

- Obtain admission weight *to establish baseline:* monitor weight qod, monitor I & O.
- Assess preoperative diet and food preferences.
- ▲ Monitor lab test results: serum albumin, protein, electrolytes, glucose, CBC.
- Observe patient during initial oral feeding for signs of aspiration: food or fluid from tracheostomy, choking.

THERAPEUTIC INTERVENTIONS

- Instruct patient on importance of adequate caloric intake *to promote incisional healing.*
- ▲ Consult speech therapy staff for swallowing evaluation as needed.
- ▲ Obtain dietician consult *to determine caloric requirements specific to patient to assess caloric intake, and to suggest enteral feedings.*
- Encourage oral intake of soft foods when allowed, with tracheostomy cuff inflated *to decrease chances of aspiration.*
- Maintain suction setup at bedside for safety. *Suction may be needed during or after feedings to keep the airway patent.*
- Assist patient in performing oral hygiene *to keep mouth fresh.*
- Instruct on need for enteral feedings if prescribed.
- Instruct on procedure for administration of home enteral feedings if prescribed.

Body Image Disturbance

RELATED FACTORS

Visible incision
Facial and neck edema
Tracheostomy
Alteration in verbal communication
Dysphagia
Life-style changes
Diagnosis of cancer

EXPECTED OUTCOMES

Patient begins to adjust to body changes as evidenced by planning for discharge, showing interest in learning, and using alternative communication methods.

ONGOING ASSESSMENT

- Assess patient's mood and behavior for signs of difficulty in coping with changes in body appearance or function.
- Assess patient's perception of life changes precipitated by radical neck surgery: occupational, interpersonal.

Continued.

Pulmonary Care Plans

RELATED FACTORS	EXPECTED OUTCOMES AND NURSING INTERVENTIONS / *RATIONALES* (■ = INDEPENDENT; ▲ = COLLABORATIVE)

DEFINING CHARACTERISTICS

Verbalization of negative feelings about body
Preoccupation with change
Refusal to look at face and neck
Withdrawal
Decreased motivation for self-care
Refusal to see visitors

THERAPEUTIC INTERVENTIONS

- Encourage patient and significant others to communicate fears/concerns, regarding diagnosis of cancer and treatment.
- Encourage visits from significant others *to help the patient feel accepted.*
- Refer to support services: Lost Cords, American Cancer Society, and International Association of Laryngectomies. *Rehabilitation after radical neck surgery is a long process, and support services can have a positive impact on the patient's recovery.*
- Arrange for a visit from a person who has had a laryngectomy *for emotional support.*

Knowledge Deficit

RELATED FACTORS

Postoperative radical neck surgery
New stoma/tracheostomy
Cancer treatment

DEFINING CHARACTERISTICS

Anxiety about discharge
Increased questioning
Expressed need for more information

EXPECTED OUTCOMES

Patient and significant others demonstrate tracheostomy care using clean technique.
Patient and significant others demonstrate tracheal suctioning using clean technique.
Patient and significant others verbalize signs and symptoms of infection and when to report.
Patient and significant others verbalize understanding of individualized course of postoperative treatment (e.g., radiation therapy).

ONGOING ASSESSMENT

- Assess knowledge of postoperative care *in order to plan teaching.*
- Assess support systems at home *to determine home care needs for discharge planning.*

THERAPEUTIC INTERVENTIONS

- Explain postoperative procedures/treatments to patient/significant other (e.g., drainage tubes, dressings, feeding tube).
- Teach patient and significant others as appropriate:
  Signs and symptoms of infection and notification of physician when present.
  Indications for suctioning.
  Procedure for tracheal suction using clean technique *to maintain a clear airway. (Use mirror for teaching.)*
  Procedure for cleaning inner cannula with soap and water and inserting and locking it in place *to decrease the incidence of a clogged tracheostomy tube.*
  Procedure for changing and maintain secure trach ties *to decrease incidence of tracheostomy dislodgment.*
- Arrange for home nursing care as needed.
- Discuss plans for radiation therapy, including what to expect, probable time schedule for the series, and possible side effects. *Postoperative radiation therapy may be used to control the patient's metastasis.*

See also:
Pre-operative:
  Anxiety, p. 5.
  Knowledge deficit, p. 41.
Postoperative:
  Fear, p. 23.
  Impaired skin integrity, p. 59.
  High risk for infection, p. 40.
  High risk for aspiration, p. 6.
  Pain, p. 49.
  Anticipatory grieving, p. 28.
  Impaired home maintenance management, p. 34.
  Impaired coping, p. 18.

By: Robin R. Young, RN, MS, CCRN

Respiratory failure, acute

Acute respiratory failure is a life-threatening inability to maintain adequate pulmonary gas exchange. Respiratory failure can result from obstructive disease (e.g., emphysema, chronic bronchitis, asthma), restrictive disease (e.g., atelectasis, ARDS, pneumonia, multiple rib fractures, postoperative abdominal or thoracic surgery, CNS depression), or ventilation-perfusion abnormalities (e.g., pulmonary embolism).

NURSING DIAGNOSES	EXPECTED OUTCOMES AND NURSING INTERVENTIONS / *RATIONALE* (■ = INDEPENDENT; ▲ = COLLABORATIVE)

Inability to Sustain Spontaneous Ventilation

RELATED FACTORS
Metabolic factors
Respiratory muscle fatigue

DEFINING CHARACTERISTICS
Shortness of breath
Increased $Paco_2$ level
Decreased Pao_2 level
Decreased O_2 saturation level
Increased restlessness and irritability
Tachycardia
Dyspnea
Tachypnea
Cyanosis
Respiratory depth changes
Decrease in level of consciousness (LOC) (may occur as respiratory insufficiency increases in severity)

EXPECTED OUTCOMES
Patient's ventilatory demand is decreased as evidenced by eupnea, no use of accessory muscles, and ABGs normal for patient.

ONGOING ASSESSMENT
- Review respiratory health history.
- Monitor vital signs with frequent monitoring of BP. *Hypoxia/hypercarbia may cause initial hypertension with restlessness and progress to hypotension and somnolence.*
- Monitor for dysrhythmias. *Cardiac dysrhythmias may result from acidosis or hypoxia.*
- Observe for changes in patient's respiratory status, including rate, depth, changes heard during auscultation, and respiratory effort.
- Observe for intercostal retractions and marked use of accessory muscles.
- Auscultate lungs and assess breath sounds for adventitious sounds: wheezing, rales (crackles), or rhonchi.
- Assess for presence of cough and if effective/productive: amount expectorated, frequency, color.
- Observe for signs of hypoxia (e.g., dyspnea, tachycardia, tachypnea, restlessness, and cyanosis). *Cyanosis is a late sign of hypoxemia because 5 g of hemoglobin must desaturate for cyanosis to occur.*
- Assess level of consciousness. *Early signs of cerebral hypoxia are restlessness and anxiety, leading on to agitation and confusion.*
- Observe for signs of increased Pco_2 (e.g., asterixis or tremors). *Elevations in $Paco_2$ result in vasodilation of cerebral blood vessels, increased cerebral blood flow, and increased ICP.*
- ▲ Monitor ABGs carefully and notify physician of abnormalities. *Increasing $Paco_2$ and/or decreasing Pao_2 is a sign of respiratory failure. However, ABG values may be acceptable initially and the patient's work of breathing may be too extreme. As the patient begins to fail, respiratory rate will decrease and $Paco_2$ will begin to rise.*

THERAPEUTIC INTERVENTIONS
- ▲ Administer O_2 as needed. For patients with severe COPD, give O_2 cautiously, preferably with a Venturi device. *(The venturi device is a high-flow O_2 delivery system with a stable Fio_2 which is unaffected by patient's respiratory rate or tidal volume). COPD patients who chronically retain CO_2 depend upon "hypoxic drive" as their stimulus to breathe. When applying O_2, close monitoring is imperative to prevent unsafe increases in patient's Pao_2, which would result in apnea.*
- Position patient with proper body alignment *for optimal chest excursion and breathing pattern.*
- Maintain adequate airway; position patient *to prevent mechanical obstruction from tongue.*
- Pace activities *to prevent fatigue.* Maintain planned rest periods.
- When necessary, prepare for intubation:
  Position patient appropriately and have necessary equipment readily available.
  Instruct patient who is awake and alert *because explanation is essential for total cooperation.*
  Stay with patient *to allay anxiety.*
  Institute suctioning via ET tube as necessary.
  See Mechanical ventilation, p. 202, as appropriate.

Continued.

Pulmonary Care Plans

NURSING DIAGNOSES	EXPECTED OUTCOMES AND NURSING INTERVENTIONS / *RATIONALES* (■ = INDEPENDENT; ▲ = COLLABORATIVE)

High Risk for Ineffective Airway Clearance

RISK FACTORS

Respiratory failure requiring intubation

EXPECTED OUTCOMES

Patient's airway is free of secretions.
Patient has clear breath sounds after suctioning.

ONGOING ASSESSMENT

- Assess for significant alterations in breath sounds (e.g., rhonchi, wheezes). After intubation, auscultate lungs for bilateral breath sounds *to assure that ET tube not in right main stem bronchus or in esophagus.*
▲ Assess for changes in ventilation rate or depth. Obtain chest x-ray study after intubation *to determine ET tube placement.*

THERAPEUTIC INTERVENTIONS

- Instruct and/or change patient's position q2hr *to mobilize secretions.*
▲ Provide humidity (when appropriate) via bedside humidifier/humidified O$_2$ therapy *(will prevent drying of secretions).*
- Instruct patient to deep breathe adequately and to cough effectively.
- Use nasotracheal suction for patients who cannot clear secretions before intubation.
After intubation:
- Institute suctioning of airway as needed, as determined by presence of adventitious sounds and/or increased ventilatory pressures.
- Use sterile saline instillations during suctioning as needed *to help facilitate removal of tenacious sputum.*

High Risk for Infection

RISK FACTORS

Suctioning of airway
Endotracheal intubation

EXPECTED OUTCOMES

Patient's risk of infection is reduced through early assessment and intervention.

ONGOING ASSESSMENT

- Monitor and document temperature and notify physician of temperature > 38.5° C. *Note: If patient is receiving steroid therapy, detecting infections may be more difficult.*
▲ Monitor WBC level.
- Observe patient's secretions for color, thickness, and amount.
- Monitor sputum cultures and sensitivities.

THERAPEUTIC INTERVENTIONS

- Practice conscientious bronchial hygiene, good handwashing techniques, and sterile suctioning. *Many infections are transmitted by hospital personnel.*
- Administer mouth care (e.g., Cepacol, mouth swabs, Chloraseptic mouth spray) q2hr and as needed. *This will help limit oral bacterial growth and promote patient comfort.*
- Institute airway suctioning as needed. *Accumulation of secretions can lead to invasive process.*
- Maintain patient's personal hygiene, nutrition, and rest *to increase natural defenses.*

Anxiety

RELATED FACTORS

Threat of death
Change in health status
Change in environment
Change in interaction patterns
Unmet needs

DEFINING CHARACTERISTICS

Restlessness
Diaphoresis
Pointing to throat (possibly unable to speak)
Uncooperative behavior
Withdrawal
Vigilant watch on equipment

EXPECTED OUTCOMES

Patient experiences absence or decrease in anxiety as evidenced by cooperative behavior, and calm appearance.

ONGOING ASSESSMENT

- Assess patient for signs indicating increased anxiety. *Respiratory failure is an acute life-threatening condition that will produce high levels of anxiety in the patient as well as significant others.*

THERAPEUTIC INTERVENTIONS

- If patient is unable to speak because of respiratory status:
  Provide pencil and pad.
  Establish some form of nonverbal communication if patient too sick to write. *Maintaining an avenue of communication is important to alleviate anxiety.*
- Anticipate questions. Provide explanations of mechanical ventilation, alarm systems on monitors and ventilators. *An informed patient who understands the treatment plan will be more cooperative.*
- Display a confident, calm manner and tolerant, understanding attitude. *Staff's anxiety may be easily perceived by patient.*
- Allow family/significant others to visit; involve them in care.
- Assure patient and significant others of close, continuous monitoring that will ensure prompt interventions. Reassure patient of staff's presence.

NURSING DIAGNOSES	EXPECTED OUTCOMES AND NURSING INTERVENTIONS / *RATIONALES* (■ = INDEPENDENT; ▲ = COLLABORATIVE)

THERAPEUTIC INTERVENTIONS—cont'd
▲ Use other supportive measures (e.g., medications, psychiatric liaison, clergy, social services) as indicated.

Knowledge Deficit

RELATED FACTORS
Unfamiliarity with disease process and treatment

DEFINING CHARACTERISTICS
Multiple questions
Lack of concern
Anxiety
Noncompliant of medication/ health care orders, e.g., smoking

See also:
ARDS, p. 183; Chest trauma, p. 188; Pneumonia, p. 211; COPD, p. 192; Asthma, p. 186; Pulmonary embolism, p. 216; Mechanical ventilation, p. 202.

EXPECTED OUTCOMES
Patient verbalizes understanding of disease process, procedures, and treatment.

ONGOING ASSESSMENT
- Evaluate patient's perception and understanding of disease process that led to respiratory failure.
- Assess patient's knowledge of O_2 therapy, deep breathing, and coughing.

THERAPEUTIC INTERVENTIONS
- Encourage patient to verbalize feelings and questions.
- Explain disease process to patient and correct misconceptions.
- Discuss need for monitoring equipment and frequent assessments. *Patient must be aware that this is an acute episode of respiratory failure.*
- Explain all tests and procedures before they occur.
- Explain necessity of O_2 therapy, including its limitations.
- Instruct patient to deep breathe and cough effectively.

By: Susan Galanes, RN, MS, CCRN

Thoracotomy

(CHEST SURGERY; THORACIC SURGERY; LOBECTOMY; PNEUMONECTOMY)

A surgical opening into the thorax for biopsy, excision, drainage, and/or correction of defects. The surgical correction may include lobectomy, segmental resection, wedge resection, or pneumonectomy.

NURSING DIAGNOSES	EXPECTED OUTCOMES AND NURSING INTERVENTIONS / *RATIONALE* (■ = INDEPENDENT; ▲ = COLLABORATIVE)

Ineffective Breathing Pattern

RELATED FACTORS
Positive pressure in pleural space secondary to surgical incision
Collapse of lung on affected side (partial or complete)
Void in thoracic cavity if pneumonectomy performed

DEFINING CHARACTERISTICS
Dyspnea
Shortness of breath
Tachypnea
Altered chest excursion
Shallow respirations
Asymmetrical chest excursion
Use of accessory muscles for breathing

EXPECTED OUTCOMES
- Patient's breathing pattern is maintained as evidenced by eupnea, normal skin color, and regular respiratory rate/pattern.

ONGOING ASSESSMENT
- Assess respiratory rate and depth by listening to breath sounds. *Respiratory rate and rhythm changes are early warning signs of impending respiratory difficulties.*
- Obtain vital signs, noting early signs of respiratory insufficiency; document and report abnormal parameters.
- Note asymmetry of chest wall movement during respirations.
▲ Assess skin color and ABGs as necessary *to determine degree to which altered breathing pattern is compromising ventilation.*
▲ Perform complete assessment of closed chest drainage system; repeat frequently:
  Check the H_2O seal for:
    Correct fluid level
    Presence/absence of fluctuation. *Absence of fluctuation indicates obstruction or lung reexpansion and must always be investigated.*
    Presence of air leaks; document and report to physician. *Bubbling in H_2O seal chamber indicates air leak, which may be present because the lung has not yet expanded or because of a persistent air leak. There may be a leak in the system before the H_2O seal drainage (e.g., loose tubing connection or air leak around entrance site of tube).*

Continued.

NURSING DIAGNOSES	EXPECTED OUTCOMES AND NURSING INTERVENTIONS / *RATIONALES* (■ = INDEPENDENT; ▲ = COLLABORATIVE)

ONGOING ASSESSMENT—cont'd

Check suction control chamber for correct fluid level as specified. *Amount of suction (negative pressure) being applied to pleural space is regulated by amount of fluid in suction control chamber, not amount dialed on Emerson/wall suction.*

Measure the output in closed chest drainage system.

Accurately report drainage of bright red blood of 100 ml/hr for 2 hr consecutive.

▲ Monitor report of postoperative chest x-ray film *to confirm chest tube placement and to see whether the lung has reexpanded.*

▪ Assess response to increasing levels of activity. *An increase in oxygen consumption and an increase in work of breathing occur as the patient begins to increase activity.*

THERAPEUTIC INTERVENTIONS

▪ Position patient so that remaining lung expansion is facilitated. *If not contraindicated, a sitting position allows for good lung excursion and chest expansion. Post pneumonectomy: position on back or with operative side dependent.*

▲ Assure that O$_2$ delivery system is applied to the patient so that the appropriate amount of oxygen is continuously delivered and the patient does not become desaturated.

▪ Encourage sustained deep breaths by:

Demonstration (emphasizing slow inhalation, holding end inspiration for a few seconds, and passive exhalation)

Use of incentive spirometer (place close for convenient patient use)

▲ Maintain chest tube drainage system:

Note: Postpneumonectomy patients generally do not have chest tubes. *The space gradually fills with serosanguinous fluid.*

Position chest drainage system below patient's chest level. *Gravity will aid in drainage and prevent backflow into chest.*

Place drainage unit in stand, tape to floor, or hang on bed *to prevent tipping of unit, maintain an upright position.*

Make sure tubing is free of kinks and clots. *This would impede air evacuation.* Milk tubing from insertion site downward.

Set suction correctly *to maintain a constant gentle bubbling in the suction control chamber. Vigorous bubbling does not produce additional suction (the water level determines the amount of suction), but it would be a "noisy" irritant to the patient and would cause earlier evaporation of the water level, with a need to refill the chamber to the correct level.*

Maintain tubing/connections:

Anchor the chest tube catheter to patient's chest wall with waterproof tape *to prevent dislodgment of the tubing.*

Secure drainage tubing connection sites with bands or tape.

Do not clamp chest tubes unless:

Physician has prescribed clamping.

Closed chest drainage system is being changed to new system.

System becomes disconnected or H$_2$O seal is disrupted. *Clamping chest tubes is dangerous because tension pneumothorax may occur*

▪ Assist patient with activity level increases daily. *Mobilizing the patient postoperatively can help to prevent pulmonary and circulatory complications.*

Ineffective Airway Clearance

RELATED FACTORS

Thoracic surgery
Incisional pain

DEFINING CHARACTERISTICS

Complaint of pain
Refusal to cough
Diminished breath sounds
Abnormal breath sounds (e.g., rhonchi, wheezes)
Splinting of respirations
Dyspnea
Fever

EXPECTED OUTCOMES

Patient's secretions are mobilized and airway is maintained free of secretions as evidenced by clear breath sounds, eupnea, and ability to cough up secretions effectively after deep breaths.

ONGOING ASSESSMENT

▪ Auscultate breath sounds every shift, noting areas of decreased ventilation and the presence of adventitious sounds. *Large FVC reductions follow thoracic surgery.*

▪ Assess cough effectiveness and productivity.

▪ Assess patient for subjective complaints of discomfort or pain. *Postoperative pain can prevent the patient from taking deep breaths and from coughing effectively to clear the airway.*

▪ Assess temperature. *Fever may develop in response to retained secretions/atelectasis.*

NURSING DIAGNOSES	EXPECTED OUTCOMES AND NURSING INTERVENTIONS / *RATIONALES* (■ = INDEPENDENT; ▲ = COLLABORATIVE)

THERAPEUTIC INTERVENTIONS

▲ Administer humidified oxygen as prescribed *to prevent drying of secretions.*

• Assist patient in performing coughing and breathing maneuvers q1hr.

• Instruct patient in:
   Use of pillow or hand splints when coughing
   Use of "huff" or stair step ventilations and/or spirometry
   Use of incentive spirometry
   Importance of early ambulation and/or frequent position changes. *These methods will help patient maintain adequate lung expansion, thus preventing buildup of secretions and atelectasis.*

• Use suctioning as needed *to clear airway.* Avoid deep tracheal suctioning in the post-pneumonectomy patient *to decrease the risk of bronchial stump suture line rupture.*

▲ Administer pain medication as needed, offering it before patient asks for it *to prevent peak periods of pain.*

• Assist patient with ambulation/position changes. *Note:* Patient with pneumonectomy should never be positioned with remaining lung in dependent position *(would compromise respiratory excursion of remaining lung).*

High Risk for Impaired Gas Exchange

RISK FACTORS

Malfunctioning chest tube drainage system
Mediastinal shift

EXPECTED OUTCOMES

Patient's optimal gas exchange is maintained through early assessment and intervention.

ONGOING ASSESSMENT

• Monitor breath sounds.

• Assess for restlessness and changes in LOC. *Altered mentation can indicate development of hypoxia.*

• Assess for presence of tachypnea and tachycardia.

• Assess for tracheal deviation. *Tracheal deviation is a sign of mediastinal shift, which in the presence of tachypnea and tachycardia is an emergency that requires immediate intervention.*

• Assess patency of chest tube drainage system.

• Assess around chest tube insertion site for crepitus or subcutaneous emphysema.

▲ Monitor ABGs

▲ Monitor serial radiograph reports *to assess progress of reexpansion of the lung.*

THERAPEUTIC INTERVENTIONS

• Maintain occlusive dressing around chest tube insertion site, using Vaseline gauze dressing as needed *to prevent air leakage into the tissues.*

• Maintain patency of chest tube drainage system; troubleshoot as necessary.

• Position pneumonectomy patient with no chest tubes on operated side. *Pooling and consolidation on the operated side are desired outcomes; dependent position facilitates this process while enhancing the remaining lung function.*

▲ If tracheal deviation is present with signs of respiratory distress, prepare for additional chest tube insertion, needle aspiration, or emergency thoracentesis.

Pain

RELATED FACTOR

Incisional pain

DEFINING CHARACTERISTICS

Patient report of pain
Guarding behavior
Relief/distraction behavior (moaning, crying, restlessness, irritability, alteration in sleep pattern)
Facial mask of pain
Autonomic responses not seen in chronic stable pain (e.g., diaphoresis, change in BP, pulse rate, pupillary dilatation, increased/decreased respiratory rate, pallor)

EXPECTED OUTCOMES

Patient's pain is relieved as evidenced by verbalization of pain relief, and relaxed facial expression.

ONGOING ASSESSMENT

• Assess pain characteristics.

• Solicit techniques patient considers useful in pain prevention/relief.

• Assess degree to which pain interferes with treatment plan.

THERAPEUTIC INTERVENTIONS

• Anticipate need for pain medications *to prevent peak episodes of pain and coincide with/facilitate ambulation and breathing exercises. Postoperative thoracotomy pain can be severe with the continued movement of respiratory muscles needed to maintain ventilation.*

▲ Respond immediately to complaints of pain by administering analgesics as prescribed, and evaluating effectiveness.

▲ Assist patient as needed with patient controlled analgesia and assess its effectiveness.

• Use nonpharmacologic methods of pain management (e.g., positioning, distraction, touch).

• Reinforce techniques to support incision during movement and breathing/coughing.

• Provide scheduled rest periods *to promote comfort, sleep, and relaxation.*

Continued.

Pulmonary Care Plans

NURSING DIAGNOSES	EXPECTED OUTCOMES AND NURSING INTERVENTIONS / *RATIONALES* (■ = INDEPENDENT; ▲ = COLLABORATIVE)

Impaired Physical Mobility: Arm on Affected Side

RELATED FACTORS
Incisional pain and/or edema
Decreased strength

DEFINING CHARACTERISTICS
Limited ROM
Reluctance to attempt movement

EXPECTED OUTCOMES
Patient experiences full ROM in affected extremity.

ONGOING ASSESSMENT
- Ask patient to raise arm on affected side laterally, assessing degree of ROM present. *During thoracotomy, muscles are incised in the chest, resulting in postoperative reluctance to move the shoulder and arm on the surgical side.*

THERAPEUTIC INTERVENTIONS
- Encourage movement of affected arm with ADL (e.g., combining hair). *Arm movement/exercising will help to maintain muscle tone and function.*
- Instruct patient to perform arm circles, with arm moving in a 360° arc *(will help maintain mobility and strength of arm on affected side).*
- Document progress.

Knowledge Deficit

RELATED FACTOR
Postoperative thoracotomy

DEFINING CHARACTERISTICS
Multiple questions
Lack of questions
Verbalized misconception(s)
Behavior(s) indicative of knowledge deficit (e.g., continued smoking)

EXPECTED OUTCOMES
Patient/significant other verbalizes understanding of postthoracotomy care.

ONGOING ASSESSMENT
- Determine knowledge of etiology of disease and need for behavior modification *to protect remaining lung.*

THERAPEUTIC INTERVENTIONS
- ▲ Collaborate with physician and reinforce postoperative surgical routine, expected recovery, and explanations.
- Instruct patient/significant other about known causes of lung cancer: cigarette smoking, air pollution, industrial pollutants.
- Stress importance of avoiding these *to protect remaining lung and improve oxygenation. Respiratory irritants can cause bronchoconstriction with resultant irritating cough and rapid shallow respiratory rate.*
- Refer patient/significant others to smoking cessation groups/support groups as appropriate.
- ▲ Instruct patient/significant others to have patient resume normal activities gradually (e.g., begin with short walks rather than stair climbing) as approved by physician.
- Instruct patient to keep follow-up appointments with physician.
- Instruct patient/significant other in administration and potential side effects of medications and/or home oxygen.
- Instruct patient/significant other to seek professional advice for dyspnea, fever/chills, unusual wound drainage/change in wound appearance, loss of appetite/unintentional weight loss.
- Reinforce need for/encourage compliance with recommended follow-up therapies.
- Refer patient to American Cancer Society for informational support.

See also:
Anxiety, p. 5.
Infection, p. 40.
Lung Cancer, p. 199.

By: Susan Galanes, RN, MS, CCRN

Tracheostomy

A surgical opening into the trachea that is used to prevent or relieve airway obstruction and/or to serve as an access for suctioning and for mechanical ventilation.

| RELATED FACTORS | EXPECTED OUTCOMES AND NURSING INTERVENTIONS / *RATIONALE* (■ = INDEPENDENT; ▲ = COLLABORATIVE) |

Ineffective Airway Clearance

Related Factors
Copious secretions
Thick secretions
Fatigue; weakness
Uncooperativeness
Confusion
Tracheostomy

Defining Characteristics
Increasing restlessness and irritability
Change in mental status
Pallor, cyanosis
Diaphoresis
Tachypnea
Increased work of breathing: use of accessory muscles, intercostal retractions, nasal flaring

Expected Outcomes
Patient's airway remains patent as evidenced by eupnea, clear breath sounds, and normal skin color.

Ongoing Assessment
- Assess for evidence of respiratory distress (tachypnea, nasal flaring, and increased use of accessory muscles of respiration).
- Assess vital signs q4hr and prn.
- Auscultate chest for normal and adventitious sounds.
- Assess for changes in mental status. *Increasing lethargy, confusion, restlessness, and/or irritability can be early signs of cerebral hypoxia.*
- Record amount, color, and consistency of secretions.

Therapeutic Interventions
- Keep suction equipment and Ambu Bag at bedside.
▲ Provide warm humidified air *to prevent drying and crusting of secretions. A tracheostomy bypasses the nose, which is the body area that humidifies and warms inspired air. A decrease in the humidity of the inspired air will cause secretions to thicken. Also, cool air may decrease ciliary function*
▲ Administer O$_2$ as needed.
- Encourage patient to cough out secretions.
- Institute suctioning of airway as needed *to clear secretions.*
  Instill 2-5 cc of sterile saline solution if secretions are thick. *This will help to loosen secretions and induce coughing.*
  Administer O$_2$ between suctioning attempts *to prevent hypoxemia.*
- Administer stoma care:
  Clean area around stoma and under phalanges of tube with a swab of half-strength hydrogen peroxide.
  If applicable, clean inner cannula with hydrogen peroxide; rinse with sterile water or saline solution. If disposable inner cannula is used, dispose of used inner cannula and replace with a new inner cannula of the correct size.
  Keep stoma clean and dry by using a sterile gauze dressing around tracheostomy site.
  Secure tracheostomy tube with twill tape, using a square knot on the side of the neck. *Twill tape will not fray and produce loose threads, which could be inhaled into the tracheostomy opening.*
- Keep spare tracheostomy tube of same size and brand at bedside.
- Keep tracheal obturator taped at HOB *for emergency use.*
- Maintain inflated tracheostomy cuff:
  Immediately after operation.
  If patient on mechanical ventilation.
  If patient prone to regurgitate and aspirate; cuff should be deflated at other times *to prevent tracheal erosion.*
- Transport patient with portable O$_2$, Ambu bag, suction equipment, and extra tracheostomy tube.

High Risk for Impaired Gas Exchange

Risk Factors
Superimposed infection
Copious tracheal secretions
Tracheostomy leak
Pneumothorax *(during insertion, apices of lungs are at risk for damage)*

Expected Outcomes
Patient's gas exchange is maintained as evidenced by normal ABGs, alert responsive mentation or no further reduction in mental status.

Ongoing Assessment
- Monitor respirations, pulse, and temperature and assess changes.
- Assess changes in orientation and behavior pattern.
- Auscultate breath sounds, assessing for decreased or adventitious breath sounds.
▲ Monitor ABGs and note changes. Use pulse oximetry as appropriate to monitor O$_2$ saturation.

Continued.

RELATED FACTORS	EXPECTED OUTCOMES AND NURSING INTERVENTIONS / *RATIONALES* (■ = INDEPENDENT; ▲ = COLLABORATIVE)

ONGOING ASSESSMENT—cont'd

- ▲ Monitor effectiveness of tracheostomy cuff. Collaborate with the respiratory therapist, as needed, to determine cuff pressure. *Maximum recommended levels range from 20 to 25 mm Hg (27 to 33 cm H_2O) or less, if the trachea can be sealed with less.* If a leak is present, try to reinflate the cuff, checking the pilot tube and valve for leaks. If unsuccessful notify physician. *If the patient is being mechanically ventilated and is losing a large portion of the tidal volume because of a cuff leak, the tracheostomy tube will need to be replaced.*
- · Assess for development of signs of impaired gas exchange: shortness of breath, tachypnea, increased work of breathing, diaphoresis, pallor. Notify physician if these occur.
- ▲ Monitor radiograph reports.

THERAPEUTIC INTERVENTIONS

- · *To decrease anxiety,* stay with the patient during episodes of respiratory distress.
- · Maintain adequate airway. If obstruction is suspected, troubleshoot as appropriate.
    Move head and neck *to correct any kinking of the tube.*
    Attempt to deflate cuff, *for possible herniated cuff.*
    Try to pass a suction catheter *in an attempt to aspirate a mucous plug.*
    Remove inner cannula *to see whether a mucous plug is lodged in the tube,* and replace with back-up inner cannula.
    Remove and replace tracheostomy tube if all else is unsuccessful.
- · Place patient in semi- to high Fowler's position *to promote full lung expansion.*
- ▲ Administer humidified O_2 as needed *to maintain oxygenation and prevent drying of mucosal membranes.*
- · If breath sounds are abnormal, use tracheal suction as needed *to clear secretions.*
- · Assist in proper positioning when portable chest radiograph is needed *so that entire lung field will be irradiated and optimal lung expansion will occur.*
- ▲ If pneumothorax is present, set up chest tube placement *to evacuate air from the pleural cavity and reexpand the collapsed lung* (see also Pneumothorax, p. 214, as appropriate).

High Risk for Infection

RISK FACTOR

Surgical incision of tracheostomy

EXPECTED OUTCOMES

Patient's risk for infection is reduced as a result of ongoing assessment and early intervention.

ONGOING ASSESSMENT

- ▲ Observe stoma for erythema, exudates, odor, and crusting lesions. If present, culture stoma and notify physician.
- · Assess vital signs, notify of abnormalities.
- ▲ Assess laboratory values of WBC and differential count.
- ▲ Assess for fever and chills; monitor blood culture results.
- · Assess skin integrity under tracheal ties every 8 hours.

THERAPEUTIC INTERVENTIONS

- · Provide routine tracheostomy care q8hr and prn *to prevent airway obstruction and infection.*
- · Do not allow secretions to pool around stoma. Suction area or wipe with aseptic technique *to keep stoma clean and dry.*
- · Keep skin under tracheostomy ties clean and dry *to prevent skin irritation.*
- · Use Reston foam or Duoderm under tracheostomy ties *to prevent breakdown* if redness is present.
- ▲ If signs of infection are present, apply topical antifungal or antibacterial agent as ordered.

RELATED FACTORS	EXPECTED OUTCOMES AND NURSING INTERVENTIONS / *RATIONALES* (■ = INDEPENDENT; ▲ = COLLABORATIVE)

Impaired Verbal Communication

RELATED FACTOR
Tracheostomy

DEFINING CHARACTERISTICS
Difficulty in making self understood
Withdrawal
Restlessness
Frustration

EXPECTED OUTCOMES
Patient uses alternative methods of communication.

ONGOING ASSESSMENT
- Assess patient's ability to understand the spoken word.
- Assess patient's ability to express ideas. *Standard tracheostomy tubes allow the vocal cords to move, but no airflow to pass over them; therefore, phonation is not possible.*

THERAPEUTIC INTERVENTIONS
- Provide call light within easy reach at all times.
- Obtain room close to nurse's station *to ensure easy observation of patient by nursing staff.*
- Provide patient with pad and pencil. Use picture or alphabet board for patient unable to write.
- Provide patient with reassurance and patience *to allay frustration.*
- ▲ Consult speech therapist for possible artificial larynx.
- ▲ Collaborate with physician on possible use of "talking" tracheostomy tube (as appropriate). *The "talking" tracheostomy tube provides a port for compressed gas to flow in above the tracheostomy tube allowing air for phonation.*
- Also see Impaired verbal communication, p. 14.

Knowledge Deficit

RELATED FACTOR
New procedure/intervention in hospital

DEFINING CHARACTERISTICS
Anxiety
Lack of questioning
Increased questioning
Expressed need for more information

EXPECTED OUTCOMES
Patient/significant others demonstrate skills appropriate for tracheostomy.

ONGOING ASSESSMENT
- Assess knowledge of tracheostomy.
- Assess ability to provide adequate home health care.
- Assess ability to respond to emergency situations.

THERAPEUTIC INTERVENTIONS
- Discuss patient's need of tracheostomy and its particular purpose.
- Begin teaching skills one at a time and reinforce daily. *Patient/significant others can begin to acquire skills at pace that is not overwhelming.*
- Provide instruction on sterile tracheostomy care and suctioning; include step-by-step care guidelines on:
  How to suction
  Use of twill tape and/or Velcro ties
  Cleaning of tracheostomy with or without disposable inner cannula
  Cleaning around tracheostomy site
  Reinsertion of tracheostomy
  Need to call physician if amount of secretions increases or change in color/characteristic occurs.
- Discuss the weaning process, as appropriate, with the use of fenestrated tracheostomy tubes, tracheostomy buttons, or progressively smaller tubes.
- Reinforce knowledge of emergency techniques.
- Provide list of resource persons to contact, including who they are and why/when they should be contacted.
- Explain importance of follow-up appointments.
- ▲ Use social services as appropriate *to attain equipment and arrange for visiting nurses.*
- Encourage a 24-hr in-hospital trial of total care before discharge.

See also:
Nutrition: less than body requirements, p. 44.
High Risk for Aspiration, p. 6.

By: Susan Galanes, RN, MS, CCRN

Tuberculosis, active

(TB)

A contagious disease of the lung caused by tubercle bacillus, which is spread by airborne droplet nuclei that are produced when an infected person coughs or sneezes. The infection can develop into clinical disease. Those at higher risk for development of clinical disease include the immunosuppressed (patients receiving cancer chemotherapy, patients with acquired immunodeficiency syndrome [AIDS], patients with diabetes mellitus, adolescents, and patients less than 2 years of age). The infection may enter a latent period in those patients who produce an effective immune response, resulting in a dormant state. However, a reactivation of the disease can later occur in patients with decreased resistance, concomitant diseases, and immunosuppression.

NURSING DIAGNOSES	EXPECTED OUTCOMES AND NURSING INTERVENTIONS / *RATIONALE* (■ = INDEPENDENT; ▲ = COLLABORATIVE)

Ineffective Breathing Pattern

RELATED FACTORS

Decreased lung volumes/ capacity
Increased metabolism as result of high fever
Frequent productive cough and hemoptysis
Nervousness, fear of suffocation

DEFINING CHARACTERISTICS

Increased work of breathing: tachypnea, use of accessory muscles, retractions, diaphoresis, tachycardia
Purulent or bloody expectoration

EXPECTED OUTCOMES

Patient's breathing pattern is maintained as evidenced by eupnea and regular respiratory rate/pattern.

ONGOING ASSESSMENT

- Assess respiratory status. Note depth, rate and character of breathing.
- Check for increased work of breathing.
- Assess cough (productive, weak, or hard). *The cough typically becomes frequent and productive.*
- Assess nature of secretions; color, amount, consistency. *Hemoptysis may be present in advanced cases.*
- Auscultate lungs for presence of normal and abnormal breath sounds.
- Monitor vital signs. Note time of temperature spikes. *Low-grade fevers occur, especially in the afternoon.*
- ▲ Monitor ABGs as indicated.

THERAPEUTIC INTERVENTIONS

- ▲ Administer O_2 as ordered *(decreases work of breathing).*
- Push fluids and promote hydration *to liquify secretions for easy expectoration.*
- Induce sputum with heated aerosol if needed *to expedite diagnosis and start early treatment.*
- Maintain semi-Fowler's position *to facilitate easy breathing.*

Actual Infection

RELATED FACTOR

Active pulmonary TB

DEFINING CHARACTERISTICS

Purulent or bloody expectoration
Temperature spikes
Positive culture report

EXPECTED OUTCOMES

Patient's infection is effectively treated as evidenced by negative culture report on reexamination and absence of fever.
Risk of spread of infection is reduced.

ONGOING ASSESSMENT

- Check amount, color, and consistency of sputum.
- Monitor temperature q4hr.
- ▲ Monitor sputum cultures. *Initially sputum cultures are obtained weekly, and then monthly, to determine whether the antimicrobial drugs are effective.*

THERAPEUTIC INTERVENTIONS

- Maintain respiratory isolation. *Respiratory isolation is indicated until the patient responds to the medication (days to weeks):*
  Keep sputum cups at bedside.
  Dispose of secretions properly.
  Keep tissues at bedside.
  Have patient cover mouth when coughing or sneezing, *to decrease airborne contaminants.*
  Use masks. *(To be effective, the masks need to be designed to filter out droplet nuclei. Other masks are of limited value):*
  Anyone entering patient's room should wear a mask.
  If patient is transported out of room, for any reason, patient should wear a mask.
  Keep door to room closed at all times and post isolation sign where visible.
  Place respiratory isolation sticker on chart.
  Assist visitors to follow appropriate isolation techniques *to prevent spread of infection.*
- Teach patient hand washing techniques to use after handling sputum.
- Refer patient contacts to be assessed for possible infection and for chemoprophylactic treatment *to prevent spread/development of infection.*
- ▲ Administer medications as ordered.

Diversional Activity Deficit

RELATED FACTOR

Isolation

DEFINING CHARACTERISTICS

Verbal expression of boredom
Preoccupation with illness
Frequent use of call light
Excessive complaints

EXPECTED OUTCOMES

Patient's boredom is reduced.
Patient participates in satisfying activities.

ONGOING ASSESSMENT

- Assess for signs of boredom/preoccupation with illness.
- Assess understanding of need for isolation.

THERAPEUTIC INTERVENTIONS

- Encourage questions, conversation, and ventilation of feelings. *The patient may feel a social stigma associated with TB and this needs to be discussed*
- Address fears about communicability of disease and need for isolation *so patient will understand need for isolation and know it is temporary, if he/she follows the prescribed treatment.*
- Encourage visitors to involve patient in activities (e.g., conversation, card games, board games).
- Arrange for television in room, when possible.
- ▲ Arrange occupational therapy in room.

Ineffective Management of Therapeutic Regimen

RELATED FACTORS

Patient value system: health and spiritual beliefs, cultural beliefs, and cultural influences
Long term therapy
Lack of knowledge of disease process
Lack of motivation
Inadequate follow-up
Patient and provider relationship

EXPECTED OUTCOMES

Patient displays optimal adherence to treatment regimen, as evidenced by regular medication schedule, reduced coughing, weight gain, or no loss.

ONGOING ASSESSMENT

- Assess patient for evidence of noncompliance: weight loss, increased coughing, thick, green-gray purulent sputum, drug-resistant organism on culture and sensitivity.
- Identify causes of noncompliance.
- ▲ Obtain sputum for culture and sensitivity studies *to determine proper combination of drugs to be reinstituted.*

Continued.

Pulmonary Care Plans

NURSING DIAGNOSES	EXPECTED OUTCOMES AND NURSING INTERVENTIONS / *RATIONALES* (■ = INDEPENDENT; ▲ = COLLABORATIVE)

DEFINING CHARACTERISTICS

TB reactivation shown on chest radiographic and sputum examination

Poor nutritional status: signs of malnutrition; not feeling well

Drug-resistant organism seen in culture and sensitivity

Verbal cue by patient/ significant others of noncompliance

THERAPEUTIC INTERVENTIONS

- Adapt respiratory isolation techniques to home environment.
- ▲ Arrange for social service involvement for patient and family.
- Discuss importance of following therapeutic regimen. *Most treatment failures result from the patient's prematurely stopping the medication, taking the medication irregularly, or failing to take the medication at all. If the patient cannot adhere to a medication regimen, a responsible person should be designated to administer the medication. The patient should be instructed of the likelihood of developing a "multiple drug resistant" strain of TB if medications are not taken as prescribed.*

Knowledge Deficit

RELATED FACTOR

Unfamiliarity with disease process and new treatment methods

DEFINING CHARACTERISTICS

Verbalization of incorrect information

Statement of lack of understanding/asking questions

Evidence of noncompliance with therapeutic regimen related to lack of information

EXPECTED OUTCOMES

Patient verbalizes basic knowledge of TB.

ONGOING ASSESSMENT

- Assess knowledge of TB.

THERAPEUTIC INTERVENTIONS

- Teach patient the following: *A patient with knowledge of disease will be more likely to be compliant with the treatment regimen:*
  Detection, transmission, signs/symptoms of relapse. *Individuals may experience relapse and so should be taught to recognize the possible recurrence of TB and to seek immediate medical attention.*
  Treatment and length of therapy
  Prevention
  Importance of compliance with therapy
  Health regimen to follow after discharge: clinic appointments, sources of free medication, ADL, resource telephone numbers.
- Reinforce respiratory isolation technique.
- Explain the importance of good nutrition while taking TB medications. *Meeting the patient's metabolic needs will decrease fatigue and help the patient to build resistance.*
- Review possible individual risk factors that may reactivate TB (e.g., malnutrition, alcoholism, immunosuppression, diabetes mellitus, and cancer).
- Encourage the patient to abstain from smoking. *Smoking would increase the possibility of bronchitis and respiratory dysfunction.*

See also:

Nutrition, less than body requirements, p. 44.
Activity intolerance, p. 2.

By: Susan Galanes, RN, MS, CCRN

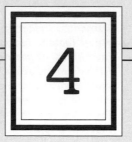

Neurologic Care Plans

Alzheimer's disease/Dementia

(MULTIINFARCT DEMENTIA [MID])

Dementia: Evidence of intellectual dysfunction related to a variety of factors, including some pathophysiologic factors. Approximately 5% of persons > 65 years of age suffer from dementia. Alzheimer's disease: An irreversible disease of the central nervous system that manifests as a cognitive disorder. The cause of Alzheimer's disease is unknown. This care plan addresses needs for patients with a wide variety of dementia, of which Alzheimer's is a type.

NURSING DIAGNOSES	EXPECTED OUTCOMES AND NURSING INTERVENTIONS / *RATIONALE* (■ = INDEPENDENT; ▲ = COLLABORATIVE)

High Risk for Violence: Self-directed or Directed at Others

RISK FACTORS

Impaired perception of reality
Impaired frustration tolerance
Decreased self-esteem
Perceived threat to self
Alteration in sleep/rest pattern
Impaired self-expression, verbal and nonverbal
Anxiety
Impaired coping skills
Decreased sense of personal boundaries
Drug intoxication or idiosyncratic reaction
Physical discomfort
Overstimulation

EXPECTED OUTCOMES

Early manifestations of violence are detected and interventional techniques applied to prevent escalation.
Patient avoids physical harm.
Caregiver avoids physical harm.

ONGOING ASSESSMENT

- Assess *cognitive* factors that may contribute to development of violent behaviors, including:
  Decreased ability to solve problems.
  Alteration in sensory/perceptual capacities.
  Impairment in judgment.
  Psychotic or delusional thought patterns.
  Impaired concentration or decreased response to redirection.
- Assess *physical* factors that may foster violence: physical discomfort, sensory overload (overstimulation).
- Assess *emotional* factors that can lead to violence: inability to cope with frustrating situations, expressions of low self-esteem, noncompliance with treatment plan, and history of aggressive behaviors as means of coping with stress. *Thorough assessment of precipitating factors is needed so preventive measures can be instituted.*

THERAPEUTIC INTERVENTIONS

- Involve patient on a cognitive level as much as possible. Begin with least restrictive measures and progress to most restrictive measures.
- ■ **Level I:** Nonaggressive behaviors: *May include wandering/pacing, restlessness/increased motor activity, climbing out of bed, changing clothes/disrobing, pulling at dressing/tubes, handwringing/handwashing.*
  - Give verbal feedback and institute interpersonal approaches.
  - Consider environmental measures to be taken. *Sensory stimulation needs to be reduced.*
  - Evaluate impact of medication regimen on behaviors in terms of contribution to agitation. *Neuroleptics may cause extrapryamidal side effects (EPSs), manifested as restlessness.* Consider use of medications prescribed for agitation.
  - Speak in slow, clear, soothing tones. Make comments brief and to the point.
  - Consider distracting the patient.
- ■ **Level II:** Verbally aggressive behaviors: *May include cursing, yelling, screaming, unintelligible/repetitive speech, and threatening/accusing.*
  - Attempt verbal control; may be feedback about behavior (for less cognitively impaired), distraction (for cognitively impaired), or limit setting (although this may increase agitation at times).
  - If feasible, allow patient more personal space. If memory span is short, leaving room briefly may decrease agitation.
  - Acknowledge fear of loss of control; evaluate use of touch and hand holding.
  - If wandering/pacing behaviors present, may need to provide visual supervision, especially if patient expresses need to leave unit. *Providing for patient's safety is priority concern.*
  - Provide diversional activity (e.g., folding towels, handling worry beads, walking with the patient).
- ■ **Level III:** Physically aggressive behaviors: *May include hitting, kicking, spitting/biting, throwing objects, pushing/pulling others, fighting.*
  - Permit verbalization of feelings associated with agitation.
  - Offer acceptable alternatives to behaviors such as undressing by suggesting that patient dress or return to room.
  - If patient poses potential threat of injury to self or others, consider use of physical restraints. *As initial measures become ineffective, more extreme measures may be indicated to ensure patient/staff safety.*

THERAPUTIC INTERVENTIONS—cont'd

▲ Use soft restraints such as cloth wrist, hand, leg, belt, or vest types (restraints always used in conjunction with full side rails secured in the up position). Refer to policy and procedure manual for application of restraints.

▲ Use leather restraints only if agitation has reached point that soft restraints are inadequate to protect patient from injury.

Bathing/grooming, feeding Self-care Deficit

RELATED FACTORS

Alteration in cognition, including impaired memory, disorientation, memory deficits, impaired judgment, impaired sense of social self

DEFINING CHARACTERISTICS

Requires assistance with at least one of the following: bathing, oral hygiene, dressing/grooming, feeding
Denies need for personal hygiene measures
Refuses to change clothes or wears more than one set
Unable to assist in personal care because of motor deficits/confusion

EXPECTED OUTCOMES

Patient participates in self-care activities, as evidenced by dressing, bathing self, feeding self.

ONGOING ASSESSMENT

- Assess cognitive deficits/behaviors that would create difficulty in bathing self, performing oral hygiene, selecting and putting on appropriate clothing, choosing food menu items and feeding self.
- Assess level of independence in completing self-care. *The patient with impaired thought processes is unable to self-monitor personal grooming, hygiene, and nutrition needs adequately.*
- Assess need for supervision/redirection during self-care.

THERAPEUTIC INTERVENTIONS

- Stay with patient during self-care activities if judgment is impaired *to promote safety and provide necessary redirection.*
- Provide simple, easy-to-read list of self-care activities to complete each day (brush teeth, comb hair, etc.) *Reminders may enhance functional abilities.*
- Assist, as needed, with perineal care each morning and evening (or after each episode of incontinence).
- Assist, as needed, in selecting clothing. Allow patient to choose if at all possible (e.g., put out 2 or 3 sets of clothing and allow to choose).
- Encourage to dress as independently as possible. Provide easy-to-wear clothes (elastic waistbands, snaps, large buttons, Velcro closures).
- Assist in selection of nutritious, high-bulk foods. Allow patient to choose food he/she prefers if possible *to promote adequate intake.*
- Assist in setup of meal as needed (opening containers, cutting food).
- If judgment is impaired, cool hot liquids to palatable temperatures before serving
- Limit number of choices of food on plate or tray *to reduce number of necessary decisions.*
- Provide easy-to-eat finger foods if motor coordination impaired.
- Provide nutritious between-meal snacks if nutritional intake inadequate.
- Follow established routines for self-care if possible.
- If patient refuses a task, use distraction techniques; break the task into smaller steps; use calm, unhurried voice to offer praise and encouragement.

Impaired Social Interaction

RELATED FACTORS

Alteration in cognition, including impaired sense of social self, memory deficits, impaired judgment, disorientation, social isolation

DEFINING CHARACTERISTICS

Change in patterns of social interaction, including language/behaviors inappropriate to social situations, lack of relationships with others

EXPECTED OUTCOMES

Patient engages in social interaction as evidenced by positive contacts with caregiver/significant other.

ONGOING ASSESSMENT

- Assess cognitive deficits/behaviors that interfere with forming relationships with others.
- Assess previous patterns of interaction. *Patient's ability and/or willingness to interact may vary with the patient's mood, perceptions, and reality orientation.*
- Assess potential to interact in community day care situation after discharge. *Confusion, disorientation, and loss of social inhibitions may result in socially inappropriate and/or harmful behavior to self or others.*

THERAPEUTIC INTERVENTIONS

- Within context of nurse-patient relationship, provide regular opportunity for frequent brief contacts.
- Discuss subjects in which patient is interested, but which do not require extensive recall.
- When discussing past experiences, assist patient in connecting them with here-and-now.
- Support participation in social activities appropriate to patient's level of cognitive functioning.
- Redirect patient when behaviors become socially embarrassing.

Continued.

Alzheimer's disease/dementia cont'd

NURSING DIAGNOSES	EXPECTED OUTCOMES AND NURSING INTERVENTIONS / *RATIONALE* (■ = INDEPENDENT; ▲ = COLLABORATIVE)

THERAPEUTIC INTERVENTION—cont'd

- If patient expresses delusional ideas, focus on reality-based interactions. Do not correct patient's ideas or confront them as delusional.
- Consider impact of milieu on social interaction. Avoid milieu that is overstimulating (noise, lights, activity, etc.). *Sensory overload aggravates cognitive thinking.*
- Involve patient in developing a daily schedule that includes time for social activity and quiet time. Consider patient's talents, interests, and abilities when developing daily program.
- Provide information on community day-care programs *that will help patient maintain social interaction. Involvement with group activities is determined by various factors, including group size, activity level and patient's tolerance level. Fluctuations in mood and affect may influence ability to respond appropriately to others.*

Impaired Home Maintenance/Management

RELATED FACTORS

Alteration in cognition: impaired memory, disorientation, memory deficits

DEFINING CHARACTERISTICS

Requires assistance with at least one of the following: food/fluid intake, personal hygiene/dressing, toileting
Disorientation in familiar surroundings
Need for supervision in potentially hazardous situations
Family caregiver concerns about caring for patient at home

EXPECTED OUTCOMES

Caregiver/family provides safe home environment.
Caregiver/family describes nursing/community resources available for home care.

ONGOING ASSESSMENT

- Assess cognitive deficits/behaviors making it difficult to:
  Prepare meals.
  Recognize signs of hunger.
  See also Bathing/Grooming/Feeding self-care deficit, p. 53.
- Assess ability to recognize danger (smoke, fire, etc).
- Assess frequency of disorientation, wandering, becoming lost in familiar surroundings.
- Assess motor, sensory, and cognitive deficits to determine safety needs.
- Assess family/caregiver's understanding of patient's needs/deficits, resources to provide adequate supervision and behavior management, ability to cope, and internal/external support systems. *Thorough assessment needed to determine potential problems/ complications.*

THERAPEUTIC INTERVENTIONS

- Involve patient/family/caregiver in all home planning.
- Identify alternate methods of meal preparation to facilitate independent feeding (e.g., finger foods, group dining if available, precooked meals, home-delivered meals).
- Discuss potential need for supervision of ADLs, including feeding.
- Discuss ways to minimize environmental hazards in home.
- Discuss need to wear identification bracelet at all times.
- Assist in developing daily schedule that allows rest and activity periods. *Fatigue makes coping difficult.*
- Suggest daily supervised exercise/walking program *to decrease wandering behavior.*
- Teach about home security devices *to decrease chances of patient's wandering from home.*
- Recommend procedure for getting help should patient become lost.
- Identify and encourage correction of obstacles/hazards in home. *Ensuring environmental safety is a priority.*
- Help family identify and mobilize available support networks *to facilitate home patient care.*
- Provide information about support groups available to family members. *Caregivers require emotional support and respite care.*
- Provide literature/references related to caring for cognitively impaired persons in home.
- Discuss available home health and community services.
- See also Home maintenance/management, impaired, p. 34.

High Risk for Urinary Incontinence or Retention

RISK FACTORS

Alteration in cognition, neurogenic bladder, lack of sensation or urge to void

EXPECTED OUTCOMES

Patient maintains normal urinary elimination pattern.

ONGOING ASSESSMENT

- Assess *physiologic* factors that may contribute to urinary difficulties. *Examples may include urinary frequency/urgency, urinary retention, distended bladder, symptoms of urinary tract infection (UTI), amount voided, color and odor of urine.*

ONGOING ASSESSMENT—cont'd

- Assess *behavioral* factors that may contribute to urinary difficulties. *Examples include impaired judgment/disorientation, agitation, depression, decreased attention span.*
- Assess for perineal skin integrity.
- Obtain specimens and residual urine as indicated.
- Maintain record of intake and output, including pattern of voiding, *to establish baseline.*

THERAPEUTIC INTERVENTIONS

- Report symptoms of UTI or urinary retention.
- Encourage and provide fluids (depending on medical status) *to promote urine flow.*
- ▲ Medicate as prescribed and assess response to medication.
- Maintain patency of external or indwelling catheters if in place.
- ▲ Administer diuretic medication in morning if prescribed; *be aware that administration of diuretics and psychotropic medications may alter urinary elimination.*
- Establish bladder program acceptable to patient/caretaker.
- Direct patient to toilet q2-3h during day. *Voiding at regular intervals prevents distention.*
- Use urinal/bedside commode at night.
- Reduce fluid intake after 6 p.m. *to reduce need to void during night.*
- *Maintain skin integrity* by assisting the patient as needed in perineal care after each voiding.
- Request and use protective skin creams as needed.
- Use protective clothing and incontinent pads as necessary during day and night. *Incontinence pads are available in several forms and sizes from simple sanitary napkin size to adult diaper size.*
- See also Urinary tract infections, p. 480; Urinary retention, p. 74.

High Risk for Bowel Incontinence

RISK FACTORS

Alteration in cognition
Spontaneous bowel evacuation
Low-bulk diet
Chronic constipation
Immobility

EXPECTED OUTCOMES

Patient achieves regular bowel evacuation pattern.

ONGOING ASSESSMENT

- Assess *physiologic* factors that may contribute to incontinence. *Examples may include constipation, diarrhea, frequent expulsion of small amounts of formed stool, alteration in frequency of bowel elimination patterns, or use of psychotropic medications. Be aware that many psychotropic medications used to control agitated behaviors may contribute to constipation.*
- Assess *behavioral* factors that may contribute to incontinence. *Examples may include impaired judgment, disorientation, agitation, depression, decreased attention span.*
- Assess skin integrity in perineal and buttock areas. *Thorough assessment needed to determine potential complications.*

THERAPEUTIC INTERVENTIONS

- Maintain daily record of bowel elimination. Note amount, consistency, and frequency.
- Consider patient's food preferences when planning diet high in bulk and fiber.
- Provide fluid intake (depending on medical status).
- Involve patient in daily exercise program.
- ▲ Establish bowel program that may include bulk laxatives, stool softeners, suppositories, or enemas if necessary.
- Locate patient near a bathroom and clearly mark the door "Bathroom."
- Take patient to toilet after breakfast *to take advantage of increased bowel motility at this time.*
- Provide privacy.
- Be aware of nonverbal cues that may indicate patient need to evacuate the bowel *(e.g., restlessness, pulling clothes, holding hand over the rectal area, and using fingers to disimpact stool from the rectum).*
- Use incontinence pads and protective clothing as necessary during daytime.

Continued.

Neurologic Care Plans

NURSING DIAGNOSES	EXPECTED OUTCOMES AND NURSING INTERVENTIONS / *RATIONALE* (■ = INDEPENDENT; ▲ = COLLABORATIVE)

Caregiver Role Strain

RELATED FACTORS

Caregiver knowledge deficit regarding management of care

Caregiver's personal and social life are disrupted by demands of caregiving

Caregiver has multiple competing roles

Caregiver has no respite from caregiving demands

Caregiver unaware of available community resources

Caregiver reluctant to use community resources

Community resources not available

Community resources not affordable

DEFINING CHARACTERISTICS

Caregiver expresses difficulty in performing patient care.

Caregiver verbalizes anger with responsibility of patient care

Caregiver states that formal and informal support systems are inadequate

Caregiver expresses problems in coping with patient's behavior

Caregiver expresses negative feeling about patient or relationship

Caregiver neglects patient care

See also:
Toileting self-care deficit, p. 53.
Sleep pattern disturbance, p. 61.
Impaired individual coping, p. 18.

EXPECTED OUTCOMES

Caregiver demonstrates competence and confidence in performing the caregiver role by meeting care recipient's physical and psychosocial needs.

Caregiver verbalizes positive feelings about care recipient and their relationship.

Caregiver reports that formal and informal support systems are adequate and helpful.

ONGOING ASSESSMENT

- Assess caregiver-care recipient relationship.
- Assess family communication pattern. *Open communication in the family creates a positive environment while concealing feelings creates problems for caregiver and care recipient.*
- Assess family resources and support systems. *Family and social support is related positively to coping effectiveness.*

THERAPEUTIC INTERVENTIONS

- Provide information on disease process and management strategies. *Accurate information increases understanding of care recipient's condition and behavior.*
- Encourage caregiver to identify available family/friends who can assist with caregiving.
- Suggest that caregiver use available community resources such as respite, home health care, adult day care, ADRDA (Alzheimer's Disease and Related Disorders Association). *Provides respite and protective services.*
- ▲ Consult social worker for referral for community resources and/or financial aid, if needed.
- Encourage caregiver to set aside time for self.
- Acknowledge to caregiver his or her role and its value.

By: Linda Arsenault, RN, MSN, CNRN

Amyotrophic lateral sclerosis (ALS)

(LOU GEHRIG'S DISEASE; MOTOR NEURON DISEASE; PROGRESSIVE BULBAR PALSY; PROGRESSIVE MUSCULAR ATROPHY)

Amyotrophic lateral sclerosis (ALS), commonly called Lou Gehrig's disease, is a progressive disease that attacks specialized nerve cells called motor neurons, which control the movement of muscles via the anterior horns of the spinal cord and the motor nuclei of the lower brain stem. Signs and symptoms of the disease include atrophic weakness of the hands and forearms (early), mild lower extremity spasticity, and diffuse hyperreflexia. Sensation and sphincter control are usually maintained. When the bulbar muscles are affected, difficulty in speech and swallowing is seen with fasciculations in the tongue. There is usually progressive paralysis, with death occurring within 5-10 yrs.

NURSING DIAGNOSES	EXPECTED OUTCOMES AND NURSING INTERVENTIONS / *RATIONALE* (■ = INDEPENDENT; ▲ = COLLABORATIVE)

Anxiety

RELATED FACTORS

Terminal disease process
Threat to self-concept
Threat to or change in health status, socioeconomic status, independence

DEFINING CHARACTERISTICS

Restlessness
Increased vigilance
Insomnia
Fearfulness
Increased tension
Scared, wide-eyed appearance
Poor eye contact
Jitteriness
Distress
Increased perspiration
Apprehension
Uncertainty
Feelings of inadequacy/ helplessness
Expressed concern about changes in life events
Trembling

EXPECTED OUTCOMES

Patient verbalizes reduction/control of anxiety.
Patient demonstrates use of at least one positive coping strategy.

ONGOING ASSESSMENT

- Assess level of anxiety (mild, severe). Note signs and symptoms, including nonverbal communication. *Patients remain alert and are aware that this is a progressive disease with no cure. They are understandably afraid of what the future holds for them.*
- Assess prior coping patterns (by interview with patient/significant others). *Prior methods may be inadequate to handle this life-threatening disease.*
- Evaluate supportive resources available to patient.

THERAPEUTIC INTERVENTIONS

- Display confident, calm manner and tolerant, understanding attitude. *The patient's feeling of stability increases in a calm and nonthreatening environment.*
- Establish rapport with patient, especially through continuity of care.
- Encourage ventilation of feelings, concerns about dependency.
   Listen carefully; sit down if possible.
   Give unhurried attentive appearance; be aware of defense mechanisms used (denial, regression, etc.).
- ▲ Use supportive measures (e.g., medications, clergy, social services, support groups).
- Provide accurate information about disease, medications, test/procedures, and self-care. *Patients need to make informed decisions about their care and future (i.e., whether to be placed on a ventilator).*
- Allow expressions of frustrations about loss and eventual outcome. *Fear/depression are normal and expected in this setting.*
- Understand that patient may have inappropriate behaviors (e.g., outbursts of laughing/ crying.) *This is known as pseudobulbar affect.*
- Try to direct patient to positive aspects of living to the maximum for the present.
- Reinforce the things the patient *can* do versus what he or she *can't.*

Ineffective Airway Clearance

RELATED FACTORS

Dysarthria, aspiration, progressive bulbar palsy, respiratory muscle weakness

DEFINING CHARACTERISTICS

Patient report of breathing difficulty
Abnormal breath sounds: rales (crackles), rhonchi, wheezes
Periods of apnea

EXPECTED OUTCOMES

Patient maintains effective airway clearance as evidenced by clear breath sounds, productive coughing, normal respiratory rate.

ONGOING ASSESSMENT

- Assess breath sounds and respiratory movement as indicated.
- Observe for signs of respiratory distress (e.g., increased respiratory rate, restlessness, rales, rhonchi, decreased breath sounds). *If increased distress is noted, patient may need artificial ventilation.*
- ▲ Monitor pulse oximetry as indicated. *If patient desaturates, will need supplemental O$_2$, possible suctioning, repositioning.*
- Evaluate cough reflex. *Allows an estimate of patient's ability to protect airway. Aspiration is a common problem.*
- ▲ Observe for signs/symptoms of infection (change in sputum color, amount, character; increased WBC).

Continued.

Amyotrophic lateral sclerosis (ALS)—cont'd

NURSING DIAGNOSES	EXPECTED OUTCOMES AND NURSING INTERVENTIONS / *RATIONALE* (■ = INDEPENDENT; ▲ = COLLABORATIVE)
	THERAPEUTIC INTERVENTIONS · Elevate head of bed (HOB); change position q2h and prn. · Encourage deep breathing exercises, use of incentive spirometry. · Encourage fluid intake to 2000 ml daily within level of cardiac reserve *to keep secretions thin.* Encourage warm liquids *(loosen secretions).* · Suction as needed. Assist patient to suction self as appropriate. ▲ Provide O$_2$ as needed. · Anticipate mechanical ventilation if signs of distress are noted.
Impaired Physical Mobility **RELATED FACTORS** Increasing motor weakness caused by paralysis Spasticity of extremities Limited ROM Fatigue Neuromuscular impairment Imposed restrictions of movement **DEFINING CHARACTERISTICS** Intolerance to activity, decreased strength and endurance Inability to move purposefully within the physical environment (including bed mobility, transfer, and ambulation) Impaired coordination, limited ROM, decreased muscle strength control, and/or muscle mass	**EXPECTED OUTCOMES** Patient maintains optimal physical mobility within limits of disease. **ONGOING ASSESSMENT** · Assess ROM, muscle strength, previous activity level, gait, coordination, and movement. · Assess patient's current level of dependence: self care ability, help in transfer from bed or chair to bathroom. · Assess patient's endurance in performing ADL. *Progressive muscle weakness and fatigue are major problems in ALS.* · Evaluate requirements for assistive devices. *Prostheses may be indicated to support weakened muscles.* **THERAPEUTIC INTERVENTIONS** · Position patient for optimum comfort, facilitation of ventilation, and prevention of skin breakdown. Reposition regularly. · Maintain exercise program: active/passive ROM *to prevent venous stasis, maintain joint mobility and good body alignment, and prevent footdrop and contractures.* · Alternate periods of activity with adequate rest periods *to prevent excessive fatigue.* ▲ Coordinate physical therapy and occupational therapy as needed. · Encourage patient's and significant other(s)' involvement in care: help them learn ways to manage problems of immobility. · Provide safety measures as indicated by individual situation. · Encourage participation in activities, occupational/recreational therapy. · Provide skin care. Wash and dry skin well; use gentle massage and lotion *to stimulate circulation.*

Urinary Retention
 	
RELATED FACTORS
Neuromuscular impairment, urinary tract infection
 	
DEFINING CHARACTERISTICS
Overflow incontinence
Frequency
Retention of > 150 cc after voiding
Dysuria
Nocturia
Urgency
	EXPECTED OUTCOMES
	Patient has residual urine volume of < 150 cc after voiding.
	
	ONGOING ASSESSMENT
	· Assess patient's ability to sense need to void.
	· Monitor amount and frequency of output.
	· Monitor for signs of urinary tract infection: burning, frequent voiding of ≤ 100 cc of foul-smelling cloudy urine.
	· Assess need for assistive devices: diapers, external catheter (males).
	· Check frequently for bladder distention; observe for overflow/dribbling *to prevent complications of infection and/or autonomic hyperflexia.*
	· Monitor I & O for at least 24 hr when indwelling catheter removed.
	
	THERAPEUTIC INTERVENTIONS
	▲ Institute appropriate bladder training program, depending on patient's amount of control. *Use* indwelling or intermittent catheter *to prevent bladder overdistention.*
	▲ Investigate alternatives (e.g., drugs, voiding maneuvers, use of diapers, external catheters) when possible.
	· Maintain acidic environment by use of vitamin C, cranberry juice *to discourage bacterial growth.*
	· Establish routine care regimen:
	   Limit fluids after 6 p.m. *(decreases need to void at night).*
	   Instruct/assist to void at precise timed intervals *to prevent overdistention and strengthen perineal muscles.*

THERAPEUTIC INTERVENTIONS—cont'd

> Wake to void at night. Agree on a scheduled time *to allow patient some control over bodily function care.*
> Respond to call light quickly if patient unable to delay voiding.
> Offer/assist with urinal/bedpan/commode.

▲ Perform catheterized postvoid residual check. If > 150 cc, insert Foley, or use intermittent catheterization.

• Anticipate genitourinary consult.

Constipation

RELATED FACTORS

Impaired neuromuscular control, physical immobility, Inadequate fluid intake

DEFINING CHARACTERISTICS

Abdominal pain/discomfort, urgency, frequency, abdominal distention, absence of stool evacuation

EXPECTED OUTCOMES

Patient maintains/reestablishes normal bowel pattern/function

ONGOING ASSESSMENT

• Inquire about usual evacuation pattern.
• Auscultate abdomen for presence, location, and characteristics of bowel sounds.
• Assess diet and nutritional status.
• Check for fecal impaction.
• Identify pathophysiologic factors which may lead to constipation: e.g., dehydration, decreased abdominal muscle strength, immobility, change in diet, infection.

THERAPEUTIC INTERVENTIONS

• Provide for changes in dietary intake that will promote bowel elimination without medications (i.e., dietary fiber, fruit, vegetables).
• Encourage oral intake of fluids (e.g., juices or commercial preparations [Gatorade]). *Note: Gatorade is high in sugar and should not be used for diabetic patients.*
• Maintain perianal skin integrity.
• Do pericare with each bowel movement as needed.
• Apply lotion/ointment/skin barrier as needed.
▲ Administer stool softeners as indicated/needed.
• Promote exercise program as patient is individually able *to increase muscle tone/strength.*
▲ Establish bowel program: regular time for defecation (usually 30 min after eating), glycerine suppositories, and/or digital stimulation.

Altered Nutrition: Less than Body Requirements

RELATED FACTORS

Progressive bulbar palsy, tongue atrophy/weakness, dysphagia
Decreased salivation
Choking during meals

DEFINING CHARACTERISTICS

Loss of appetite
Loss of weight

EXPECTED OUTCOMES

Patient maintains weight or does not lose weight.

ONGOING ASSESSMENT

• Assess swallowing, presence/absence of gag reflex daily.
• Assess nutritional status. *Total protein, serum albumin levels will provide some index of nutritional state.*
• Inquire about food and fluid preferences.
• Assess weight loss; inquire about weight gain/loss over past few weeks/months.
• Assess tissue turgor, mucous membranes, muscular weakness, and tremors.

THERAPEUTIC INTERVENTIONS

• Encourage intake of food patient can swallow; provide frequent small meals and supplements.
• Instruct patient not to talk while eating.
• Encourage patient to chew thoroughly and eat slowly.
• Maintain patient in high Fowler's position during and after meals *to minimize risk of aspiration.*
• Provide sufficient fluids with meals. *Decreased salivation makes swallowing of certain foods difficult.*
• Prepare environment so that it will be well ventilated, uncluttered, cheerful, distraction-free.
▲ Coordinate speech therapy consultation as appropriate to evaluate swallowing. *Special techniques can be taught to facilitate muscle control.*
• Anticipate need for N/G or gastrostomy tube *to maintain adequate nutritional state and weight.*

Continued.

Neurologic Care Plans

NURSING DIAGNOSES	EXPECTED OUTCOMES AND NURSING INTERVENTIONS / *RATIONALE* (■ = INDEPENDENT; ▲ = COLLABORATIVE)

Impaired Verbal Communication

RELATED FACTORS

Dysarthria
Tongue weakness
Nasal tone to speech

DEFINING CHARACTERISTICS

Difficulty in articulating words
Inability to express self clearly

EXPECTED OUTCOMES

Patient uses language or an alternative form of communication, as evidenced by effective use of language to communicate needs.

ONGOING ASSESSMENT

- Determine the degree of speech difficulty by assessing ability to speak spontaneously, endurance of ability to speak.
- Assess patient's ability to use alternative methods of communication (i.e., spelling board, finger writing, eye blinks, signal system, word cards).
- See Impaired communication, p. 14.

THERAPEUTIC INTERVENTIONS

- Use close-ended questions requiring only yes/no response *to minimize effort, conserve energy, and decrease anxiety.*
- Allow patient time to respond. *It is difficult to respond under pressure; allow time to organize responses.*
- Anticipate needs *to decrease feelings of helplessness.*
▲ Consult speech therapist for additional help.
- Praise accomplishments.
- Provide with writing pad, spelling board, etc. as indicated.
- Inform patient/family about dysarthria and its effects on speech and language ability.

Knowledge Deficit

RELATED FACTORS

Unfamiliarity with disease process and management

DEFINING CHARACTERISTICS

Lack of questions
Multiple questions
Misconceptions

EXPECTED OUTCOMES

Patient/family demonstrates knowledge of ALS, progressive course, nutritional and respiratory needs, and available community resources.

ONGOING ASSESSMENT

- Assess knowledge of disease process, diagnostic tests, treatment, outcome.
- Evaluate knowledge/awareness of community support groups.

THERAPEUTIC INTERVENTIONS

- Provide information about:
    Disease process: *Progressive degenerative motor disease of unknown cause that interferes with motor activities (may include lower cranial nerves: swallowing, speech, and respiration).*
    Diagnostic testing: EMG, muscle biopsy, pulmonary function, etc. *To R/O other muscle diseases. At this time there is no definitive test for ALS.*
    Home care planning: nutrition, communication aids. *Patients have major self-care problems. Some patients use ventilators at home for respiratory support.*
- Provide information on ALS support groups:
    ALS Society of America,
    15300 Ventura Blvd., Ste. 315
    Sherman Oaks, CA 91403

    National ALS Foundation, Inc.
    185 Madison Ave.
    New York, NY 10016

    Muscular Dystrophy Assoc., Inc.
    810 Seventh Ave.
    New York, NY 10019

See also:
Impaired individual coping, p. 18.
Hopelessness, p. 36.
Powerlessness, p. 52.
High risk for aspiration, p. 6.
Impaired gas exchange, p. 27.
High risk for impaired skin integrity, p. 59.
Care giver role strain, p. 13.

By: Lela Starnes, RN

Cerebral artery aneurysm: preoperative/unclipped

(SUBARACHNOID HEMORRHAGE [SAH];
INTRAPARENCHYMAL HEMORRHAGE;
INTRACRANIAL ANEURYSM)

Thin-walled blisters, 2 mm to 3 cm in size, protruding from the arteries of the circle of Willis or its major branches, located predominantly at bifurcation of vessels. Intracranial aneurysm may be congenital, traumatic, arteriosclerotic, or septic in origin. Approximately 90% are congenital. It is presumed to be the result of developmental defects in the media and elastica. The intima bulges outward, covered only by adventitia, and eventually rupture may occur.

Subarachnoid hemorrhage (SAH) occurs in about 15,000 Americans/yr, in females more than males. Upon admission to the hospital, most patients are classified according to Hunt and Hess's graded scale based on clinical status as follows: (I) asymptomatic, minimal headache, slight/mild nuchal rigidity; (II) moderate-severe headache, nuchal rigidity, no neurologic deficit other than third nerve palsy; (III) drowsiness, confusion, mild focal deficit; (IV) stupor, moderately severe hemiparesis; (V) coma. After subarachnoid hemorrhage, patients are at risk for rebleed, vasospasm (stroke), and hydrocephalus.

NURSING DIAGNOSES

EXPECTED OUTCOMES AND NURSING INTERVENTIONS / *RATIONALE*
(■ = INDEPENDENT; ▲ = COLLABORATIVE)

Altered Cerebral Tissue Perfusion

RELATED FACTORS

Subarachnoid/intracerebral
  hemorrhage
Ruptured aneurysm
Vasospasm (ischemia)
Cerebral edema
Increased intracranial pressure
  (ICP)

DEFINING CHARACTERISTICS

Severe headache (unlike any
  experienced before)
Unconsciousness: transitory or
  lasting
Nuchal rigidity
Mental confusion, drowsiness
Seizures
Transitory or fixed neurologic
  signs (numbness, speech
  disturbance, paresis)
Hypertension, *which may accentuate or aggravate any vascular weakness, although not necessarily a causative factor in aneurysm development or rupture*

EXPECTED OUTCOMES

Patient maintains optimal cerebral perfusion as evidenced by intact orientation (Glasgow Coma Scale [GCS] > 13).
Potential complications related to SAH are detected early, allowing prompt medical and surgical intervention.

ONGOING ASSESSMENT

- Complete an initial assessment of patient's symptoms. *Time of onset is important in assessing time of initial bleed and subsequent hemorrhage, and it may influence timing of surgery.*
- Complete baseline assessment of neurologic status and deficits, with attention to LOC, mental status, pupils, speech and motor function.
- Assess for seizure activity, noting time of onset, localization of seizure, postictal state.
- Assess for meningeal signs: nuchal rigidity, photophobia.
- Monitor vital signs *(antihypertensive medication may be needed to prevent rebleeding).*

THERAPEUTIC INTERVENTIONS

- Place patient on bed rest in private room if possible *to allow quite environment; minimize startling noises that may increase BP.*
- Keep lighting subdued *because of photophobia associated with subarachnoid hemorrhage.*
- ▲ Administer anticonvulsants as ordered:
    Dilantin: PO/IV. Give slow IV push *(not faster than 50 mg/min). Cannot be given in D_5W (precipitation occurs). Must be given slowly to prevent cardiac dysrhythmias/arrest.*
    Valium: Give slow IV infusion, *no faster than 10 mg/min, to prevent respiratory arrest. Also monitor heart rate and BP (short acting).*
    Phenobarbital: PO/IV/IM 100-200 mg/day in divided doses. *May cause drowsiness.*
- ▲ Administer antihypertensive agents as prescribed.
- Encourage liquid intake if cardiovascular status and electrolytes within normal limits. *Dehydration has an adverse effect on cerebral vasospasm.*
- Limit visitors.
- ▲ Administer stool softeners *to prevent straining, which may increase intracranial pressure.*

Altered Levels of Consciousness

RELATED FACTORS

Vascular spasm/ischemia,
  hemorrhage or rebleed, cerebral edema, hydrocephalus

EXPECTED OUTCOMES

Patient maintains optimal state of consciousness as evidenced by GCS > 13, mental alertness.

ONGOING ASSESSMENT

- Assess for signs of altered levels of consciousness.
- Record serial assessments (See Defining Characteristics.) *LOC is most sensitive and reliable index of change in patient with neurologic disease or injury.*

Continued

NURSING DIAGNOSES	EXPECTED OUTCOMES AND NURSING INTERVENTIONS / *RATIONALE* (■ = INDEPENDENT; ▲ = COLLABORATIVE)
DEFINING CHARACTERISTICS Change in alertness, orientation, verbal response, eye opening, motor response, memory impairment, judgment impairment, agitation, inappropriate affect, impaired thought processes, Glasgow Coma Scale < 11	**THERAPEUTIC INTERVENTIONS** • Maintain airway patency. *Hypoxia and/or hypercapnea can cause increased cerebral blood flow and intracranial pressure.* • See Consciousness, altered level of, p. 252.
High Risk for Injury: Rebleed **RISK FACTORS** Alterations in autoregulation, elevated BP	**EXPECTED OUTCOMES** Risk for rebleed is reduced, as evidenced by blood pressure within acceptable parameters, and stable neurologic status. **ONGOING ASSESSMENT** • Monitor neurologic signs for changes which may indicate deterioration (change in LOC, new focal signs). • Closely monitor BP. Report if Systolic BP < 100 or > 150 mm Hg; Diastolic BP < 60 or > 90 mm Hg; Mean BP < 90 or > 100 mm Hg. ▲ Monitor other hemodynamics, including central venous pressure (CVP), PCWP, cardiac output. **THERAPEUTIC INTERVENTIONS** • Provide bed rest and quiet environment by closing doors, keeping lights low and noise level minimum, and limiting visitors. Provide private room if possible. ▲ Administer antihypertensives as ordered; keep BP in prescribed range. *Sodium nitroprusside may be used initially. Changing to oral antihypertensives requires caution (possibility of sudden hypotension with methyldopa or clonidine therapy).*
High Risk for Injury: Ischemia **RISK FACTOR** Vasospasm	**EXPECTED OUTCOME** Patient exhibits minimal/no effects of vasospasm as evidenced by stable clinical status, absence of headache, and absence of neurologic deficits. **ONGOING ASSESSMENT** • Monitor patient closely for signs of ischemia: impaired mental status, change in LOC, focal abnormalities, speech difficulties, motor deficit, headache, fever. *Following SAH, vasospasm is the most important cause of death/disability. The more severe the hemorrhage, the greater the risk. The usual onset is 3 days after hemorrhage; lasts up to 2 or more weeks.* ▲ Monitor serum electrolyte, BUN, creatinine, serum OSM, urine specific gravity, and I & O closely for signs of dehydration, *which is thought to aggravate vasospasm.* **THERAPEUTIC INTERVENTIONS** ▲ Administer IV fluids as prescribed (often at rate of 125-150 ml/hr). ▲ Administer nimodipine (Nimotop) as prescribed. *This calcium channel blocker is given to prevent/minimize cerebral vasospasm. Initial dose is given as soon as possible after the initial bleed. Medication comes in 30 mg capsules. The dose is 60 mg q4h times 21 days. This is very costly, at around $5/per pill, or $1260 for full course.*

High Risk for Injury: deep vein thrombosis/pulmonary embolus
 	
RISK FACTOR
Complications of antifibrinolytic therapy (Epsilon aminocaproic acid [Amicar])
	EXPECTED OUTCOME
	Risk of complications of antifibrinolytic therapy is reduced.
	
	ONGOING ASSESSMENT
	• Monitor patient for side effects of drug.
	▲ Monitor coagulation studies.
	• Monitor for signs/symptoms of:
	  Deep vein thrombosis: pain in lower extremities, positive Homan's sign, increased extremity circumference, increased temperature.
	  Dehydration: decreased CVP (< 5 cm H_2O), poor skin turgor, dry mucous membranes.

NURSING DIAGNOSES	EXPECTED OUTCOMES AND NURSING INTERVENTIONS / *RATIONALE* (■ = INDEPENDENT; ▲ = COLLABORATIVE)

ONGOING ASSESSMENT—cont'd

Pulmonary emboli: dyspnea, tachycardia, wheezing, chest pain, hemoptysis, right axis deviation on ECG. If pulmonary infarct occurs, pleural effusion, friction rub, and fever may be noted.

THERAPEUTIC INTERVENTIONS

▲ Apply TED hose and sequential compression devices to lower extremities as ordered.

▲ Administer antifibrinolytic agents as prescribed. *In patients who cannot tolerate or refuse early surgery to clip/wrap the aneurysm, Amicar may be given to inhibit fibronolysis; prevent clot degradation and potential rebleed:*
   Epsilon aminocaproic acid: initial dose 5 g orally or by *slow* IV infusion followed by 1-2 g/hr. Total daily dose 24-36g/24:

▲ Administer IV/PO fluids, as prescribed, *to prevent dehydration. Hourly rate may be ≥ 125 ml/hr.*

▲ Monitor electrolytes, BUN/creatinine, serum OSM, CVP/PCWP carefully during hydration.

▪ Explain purpose of drug therapy to patient/significant others.

▪ Explain possible side effects of drug to patient/significant others: nausea, cramps, diarrhea, dizziness, headache, rash, deep vein thrombosis, pulmonary emboli.

Impaired Physical Mobility

RELATED TO

Prolonged bed rest

DEFINING CHARACTERISTICS

Inability to move purposefully within physical environment
Decreased muscle strength
Imposed restriction of movement (e.g., medical protocol)

EXPECTED OUTCOMES

Patient maintains optimal physical mobility as evidenced by performance of ROM exercises, participation in appropriate self-care activities.

ONGOING ASSESSMENT

▪ Assess muscle strength and coordination.
▪ See Impaired physical mobility, p. 47.

THERAPEUTIC INTERVENTIONS

▪ Encourage deep breathing exercises 10 times/hr while awake.
▪ Encourage foot plantar flexion and dorsiflexion exercises 10 times/hr when awake. *These exercises stimulate antagonistic muscle groups, promote venous flow, and help decrease bone demineralization.*
▪ Instruct patient and family to avoid Valsalva's maneuver. As patient is turned or pulled up in bed, instruct to exhale *to prevent straining and increased ICP, increased BP.*
▪ Instruct to avoid isometric and vigorous active ROM exercises *in preoperative period to minimize possibility of increasing BP and potential rebleed.*
▪ Instruct patient and family in activity restrictions.

Knowledge Deficit Regarding Diagnostic Tests, Potential Complications, Treatment

RELATED FACTOR

Lack of exposure

DEFINING CHARACTERISTICS

Multiple questions
Lack of questions
Misconceptions

EXPECTED OUTCOMES

Patient verbalizes understanding of extent and cause of bleed; potential for rebleed, vasospasm (stroke), and elevated ICP; diagnostic testing; treatment.

ONGOING ASSESSMENT

▪ Assess level of understanding.

THERAPEUTIC INTERVENTIONS

▪ Explain possible causes of intracranial hemorrhage, aneurysmal rupture. Explain potential complications (rebleed, vasospasms [stroke], and increased intracranial pressure secondary to hydrocephalus or cerebral edema).
▪ Explain rationale for limitation of length and frequency of visits *to provide most quiet and restful environment possible to prevent excitement/stimulation associated with changes in BP and ICP.*
▪ Explain necessity to avoid Valsalva's maneuver. Stress importance of exhaling when pulled up in bed and avoiding coughing and straining at stool. Provide stool softener if necessary.
▪ Discuss studies (e.g., computed axial tomography [CT], cerebral angiography, cerebral blood flow) ordered.
▪ Explain need to avoid nicotine. *Nicotine has vasospastic effect on blood vessels; thus increases risk of hemorrhage or vasospasm.*
▪ When possible, coordinate time for patient/family to ask the neurosurgeon questions about condition, treatment plan, surgery.
▪ Teach patient/family about diet (low-salt, low-fat); and stress management.
▲ Involve social worker if anticipate prolonged hospitalization, need for rehabilitation post discharge, or need for assistance to obtain Nimodipine on discharge.

By: Linda Arsenault, RN, MSN, CNRN

Cerebrovascular accident

(CVA, HEMIPLEGIA STROKE)

A sudden neurologic incident related to impaired cerebral blood supply, which may be caused by hemorrhage, embolism, or thrombosis resulting in ischemia to the brain. It is the third leading cause of death in the United States. The clinical manifestations of stroke vary, depending on the area of the brain affected.

NURSING DIAGNOSES	EXPECTED OUTCOMES AND NURSING INTERVENTIONS / *RATIONALE* (■ = INDEPENDENT; ▲ = COLLABORATIVE)

High Risk for Injury: Alteration in Integrated Regulation

Risk Factors

Strokes occurring in areas of the brain and brain stem that control systemic functions

Expected Outcomes

Patient maintains patent airway.
Patient maintains normal ECG pattern and rhythm.
Patient maintains normal rate and rhythm of respiration.
Patient maintains normal ABGs.
Patient is normothermic.
Patient is normovolemic with electrolyte balance.

Ongoing Assessment

- Assess past history of systemic problems: previous cardiac disease, hypertension, smoking, previous pulmonary disease.
- Monitor vital signs as needed.
- ▲ Monitor baseline ECG and observe for changes *as stroke can produce cardiac electrical changes and dysrhythmias.*
- Monitor respiratory rate, rhythm, breath sounds, and ability to handle secretions. *Strokes may interfere with normal pattern. Maintaining a patent airway is crucial.*
- Check presence of gag reflex. *Brainstem strokes may diminish cranial nerve function.*
- Observe for evidence of respiratory distress that may result from neurogenic pulmonary edema: patient complaints, cyanosis, restlessness, shortness of breath, nasal flaring.
- Monitor intake and output, urine specific gravity. *Because of cerebral edema, fluid balance must be regulated.*
- Monitor weight daily.
- ▲ Monitor hemodynamic status if at risk for compromise (requires pulmonary arterial catheter).
- ▲ Monitor electrolytes, arterial blood gases.

Therapeutic Interventions

- Position upright *to facilitate work of breathing*: monitor blood pressure closely during any position change.
- *Prevent pooling of secretions*: change position q2-4h, encourage deep breathing, add humidity to the environment.
- ▲ Provide respiratory support:
    Administer supplemental oxygen as prescribed.
    Provide endotracheal or tracheal care if warranted. *Maintenance of patent airway is first priority.*
    Oversee ventilatory support if used.
    Avoid respiratory measures that increase intracranial pressure.
    Instruct in deep breathing techniques, incentive spirometry.
- Restrict physical activity initially; patient gradually resumes activity as tolerated. *To reduce myocardial O_2 consumption.*
- ▲ Control body temperature: administer antipyretics, initiate topical cooling methods, administer hypothalamic depressants as prescribed *To reduce metabolic demands of the brain.*
- Review medications for effects on fluid and electrolyte balance. Explain medications to patient.
- ▲ Maintain volume status by replacing or restricting fluids as prescribed. Explain pathophysiologic disorder underlying abnormalities in production of antidiuretic hormone, need for fluid replacement or restriction.
- ▲ Administer vasopressin as prescribed.

NURSING DIAGNOSES	EXPECTED OUTCOMES AND NURSING INTERVENTIONS / *RATIONALE* (■ = INDEPENDENT; ▲ = COLLABORATIVE)

Impaired Physical Mobility

RELATED FACTORS

Paresis or paralysis, loss of balance and coordination, increased muscle tone

DEFINING CHARACTERISTICS

Inability to move purposefully within physical environment
Limited range of motion
Decreased muscle strength, control, and/or mass

EXPECTED OUTCOMES

Patient maintains maximum level of function within limits of disease.
Patient maintains ROM in spastic extremities.
Patient's ability to perform fine and gross motor activities is increased
Patient learns how to identify where the extremities and center of balance are located in relation to the environment.

ONGOING ASSESSMENT

- Assess patient's degree of weakness in both upper and lower extremities. *There may be differing degrees of involvement on the affected side.*
- Assess ability to move and change position.
- Assess ability to transfer and walk.
- Assess ability for fine muscle movement.
- Assess ability for gross muscle movements.
- Determine active and passive range of motion capabilities. *Initially muscles demonstrate hyporeflexia, which later progresses to hyperreflexia.*
- Assess for activities or situations that increase or decrease tone.

THERAPEUTIC INTERVENTIONS

- Change position of patient at least q2h, keeping track of position changes with a turning schedule. *Patients may not feel increases in pressure or have the ability to adjust position.*
- Perform active and passive range of motion exercises in all extremities several times daily *to improve muscle strength and prevent contractures.*
- Increase functional activities as strength improves and the patient is medically stable.
- Teach patient and family exercises and transfer techniques.
- Monitor skin integrity for areas of blanching or redness as signs of potential breakdown.
- If patient is at high risk for pressure ulcer development, use pressure-relieving devices on the bed and chair.
For balance and coordination problems:
- Assist patient in performing movements or tasks; begin with small range of movements and encourage control. *Patients may have tremors.*
- Encourage focusing on proximal muscle control initially and then distal muscle control. *This especially helps patients who have ataxia.*
- Ensure center of gravity is over pelvis or equally distributed over stance for sitting and standing activities; provide safe environment for these activities *as patients may have impaired righting reflexes and wide base stance.*
- Teach patient and family exercises and techniques to improve balance and coordination.
- Reinforce safety precautions with patient and family.
For increased muscle tone (spasticity):
- Perform activities in quiet environment with few distractions.
- Apply heat or cold to the extremities *in an effort to reduce tone before initiating movement.*
- Perform muscle stretching activities in gentle, rhythmical motions *to provide input into the central nervous system.*
- ▲ Integrate inhibiting patterns for reducing spasticity as instructed by physical therapy.
- ▲ Give medications to reduce spasticity as prescribed.
- ▲ Apply splinting devices to spastic extremities as prescribed, with ongoing assessment for increasing tone.
- Instruct family in concepts of spasticity and ways to reduce tone.

High Risk for Impaired Verbal Communication

RISK FACTORS

Left brain hemisphere stroke

EXPECTED OUTCOMES

Patient effectively communicates basic needs.
Patient maximizes remaining communication ability.
Patient and family verbalize understanding of communication impairment.
Patient and family are involved in measures to promote communication.

ONGOING ASSESSMENT

- Assess speech-language history: ability to read, write, and understand English; level of education.
- Assess speech-language function: automatic speech, auditory comprehension, comprehension of written language, expressive ability, ability to write. *Depending on the area of brain involvement, patients may experience aphasia (receptive or expressive), dysarthria, or both.*

Continued.

Cerebrovascular accident—cont'd

NURSING DIAGNOSES	EXPECTED OUTCOMES AND NURSING INTERVENTIONS / *RATIONALE* (■ = INDEPENDENT; ▲ = COLLABORATIVE)

THERAPEUTIC INTERVENTIONS

- Approach the patient as an adult. *Inability to express needs/feelings is most distressing to patients. Staff need to be sensitive to the dignity of the patient.*
- Enhance the environment to facilitate communication and minimize distractions.
- Modulate personal communication, controlling body language and providing clear, simple directions.
- Incorporate multimodality input *to enhance function in intact speech-language areas.*
- Use written materials *to supplement auditory input.*
- Use prompting clues.
- Allow adequate time for patient response.
- Provide opportunities for spontaneous conversation.
- Anticipate patient needs until alternative means of communication can be established.
- Provide reality orientation and focus attention.
- ▲ Collaborate with speech-language pathologist *to implement a comprehensive plan of care.*
- Encourage family to attempt communication with patient.
- Demonstrate to patient progress made. *Will increase confidence and facilitate ongoing efforts.*

High Risk for Sensory/Perceptual Alterations (Tactile)

RISK FACTORS

Stroke within the sensory transmission and/or integration pathways of the brain

EXPECTED OUTCOMES

Patient and family demonstrate skill in therapeutic interventions.
Patient's skin will remain free of injuries, including pressure ulcers.
Patient learns to use compensatory methods.

ONGOING ASSESSMENT

- Assess patient's ability to sense light touch, pinprick, temperature.
- Using patient's toes or fingers, assess ability to sense joint position.
- Check for hypersensitivity reactions.

THERAPEUTIC INTERVENTIONS

- Perform regular skin inspections and instruct patient in techniques to do the same. Explain consequences of excess pressure on the skin.
- Provide tactile stimulation to affected limbs using rough cloth or hand and instruct patient/family in methods used.
- Explain how stimulus might feel (e.g., cool water, soft flannel).
- Teach patient to check temperature of water with unaffected side before using water (thermal screening).
- Regularly move affected limbs.
- Enhance environment for optimum safety.

Sensory/Perceptual Alterations/Unilateral Neglect

RISK FACTORS

Stroke causing interruption in normal perceptual abilities

EXPECTED OUTCOMES

Patient incurs no injuries.
Patient can cross midline with eyes and unaffected arm.
Patient observes and touches affected side during ADL activities.
Patient begins to wash, dress, and eat with attention to both sides.
Patient and family verbalize cognitive awareness of deficit.

ONGOING ASSESSMENT

- Conduct sensory assessment.
- Perform visual fields confrontation test.
- Observe patient's performance of ADL.
- Observe patient's response to sounds from affected side.
- Conduct paper drawing test to test for distorted spatial relationships.
- Observe for remark of denial of body parts (anosognosia) and degree to which patient confuses objects in space. *Diminished awareness is a safety hazard.*
- Have patient point to various body parts (somatognosia).
- Assess safety practices.

NURSING DIAGNOSES	EXPECTED OUTCOMES AND NURSING INTERVENTIONS / *RATIONALE* (■ = INDEPENDENT; ▲ = COLLABORATIVE)

See also:

THERAPEUTIC INTERVENTIONS

- Approach patient from unaffected side during the *acute* phase; approach patient from the *affected* side during the rehabilitation phase. *This will encourage the patient to use affected side of body and environment.*
- Ensure safe environment with call bell on patient's unaffected side.
- Provide tactile stimulation to affected side and approach patient from affected side, calling patient's name to encourage overcoming neglect.
- Place all food in small quantities, arranged simply on plate.
- Attach watch or bright bracelet to affected arm *to draw patient's attention.*
- Provide a mirror for visual cues with ADLs; assist with verbal cues.
- Practice with patient manipulating objects.
- Practice drawing and copying figures with patient.
- Draw bright mark on sides of paper when patient is reading to give cue to read entire line and return for next line.
- Teach compensatory strategies such as visual scanning *to reduce chance of injury.*

(adapted from Promoting Stroke Recovery: A Research Based Approach for Nurses, Mosby, 1991).
By: Kathryn Bronstein, Ph.D., R.N.; Judith Popovich Ph.D., R.N.; Christina Stewart-Amidei, M.S.N., R.N.

Consciousness, altered level of

(COMA; IMPAIRED MENTAL STATUS; UNRESPONSIVENESS)

Normal consciousness can be defined as the condition of the normal person when awake. In this state, the patient is fully responsive to stimuli and indicates by behavior and speech that he/she has an accurate awareness of himself/herself and the environment. There are two components of consciousness: (1) arousal or wakefulness, which reflects the integrity of the reticular activating system (RAS) located in the upper brain stem and diencephalon; and (2) cognition or awareness, which reflects the integrity of the cortical cerebral hemisphere.

| NURSING DIAGNOSES | EXPECTED OUTCOMES AND NURSING INTERVENTIONS / *RATIONALE* (■ = INDEPENDENT; ▲ = COLLABORATIVE) |

Altered Level of Consciousness

RELATED FACTORS

Structural: stroke, head trauma, tumor, cerebral edema, increased ICP
Infectious: meningitis, encephalitis, abscess
Metabolic: anoxia, profound hypoglycemia, hypercalcemia (>12 mg%), profound hyponatremia or hypernatremia toxic agents

DEFINING CHARACTERISTICS

Change in alertness, orientation, verbal response, eye opening, response to command, motor response
Impaired memory
Impaired judgment
Agitation
Inappropriate affect
Impaired thought processes
Glasgow Coma Scale < 11

EXPECTED OUTCOMES

Patient maintains optimal level of consciousness, as evidenced by appropriate response, GCS > 13, absence of deterioration.

ONGOING ASSESSMENT

- Assess level of consciousness/responsiveness as indicated.
- Determine contributing factors to any change (e.g., anesthesia, medications, awakening from sound sleep, not understanding questions).
- Assess patient's/significant others' understanding of events surrounding change in LOC.
- Assess potential for physical injury.
- Assess vital signs, especially respiratory status.
- ▲ Monitor ABGs, pulse oximetry, electrolytes, glucose, calcium levels.
- Review current medications.

THERAPEUTIC INTERVENTIONS

- Record serial assessments.
- Report/record change or deterioration.
- Keep side rails up at all times, bed in low position, and functioning call light within reach.
- If restraints are needed, patient must be positioned on side, never on back. *(Reduces risk of aspiration). Restraints should be used judiciously (may increase agitation/anxiety and contribute to increased ICP).*
- Reorient to environment as needed *to decrease apprehension and anxiety. Short-term memory may be affected by pathologic cause.*
- Explain all nursing activities before initiating.
- Protect patient from possible injury (seizure activity, decreased corneal reflex, decreased blink, decreased gag reflex, airway obstruction/aspiration).
- Avoid contributing to confusion/disorientation by agreeing with misinterpretations. *Reality orientation decreases false sensory perception and enhances patient's sense of personal dignity and self-esteem.*
- Use calendars, television, radio, clocks, lights *to help with reorientation.*
- ▲ Call neurologic resource personnel if instructions needed.
- Involve patient/significant others in goal setting and care planning.
- Encourage significant others to provide familiar objects (e.g., pictures, pajamas).
- ▲ Consult rehabilitation medicine and social service departments as needed.
- Encourage and support verbalization by patient and significant others.

By: Linda Arsenault, RN, MSN, CNRN

Craniotomy

(CRANIECTOMY; BURR HOLE; TREPHINATION)

Surgical opening of a part of the cranium to gain access to disease or injury affecting the brain, ventricles, or intracranial blood vessels. Craniectomy is removal of part of the cranium if needed for compound fractures or infection.

NURSING DIAGNOSES	EXPECTED OUTCOMES AND NURSING INTERVENTIONS / *RATIONALE* (■ = INDEPENDENT; ▲ = COLLABORATIVE)

Altered Cerebral Tissue Perfusion

RELATED FACTORS

Cerebral edema, intracranial bleeding
Cerebral ischemia/infarction
Increased ICP
Metabolic abnormalities
Hydrocephalus

DEFINING CHARACTERISTICS

Changed LOC
Changed pupillary size, reaction to light, deviation
Focal or generalized motor weakness
Presence of pathologic reflexes (Babinski)
Seizures
Increased BP and bradycardia
Changed respiratory pattern

EXPECTED OUTCOMES

Optimal cerebral perfusion is maintained, as evidenced by GCS > 13, absence of new neurologic deficit.

ONGOING ASSESSMENT

- Assess and document baseline level of consciousness: pupillary size, position, reaction to light; motor movement and strength of limbs; and vital signs. *Early detection of changes is necessary to prevent permanent neurologic dysfunction.*
- Compare current assessment to previous assessment. Report any deviations. (Worrisome signs include change in LOC, pupillary asymmetry, new focal deficits, respiratory changes, speech changes, increased complaint of headache, yawning/hiccuping. Increased blood pressure and bradycardia are late signs usually associated with medullary ischemia/compression.)
- Evaluate contributing factors to change in responsiveness; reevaluate in 5-10 min. *to see whether change persists as a result of such factors as anesthesia, medications, awakening from sound sleep, not understanding question.*
- Check head dressing for presence of drains. *Intraventricular drains, self-contained bulb suction and drainage systems are most commonly used. All drains and catheters should be secured to patient/bed to prevent falls to floor, negative gravity suctioning, and increased risk of bleeding or dislodging of drain.*
- Evaluate function of catheter used to monitor ICP (Normal ICP < 15 mm Hg).
- Evaluate for lash reflex.
- Assess current medications and compare to preoperative medications, with specific attention to thyroid replacement, anticonvulsants, and steroids.
- ▲ Monitor CBC, electrolytes, and ABGs. Report:
  Po_2 < 80 mm Hg.
  Pco_2 > 45 mm Hg.
  CBC: Hct < 30.
  Electrolytes: Na <130, >150.
  Glucose <80 or >200.
  Osmolarities <185 >310 mOsm/L.

THERAPEUTIC INTERVENTIONS

- ▲ Report temperature >39° C (102.2° F). Maintain normothermia with tepid sponge bath/antipyretics or hypothermia blanket as ordered. Turn blanket off at temperature of 100° F rectally (38° C).
- Maintain HOB at 30 degrees unless contraindicated (e.g., hemodynamically unstable, following insertion of ventricle-peritoneal shunt or drainage of chronic subdural hematoma. *In these patients it is usually preferable that patients be nursed with the head of the bed flat to minimize risk of new/recurrent subdural hemorrhage.*
- Turn and reposition patient on side, with head supported in neutral alignment, q2h. Avoid neck flexion/rotation *to prevent venous outflow obstruction and increased ICP.*
- Reorient patient to environment as needed.
- If soft restraints needed, position patient on side, never on back.
- Avoid nursing activities that may trigger increased ICP (straining, strenuous coughing, positioning with neck in flexion, head flat).
- If patient has difficulty closing eye (cranial nerve VII palsy), administer artificial tears (methyl-cellulose drops) q2h. Glad plastic wrap or Saran or facsimile can be applied over eyelid or the eyelids may be taped closed *to protect exposed cornea and prevent dryness.*
- See Altered level of consciousness, p. 252.

Continued.

Craniotomy—cont'd

NURSING DIAGNOSES	EXPECTED OUTCOMES AND NURSING INTERVENTIONS / *RATIONALE* (■ = INDEPENDENT; ▲ = COLLABORATIVE)
High Risk for Fluid Volume Deficit **RISK FACTORS** Neurogenic diabetes insipidus Dehydration secondary to use of hyperosmotic agents, high fever, profuse diaphoresis, emesis	**EXPECTED OUTCOMES** Optimal fluid volume is maintained as evidenced by normal Na Osm, SG < 1.025. **ONGOING ASSESSMENT** • Monitor I & O q1h with specific attention to fluid volume infused over output. Report urine output >200 ml/hr for 2 consecutive hours. • Check urine specific gravity q2-4h. *Specific gravity is decreased to <1.005 with diabetes insipidus.* ▲ Monitor serum and urine electrolytes and osmolarity. • Assess for signs of dehydration (tachycardia, hypotension, poor skin turgor). • Weigh daily if possible. **THERAPEUTIC INTERVENTIONS** ▲ Replace fluid output as directed. ▲ Administer vasopressin (Pitressin) *(exogenous synthetic antidiuretic hormone that causes decreased urinary output)* as prescribed. • Record urinary output response to administration of vasopressin. • Record any side effects related to vasopressin administration: change in heart rate, abdominal cramping. • See Fluid volume deficit, p. 25. • See Diabetes insipidus, p. 488.
High Risk for Fluid Volume Excess **RISK FACTORS** Syndrome of inappropriate antidiuretic hormone secretions (SIADH)	**EXPECTED OUTCOMES** Patient maintains optimal fluid balance, as evidenced by normal Na, OSM, urine SG >1.005. **ONGOING ASSESSMENT** • Assess patient for fluid volume excess *(usually determined by hyponatremia/ hyposmolarity). Edema is usually not present in syndrome of inappropriate antidiuretic hormone (SIADH).* ▲ Monitor serum and urine electrolyte levels and osmolarity daily. • Monitor I & O. • Monitor for clinical signs of hyponatremia. **THERAPEUTIC INTERVENTIONS** ▲ Restrict PO/IV fluids as ordered. *Fluid restriction of 1-1.2 L/day usually corrects hyponatremia associated with SIADH. Intravenous D_5 W is inappropriate because of excess free water and should not be used for piggyback medications. Additionally normal saline solution can be used to flush NG tube after feedings.* • Weigh patient daily. ▲ If fluid restriction fails, 3% saline solution with the concomitant use of K+ and IV furosimide (Lasix) may be ordered. In this event, serial Na, K+, and serum Osm should be monitored q6h. • See also SIADH, p. 499; Seizure activity, p. 281.
High Risk for Impaired Physical Mobility **RISK FACTORS** Decreased LOC Weakness/paralysis of extremities Imposed restrictions	**EXPECTED OUTCOMES** Patient achieves optimal mobility as evidenced by absence of contractures, preservation of ROM to all joints, absence of atrophy. **ONGOING ASSESSMENT** • Assess for alteration in mobility. **THERAPEUTIC INTERVENTIONS** • Do not position patient in prone or semiprone position *(increases intrathoracic pressure; may increase ICP).* • Encourage active ROM of affected joints *to maintain muscle strength and prevent contractures.* • Establish turning schedule *to prevent skin breakdown, respiratory complications, bone demineralization, and muscle wasting.* • See also Impaired physical mobility, p. 47.

NURSING DIAGNOSES	EXPECTED OUTCOMES AND NURSING INTERVENTIONS / *RATIONALE* (■ = INDEPENDENT; ▲ = COLLABORATIVE)

Ineffective Airway Clearance

RELATED FACTORS

Decreased LOC, prolonged surgical procedure with lengthy general anesthesia, postoperative atelectasis, pain

DEFINING CHARACTERISTICS

Abnormal breath sounds (rhonchi, rales, wheezing)
Change in rate, depth of respirations; tachypnea/apnea
Ineffective cough, cyanosis
Change in respiratory rhythm
Nasal flaring
Tachycardia
Increased secretions
Dyspnea

EXPECTED OUTCOMES

Patient maintains airway free of secretions on auscultation; patient has normal ABGs.

ONGOING ASSESSMENT

- Assess for signs of ineffective airway clearance.

THERAPEUTIC INTERVENTIONS

- Suction prn. *However, nasotracheal suctioning is contraindicated for patient having surgery proximal to frontal sinuses (i.e., pituitary tumor, basal frontal meningioma, basal skull fracture). This can result in introduction of catheter tip into brain or allow bacterial communication.*
- See Airway clearance, ineffective, p. 3.
- See Breathing pattern, ineffective, p. 10.

High Risk for Injury: Seizures

RISK FACTORS

Intracranial bleeding, infarction, tumor, trauma

EXPECTED OUTCOMES

Patient is free of injury during seizures, through maintenance of seizure precautions and delivery of appropriate interventions.

ONGOING ASSESSMENT

- Observe for seizure activity. Record and report observations:
  Note time and signs of seizures.
  Observe body parts involved; order of involvement and character of movement.
  Check deviation of eyes; note change in pupillary size.
  Assess for incontinence.
  Note duration of seizure.
  Note tonic-clonic stages.
  Assess postictal state (e.g., loss of consciousness, loss of airway).
- Monitor for signs of respiratory distress.

THERAPEUTIC INTERVENTIONS

- To ensure safety, protect head from injury. Pad side rails.
- Keep bed in low position.
- Keep side rails up.
- Maintain airway during postictal state. Turn patient on side; suction as needed.
- Maintain minimal environmental stimuli: noise reduction, curtains closed, private room (when available/advisable), dim lights.
- ▲ Administer anticonvulsants as indicated. *Phenytoin (Dilantin) can only be administered PO/IV. When given IV it should be administered in NS. It will precipitate in any dextrose solution. Infuse no faster than 50 mg/min to prevent hypotension. IV diazepam (Valium) is often used to control recurrent seizures and should not be administered any faster than 10 mg/min to prevent respiratory compromise. Latter agent is short acting.*
- If seizure occurs, remain with patient and do not attempt to introduce anything in his/her mouth during the seizure. *This could result in increased risk of aspiration, broken teeth, or soft tissue injury.*
- If indicated, wipe/suction secretions and administer oxygen.

Knowledge Deficit

RELATED FACTOR

New procedures and treatments

EXPECTED OUTCOMES

Patient/significant others describe postoperative expectations and usual length of recovery.

ONGOING ASSESSMENT

- Assess patient's/significant others' knowledge and readiness for learning.
- Assess for barriers to learning.

Continued.

Craniotomy—cont'd

NURSING DIAGNOSES	EXPECTED OUTCOMES AND NURSING INTERVENTIONS / *RATIONALE* (■ = INDEPENDENT; ▲ = COLLABORATIVE)

DEFINING CHARACTERISTICS

Patient/significant others verbalize questions and concerns

THERAPEUTIC INTERVENTIONS

- Discuss change in body image related to head dressing and loss of hair, potential for and duration of facial edema. *The edema usually peaks about 3 days after surgery and then gradually diminishes.*
- Discuss need for monitoring equipment and frequent assessments.
- Explain unit visiting hours and reasons for restrictions.
- Instruct in deep breathing and leg exercises.
- Explain use of medications such as dexamethasone (Decadron), anticonvulsants, antibiotics.
- Discuss need for frequent assessment, reorientation, etc.
- Encourage significant others to participate in reorientation, rehabilitation.
- Reinforce discussion of neurologic definitions/progress given by physician to significant others.

By: Linda Arsenault, RN, MSN, CNRN

Guillain Barré syndrome

(POLYNEURITIS; GBS, DEMYELINATING POLYNEUROPATHY)

A rapidly evolving reversible paralytic illness of unknown origin. The disease is thought to be autoimmune in origin and has been reported to be related to the occurrence of varicella, the Epstein-Barr virus, swine flu vaccines, or following respiratory or gastrointestinal illnesses, mumps, or mycoplasma pneumonia. The disease occurs as a result of destruction of peripheral nerve myelin sheaths. The onset of neurological symptoms is abrupt, with a tendency for the paralysis to ascend the body symmetrically. Acute GBS typically begins with parathesia in the toes or fingertips followed within days by leg weakness. Arm, facial, and oropharyngeal weakness ensues. In severe cases the disease progresses to affect respiration, eye movements, and swallowing. Weakness/paralysis stops advancing in 1-3 weeks and slowly improves following a plateau phase of several weeks.

NURSING DIAGNOSES	EXPECTED OUTCOMES AND NURSING INTERVENTIONS / *RATIONALE* (■ = INDEPENDENT; ▲ = COLLABORATIVE)

High Risk for Ineffective Breathing Pattern

RISK FACTORS

Respiratory muscle weakness
Ascending muscle paralysis
Respiratory insufficiency
Loss of cough/sigh/gag reflexes

EXPECTED OUTCOMES

Patient maintains optimal oxygenation, as evidenced by $Po_2 > 80$ mm Hg, Pco_2 35-45 mm Hg, O_2 SAT $> 95\%$, vital capacity > 18 ml/kg body weight.

ONGOING ASSESSMENT

- Assess respiratory rate, pattern, and depth. *Respiratory failure is the most serious complication.*
- Auscultate breath sounds.
- ▲ Monitor tidal volume and vital capacity daily and prn. *A significant amount of respiratory muscle insufficiency may exist without being clinically obvious in the early stages.*
- ▲ Monitor ABGs for the development of hypercapnia and hypoxia.
- Monitor for ability to cough, sigh, gag. *Chest PT, deep breathing exercises, and incentive spirometry may be helpful to minimize ongoing atelectasis.*
- Assess for dysphagia, especially before feeding. *Paralysis of the IX and X cranial nerves may occur and result in dysphagia or aspiration.*
- Observe for mental status changes *that may be indicative of cerebral oxygenation.*
- Assess for ascending paralysis involving abdominal, respiratory, and diaphragmatic innervation. *Many patients will develop clinical signs of fatigue such as paradoxical movement of the diaphragm, diaphoresis, and tachycardia. If vital capacity decreases to 18 ml/kg body weight, ICU monitoring is warranted and elective intubation may be indicated.*

THERAPEUTIC INTERVENTIONS

- Elevate head of bed *to promote optimal ventilatory excursion.*
- Encourage coughing and deep breathing exercises when possible.
- Notify physician of noted decreases in cough and gag reflexes or any difficulty in swallowing. *Early intervention such as incentive spirometry and chest PT may be helpful to minimize atelectasis. Additional respiratory parameters may also need to be assessed (e.g., ABGs, O$_2$ SAT, TV, VC).*
- Use oropharyngeal or orotracheal suctioning as needed.
- ▲ Anticipate the need for intubation and mechanical ventilation if respirations become labored, shallow, or rapid with decreased TV and VC. *Intercostal and diaphragmatic paralysis produces progressive alveolar hypoventilation, which can occur within 36 hr. The patient may not be clinically symptomatic because of the gradual onset and insidious progression.*
- See also Mechanical ventilation, p. 202.

Anxiety/Fear

RELATED FACTORS

Change in health status
Fear of unknown
Communication difficulties
Deteriorating motor strength

DEFINING CHARACTERISTICS

Restlessness
Fear
Crying
Withdrawal
Facial tension
Expressions of fear
Anxiety

EXPECTED OUTCOMES

Patient appears relaxed.
Patient verbalizes concerns and demonstrate a positive coping mechanism.

ONGOING ASSESSMENT

- Assess level of fear/anxiety. *Abrupt onset of symptoms with tendency for paralysis is extremely frightening.*
- Assess normal coping patterns (by interview with patient/significant other).

THERAPEUTIC INTERVENTIONS

- Allow time for patient to communicate feelings and express concerns and fears while verbal communication is still possible.
- Assist patient to verbalize feelings through writing or using alphabet board. *Creative methods of communication may be indicated as disease progresses.*
- Reduce distracting stimuli *to provide quiet environment.*
- Plan adequate rest periods for patient *to prevent sensory overload and depletion of energy reserves.*
- Provide diversional activities (e.g., television, books, radio, magazines) as appropriate. Encourage family/significant other to bring in tapes of patient's favorite music, messages from friends, book tapes as appropriate. *May assist in making medical environment less threatening.*
- Reinforce explanations regarding disease progression, treatment (which is predominantly supportive), and potential for recovery (slow but often complete).
- Display a confident, calm manner *to reassure patient.*
- ▲ Consult social worker, chaplain services, as appropriate.
- ▲ Coordinate psychological/psychiatric consultative services as needed *to help patient develop/maintain needed coping mechanisms and to provide emotional support.*

High Risk for Decrease in Cardiac Output

RISK FACTORS

Vasomotor instability
Autonomic dysfunction, which reflects conduction deficits through the myelinated preganglionic fibers and the ganglia

EXPECTED OUTCOMES

Patient maintains adequate cardiac output, as evidenced by heart rate 60-100beats/min, BP within normal limits, strong peripheral pulses, lack of dysrhythmias.

ONGOING ASSESSMENT

- Monitor BP and heart rate continuously. *Autonomic dysfunction causes sinus tachycardia, hypertension. Hypotension may occur.*
- Monitor ECG for dysrhythmias.
- Assess peripheral pulses.
- Observe for profuse diaphoresis or loss of sweating. *Diaphoresis is related to sympathetic preponderance; sweating to parasympathetic preponderance.*
- Observe for mental status changes, signs of fatigue/lethargy.
- ▲ Monitor pulmonary artery wedge pressure and cardiac output, as available.

THERAPEUTIC INTERVENTIONS

- ▲ Administer inotropic medications as prescribed *to maintain hemodynamic parameters* (heart rate, BP, cardiac output, CVP, pulmonary artery pressures).
- ▲ Apply sequential compression devices and antiembolic stockings *to promote increased venous return, decreased peripheral pooling of blood, and decreased risk of thrombosis.*

Continued.

Guillain Barré syndrome—cont'd

NURSING DIAGNOSES	EXPECTED OUTCOMES AND NURSING INTERVENTIONS / *RATIONALE* (▪ = INDEPENDENT; ▲ = COLLABORATIVE)

Impaired Physical Mobility

RELATED FACTORS

Muscle weakness or total paralysis as a result of the disease process
Paresthesia
Sensory loss

DEFINING CHARACTERISTICS

Inability to move purposefully as desired/needed
Reluctance to attempt movement
Limited range of motion

EXPECTED OUTCOMES

Patient maintains optimal physical mobility, as evidenced by lack of contractures, good ROM.

ONGOING ASSESSMENT

- Assess motor strength and reflexes, checking for level of progression of ascending paralysis, paresthesia.
- Assess ROM.
- Assess previous activity level, and preillness pattern of exercise.
- Assess requirements for assistive devices, help needed to turn/transfer and perform ADL activities.

THERAPEUTIC INTERVENTIONS

- Turn and reposition q2h as needed.
- Maintain limbs slightly extended and begin passive range of motion *to prevent contractures, and maintain function. Some patients with limb pain are intolerant of exercises during the first few weeks of illness. Active strengthening generally can begin during the plateau stage of illness.*
- ▲ Coordinate and work with physical therapist *to assist in maintaining muscle tone.*
- ▲ Coordinate and work with occupational therapist *to assist in maintaining position of upper and lower extremities, e.g., hand rolls; ankle, foot, and wrist splints.*
- Schedule times when the assistive devices (splints) should be on or off.

High Risk for Aspiration

RISK FACTORS

Muscle paralysis, cranial nerve involvement (especially IX, X)

EXPECTED OUTCOME

Patient maintains absence of aspiration, as evidenced by normal breath sounds, respiratory rate 18-24/min.

ONGOING ASSESSMENT

- Assess for presence of gag and cough reflexes every shift.
- Assess for difficulty in swallowing every shift and before oral intake. *Paralysis of the ninth and tenth cranial nerves may occur.*
- Assess breath sounds and respiratory status for clinical evidence of aspiration. *Dyspnea, SOB, tachypnea, and cyanosis indicate need for intervention.*

THERAPEUTIC INTERVENTIONS

- Notify physician immediately of noted decreases in cough and gag reflexes or difficulty in swallowing. *Early intervention protects airway and prevents aspiration.*
- Assist patient with oral intake *to detect abnormalities early.*
- Remain with patient during feeding.
- Suction as needed. *With impaired swallowing and reflexes, secretions can accumulate in posterior pharynx and upper trachea, increasing the risk of aspiration.*

High Risk for Impaired Skin Integrity

RISK FACTORS

Complete bed rest, impaired physical mobility, paresthesia

EXPECTED OUTCOME

Patient maintains intact skin, as evidenced by absence of breakdown.

ONGOING ASSESSMENT

- Assess skin integrity every shift, noting color, moisture, texture, and temperature.

THERAPEUTIC INTERVENTIONS

- Maintain good skin care, keeping skin clean and lubricated with lotion/emollient as needed.
- Turn q2h according to an established turning schedule.
- Use turn sheet and lift and turn patient when repositioning. *This will reduce the shearing and abrading of the patient's skin across sheets when repositioning.*
- Keep bed clothing free of wrinkles, crumbs, etc.
- Provide prophylactic use of egg crate, air/water mattresses/pads *to help in preventing skin breakdown.*

NURSING DIAGNOSES	EXPECTED OUTCOMES AND NURSING INTERVENTIONS / *RATIONALE* (■ = INDEPENDENT; ▲ = COLLABORATIVE)

Knowledge Deficit

RELATED FACTORS

Disease of sudden onset, lack of resources

DEFINING CHARACTERISTICS

Request for information
Multiple questions
Lack of questions

EXPECTED OUTCOME

Patient verbalizes understanding of the disease process, treatment, prognosis.

ONGOING ASSESSMENT

- Assess patient for current status of disease/stability of condition (in early stages may be deteriorating).
- Assess knowledge of illness.
- Assess understanding of therapeutic regimen.

THERAPEUTIC INTERVENTIONS

- Explain diagnostic tests: CSF analysis, EMG, nerve conduction tests.
- Explain the disease process as simply as possible:
  A rapidly progressive illness that may be mild or severe.
  It usually begins with numbness/tingling in the extremities followed by a variable degree of weakness, which may become severe.
  Cause is unknown, but probably an autoimmune reaction.
  A severe case results in total paralysis with breathing and swallowing problems in which the patient may need mechanical ventilation up to a year.
  Recovery is over a period of weeks or months. Permanent weakness or imbalance occurs in 5%-10% of cases. Rehabilitation is usually required. *Patient/significant other must be aware that prognosis for recovery is good, but recovery tends to be slow.*
- If newly diagnosed, explain possible treatments. *Pooled gamma globulin may be administered during the first 2 weeks of the disease. Usual dose = 0.4 g/kg/day.*
- Explain the use of plasmapheresis to *minimize the immune response of cells to the offending virus. It is believed that the immune response causes the demyelination of peripheral nerves. Usually 200-250 ml of plasma/kg is removed in 4-6 treatments on alternate days. Saline solution and albumen are usually used as replacement fluid.*
- ▲ Coordinate social service, financial counselor involvement as soon as possible *to help with supportive care, insurance concerns/disability planning, and discharge planning.*
- Provide information about additional resources, such as the
  Gullian Barré Syndrome Foundation International
  P.O. Box 262
  Wynnewood, PA 19006
  Telephone: 215-667 0131

See also:
Impaired individual coping, p. 18.
Self-care deficit, p. 53.
Ineffective airway clearance, p. 3.
Body image disturbance, p. 7.
Constipation, p. 16.
Urinary retention, p. 74.
Altered nutrition, p. 44.
Mechanical ventilation, p. 202.

By: Linda Arsenault, RN, MSN, CNRN

Head trauma

Head injuries are the leading cause of death in the United States for persons aged 1 to 42. About two thirds of all severe head injuries result from motor vehicle accidents. The severity of the head injury is defined by the traumatic coma data bank on the basis of the Glasgow Coma Score (GCS): Severe head injury = GCS 8 or less; moderate head injury = GCS 9-12. Most head injuries are blunt (closed) trauma to the brain. Damage to the scalp, skull, meninges, and brain runs the gamut of skull fracture, concussion, and/or extracerebral or intracerebral pathological conditions.

NURSING DIAGNOSES	EXPECTED OUTCOMES AND NURSING INTERVENTIONS / *RATIONALE* (■ = INDEPENDENT; ▲ = COLLABORATIVE)

Altered Tissue Perfusion: Cerebral

RELATED FACTORS

Increased intracranial pressure (ICP)
Cerebral edema
Decreased cerebral perfusion pressure (CPP)
Impaired autoregulation
Cortical laceration
Intracranial hemorrhage

DEFINING CHARACTERISTICS

Decreased level of consciousness (confusion, disorientation, somnolence, lethargy, coma)
Headache
Vomiting
Pupillary asymmetry
Changes in pupillary reaction
ICP > 15 mm Hg
CPP <60 mm Hg

EXPECTED OUTCOMES

Patient maintains optimal cerebral tissue perfusion, as evidenced by GCS > 13, absence of new neurologic deficit.

ONGOING ASSESSMENT

- Assess neurological status as follows:
    Level of consciousness (Glasgow Coma Score).
    Orientation to person, place, and time.
    Motor signs: drift, decreased movement, abnormal or absent movement, increased reflexes. *Focal signs of neurologic dysfunction suggest structural versus metabolic abnormality.*
    Pupil size, symmetry, and reaction to light.
    Extraocular movement, deviation.
    Speech, thought processes, and memory changes.
- Monitor vital signs. *Increased blood pressure associated with bradycardia is a late sign of increased ICP that suggests medullary ischemia/compression.*
- Evaluate presence/absence of protective reflexes: corneal, gag, blink, cough, startle, grab, Babinski.
- ▲ Monitor ICP via institutional preference device. *Normal ICP should be below 15 mm Hg with patient at rest.*
- Calculate the cerebral perfusion pressure (CPP) (CPP = mean systemic arterial pressure − ICP). *CPP should be 80-100 mm Hg.*
- ▲ Monitor oxygen and CO_2 levels via an arterial blood gas assessment. *Normal levels are Po_2 >80 mm Hg and Pco_2 <35 mm Hg. Goal of hyperventilation is Pco_2 25-30 mmHg. Secondary insults such as hypoxia, hypercapnia, and hypotension are significant causes of mortality and morbidity in head injury patients.*
- Monitor I & O q1-2h or more frequently when needed. Assess urine specific gravity and urine glucose.
- Assess for pain, fever, and shivering.
- ▲ Monitor serum electrolytes, BUN, creatinine, osmolarity, glucose, and hemoglobin and hematocrit.
- Monitor closely when inducing treatment and when titrating treatment.

THERAPEUTIC INTERVENTIONS

- Record serial assessment of LOC (GCS), neurologic signs, and vital signs q1-4h or as needed.
- If ICP is above 15 mm Hg, postpone nursing care activities that can be deferred (e.g., routine care, invasive procedures).
- Report ICP > 15 mm Hg sustained for more than 5 min.
- Elevate HOB 30 degrees unless the patient is in shock (MAP less than 80) or with concomitant spinal cord injury. In these situations, place patient supine.
- Position head in neutral position *to promote venous drainage.*
- If patient is intubated, ensure that tapes securing ET tube are not too tight, thereby impeding jugular venous outflow.
- ▲ Administer hyperosmotic agents such as Mannitol as ordered. Infuse Mannitol through a filter. Insert a Foley catheter *to allow for accurate measurement of diuretic response (20-30 min after infusion).*
- ▲ During course of treatment with hyperosmotics, check serum electrolytes, glucose, and serum Osm q6-8h.

NURSING DIAGNOSES	EXPECTED OUTCOMES AND NURSING INTERVENTIONS / *RATIONALE* (■ = INDEPENDENT; ▲ = COLLABORATIVE)

THERAPEUTIC INTERVENTIONS—cont'd

- If neuromuscular blocking agents are used (pancuronium [Pavulon]), remember that cerebration is still intact and that pain is perceived.
- Avoid or counteract maneuvers that would increase intrathoracic pressure and ICP (e.g., Valsalva's maneuver, vomiting, coughing, straining against ET tube).
- Hyperventilate and hyperoxygenate before suctioning ET tube/trach.

Decreased Level of Consciousness

RELATED FACTORS

Head trauma, cerebral edema, increased ICP

DEFINING CHARACTERISTICS

Change in alertness, orientation, verbal response, eye opening, motor response
Agitation
Inappropriate affect
Reduced awareness
Decreased response to stimulation
Lethargy

EXPECTED OUTCOMES

Patient maintains optimal state of consciousness, as evidenced by GCS > 13, stable GCS.

ONGOING ASSESSMENT

- Assess LOC and perform neurological assessment q1-2h.
- Assess for contributing factors that may affect LOC (e.g., anesthesia, medications).
- Assess vital signs.
- Assess for communication barriers.
- Assess for rhinorrhea (CSF drainage from nose), otorrhea (CSF drainage from ear), battle sign (ecchymosis over the mastoid process). *These signs may occur with basal skull fractures.*

THERAPEUTIC INTERVENTIONS

- Record all assessment changes and/or deteriorations. *The Glasgow Coma Scale uses the same parameters for eye opening and motor movement. Verbal response must be evaluated by smiles, orientation to sound, appropriate interactions.*
- Protect patient from secondary injury by:
   Maintaining side rails in high position; bed in low position.
   Protecting for decreased corneal and gag reflex.
   Protecting from seizure activity.
- If restraints are needed, position patient on side. *Restraints should be used judiciously, since they may increase agitation and anxiety, thereby increasing ICP.*
- Reorient to environment as needed *to decrease anxiety.* Provide familiar objects, pictures.
- Explain all nursing activites. Do not try to explain the whole procedure at once. Take one step at a time before proceeding to the next step.
- See also Altered level of consciousness, p. 252.

High Risk for Fluid Volume Deficit

RISK FACTORS

Diabetes insipidus
Administration of hyperosmotic agents such as mannitol or high protein tube feedings
High fever
Profuse diaphoresis
Vomiting
Diarrhea

EXPECTED OUTCOME

Patient maintains optimal fluid volume, as evidenced by normal skin turgor, urine specific gravity between 1.005-1.0025.

ONGOING ASSESSMENT

- Monitor I & O every hour.
- Assess urine specific gravity q2-4h.
- ▲ Monitor serum and urine electrolytes and osmolarity.
- Monitor for signs of dehydration (decreased skin turgor, weight loss, increased heart rate, decreased BP).
- Monitor vital signs every hour.
- Assess urine for glucose.
- Monitor daily weights.

THERAPEUTIC INTERVENTIONS

- Notify physician of urine output >200 ml/hr for 2 consecutive hours. Maintain an indwelling Foley catheter *to provide accurate assessment of urine output.*
- Replace fluid output as directed.
- Notify physician of urine specific gravity <1.005. *Diabetes insipidus will result in a decrease in urine specific gravity.*
- Notify physician of positive urine glucose finding, *Glucosuria may lead to dehydration and increased urine output, mimicking diabetes insipidus.*
- ▲ Administer vasopressin as ordered. *Vasopressin is a synthetic antidiuretic hormone that will induce concentration and decrease urine output. Careful monitoring of the urine output and serum Na and osmolarity is mandatory when vasopressin is administered.*
- Keep accurate records of all fluid losses (blood draws, vomiting, diarrhea).

Continued.

NURSING DIAGNOSES	EXPECTED OUTCOMES AND NURSING INTERVENTIONS / *RATIONALE* (■ = INDEPENDENT; ▲ = COLLABORATIVE)

High Risk for Fluid Volume Excess

RISK FACTORS

Free water excess
Syndrome of inappropriate secretion of antidiuretic hormone (SIADH) (seen in 5% of head injury patients)

EXPECTED OUTCOMES

Patient maintains optimal fluid balance, as evidenced by normal serum Na, normal osmolarity, urine specific gravity 1.005-1.0025.

ONGOING ASSESSMENT

- Assess intake and output.
- ▲ Assess electrolytes and osmolality at least daily.
- Monitor vital signs and neurological status q1-2h.
- Monitor weight daily.

THERAPEUTIC INTERVENTIONS

- ▲ Restrict fluid intake as directed (*usually 1L/day combined with PO/IV/nasogastric tube liquids).*
- ▲ Limit free water intake. Use 0.9% NS for medication piggyback or nasogastric tube.
- ▲ If fluid restriction fails to correct hyponatremia, anticipate order for 3% saline solution infusion given with potassium and furosemide (Lasix). In this event, monitor serial Na, K, and serum Osm q6h.

Ineffective Airway Clearance

RELATED FACTORS

Decreased LOC
Possible mechanical obstruction resulting from facial trauma
Facial edema
Use of neuromuscular paralytic agents
Concomitant cervical/high thoracic spinal cord injury

DEFINING CHARACTERISTICS

Abnormal or ineffective breathing pattern
Decreased Po_2 or increased Pco_2
Change in rate of respiration (tachypnea or apnea)
Change in heart rate (tachycardia or bradycardia)
Cyanosis
Use of accessory muscles of respiration
Nasal flaring, grunting
Intercostal retractions

EXPECTED OUTCOMES

Patient maintains patent airway, as evidenced by clear breath sounds, normal respiratory rate, normal ABGs, normal cardiac rate and rhythm.

ONGOING ASSESSMENT

- Assess rate and quality of respirations q1-2h.
- Monitor breath sounds q2h.
- Monitor neurological status q2-4h.
- ▲ Monitor ABGs as needed.
- Assess ability to cough.
- Check for swallowing ability (gurgling/cough).
- Check for gag reflex.

THERAPEUTIC INTERVENTIONS

- Encourage deep breathing exercises (slow deep breaths at least 10 times/hr).
- ▲ Administer oxygen as directed.
- Suction secretions prn. *Nasotracheal suctioning is contraindicated with head trauma resulting from possible basilar skull fracture. This could result in the introduction of the catheter tip into the brain.*
- Turn frequently side to side.
- If patient is at risk for increased ICP or if ICP is elevated above baseline, hyperoxygenate and hyperventilate before and after suctioning.

High Risk for Seizures

RISK FACTORS

Cortical laceration
Temporal lobe contusion
Acute intracranial bleeding
Hyponatremia/hypoglycemia
Hypoxia
Multiple contusions
Penetrating injuries to brain
Early seizure in the 1st week of head injury

EXPECTED OUTCOME

Patient does not experience additional injury secondary to maintenance of appropriate seizure precautions.

ONGOING ASSESSMENT

- Observe for seizure activity. Record and report observations:
  Length of seizure.
  Body part involved, pattern and order of movement.
  Preictal activity.
  Direction of eye deviation and change in pupil size.
  Airway and respiratory pattern.
  Length of postictal state and characteristics.
  Incontinence.

NURSING DIAGNOSES	EXPECTED OUTCOMES AND NURSING INTERVENTIONS / *RATIONALE* (■ = INDEPENDENT; ▲ = COLLABORATIVE)

THERAPEUTIC INTERVENTIONS

- Protect head from injury.
- Pad side rails.
- Maintain patent airway during the postictal state. Turn head to the side and suction secretions as necessary.
- Administer anticonvulsants as directed. *Phenytoin (Dilantin) can only be mixed in NS. Precipitation will be noted when mixed with D_5W. Observe for hypotension during the administration and administer <50 mg/min IVP.*
- If seizure occurs, protect the head and body from injury. Do not attempt to put anything into the mouth.
- Suction as indicated.
- Keep bed in low position.
- Keep side rails up.

High Risk for Altered Nutrition: Less than Body Requirements

RISK FACTORS

Facial trauma, restriction of intake, physical immobility, impaired LOC, multisystem trauma

EXPECTED OUTCOME

Patient maintains optimal nutritional status, as evidenced by good skin turgor, normal electrolyte levels, weight gain.

ONGOING ASSESSMENT

- Monitor albumin, protein, urea nitrogen levels, glucose, electrolytes.
- Assess skin color, turgor, and muscle mass.
- Assess rate and quality of wound healing.
- Observe for signs of infection and local infection at catheter insertion site. *Wound healing and immunocompetence depend on good nutrition.*
- Monitor daily weights.
- Verify placement of gastric tube before initiation of tube feedings. Avoid insertion of feeding tube through the nose in a patient with head injury unless the possibility of a basal skull fracture has been excluded.

THERAPEUTIC INTERVENTIONS

- Administer tube feedings or total parenteral nutrition (TPN) as directed. *Patients with head injury need about 2000 kcal/day. Patients with multiple trauma may need 2-3 times (or more) that. Note: 1 L of IV solution contains an average of 200 cal*
- Maintain head of bed at 30 degrees *to prevent risk of aspiration.*

Knowledge Deficit Regarding Diagnosis, Treatment, Outcome

RELATED FACTORS

Lack of prior experience with head injury

DEFINING CHARACTERISTICS

Questioning members of health care team or other family members
Verbalization of incorrect information
Withdrawal from environment
Frustration with health care and family members

EXPECTED OUTCOME

Patient/family describes the illness, treatment, and expected outcome.

ONGOING ASSESSMENT

- Assess knowledge of equipment and health care status.

THERAPEUTIC INTERVENTIONS

- Prepare family for the equipment and monitors used in the environment.
- Reinforce information given to patient/family about type of head injury, results of CT scan, and plan of care.
- If patient has impaired LOC, instruct family/significant other to avoid discussions at bedside they would not want patient to hear. *Though patient may be unresponsive, ability to hear may be intact.*
- Encourage family/significant other to bring in pictures, tapes of favorite music, messages from children and friends.
- Keep family up to date with any new changes in condition.
- Discuss role of physical, occupational, or speech therapist. *Specialized services may be required for present/future recovery.*
- Discuss need for rehabilitation if anticipated after discharge.
- Provide family with name and number of local support group if available. *Groups that come together for mutual support can be beneficial.*
- Refer family to social service, financial counselor as appropriate.

By: Jan Colip, RN, MSN, CCRN and Linda Arsenault, RN, MSN, CNRN

Hydrocephalus

A condition in which cerebrospinal fluid (CSF) production exceeds absorption. Noncommunicating hydrocephalus refers to an obstruction in or proximal to the ventricular system between the lateral ventricles, third ventricle, fourth ventricle, or outflow ports of the fourth ventricle. Communicating hydrocephalus usually connotes a problem with flow and absorption within the subarachnoid pathway and superior sagittal sinus.

| NURSING DIAGNOSES | EXPECTED OUTCOMES AND NURSING INTERVENTIONS / *RATIONALE* (■ = INDEPENDENT; ▲ = COLLABORATIVE) |

Altered Tissue Perfusion: Cerebral

RELATED FACTORS

Increased intracranial pressure (ICP)
Decreased cerebral perfusion pressure (CPP)
Untreated hydrocephalus
Obstructed shunt
Subdural hematoma after shunt complication

DEFINING CHARACTERISTICS

Decreased level of consciousness (lethargy, decreased Glasgow Coma Scale, coma)
Headache
Vomiting
Parinaud's sign (sunsetting, failure of upward gaze)
Impaired thought processes
Increased blood pressure with bradycardia
Motor weakness

EXPECTED OUTCOMES

Patient maintains optimal cerebral tissue perfusion, as evidenced by one or more of the following: stability in LOC, normal ICP, normal CPP, neurologically intact, absence of neurologic deterioration.

ONGOING ASSESSMENT

- Obtain presenting signs and symptoms.
- Assess for signs/symptoms of increased ICP by evaluation of the following: LOC (Glasgow Coma Scale); extraocular movements; speech, thought processes; vital sign changes: increased BP and bradycardia; motor strength; headache/emesis.
▲ If patient has a ventricular shunt in place, locate reservoir pump and press down in pumping fashion—should depress and refill within seconds. *If unable to depress or fails to refill, shunt may be obstructed.*

THERAPEUTIC INTERVENTIONS

- Document serial assessment q1-4hr as indicated.
- Report deterioration in assessment (e.g., increased lethargy, sunsetting, vital sign changes, respiratory distress).
▲ Administer medications as ordered, e.g., furosemide (Lasix), mannitol *used to decrease ICP.*
▲ Maintain head of bed as prescribed. *It is not uncommon for patient to be kept flat (with one pillow and frequent turning side to side) for 1-2 days to prevent sudden drop in intraventricular pressure with subsequent intracranial hemorrhage.*
- See also Increased intracranial pressure, p. 268.

High Risk for Fluid Volume Deficit

RELATED FACTORS

Externalization of ventricular shunt for CSF drainage
Use of diuretics/hyperosmotic agents to control ICP
Vomiting
Fluid restriction

DEFINING CHARACTERISTICS

Thirst
Polyuria
Poor skin turgor
Weight loss
Tachycardia, hypotension
Weak peripheral pulses
Decreased urine output <0.5 ml/kg/hr
Urine specific gravity >1.025
Serum Na >155 mEq/L
Serum Osm >310 mOsm/L

EXPECTED OUTCOMES

Patient is adequately hydrated, as evidenced by one or more of the following: normal Na, normal Osm, urine specific gravity < 1.025, absence of thirst, normal skin turgor.

ONGOING ASSESSMENT

- Monitor I & O hourly. *Urine output should normally be >0.5 ml/kg/hr. CSF drainage will vary, depending on external drainage bag position. Normal CSF production approximately 20 ml/hr (500 ml/day).*
▲ Monitor serum Na, osmolality, and urine specific gravity as indicated.
- Monitor for signs of dehydration (see Defining Characteristics).

THERAPEUTIC INTERVENTIONS

▲ Administer IV fluids as prescribed.
▲ If ventricular shunt is externalized, secure collection bag to head of bed/IV pole at prescribed level. *If drainage bag were to fall to the floor, the CSF would be drained by gravity with the potential for intraventricular hemorrhage/subdural hemorrhage.*
▲ Document amount of CSF output hourly in externalized shunt.

NURSING DIAGNOSES	EXPECTED OUTCOMES AND NURSING INTERVENTIONS / *RATIONALE* (■ = INDEPENDENT; ▲ = COLLABORATIVE)

Pain/Discomfort

RELATED FACTORS

Rapid decrease in cerebrospinal fluid volume and pressure by shunting
Revision of shunt or externalization of shunt
Incisional discomfort

DEFINING CHARACTERISTICS

Headache
Dizziness
Vomiting
Restlessness
Lethargy

EXPECTED OUTCOMES

Patient verbalizes comfort.

ONGOING ASSESSMENT

- Assess for signs of disequilibrium related to sudden drop in CSF pressure after shunting: headache that worsens when patient sits up, dizziness, emesis with or without nausea, restlessness.

THERAPEUTIC INTERVENTIONS

▲ Administer IV fluids as prescribed.
▲ Administer medication (light analgesics, antiemetics) as prescribed.
- If complaint of headache when sitting up, keep head of bed flat with gradual elevation as tolerated over several days.
- Encourage oral fluids as tolerated (Gatorade, juices, water).
- Explain need for CT scan. *A CT scan may be prescribed to evaluate ventricular size, establish a baseline, and rule out subdural hematoma following shunting or revision of shunt.*

Knowledge Deficit

RELATED FACTORS

New shunt, lack of prior experience

DEFINING CHARACTERISTICS

Questioning of health care members
Verbalization of incorrect information
Expressions of frustration
Expressions of apprehension, anxiety, fear

EXPECTED OUTCOMES

Patient/caregivers discuss hydrocephalus, shunting treatment, and possible signs of shunt malfunction before discharge.

ONGOING ASSESSMENT

- Assess knowledge of hydrocephalus cause and treatment (ventriculoperitoneal or atrial shunting).
- Evaluate caregiver knowledge of signs and symptoms of shunt obstruction and follow-up care before discharge.

THERAPEUTIC INTERVENTIONS

- Reinforce explanation of shunt insertion *(usually right frontal into anterior horn of right lateral ventricle; tubing tunneled subcutaneously to peritoneum).*
- Provide written information regarding shunt malfunction: vomiting; decreased appetite; unusual irritability or restlessness; persistent headache; difficulty walking; blurred/double vision; inability to retain urine; fever, puffiness, redness, swelling at incisions or along shunt tubing; and unusual sleepiness.
- Discuss wound care after removal of sutures/staples. *(Can wash over incisions. Okay to apply small amount of Vaseline/vitamin E cream/cocoa butter to treat dry skin).*
- Instruct to notify physician if drainage/leakage from any of the incisions develops.
- Provide follow-up appointments and information for emergency access to health care system.
▲ Involve social worker as indicated.

By Linda Arsenault, RN, MSN, CNRN

Increased intracranial pressure

Intracranial pressure (ICP) reflects the pressure exerted by the intracranial components of blood, brain, cerebrospinal fluid (CSF), and any other fluid/mass (subdural, tumor, abscess, etc.). Increases in ICP occur when compensation mechanisms fail (mostly blood and CSF buffering). The normal range of ICP is up to 15 mm Hg; excursions above that level occur normally, but readily return to baseline parameters. In the event of disease, trauma, or a pathological condition, a disturbance in autoregulation occurs and ICP is increased and sustained.

NURSING DIAGNOSES

EXPECTED OUTCOMES AND NURSING INTERVENTIONS / *RATIONALE*
(■ = INDEPENDENT; ▲ = COLLABORATIVE)

Altered Tissue Perfusion: Cerebral

RELATED FACTORS

Increased ICP
Increased cerebral blood flow (CBF)
Cerebral edema
Decreased CBF and cerebral perfusion pressure (CPP)

DEFINING CHARACTERISTICS

Decreased LOC (confusion, disorientation, somnolence, lethargy, coma)
Headache
Vomiting
Papilledema
Pupil asymmetry
Decreased pupil reactivity
Impaired memory, judgment, thought processes
Glasgow Coma Scale <11
Unilateral or bilateral VI nerve palsy

EXPECTED OUTCOME

Patient maintains optimal cerebral tissue perfusion, as evidenced by normal ICP, GCS > 13, normal CPP.

ONGOING ASSESSMENT

- Assess neurological status as follows: LOC per Glasgow Coma Scale; pupil size, symmetry, reaction to light; extraocular movement (EOM); gaze preference; speech, thought processes, memory; motor-sensory signs—drift, increased tone, increased reflexes, Babinski.
- Monitor vital signs.
- ▲ Monitor ICP if ICP monitor in place. Report ICP > 15 mm Hg for 5 min.
- Evaluate presence/absence of protective reflexes: swallow, gag, blink, cough, etc.
- ▲ Monitor ABGs. *Recommended parameters of Po_2 >80 mm Hg and Pco_2 <35 mm Hg with normal ICP. If patient's lungs are being hyperventilated to decrease ICP, Pco_2 should be between 25 and 30 mm Hg. A Pco_2 < 20 mm Hg may decrease CBF because of profound vasoconstriction → that produces hypoxia. pco_2 > 45 mm Hg induces vasodilation with increase in CBF, which may trigger increase in ICP.*
- Monitor I & O q1-2h with urine specific gravity. Report urine specific gravity >1.025 or urine output <½ ml/kg/hr.
- Calculate CPP. *Should be ~90-100 mm Hg and not <50 mm Hg to ensure blood flow to brain.* Calculate CPP by subtracting ICP from the mean systemic arterial pressure (MSAP): CPP = MSAP − ICP. *To calculate MSAP, use the following formula:*

$$\left(\frac{\text{Systolic BP} - \text{Diastolic BP}}{3}\right) + \text{Diastolic BP}$$

- ▲ Monitor serum electrolytes, BUN, creatinine, glucose, osmolality, Hb, and Hct as indicated.
- Monitor closely when treatment of increased ICP begins to be tapered, i.e., once ICP is stabilized at normal pressure for 48 hours.
- ▲ Serially monitor ICP pressure and waveforms. Types of ICP waveforms:
   Lundberg A waves (plateau waves) *are increased in ICP > 50 mm Hg sustained for > 5 min.*
   B waves *are increased ICP, usually between 20-40 mm Hg, and may preceed an A wave.*
   C waves *are nonpathologic and often correlate with heart rate and respiratory rate.*

THERAPEUTIC INTERVENTIONS

- ▲ Elevate head of bed 30 degrees and keep head in neutral alignment *to prevent decrease in venous outflow with increase in ICP.* (Exceptions include shock, cervical spine injuries).

- Avoid Valsalva's maneuver, *which increases intrathoracic pressure and CBF, thereby increasing ICP.*
▲ If ICP increases and fails to respond to repositioning of head in neutral alignment and head elevation, recheck equipment. If ICP is increased, one or more of the following may be prescribed by the physician:
    Hyperventilate the patient *to decrease Paco$_2$ to between 25 and 30 mm Hg; this induces vasoconstriction and decrease in CBF.*
    Administer mannitol 0.25 g/kg-1 g/kg given over 30-60 min. *This is a hyperosmotic agent and needs to be given with caution; it is contraindicated with hypovolemic symptoms: hypotension, tachycardia, CHF, renal failure, hypernatremia. A diuretic response can be anticipated within 30-60 min. A Foley catheter should be in place. An IV filter should be used when mannitol is infused. Electrolytes, osmolality, and serum glucose must be monitored q4-6h during mannitol infusion.*
▲ Administer barbiturates, additional diuretics such as furosemide as prescribed by physician if ICP is refractory to hyperventilation/mannitol regimen.
▲ If patient is intubated, administer neuromuscular blocking agent as prescribed q1-4h *to reduce shivering, coughing, bucking, Valsalva's maneuver. Remember, however, that neuromuscular blocking agents have no effect on cerebration; therefore, patient should receive short-acting sedation before noxious stimulation.*
▲ Administer a short-acting pain reliever, e.g., morphine, midazolam (Versed), before painful stimulation or stress-related care such as suctioning, IV line changes.
- If ICP elevated 12-15 mm Hg, reduce nursing and medical procedures to those absolutely necessary. *Counteract noxious stimulation with preoxygenation, hyperventilation, analgesia.*
- Maintain normothermia with antipyretics, tepid sponges, cooling blanket. *Fever increases cerebral metabolic demand; may increase cerebral blood flow and increase intracranial pressure.*

Knowledge Deficit

RELATED FACTOR

Lack of prior experience

DEFINING CHARACTERISTICS

Questioning of members of
    health care team
Verbalization of incorrect information
Anger/hostility
Depression
Withdrawal from environment
Expressions of frustration

EXPECTED OUTCOMES

Patient/family discuss illness, treatment, and expected outcome if known.

ONGOING ASSESSMENT

- Assess knowledge of increased ICP, causes, treatment, and outcome.

THERAPEUTIC INTERVENTIONS

- Define increased ICP (e.g., increased pressure against the brain).
- Discuss cause if known.
- Reinforce discussions related to treatment (e.g., HOB elevated, medication, intubation, and hyperoxygenation).
- Offer family frequent feedback regarding patient's status.

By: Linda Arsenault, RN, MSN, CNRN

Intracranial infection

(ENCEPHALITIS; BRAIN ABSCESS; CENTRAL
NERVOUS SYSTEM INFECTION; MENINGITIS,
VENTRICULITIS, EMPYEMA, CEREBRITIS)

Intracranial infection may be the result of meningitis, encephalitis, ventriculitis, brain abscess, or empyema. Meningitis is an inflammation/infection of the membranes of the brain or spinal cord caused by bacteria, viruses, or other organisms. Encephalitis is an inflammation/infection of the brain and meninges. Ventriculitis is an infection that establishes itself in the ventricular system. An abscess is a localized purulent collection in the brain. Empyema is an infection that forms in a preexisting space such as the subdural space of the brain. It may also form in the epidural space of the spine.

NURSING DIAGNOSES	EXPECTED OUTCOMES AND NURSING INTERVENTIONS / *RATIONALE* (■ = INDEPENDENT; ▲ = COLLABORATIVE)

Hyperthermia

RELATED FACTORS

Brain infection
Encephalitis
Brain abscess

DEFINING CHARACTERISTICS

Fever > 39° C (102° F)
Increased WBC
Nuchal rigidity
Altered level of consciousness (LOC)
Irritability
Motor-sensory abnormalities
Chills
Malaise
Headache
Localized redness/swelling (e.g., along a suture line or area of injury)

EXPECTED OUTCOME

Patient maintains normal temperature of 37° C.

ONGOING ASSESSMENT

- Monitor temperature q4h.
▲ Monitor WBC daily or as prescribed.
- Evaluate LOC. *Symptoms provide a clinical picture on which treatment will be based.*
- Evaluate motor-sensory status.
- Evaluate for signs of CSF otorrhea/rhinorrhea. *After basal skull fracture, CSF leakage may lead to intracranial infection.*
▲ Monitor peak/trough levels of antibiotics as prescribed.
▲ Monitor serum Na and osmolality *(index of hydration/dehydration)* as prescribed.
- Check and record urine specific gravity. *Patient may become dehydrated because of fever and conservative fluid administration with concern for cerebral edema.*
- Monitor IV insertion site closely for signs of infiltration, thrombosis, phlebitis.

THERAPEUTIC INTERVENTIONS

- Administer tepid sponge baths prn for temperature > 39° C.
- Apply cooling blanket for temperature > 39.5° C.
▲ Administer antipyretics as prescribed; document patient response. *Fever increases cerebral metabolic demand.*
- Provide mouth care and lubrication q1h.
▲ Administer antibiotics on strict administration schedule *to maintain therapeutic blood levels, reduce virulence, eradicate pathogen, and prevent swings in antibiotic blood levels.*
- Change IV site per hospital policy.

High Risk for Seizures

RISK FACTORS

Cerebral irritation, focal edema, cerebritis, ventriculitis

EXPECTED OUTCOMES

Patient does not experience seizure activity.
If patient experiences seizure, early assessment and treatment are initiated to prevent injury.

ONGOING ASSESSMENT

- Monitor level of consciousness. *Change in alertness, orientation, verbal response, eye opening, motor response provides basis for further treatment.*
- Monitor for seizure activity. *May exhibit as involuntary repetitive motor/sensory movement/spasticity or repetitive psychomotor activity.*
- Document seizure pattern and frequency of occurrence. Notify physician as appropriate *(i.e., first seizure, repetitive seizures; seizure pattern that varies may indicate need for anticonvulsant medications, reevaluation and/or further neurologic evaluation).*
▲ Monitor anticonvulsant levels.
- Evaluate patency of airway; monitor rate and rhythm of respirations.

THERAPEUTIC INTERVENTIONS

- After motor activity has ceased, roll patient to side/semiprone position *to promote gravity drainage of secretions.*
- Suction prn *to prevent aspiration.*
▲ Administer anticonvulsants as prescribed.
- See also Seizure activity, p. 281.

NURSING DIAGNOSES	EXPECTED OUTCOMES AND NURSING INTERVENTIONS / *RATIONALE* (■ = INDEPENDENT; ▲ = COLLABORATIVE)

High Risk for Altered Cerebral Tissue Perfusion

RISK FACTORS

Cerebral edema, increased intracranial pressure, hydrocephalus

EXPECTED OUTCOMES

Patient maintains optimal tissue perfusion, as evidenced by alertness, normal pupillary reaction, absence of seizures, GCS > 13, absence of meningeal signs.

ONGOING ASSESSMENT

- Evaluate neurologic parameters as follows:
  Assess LOC, Glasgow Coma Score. Record serially.
  Determine factors contributing to LOC change (i.e., *awakening from sleep, sedation, seizure*).
  Monitor pupillary size, reaction to light.
- Report persistent deterioration in LOC. *If LOC decreases, treatment may need to be changed, new treatment instituted, or additional tests obtained. Change in mentation seizures, increased BP, bradycardia, or respiratory abnormalities may indicate increasing ICP with decreased CPP.*
- Monitor motor strength and coordination.
- Assess ability to follow simple/complex commands.
- Evaluate presence/absence of protective reflexes: swallow, gag, blink, cough, etc.
- Assess for meningeal signs: nuchal rigidity, headache, photophobia, Brudzinki's sign *(flexion of neck onto chest causes flexion of both legs and thighs)*, Kernig's sign *(resistance to extension of the leg at the knee with the hip flexed). Symptoms provide a clinical picture on which further diagnosis and treatment are based.*

THERAPEUTIC INTERVENTIONS

- Reorient to environment prn.
- Position with HOB elevated 30-45 degrees with head in neutral alignment. *If actual/potential increased ICP, positioning with elevated HOB will promote venous outflow from brain and help decrease ICP.*
- See also Altered level of consciousness, p. 252.

Pain

RELATED FACTORS

Meningeal irritation, increased ICP

DEFINING CHARACTERISTICS

Headache
Photophobia
Nuchal rigidity
Irritability
Diaphoresis

EXPECTED OUTCOMES

Patient verbalizes relief from pain/comfort.
Patient appears comfortable.

ONGOING ASSESSMENT

- Assess for headache, photophobia, restlessness, irritability, diaphoresis.
- Evaluate response to analgesics.

THERAPEUTIC INTERVENTIONS

- Restrict visitors as appropriate.
- Reduce noise in environment.
- Keep patient's room darkened and ask family to bring in sunglasses *to minimize effects of photophobia.*
- ▲ Administer analgesics as prescribed.
- Discourage Valsalva's maneuver *(e.g., instruct patient to exhale when moving up in bed; provide stool softeners to prevent straining and subsequent increased cerebral blood flow and increased ICP).*
- See also Pain, p. 49.

High Risk for Fluid Volume Deficit

RISK FACTORS

Reduced LOC, lack of oral intake, fever, vomiting, diarrhea

EXPECTED OUTCOMES

Patient maintains optimal fluid volume, as evidenced by good skin turgor, normal specific gravity, and normal serum sodium and osmolality.

ONGOING ASSESSMENT

- Assess skin turgor. *Loss of interstitial fluid causes loss of skin elasticity.*
- Monitor intake and output.
- Monitor weight. *Changes may reflect fluid volume changes.*
- ▲ Monitor serum electrolytes, urine specific gravity, and blood urea nitrogen (BUN).
- Document and report changes in BP, heart rate. *Reduction in circulating blood volume can cause changes in vital signs.*
- ▲ Record urine specific gravity and check laboratory results that may reflect dehydration: *urine specific gravity > 1.025, serum sodium > 150 mEq/L, serum osmolality > 310 Osm/L, BUN > 18 mg/dl, creatinine > 0.4 mg/dl.*

Continued.

Neurologic Care Plans

NURSING DIAGNOSES	EXPECTED OUTCOMES AND NURSING INTERVENTIONS / *RATIONALE* (■ = INDEPENDENT; ▲ = COLLABORATIVE)

THERAPEUTIC INTERVENTIONS

- Encourage fluid intake as appropriate. *Patient may require intravenous or nasogastric feedings to ensure hydration. Average daily fluid loss is 1500 cc urine, 200 cc stool, and 700-1300 cc perspiration/respiration/insensible water loss.*
- Provide oral care, lubrication to lips.
- See also Fluid Volume Deficit, p. 25.

High Risk for Altered Nutrition: Less than Body Requirements

RISK FACTORS

Altered level of consciousness
Infection with increased metabolic activity
Reduced oral intake
Vomiting
Loss of appetite

EXPECTED OUTCOMES

Patient maintains adequate caloric intake, as evidenced by maintenance of body weight.

ONGOING ASSESSMENT

- Assess patient's ability to swallow. *Altered neurologic status may place patient at risk for aspiration.*
- Assess admission weight. Compare normal caloric requirements for body weight to present weight.
- Monitor caloric intake and food; record every meal. *Provides objective data on types, amounts consumed.*
- ▲ Monitor appropriate laboratory parameters (i.e., serum albumin, iron, total protein, and electrolytes) 2-3 times/wk.
- Monitor I & O every shift.

THERAPEUTIC INTERVENTIONS

- Assist with meals prn. *Smaller meals may facilitate gastric emptying and improve appetite.*
- Elevate HOB for meals and for 1 hr after meals. *Helps prevent epigastric discomfort/feeling of fullness and minimize potential for aspiration.*
- Provide adaptive/assistive devices (plate guard, special padded utensils, splints).
- Encourage family/friends to visit. *Being with others may promote oral intake; others may be able to encourage/assist.*
- ▲ Consult dietitian as appropriate.
- See also Altered nutrition: less than body requirements, p. 44.

Knowledge Deficit

RELATED FACTORS

New treatment, possible surgical drainage

DEFINING CHARACTERISTICS

Patient/significant others verbalize questions/concerns
Incorrect/inaccurate information conveyed

EXPECTED OUTCOME

Patient/significant others can discuss current infection, possible causes, tests, treatment, and follow-up care.

ONGOING ASSESSMENT

- Assess patient's/significant others' knowledge base about current CNS infection.
- Assess patient's mental status (orientation, thought processes, memory, insight, judgment). *Altered mental status is barrier to learning; family/significant others will need to be more actively involved.*

THERAPEUTIC INTERVENTIONS

- Provide explanations of disease process, cause if known, diagnostic testing (e.g., CT scan, MRI, lumbar puncture).
- Instruct patient/significant others in principles of antibiotic therapy, effects and possible side effects, maintenance of therapeutic levels, and duration of treatment. *This involves patient/significant others, making them educated consumers, and helps decrease anxiety/fear.*
- If patient is to be discharged on medications (e.g., antibiotics, anticonvulsants), instruct caregiver in dose, frequency, route, and possible side effects. *It is best to provide written instructions for reference at home.*
- Provide information about adjunct treatments that may be indicated: physical, occupational, speech therapy.
- Determine need for social service consultation *in anticipation of discharge planning needs.*

By: Linda Arsenault, RN, MSN, CNRN

Multiple sclerosis (MS)

(DISSEMINATED SCLEROSIS; DEMYELINATING DISEASE)

A chronic progressive nervous system disease characterized by scattered patches of demyelination and glial tissue overgrowth in the white matter of the brain and spinal cord leading to decreased nerve conduction. As the inflammation/edema diminishes, some remyelination may occur, and nerve conduction returns. Among the clinical symptoms associated with multiple sclerosis are extremity weakness, visual disturbances, ataxia, tremor, uncoordination, sphincter impairment, and impaired position sense. Remissions and exacerbations are associated with the disease.

NURSING DIAGNOSES	EXPECTED OUTCOMES AND NURSING INTERVENTIONS / *RATIONALE* (■ = INDEPENDENT; ▲ = COLLABORATIVE)

Impaired Physical Mobility

RELATED FACTORS

Motor weakness
Tremors
Spasticity

DEFINING CHARACTERISTICS

Unsteady gait
Limited ROM
Lack of coordination
Inability to move purposefully
Reluctance to attempt movement

EXPECTED OUTCOMES

Patient uses adaptive techniques to maximize mobility.
Patient verbalizes ability to move appropriately within limits of disease.

ONGOING ASSESSMENT

- Assess patient's girth, muscle strength, weakness, coordination, and balance. *There may be periods of remission during early course of disease.*
- Inquire about falls, use of assistive devices, and decrease in muscle strength.
- Inquire about prior use of adaptive techniques/devices.
- Assess endurance level and stamina (e.g., how many stairs can climb; how far can walk).

THERAPEUTIC INTERVENTIONS

- Encourage ambulation with assistance/supervision *to keep patient as functionally active as feasible.*
- Encourage self-care as tolerated; assist when necessary; avoid rushing patient.
- Place belongings within reach.
- Schedule rest periods *to decrease fatigue.*
- ▲ Consult physical therapist and occupational therapist *for use of assistive/ambulatory devices and ADL evaluation.*
- Use adaptive techniques and equipment with patient. These may include: wrist weight, use of proximal rather than upper extremities, adaptive equipment such as stabilized plates and nonspilling cups, stabilization of extremity and training of patient to use trunk and head to compensate for impaired function.
- Encourage stretching exercises daily. Assist with ROM.
- ▲ Administer antispasmodics as prescribed. *May be required if spasticity is a problem.*

High Risk for Sensory Perceptual Alterations: Visual

RISK FACTOR

Optic nerve demyelination

EXPECTED OUTCOME

Patient uses adaptive techniques to cope with visual impairment.

ONGOING ASSESSMENT

- Assess for visual impairment. *Common symptoms include diplopia, blurred vision, nystagmus, visual loss, scotomas (blind spots).*
- Assess patient's ability to perform ADL.

THERAPEUTIC INTERVENTIONS

- Orient patient to environment as appropriate.
- Place objects within reach.
- Provide eyepatch for diplopia; encourage alternating patch from eye to eye.
- Instruct patient to rest eyes when fatigued.
- Advise of availability of large-type reading materials and talking books.
- Place call light within reach with side rails up and bed in low position *to prevent injury.*
- Place sign over the bed; indicate visual impairment in chart.
- See also Visual impairment, p. 56.

Continued.

NURSING DIAGNOSES	EXPECTED OUTCOMES AND NURSING INTERVENTIONS / *RATIONALE* (■ = INDEPENDENT; ▲ = COLLABORATIVE)

High Risk for Altered Pattern of Elimination: Urinary Retention/ Frequency

RISK FACTORS
Neurogenic bladder

EXPECTED OUTCOMES
Patient maintains urine output of ~ 30 ml/hr.
Patient maintains residual urine of < 100 ml/hr.
Patient does not experience urinary tract infection.

ONGOING ASSESSMENT
- Inquire about symptoms of urinary retention, abdominal distention, frequency, urgency, pain. *Patients may experience either a spastic bladder characterized by frequency, dribbling, or a flaccid bladder, in which an absence of sensation to void results in urine retention.*
- Assess for signs of urinary tract infection. *Retention predisposes to infection.*

THERAPEUTIC INTERVENTIONS
- Measure urine output; catheterize for residual urine as indicated. *Note: Residual urine > 100 ml predisposes patient to urinary tract infections.*
- Initiate individualized bladder training program; instruct patient about Credé method, intermittent catheterization, signs and symptoms of urinary tract infection, time of voiding.
- ▲ Administer medications as prescribed. *Cholinergic drugs are indicated for flaccid bladder, and anticholinergic for spastic bladder.*
- Recommend vitamin C and liberal intake of cranberry juice *to acidify urine and reduce bacterial growth.*
- See also Urinary retention, p. 74; Urinary incontinence, p. 71.

High Risk for Impaired Skin Integrity

RISK FACTORS
Sensory changes, immobility

EXPECTED OUTCOME
Patient maintains intact skin as evidenced by absence of breakdown, burns, or decubitus formation.

ONGOING ASSESSMENT
- Assess skin integrity. *Sensory changes may result in hypoalgesia, paresthesia, and loss of position sense, which can lead to trauma, injury, and skin integrity changes.*
- Inquire about areas of body with decreased sensation.

THERAPEUTIC INTERVENTIONS
- Avoid heat, cold, and pressure.
- Instruct patient to test bath water with unaffected extremity.
- Instruct patient to notice foot placement when ambulating *to compensate for decreased position sense.*
- Instruct to change position q2h.
- See also Potential impaired skin integrity, p. 59.

Body Image Disturbance

RELATED FACTORS
Physical and psychosocial changes
Negative feelings about self
Negative feelings about body
Change in social involvement
Feelings of hopelessness, powerlessness

DEFINING CHARACTERISTICS
Poor eye contact
Refusal to participate in care/ treatment

EXPECTED OUTCOMES
Patient verbalizes positive coping mechanisms.
Patient expresses positive attitude about self.

ONGOING ASSESSMENT
- Assess quality and quantity of verbalizations about body and self-image.
- Observe for changes in behavior and/or level of functioning. *Persons with muscular sclerosis may also experience depression, anger, and emotional lability.*
- Inquire about coping skills used before illness.

THERAPEUTIC INTERVENTIONS
- Make frequent, unhurried patient contact.
- Provide opportunity to ask questions and talk about feelings. *Verbalization provides an outlet for concerns.*
- Include patient in care planning. *May foster positive self-concept/body image.*
- Support patient's efforts to maintain independence.
- ▲ Use referral sources (e.g., liaison psychiatry service) when appropriate *to facilitate patient's attempts at coping.*
- Refer to support group. *Groups that come together for mutual goals and information exchange can provide valuable education and emotional support.*

| NURSING DIAGNOSES | EXPECTED OUTCOMES AND NURSING INTERVENTIONS / *RATIONALE*
(■ = INDEPENDENT; ▲ = COLLABORATIVE) |

Knowledge Deficit

RELATED FACTOR

Unfamiliarity with the disease process and management

DEFINING CHARACTERISTICS

Verbalization of misconceptions

Questioning

Noncompliance

EXPECTED OUTCOME

Patient/significant others discuss disease process, medications used, adverse effects, follow-up care.

ONGOING ASSESSMENT

- Assess knowledge of disease, exacerbations, remissions, medical regimen, resources.

THERAPEUTIC INTERVENTIONS

- Discuss disease process in simple, straightforward manner:

  MS is a chronic, slowly progressive nervous system disease that affects nerve conduction.

  There is no definitive diagnostic test.

  There is no specific cure.

  It can result in weakness, visual disturbance, walking unsteadiness, and sometimes urine or bowel problem.

- Instruct patient/significant others when to contact health team (e.g., urinary symptoms; exacerbations; motor, sensory, visual disturbances).

- Instruct patient/significant others about steroid therapy (*decreases edema and acute inflammatory response within evolving plaque):*

  Side effects (e.g., sodium retention, fluid retention, pedal edema, hypertension, gastric irritation).

  Measures to control side effects (e.g., low-sodium diet, daily weighing, leg elevation, support hose, blood pressure monitoring, antacids, adequate rest, and avoidance of contact with persons with infectious disease).

- Instruct of:

  Importance of maintaining most normal activity level possible *to maintain functional limits and body image.*

  Avoidance of hot baths (*increase metabolic demands and may increase weakness).*

  Sleeping in a prone position *to decrease flexion spasms.*

  Need to inspect areas of impaired sensation for serious injuries.

  Need to use energy conservation techniques.

- Instruct to avoid potentially exacerbating activities: emotional stress, physical stress/fatigue, infection, pregnancy, physically "run down" condition.

See also.

Self-care deficit, p. 53.

Constipation, p. 16.

Powerlessness, p. 52.

Anticipatory grieving, p. 28.

Altered sexuality patterns, p. 58.

By: Linda Arsenault, RN, MSN, CNRN

Myasthenia gravis: acute phase

(MYASTHENIC CRISIS; CHOLINERGIC CRISIS)

Myasthenia gravis is a chronic autoimmune disease of the neuro-muscular junction. It is characterized by motor muscle weakness that is aggravated by repetitive activity and is improved with rest and/or administration of anticholinesterase agents. The muscles most frequently affected are the oculomotor (affecting eye movements and lid elevation), facial, pharyngeal and laryngeal and muscles of the neck, shoulders, and limb. Although symptoms may vary in severity from person to person, disruptions can occur in vision, facial appearance, walking, talking, and swallowing. Myasthenia gravis is more common in women of childbearing age, and in men during or after the fifth decade of life. The goal of treatment is to induce remission if possible and/or to control the muscle weakness with anticholinesterase agents. Thymectomy may be performed early in the disease to eliminate the possibility that antiacetylcholine antibodies will be produced in the thymus gland. Chemical immunosuppression to decrease antibody binding to acetylcholine receptor sites at the muscular endplate is also used (prednisone, imuran, cyclosporine).

NURSING DIAGNOSES	EXPECTED OUTCOMES AND NURSING INTERVENTIONS / *RATIONALE* (■ = INDEPENDENT; ▲ = COLLABORATIVE)

High Risk for Aspiration

RISK FACTORS

Facial, pharyngeal, laryngeal, respiratory muscle weakness

EXPECTED OUTCOMES

Patient swallows food/fluids without choking.
Patient maintains clear lungs and avoids aspiration.

ONGOING ASSESSMENT

- Ask the patient about prior episodes of/problems with choking, nasal regurgitation of foods or fluids, difficulty swallowing foods or fluids.
- Assess mental status. *If the patient is inattentive, swallowing problems are an increased possibility.*
- Assess for signs of a facial droop, drooling, weak or hoarse voice. *Some patients will not show signs of choking or aspiration acutely; however, if any of these signs are present, a formal swallowing evaluation would be prudent.*
- Assess ability to clench jaw and tighten facial muscles, frown, smile, whistle, raise eyebrows, wrinkle forehead, and close eyes. Also evaluate whether able to shrug shoulders, turn chin to the side against your hand, stick out tongue, and move tongue side to side. *All of these functions reflect integrity of cranial nerves V, VII, IX, X, and XII and are important for swallowing.*
- Assess oral secretions for color, amount, consistency. *Patients with thick tenacious secretions are at increased risk for choking.*
- Assess respiratory rate and rhythm.
- Monitor breath sounds for rales, rhonchi, and decreased/absent breath sounds.

THERAPEUTIC INTERVENTIONS

- Try to plan for a period of 20-30 min of rest before meals. *These patients tire very easily.*
- Coordinate patient's meals with peak drug action. *For example, neostigmine (Prostigmine) given 40-60 min before meals will provide peak action over the mealtime.*
- Sit the patient upright in a chair or bed for meals or when giving any oral agent.
- Try to eliminate any distractions. *For example, keep conversations at a minimum because the same muscles are used for talking and eating.*
- Supervise the patient closely; avoid rushing.
- Encourage the patient to concentrate on swallowing.
- Give small amounts of food at one time and allow time to swallow 2-3 times.
- ▲ Consult the dietitian for help in meal planning. *Semisolid foods like custard, scrambled eggs are easier to swallow than sticky mucus-forming foods such as peanut butter, chocolate, white bread.*
- ▲ Consult occupational therapist if built-up lightweight utensils are needed for eating.
- Keep patient's head up with the neck bent slightly forward.
- Keep patient upright for 30-60 min after meals *to reduce risk of aspiration.*
- Keep suction equipment at bedside and suction patient as needed.

High Risk for Impaired Gas Exchange

Risk Factor

Respiratory failure secondary to myasthenic or cholinergic crisis

Expected Outcome

Patient maintains adequate gas exchange, as evidenced by normal heart rate, ABGs within normal range, $Po_2 > 80$ mm Hg, $Pco_2 < 45$ mm Hg.

Ongoing Assessment

- Inquire about medication regimen: medications, dose, time last taken.
- Inquire about recent stress, menses, URI. *All of these can increase symptoms and may necessitate a slight increase in drug dosage.*
- Assess respiratory rate/rhythm, breath sounds.
- ▲ Monitor oxygen saturation/ABGs as indicated.
- ▲ Monitor vital capacity serially. *Weakness of the diaphragm and intercostal muscles reduces vital capacity. If below 18 ml/kg body weight, intubation and ventilatory support may be indicated.*
- Monitor for increased muscle weakness, twitching muscle groups (fasciculations). *They may be most noticeable around the mouth.*
- Monitor for mental status changes. *They may reflect inadequate oxygen delivery to the brain.*

Therapeutic Interventions

- Position patient with HOB elevated *to facilitate breathing. Weakness of the neck muscles may prevent patient from elevating head.*
- Suction as needed.
- ▲ Provide supplementary oxygen as needed.
- Instruct patient in deep breathing and coughing exercises if feasible, especially after taking medication, when the muscles are stronger.
- Avoid unnecessary activities that may increase fatigue.
- Have intubation equipment available. *Respiratory distress may occur rapidly.*
- ▲ Assist physician in the event a Tensilon test is performed to differentiate state/cause of crisis. *If the patient is in myasthenic crisis, the response should be an increase in strength. If the patient is in cholinergic crisis, he or she may become suddenly worse and need respiratory resuscitation.*

High Risk for Impaired Verbal Communication

Risk Factors

Muscle weakness, tracheal intubation

Expected Outcome

Patient communicates his/her needs adequately by verbal/alternative means.

Ongoing Assessment

- Assess ability to communicate verbally.
- Assess ability to use alternative method of communication.

Therapeutic Interventions

- Have some form of communication system for patients with severe dysarthria and/or tracheal tubes (e.g., paper, pencil; letter, number, picture board; blinking of eyes to indicate yes/no). *This will help alleviate anxiety related to inability to communicate verbally.*
- Encourage patient who is able to speak to ventilate his/her feelings.
- Have call light readily available at all times.
- Explain all procedures to patient beforehand.
- If patient is intubated, explain reason for ventilator alarms (*one of patients' major fears is malfunctioning ventilator*).
- Reassure patient with endotracheal intubation that he/she will be able to speak after extubation. *Patient needs to know inability to communicate verbally is temporary, caused by endotracheal tube's passing through vocal cords.*
- See also Impaired verbal communication, p. 14.

Continued.

NURSING DIAGNOSES	EXPECTED OUTCOMES AND NURSING INTERVENTIONS / *RATIONALE* (■ = INDEPENDENT; ▲ = COLLABORATIVE)

High Risk for Altered Nutrition: Less than Body Requirements

RISK FACTORS

Inability to swallow or chew because of weakness of bulbar muscles

Lack of appetite resulting from side effects of anticholinesterase medications (i.e., abdominal cramping, nausea, vomiting, and diarrhea)

EXPECTED OUTCOME

Patient maintains optimal nutritional status, as evidenced by weight gain, adequate oral intake.

ONGOING ASSESSMENT

- Assess patient's ability to swallow and chew. *These patients are at risk for aspiration.*
- Assess for presence of nausea, vomiting, abdominal cramping, or diarrhea.

THERAPEUTIC INTERVENTIONS

- Withhold meal if swallowing is impaired. Plan meal around peak action of medication (usually 1 hr after dose). *Anticholinesterase medications improve neuromuscular transmission, thereby increasing muscle strength. Chance of aspiration is lessened by giving meals during peak medication action.*
- Give atropine or anticholinergic drug (i.e., Donnatal) as prescribed *to decrease side effects of anticholinesterase medication (be aware that anticholinergic drugs can mask symptoms of overdosage and therefore precipitate cholinergic crisis).*
- Instruct patient in side effects of anticholinesterase: diarrhea, urinary frequency, abdominal cramps, muscle twitching/fasciculations, insomnia, sweating, increased salivation, muscle spasms, nausea, irritability.
- Instruct patient of side effects of prednisone: weight gain, increased appetite, GI distress, swelling in ankles/feet, depression, hypokalemia, acne.
- Encourage patient to eat well-balanced diet when possible and space meals during periods of optimal muscular strength.
- Assist patient to sit upright.
- Reduce distractions *to decrease risk of aspiration.*
- Instruct patient to report significant changes in swallowing ability *to enable early detection of difficulties and prevent aspiration.*
- If patient is intubated or unable to swallow effectively, prepare to feed patient via nasogastric tube. See also Altered nutrition: less than body requirements, p. 44; Enteral tube feeding, p. 303.

Knowledge Deficit

RELATED FACTORS

Unfamiliarity with disease process, treatment

DEFINING CHARACTERISTICS

Multiple questions
Lack of questions
Misconceptions

EXPECTED OUTCOMES

Patient verbalizes understanding of disease process, cholinergic/myasthenic crisis, precipitating factors, medication regimen, and possible side effects.

ONGOING ASSESSMENT

- Assess knowledge of disease progress and treatment regimen.

THERAPEUTIC INTERVENTIONS

- Provide information on cause of disease, course of disease. *Varies, may have short remissions or severe involvement. Muscle weakness may be so severe that patient needs assistance with breathing.*
- Discuss diagnostic methods: EMG, Tensilon test.
- Discuss possible treatment regimens:
    - Anticholinesterase drugs.
    - Corticosteroids.
    - Nonsteroidal immunosuppressants.
    - Plasmapheresis: *To remove antiacetylcholine antibodies in plasma from circulatory system. Exchanges may be performed for crisis Rx/prevention, or may be done on a more regular basis.*
    - Surgery to remove thymoma: *to induce remission since it is thought that antiach antibodies are present in the thymus gland. Remission rates vary from <20% to 50%.*
- Instruct patient in difference between cholinergic and myasthenic crisis:
    - Cholinergic *(caused by excess medication):* increased muscle weakness; fasciculations, especially around mouth and eyes; diarrhea/cramping; sweating; increased salivation/drooling.
    - Myasthenic *(caused by insufficient/ineffective medication):* increased muscle weakness, anxiety/apprehension, shortness of breath.
- Teach patient factors precipitating crisis and ways to avoid them: stress, change in medication schedule, skipping medication, alcohol intake, inadequate sleep.
- Instruct in signs and symptoms of pending or recurring pulmonary problems and ways to avoid precipitating factors (e.g., avoiding those with upper respiratory infection/smokers).

NURSING DIAGNOSES	EXPECTED OUTCOMES AND NURSING INTERVENTIONS / *RATIONALE* (■ = INDEPENDENT; ▲ = COLLABORATIVE)

THERAPEUTIC INTERVENTIONS—cont'd

- Instruct patient to avoid drugs that could cause problems: quinidine, mycinantibiotics, procainamide, quinine, phenothiazides, barbiturates, tranquilizers, narcotics, alcohol *(may precipitate crisis).*
- Discuss possible side effects of anticholinesterase agents (see preceding list).
- Aid patient in identifying/documenting for own use those situations that may aggravate side effects of anticholinesterase agents: taking on empty stomach, concomitent use of alcohol, hot weather.
- Teach importance of adjusting dose as symptoms of weakness vary.
- Instruct to take medications on time. *Delay may cause muscle weakness, which impedes swallowing of medications.*
- Teach to prioritize activities/pace self. Instruct in energy conservation principles.
- Instruct to wear Medic-Alert tag.
- Evaluate whether patient should live alone. *Respiratory distress can be a life-threatening complication.*
- Recommend referral to Myasthenia Gravis Foundation for educational materials/ information.
- Refer to support group.

See also:
Activity intolerance, p. 2.
Impaired physical mobility,
  p. 47.
Impaired coping, p. 18.
Body image disturbance,
  p. 7.
Self-care deficit, p. 53.
Sensory/perceptual alteration:
  visual, p. 56.

By: Linda Arsenault, RN, MSN, CNRN

Parkinsonism

(PARALYSIS AGITANS)

Is a movement disorder associated with dopamine deficiency in the brain. Other neurotransmitter alterations may also contribute to the disease process. This chronic neurologic disorder affects the extrapyramidal system of the brain responsible for control/ regulation of movement. The clinical manifestations are tremor at rest, rigidity, slowness of movement, bent posture, shuffling gait, masklike facial expressions, and muscle weakness affecting writing, speaking, eating, chewing, and swallowing.

NURSING DIAGNOSES	EXPECTED OUTCOMES AND NURSING INTERVENTIONS / *RATIONALE* (■ = INDEPENDENT; ▲ = COLLABORATIVE)

Impaired Physical Mobility

RELATED FACTORS

Neuromuscular impairment,
  decreased strength and endurance

DEFINING CHARACTERISTICS

Tremors
Muscle rigidity
Decreased ability to initiate
  movements (akinesis)
Impaired coordination of
  movement
Limited ROM
Impaired ability to carry out
  ADL
Postural disturbances

EXPECTED OUTCOMES

Patient achieves optimal level of functioning.

ONGOING ASSESSMENT

- Evaluate baseline activity level.
- Assess tremors. *Typically they are more prominent at rest and are aggravated by emotional stress.*
- Assess posture, coordination, and movements. *Clinical manifestations may range from only a slight limp to the typical shuffling, propulsive gait with rigidity.*
- Assess adaptions to impaired mobility.

THERAPEUTIC INTERVENTIONS

- Allow sufficient time for ADL. *Nursing staff/family frequently want to perform task rather than enable patient to do it.*
- Encourage ROM to all joints twice daily.
- Supervise and assist with ambulation. *Activity is important to reduce hazards of immobility.*

Continued.

NURSING DIAGNOSES	EXPECTED OUTCOMES AND NURSING INTERVENTIONS / *RATIONALE* (■ = INDEPENDENT; ▲ = COLLABORATIVE)
	THERAPEUTIC INTERVENTIONS—cont'd • Encourage patient to lift feet and take large steps while walking *to improve balance and minimize shuffling. A broad-based gait helps improve balance.* ▲ Consult physical and occupational therapists about aids *to facilitate ADL and safe ambulation, and promote muscle strengthening.* • Remove environmental barriers. • Provide tips for getting in and out of chair.
Impaired Verbal Communication **RELATED FACTOR** Dysarthria **DEFINING CHARACTERISTICS** Difficulty in articulating words Monotonous voice tones Slow, slurred speech Stammered speech	**EXPECTED OUTCOMES** Patient communicates needs adequately. Patient uses alternative methods of communication as indicated. **ONGOING ASSESSMENT** • Evaluate ability to communicate and understand spoken words. • Assess ability to write/understand written words/pictures. **THERAPEUTIC INTERVENTIONS** • Place call light and other articles (tissues, water, glasses) within reach. • Maintain eye contact when speaking *(promotes focus and attention and encourages patient).* • Allow patient time to articulate. • Encourage face and tongue exercises *to reduce rigidity.* • Avoid speaking loudly unless patient is deaf. ▲ Consult speech therapist if indicated. • Encourage patient to practice reading aloud. • Provide alternative communication aids as needed.
Altered Nutrition: Less than Body Requirements **RELATED FACTORS** Difficulty swallowing Choking spells Drooling Regurgitation of food/fluids through nares **DEFINING CHARACTERISTICS** Documented intake below required caloric level Weight loss	**EXPECTED OUTCOMES** Patient maintains optimal nutritional status, as evidenced by weight gain, adequate oral intake. **ONGOING ASSESSMENT** • Assess degree of swallowing difficulty (fluids, solids, medications). • Inquire about episodes of choking/nasal regurgitations. • Assess nutritional status. • Weigh patient three times per week. • Monitor I & O. **THERAPEUTIC INTERVENTIONS** • Place patient in a high Fowler's position for eating and drinking. • Supervise patient during meals. Avoid distractions *to help patient focus on swallowing.* • *Allow time for meals; avoid rushing patient to avoid frustration.* Offer high-calorie, low-volume supplements between meals *to provide additional caloric intake.* • Offer small bites of food, *which may be easier to swallow.* Encourage patient to swallow 2-3 times after taking a bite of food. • Provide thickened rather than watery fluids/food. ▲ Consult dietitian for needed changes in food consistency and for caloric counts. • Assist with oral hygiene after meals. ▲ Consult the speech therapist to evaluate swallowing.
High Risk for Urinary Incontinence **RISK FACTORS** Inability to get to bathroom in time secondary to gait disturbance	**EXPECTED OUTCOMES** Patient voids at regular intervals. Patient will be continent of urine. **ONGOING ASSESSMENT** • Evaluate previous pattern of voiding. Evaluate intervals between voiding. • Assess amount, frequency, character, color, odor, specific gravity. • Evaluate current medications that may contribute to urinary problems. • Evaluate I & O.

NURSING DIAGNOSES	EXPECTED OUTCOMES AND NURSING INTERVENTIONS / *RATIONALE* (■ = INDEPENDENT; ▲ = COLLABORATIVE)

THERAPEUTIC INTERVENTIONS

- Place bedpan/urinal/bedside commode within reach.
- Assist patient in identifying regular intervals to go to bathroom, and assist to do so.
- Decrease fluid intake after 6 p.m. *to reduce need for frequent nighttime urination.*
- ▲ Institute intermittent catheterization or Foley catheter as indicated.

Self-esteem Disturbance

RELATED FACTORS

Changes in body image, dependence

DEFINING CHARACTERISTICS

Minimal eye contact
Self-deprecating statements
Anger
Expression of shame
Rejection of positive feedback

EXPECTED OUTCOME

Patient recognizes self-maligning statements and begins to verbalize positive expression of self-worth.

ONGOING ASSESSMENT

- Assess perception of self. Note verbalizations regarding self.
- Assess degree to which patient feels loved and respected by others.
- Evaluate support system.

THERAPEUTIC INTERVENTIONS

- Encourage patient to verbalize fears and concerns. Listen attentively *to facilitate development of trust.*
- Discuss feelings about symptoms: tremors, drooling of saliva, slurred speech.
- Discuss "normal" impact of alteration in health status on self-esteem. *Use of lay support groups/individuals may help patient to recognize positives even in face of disease.*
- Explore strengths and resources with patient.
- Advise of realistic need for additional support in coping with lifelong illness.
- Avoid overprotection of individual; promote social interaction as appropriate.
- Clarify patient's misconceptions and provide accurate information.
- Provide privacy as needed, especially when performing ADL, eating.
- Teach patient necessary self-care measures related to disease. *Each success will reinforce positive self-esteem.*
- Teach patient the harmful effects of negative talk about self.

Knowledge Deficit

RELATED FACTOR

Uncertainty about cause of disease and its treatment

DEFINING CHARACTERISTICS

Multiple questions
Lack of questions
Apparent confusion over condition

EXPECTED OUTCOME

Patient/significant others verbalize disability and special needs with regard to disease process, activity, exercises, ambulation, medication, diet, and elimination.

ONGOING ASSESSMENT

- Evaluate patient's/significant others' understanding of disease process, diagnostic tests, treatments, and outcomes.

THERAPEUTIC INTERVENTIONS

- Reinforce explanation of disease and treatment:
  Disease: has a gradual onset, progresses gradually, has no known cure.
  Treatment: therapy aimed at relieving symptoms and preventing complications.
- Encourage independence and avoid overprotection by permitting patient to do things for self: self-care, feeding, dressing, ambulation.
- Discuss with patient, family/significant others:
  Medication:
  Potential side effects of common medications:

Medications	Potential Side Effects
Anticholinergics	
Artane	constipation
Cogentin	dry mouth
Kemadrin	confusion
Parsidol	blurred vision
Antihistamines	lethargy
	dry mouth
	confusion
	sleepiness
Dopaminergics	
Symmetrel	edema in legs
Sinemet	nausea
	dystonia
Dopamine Agonists	
Parlodel	orthostatic hypotension
Permax	confusion
	nausea
	insomnia

Continued.

NURSING DIAGNOSES	EXPECTED OUTCOMES AND NURSING INTERVENTIONS / *RATIONALE* (■ = INDEPENDENT; ▲ = COLLABORATIVE)

THERAPEUTIC INTERVENTIONS—cont'd

Medications (especially Sinemet) should generally be taken 20-30 min before meals.

For patients taking levodopa, high-protein foods such as milk, meat, fish, cheese, eggs, peanuts, grains, and soybeans should be limited. *They delay absorption of medication.*

Diet:

A high-caloric, soft diet, is recommended.

Finger food is easier for patient to manage independently.

Utensils should be within easy reach.

Use blender for thick foods.

Use brace for severe tremors occurring during meals.

Maintain 2000-ml/day liquid intake.

Offer frequent small feedings.

Use straws and bibs for excessive drooling.

Instruct patient to swallow slowly and take small bites of food.

Activity:

Plan rest periods.

Encourage passive and active ROM exercises to all extremities.

Encourage family/significant others to participate in physical therapy exercises of stretching and massaging muscles.

Encourage daily ambulation outdoors but avoidance of extreme hot and cold weather.

Encourage patient to practice lifting feet while walking, using heel-toe gait, and swinging deliberately while walking. *A wide base of support is best for balance.*

Avoid sitting for long periods. *Stiffness may occur.*

Encourage patient to dress daily, avoid clothing with buttons (use zippers or Velcro instead) and shoes with laces or snaps or Velcro.

Offer diversional activities depending on extent of tremors and disability: read, watch television, hobbies.

Prevent falls by clearing walkways of furniture and throw rugs and provide side rails on stairs.

Speech therapy:

Instruct patient to speak slowly and practice reading aloud in an exaggerated manner.

Oral hygiene: Perform q2-4h and prn *(especially if drooling)* and have tissues accessible to patient.

Elimination:

Institute voiding measures as needed.

Institute bladder control program as needed.

Raise toilet seats with side rails at home *to facilitate sitting or standing.*

Avoid constipation; encourage fluids, use of natural laxatives (prune juices and roughage) and stool softeners as needed.

See also:

Constipation, p. 16.
Diarrhea, p. 19.
Self-care deficit, p. 53.
Activity intolerance, p. 2.
High risk for aspiration, p. 6
Caregiver role strain, p. 13.

By: Marian D. Cachero-Salavrakos, RN, BSN
Linda Arsenault, RN, MSN, CNRN

Seizure activity/status epilepticus

(CONVULSION; EPILEPSY; SEIZURE DISORDER)

A seizure is an occasional, excessive disorderly discharge of neuronal activity. Recurrent seizures (epilepsy) may be classified as partial, generalized, or partial complex. Status epilepticus is characterized by recurrent seizures that fail to allow recovery from previous seizure and in which the level of consciousness is not regained, or a series of seizures that last longer than 30 minutes. Status epilepticus is a medical emergency, with mortality ranging from 6% to 30% and high morbidity, both of which are duration dependent; therefore, prompt intervention is imperative. Factors that contribute to high morbidity are hypoxia, fractures, aspiration, cardiac dysrhythmias, and acidosis.

NURSING DIAGNOSES	EXPECTED OUTCOMES AND NURSING INTERVENTIONS / *RATIONALE* (■ = INDEPENDENT; ▲ = COLLABORATIVE)

High Risk for Injury

RISK FACTORS

Seizure activity
Postictal state
Altered level of consciousness
Impaired judgment

DEFINING CHARACTERISTICS

Increased rhythmic motor activity—jerking of arms and legs
Repetitive psychomotor activity
Tonic-clonic movements
Change in alertness, orientation, verbal response, eye opening, motor response
Aspiration of oral secretions

EXPECTED OUTCOMES

Risk for physical injury is reduced, as evidenced by maintenance of seizure precautions/appropriate interventions.

ONGOING ASSESSMENT

- Assess frequency, duration, and type of seizure activity.
- Inquire about warnings before seizure (e.g., aura).
- Note the following: change in LOC preceding seizure activity, where seizure started, epileptic cry, automatism, length of seizure, head and eye turning, pupillary reaction, associated falls, oral secretions, urinary or fecal incontinence, cyanosis, postictal state, any postseizure focal abnormality (e.g., Todd's paralysis).
- Document observations and frequency of seizures; notify physician as indicated.

THERAPEUTIC INTERVENTIONS

- Roll patient to side after cessation of muscle twitching *to prevent aspiration.*
- If patient is in bed: pad side rails and keep up; remove sharp objects from bed; keep bed in low position.
- If patient is on floor, remove furniture or other potentially harmful objects from area.
- Do not restrain. *Physical restraint applied during seizure activity can cause pathogenic trauma.*
- Allow patient to have seizure. Do *not* place tongue blade or other objects in mouth. *Often inserting objects will cause more harm, such as dislodging teeth, causing lacerations, and obstructing airway.*
- If airway is occluded, open airway, then insert oral airway.
- ▲ Administer anticonvulsants as prescribed.
- Keep suction equipment and oxygen available for high-risk/seizure-prone patients.

Impaired Gas Exchange

RELATED FACTORS

Aspiration related to prolonged seizure activity
Hypoxia during seizure activity
Hypoventilation secondary to prolonged muscle contraction

DEFINING CHARACTERISTICS

Increased secretions
Grunting
Tachypnea
Irregular respirations
Choking
Dyspnea
Cyanosis
Hypoxia
Hypercapnea
Restlessness

EXPECTED OUTCOMES

Patient maintains adequate ventilation and oxygenation as evidenced by normal ABGs, clear breath sounds, regular respiration.

ONGOING ASSESSMENT

- Assess respirations during and after seizure activity.
- Monitor for presence of any of the defining characteristics during and after seizure activity.
- Monitor breath sounds hourly as indicated.
- Monitor closely during administration of medications to halt seizures. *Most common side effects are depressed respirations, apnea, hypotension. The combination of prolonged seizure activity and administration of medications intravenously to stop them may precipitate sudden respiratory failure and necessitate rapid intubation.*
- ▲ Monitor arterial blood gases as indicated.
- ▲ Monitor ECG as needed.

Continued.

Seizure activity/status epilepticus—cont'd

NURSING DIAGNOSES	EXPECTED OUTCOMES AND NURSING INTERVENTIONS / *RATIONALE* (■ = INDEPENDENT; ▲ = COLLABORATIVE)

THERAPEUTIC INTERVENTIONS

▲ During seizure:
  Stay with the patient.
  Loosen clothing.
  Try to roll onto a side-lying position *to facilitate drainage of secretions.*
  Administer oxygen if necessary.
  Suction as indicated.
  Assist with intubation.
  Apply pulse oximeter if possible.

▲ Administer medications to stop seizures as prescribed. The following medications are generally used:
  Lorazepam (Ativan) 0.05 mg/kg IV over 2 min; may be repeated every 2-3 min × 3 doses total.
  Diazepam (Valium) 0.2-0.5 mg/kg/dose/min with maximum 10 mg.
  Simultaneous administration of phenytoin (Dilantin): 18 mg/kg at no faster than 50 mg/min in saline solution. *Dilantin will precipitate in any dextrose solution.*
  Alternate medication to phenytoin is phenobarbital 5-10 mg/kg q20-30min to maximum dose of 30-40 mg/kg.
  If seizures persist, anticipate need for a general inhalation anesthetic agent.
  Additional medications that may be used: lidocaine, valproic acid, and carbamazepine (Tegretol).

▪ See also Potential for aspiration, p. 6.

Altered Tissue Perfusion: Cerebral

RELATED FACTORS

Cerebral hypoxia secondary to prolonged seizure activity
Cerebral edema

DEFINING CHARACTERISTICS

Impaired LOC
Confusion, disorientation
Impaired memory, judgment, speech
Glasgow Coma Scale < 11
Motor-sensory impairment
Incontinence
Pupillary asymmetry, dilation, decreased light activity
Gaze preference

EXPECTED OUTCOMES

Patient maintains optimal cerebral perfusion, as evidenced by GCS > 13, alertness, appropriate speech, pupils equal and reactive to light.

ONGOING ASSESSMENT

▪ Once seizure has ceased, assess for level of orientation; memory, judgment; speech appropriateness; motor-sensory integrity; incontinence; Glasgow Coma Scale; pupillary size, reaction to light.
▪ Monitor for signs of cyanosis, emesis, respiratory difficulties.
▲ Monitor arterial blood gases.

THERAPEUTIC INTERVENTIONS

▪ Remain with patient.
▪ Turn onto side with head down *to promote drainage of secretions and maintain open airway.*
▪ Remove restrictive clothing.
▪ Support head.
▪ Suction as needed.
▲ Provide oxygen as indicated.

NURSING DIAGNOSES	EXPECTED OUTCOMES AND NURSING INTERVENTIONS / *RATIONALE* (■ = INDEPENDENT; ▲ = COLLABORATIVE)
High Risk for Disturbance in Self-Concept **RISK FACTORS** Seizure activity, dependence on medications	**EXPECTED OUTCOMES** Patient verbalizes some positive statements about self in relation to living with seizure disorder. **ONGOING ASSESSMENT** ▪ Assess feelings about self and disorder. ▪ Assess perceived implications of disorder and need for long-term therapy. **THERAPEUTIC INTERVENTIONS** ▪ Encourage ventilation of feelings. ▪ Incorporate family and significant others in care plan. *May be helpful in assisting/giving support.* ▪ Assist patient and others in understanding nature of disorder. ▪ Dispel common myths and fears about convulsive disorders. ▪ Refer to support group if possible. ▲ Consult social worker, psychologist as indicated.

Knowledge Deficit Regarding Symptoms, Causes, and Treatment
 	
RELATED FACTORS
Lack of exposure, information misinterpretation, unfamiliarity with information resources
 	
DEFINING CHARACTERISTICS
Verbalization of problem
Inappropriate or exaggerated behavior
Request for information
Statement of misconception
	EXPECTED OUTCOMES
	Patient discusses the disease process, treatment, and safety measures.
	
	ONGOING ASSESSMENT
	▪ Assess knowledge concerning disorder and treatment.
	▪ Assess readiness for learning, *so that information is presented at a time when comprehension will be optimal.*
	▪ Evaluate barriers that may interfere with patient's ability to obtain medication/return for follow-up check-ups.
	
	THERAPEUTIC INTERVENTIONS
	▪ Discuss disease process.
	▪ Review need for medication and schedule: right medication at right time and dosage, drug levels, danger of seizure activity with abrupt withdrawal, possible side effects and interactions of medication.
	▪ Discuss need for periodic check on anticonvulsant blood levels and possibly CBC. Instruct patient to discuss frequency/time intervals with physician.
	▪ Educate about safety measures:
	    Driving *(laws vary state to state: must be seizure free for 6 mo to 2 yr in most states).*
	    Home safety.
	    Climbing, e.g., on ladders.
	    Construction work.
	    Diving/swimming with companion.
	    Effect of alcohol/drugs. *There is an increased risk of seizures produced by interaction with anticonvulsants.*
	    Medic-Alert tag.
	▪ Refer to Epilepsy Foundation of America, Landover, MD 20785.

See also: High risk for impaired home maintenance management, p. 34.	

By: Linda Arsenault, RN, MSN, CNRN

Spinal cord injury (SCI)

Damage to the spinal cord from C1 to L1-2, where spinal cord ends. Injury may result in (a) concussion (transient loss of function), (b) complete cord lesion (no preservation of motor and sensory function below the level of injury; irreversible damage), (c) incomplete lesion (residual motor/sensory function below level of injury with some potential for improvement in function). Complete cord injury above C7 results in quadriplegia; from C7 to L1 causes paraplegia. Spinal shock follows complete SCI. It results in (a) total loss of all motor and sensory function below injury; (b) sympathetic disruption resulting in loss of vasoconstrictions and leaving parasympathetics unopposed, leading to bradycardia and hypotension; (c) loss of all reflexes below injury; (d) inability to control body temperature, secondary inability to sweat/shiver/vasoconstrict below level of injury; (e) ileus; (f) urinary retention. Shock persists for a variable duration, to be followed by a stage of spasticity. Primary causes of SCI are motor vehicle accidents (MVAs), followed by sporting accidents, falls, and penetrating injuries (gunshot/knife wounds). Approximately 10,000 new SCIs occur per year; about 80% occur in men < 40 years of age.

NURSING DIAGNOSES	EXPECTED OUTCOMES AND NURSING INTERVENTIONS / *RATIONALE* (■ = INDEPENDENT; ▲ = COLLABORATIVE)

High Risk for Inability to Sustain Spontaneous Ventilation

RISK FACTOR
High cervical SCI

EXPECTED OUTCOME
Patient maintains adequate ventilation, within limits, as evidenced by $Po_2 > 80$ Hg, $Pco_2 < 45$ mm Hg, O_2 saturation > 95%.

ONGOING ASSESSMENT
- Assess patient's ability to speak and swallow.
- Assess patient's ability to cough. *If patient has cervical–high thoracic cord injury, abdominal and intercostal muscle innervation will be absent/diminished and patient will be unable to take a deep breath and cough.*
- Monitor respiratory rate, depth, effort.
- Auscultate lungs and note breath sounds.
- ▲ Monitor serial ABGs: Po_2, Pco_2.
- ▲ Apply pulse oximeter to monitor O_2 saturation.
- Evaluate patient's ability to shrug shoulders and bend arms at elbow. *These muscles are innervated by C3-4 and C5-6, respectively. If impaired, phrenic nerve to diaphragm may be interrupted and patient will be at risk for apnea.*

THERAPEUTIC INTERVENTIONS
- ▲ Administer O_2 as needed.
- ▲ Assist with intubation if indicated. *Patients with high cervical cord injury (above C4-5) are at greatest risk. Blind nasotracheal intubation/fiberoptic endotracheal intubation without neck involvement will be performed.*
- Suction patient as needed.
- Avoid neck movement in positioning patient. *If patient has unstable fracture, important to prevent further injury and loss of function.*

Altered Systemic Tissue Perfusion

RELATED FACTOR
Neurogenic shock (traumatic sympathectomy) as a result of SCI

DEFINING CHARACTERISTICS
Bradycardia
Hypotension
Restlessness
Reduced peripheral pulses
Fluid overload

EXPECTED OUTCOME
Patient maintains heart rate of 60-100 beats/min and BP >90 mm Hg.

ONGOING ASSESSMENT
- Assess heart rate and BP closely. *Bradycardia and hypotension are common complications.*
- Monitor I & O. *Urine output should be ~0.5 ml/kg/hr.*
- ▲ Assess CVP. *Because of abnormal autonomic hemodynamics, overhydration may lead to pulmonary edema.*
- Assess mental status.
- Assess peripheral pulses, capillary refill.

NURSING DIAGNOSES	EXPECTED OUTCOMES AND NURSING INTERVENTIONS / *RATIONALE* (■ = INDEPENDENT; ▲ = COLLABORATIVE)

THERAPEUTIC INTERVENTIONS

▲ Administer IV fluids as ordered with attention to CVP/PA/PCWP.

▪ Keep patient immobilized.

▪ Avoid elevating HOB. *Because of sympathetic disruption and resultant loss of vasoconstrictor tone below the injury, head elevation will result in further drop of BP.*

▲ Administer pressors as ordered. *Dopamine is the usual agent of choice. Phenylephrine (which is noninotropic with possible reflex increase in vagal tone) should be avoided.*

▲ Apply MAST suit as ordered. *Helps to compensate for lost muscle tone and decreases venous pooling.*

▲ Insert Foley catheter. *Facilitates monitoring of I & O and prevents distention from urinary retention.*

High Risk for Injury: Impaired Neurologic Functioning

RISK FACTOR

Spinal Cord Injury

EXPECTED OUTCOMES

Patient's neurologic status is stabilized.

Early signs of deterioration are detected and treated appropriately.

ONGOING ASSESSMENT

▪ Inquire about history of present illness: mechanisms of injury, history of loss of consciousness, presence/absence of weakness in the arms/legs post trauma, numbness/tingling after injury.

▪ Assess for pain or tenderness in spine.

▪ Evaluate movement of major muscle groups in upper and lower extremities: at toes, ankles, knees, hips, fingers, elbows, and shoulders.

▪ Check for voluntary sphincter contraction and perianal sensation, *e g , sacral sparing.*

▪ Evaluate sensation to pinprick (spinothalamic tract). Start at toes and ascend gradually up to face. If sensation changes, mark skin. *Necessary to localize dermatome.*

▪ Assess light touch (anterior spinothalamic track). Start at toes and ascend as described.

▪ Check for proprioception (joint position sense that reflects posterior columns). Ask patient to close eyes. Use toes and fingers and move them up and down slowly to see whether patient can perceive motion.

▪ Evaluate deep tendon reflexes: biceps, triceps, knee, ankle.

▪ Serially monitor patient for any deviation from initial baseline exam findings, noting whether signs of complete versus incomplete injury. *If patient has a worsening deficit or higher evolving sensory deficit, additional studies such as MRI or myelography are indicated.*

> *Complete SCI:* above C7: quadriplegia, C7-T12/L1: paraplegia, total loss of sensation below level of injury, paralytic ileus, urinary retention, total loss of reflexes below lesion.

> *Incomplete SCI:* sacral sparing, variable loss of motor sensation below lesion, paresthesia, pain.

THERAPEUTIC INTERVENTIONS

▪ Apply a foam/egg crate–type mattress to bed before patient is placed in bed. If patient requires traction to stabilize/reduce fracture/subluxation, keep weights off floor and hanging free.

▪ Immobilize patient. Maintain in collar and on backboard *to prevent active/passive movements of the spine.*

▪ Once all studies are complete and patient is placed into bed, remove from backboard. *Early removal from board reduces potential for decubitus ulcer formation.*

▲ Insert nasogastric tube if appropriate *to prevent vomiting and aspiration; paralytic ileus after SCI is common.*

▲ Insert Foley urinary catheter *to allow accurate monitoring of I & O and prevent overdistention secondary to urinary retention.*

▲ Administer methylprednisolone as prescribed *to minimize edema and enhance microcirculation. Suggested dose is 30 mg/kg. Initial dose is given over 15 minutes followed by 5.4 mg/kg/hr for 23 hours starting 45 min after initial dose.*

Impaired Physical Mobility

RELATED FACTORS

Neuromuscular impairment, muscle weakness or paralysis, imposed immobilization by traction

EXPECTED OUTCOME

Patient maintains full ROM as evidenced by absence of contractures and absence of foot drop.

ONGOING ASSESSMENT

▪ Assess patient's ability to carry out ADL.

▪ Assess motor strength, checking for level of progression, symmetry/asymmetry, ascending/descending paralysis, paresthesia.

▪ Assess baseline ROM.

Continued.

Spinal cord injury (SCI)—cont'd

NURSING DIAGNOSES	EXPECTED OUTCOMES AND NURSING INTERVENTIONS / *RATIONALE* (■ = INDEPENDENT; ▲ = COLLABORATIVE)
DEFINING CHARACTERISTICS Inability to move purposely within environment Limited ROM Decreased muscle strength	**THERAPEUTIC INTERVENTIONS** • If spine is stable, log roll and reposition at least q2h. • Begin ROM exercises *to minimize potential for contractures, which may occur once spinal shock advances to next stage of spasticity.* • Provide support to foot to prevent foot drop. *A high top sneaker or special device may be helpful.* ▲ Consult and work with physical and occupational therapists. • See also Impaired physical mobility, p. 47.
High Risk for Impaired Skin Integrity **RISK FACTORS** Impaired physical mobility, complete bed rest, sensory disturbance	**EXPECTED OUTCOME** Patient maintains intact skin. **ONGOING ASSESSMENT** • Assess skin integrity q2-4h, noting color, moisture, texture, and temperature. **THERAPEUTIC INTERVENTIONS** • Keep skin clean and dry. • Keep skin lubricated to *prevent dryness/cracking.* • Turn q2h. • If patient is up in a wheelchair, instruct to shift position q20-30min *to prevent pressure area from developing.* • Provide appropriate prophylactic use of pressure-relieving devices *to help in preventing skin breakdown.* • See also: Impaired skin integrity, p. 59.
Body Image Disturbance **RELATED FACTOR** Paralysis secondary to SCI **DEFINING CHARACTERISTICS** Verbalization of functional alteration of body part Denial of injury outcome Withdrawal, isolation Focused behavior/verbal preoccupation with body part/function	**EXPECTED OUTCOMES** Patient discusses feelings about impairment. Patient identifies/uses positive coping mechanisms. **ONGOING ASSESSMENT** • Assess perception of dysfunction. *Patient may perceive changes that are not present/real.* • Assess perceived impact on ADL, personal relationships, occupational activity. • Inquire about coping skills used before injury. **THERAPEUTIC INTERVENTIONS** • Acknowledge normality of emotional response to change in body function. *Stages of grief over loss of body function are normal.* • Help patient identify positive/negative feelings regarding impairment. • Help patient identify appropriate coping mechanisms. *As a result of the overwhelming nature of SCI, prior coping skills may not be effective.* ▲ Refer for counseling as needed. • Encourage use of support groups. *Groups that come together for mutual support and information exchange can be beneficial.*

See also:
Altered sexuality patterns, p. 58.
Feeding self-care deficit, p. 53.
Bathing/hygiene self-care deficit, p. 53.
Hopelessness, p. 36.
Caregiver role strain, p. 13
Bowel incontinence, p. 19.
Urinary retention, p. 74.
Ineffective individual coping, p. 18.
High risk for infection, p. 40.
Anxiety/fear, p. 5, 23.

By: Linda Arsenault, RN, MSN, CNRN

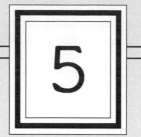

5

Gastrointestinal and Digestive Care Plans

Abdominal surgery

Open surgery of the abdomen may be done for the following: gastrectomy (removal of all or part of the stomach), splenectomy (removal of the spleen), pancreatectomy (partial or total removal of the pancreas), liver resection, cholecystectomy (removal of the gallbladder), removal of biliary stones or resection of biliary structures, prostatectomy (removal of the prostate gland), cystectomy (removal of the bladder), appendectomy (removal of the appendix), hysterectomy (removal of the uterus), nephrectomy (removal of a kidney), resection/repair of abdominal aortic aneurysms, small and large bowel resection, and repair of trauma to any abdominal structure resulting from blunt or penetrating trauma, commonly referred to as an exploratory laparotomy. Nursing care interventions are similar for all patients having all abdominal surgery, regardless of the type.

NURSING DIAGNOSES	EXPECTED OUTCOMES AND NURSING INTERVENTIONS / *RATIONALE* (■ = INDEPENDENT; ▲ = COLLABORATIVE)

Knowledge deficit: preoperative

RELATED FACTORS
Proposed surgical experience
Lack of previous similar surgical procedure

DEFINING CHARACTERISTICS
Questions
Lack of questions
Verbalized misconceptions

EXPECTED OUTCOMES
Patient verbalizes understanding of proposed surgical procedure and realistic expectations for the postoperative course.

ONGOING ASSESSMENT
- Assess patient's knowledge of proposed surgical procedure. *Patient should be aware of the nature of the surgical procedure, the reason it is being done, and whether the surgeon plans an open abdominal procedure or a laparoscopic procedure.*
- Assess patient's previous experience with surgery. *Patients who have had surgery in the past may have negative feelings related to side effects of anesthesia, postoperative pain, and lengthy recovery.*

THERAPEUTIC INTERVENTIONS
- Explain and reinforce surgeon's explanations regarding proposed surgical procedure.
- Prepare patients having open abdominal surgery to expect a 4- to 7-day postoperative hospitalization including the following:
    An incision in the abdomen *(size and location depend on the nature of the surgical procedure)* either stapled or sutured closed, with a dressing in place.
    Surgical drains near the surgical incision *to drain lymphatic fluid from the operative site.*
    IVs *to provide fluid and electrolytes until bowel peristalsis returns, usually 72-96 hours postoperatively.*
    Nasogastric tube *to keep the stomach free of fluid and to prevent distention, nausea, and vomiting.*
    Early ambulation, usually out of bed the first postoperative day, *to prevent pulmonary atelectasis and deep vein thrombosis.*
    Antiembolic stockings or sequential compression devices *to prevent deep vein thrombosis.*
    Need for aggressive turning, coughing, and deep-breathing *to prevent pulmonary atelectasis and stasis of secretions, which could lead to pneumonia. Patients should be instructed in the use of incentive spirometer and coughing using splinting techniques preoperatively; provide an opportunity for return demonstration.*
    Need for pain management. *Adequate pain management allows patients having abdominal surgery to participate actively in ambulation and pulmonary hygiene. The patient has a right to aggressive management of postoperative pain and should be involved in selecting the type of pain management used. See also Pain, p. 49.*

| NURSING DIAGNOSES | EXPECTED OUTCOMES AND NURSING INTERVENTIONS / *RATIONALES*
 (■ = INDEPENDENT; ▲ = COLLABORATIVE) |

Ineffective Breathing Pattern

RELATED FACTORS

Abdominal incision pain
Abdominal distention compromising lung expansion
Sedation

DEFINING CHARACTERISTICS

Poor coughing effort
Shallow breathing
Splinting respirations
Refusal to use incentive spirometer

EXPECTED OUTCOMES

Patient maintains an effective breathing pattern as evidenced by ability to use incentive spirometer correctly, clear breath sounds.

ONGOING ASSESSMENT

- Assess rate and depth of respirations. *Respirations are typically shallow, because the least amount of excursion is least painful when an abdominal incision is present. Also, the higher the incision, the more breathing is affected.*
- Auscultate breath sounds at least q4h for the first 48 hours postoperatively. *The bases of the lungs are least likely to be ventilated; therefore breath sounds may be diminished over the bases.*
- Observe for splinting. *Splinting refers to the conscious minimization of an inspiration to reduce the amount of discomfort caused by full expansion.*
- Assess ability to use incentive spirometer. *In incentive spirometry the patient takes and holds a deep breath for a few seconds. Incentive spirometry encourages deep-breathing, and holding the breath allows for full expansion of alveoli.*
- Assess for abdominal distention, *which can impair excursion.*

THERAPEUTIC INTERVENTIONS

- ▲ Manage pain using whatever plan for pain management has been prescribed. *Patient using patient-controlled analgesia (PCA) may need reinstruction or reminders to "push the button" during the early postoperative phase when they are still under the effects of anesthesia.*
- Position patient with HOB elevated 30 degrees. *This position puts the least strain on abdominal muscles.*
- Encourage/assist the patient to turn side to side q2h *to mobilize secretions.*
- Encourage the patient to do deep-breathing a minimum of 10 times every hour.
- Encourage coughing q1h *to clear the bronchial tree of secretions.*
- Help patient splint abdominal incision by using hands or a pillow. *Splinting the incision eases the discomfort of coughing and taking deep breaths.*
- Encourage use of incentive spirometer.
- Encourage ambulation as tolerated.

Pain

RELATED FACTORS

Abdominal incision
Presence of drains, tubes

DEFINING CHARACTERISTICS

Subjective complaint of pain
Guarded movement

EXPECTED OUTCOMES

Patient requests pain medications or demonstrates effective use of other pain-control measures.
Patient verbalizes relief of pain or ability to tolerate pain.

ONGOING ASSESSMENT

- Assess nature of pain (location, quality, duration).
- Monitor change in perception of pain associated with abdominal distention. *Distention of the abdomen by accumulation of gas and fluid occurs postoperatively because normal peristalsis does not return until the third or fourth day after surgery; distension stresses the suture line(s) and causes pain.*
- Check abdomen for rigidity and rebound tenderness *(may indicate peritonitis).*

THERAPEUTIC INTERVENTIONS

- Assist patient to comfortable position.
- Use nonpharmacologic measures to reduce perception of pain (distraction, relaxation).
- ▲ Administer analgesics or assist patient in using PCA before pain becomes too severe. *It is more difficult to control pain once it becomes severe.*
- ▲ Administer pain medication, before painful procedures (e.g., dressing changes, ambulation) *to maximize patient's ability to tolerate/participate.*
- ▲ Document patient's response to pain-relieving measures and advocate additional medication if patient is not comfortable. *Patients have very individualized pain tolerance levels, and all patients will not be made comfortable with standard doses.*
- Ensure function of suction machines *(protects gastric suture line from tension).*
- See also Pain, p. 49.

Continued.

Gastrointestinal and Digestive Care Plans

NURSING DIAGNOSES	EXPECTED OUTCOMES AND NURSING INTERVENTIONS / *RATIONALES* (■ = INDEPENDENT; ▲ = COLLABORATIVE)

High Risk for Fluid Volume Deficit

RISK FACTORS

Nasogastric suctioning
Intestinal or space drains
Wound drainage
Blood loss in surgery
NPO status
Vomiting

EXPECTED OUTCOMES

Patient maintains normal fluid volume balance as evidenced by stable B/P and heart rate and by urine output at least 30 ml/hour.

ONGOING ASSESSMENT

- Monitor for postoperative bleeding:
  Intraabdominal: *May occur from any vessel in the dissected area; usually shows as increased bloody drainage on dressing.*
  Intraluminal: *Usually from anastomosis; shows as increased blood drainage from tubes.*
  Incisional: *Usually from subcutaneous tissue; shows as increased bloody drainage on dressings.*
- Mark extension of drainage from incisions. *Outlining the stain on the surface of the dressing and indicating the time of the assessment allow staff to quantify amount of drainage, severity of bleeding later.*
- ▲ Assess hydration status:
  Check central venous pressure (CVP): *CVP is an indication of circulating blood volume.*
  Monitor blood pressure, heart rate.
  Check mucous membranes and skin turgor; *moist mucous membranes and good skin turgor are signs of adequate hydration.*
  Monitor urine output: *Output of 30 ml/hr indicates adequate hydration.*
- Monitor and record I & O, including urinary output, emesis, nasogastric (NG) tube output, output from surgical drains (check for drainage around drains, as well), and incisional drainage.
- ▲ Monitor Hb and Hct. *Dropping Hb and Hct may indicate internal bleeding.*
- ▲ Monitor coagulation profile. *Excessive post-operative bleeding may result from coagulopathy.*
- Weigh patient daily, using same scale.

THERAPEUTIC INTERVENTIONS

- ▲ Administer IV fluid as ordered; be prepared to increase fluids if signs of fluid volume deficit appear.
- Report any unusual or new bleeding.
- Report dramatic increases in NG output.
- ▲ Provide oral fluids of patient's choice as allowed. *Oral fluids are usually restricted until peristalsis returns and NG tube is removed, because swallowed fluids will be sucked out by the NG tube along with electrolytes; this puts the patient at risk for electrolyte imbalance, especially hypokalemia. However, patients may be allowed ice chips, or small sips of fluids.*
- Provide oral hygiene. *NPO status and/or fluid volume deficit will cause a dry, sticky mouth.*

High Risk for Infection

RISK FACTORS

Abdominal incision
Indwelling urinary catheter
Venous access devices
Presence of tubes/drains
Invasion of pathogens through inadvertent interruption of closed drainage systems

EXPECTED OUTCOMES

Patient is free of infection, as evidenced by:
  Healing wound/incision, free of redness, swelling purulent discharge, pain.
  Normal body temperature within 72 hours post-op.
  Venous access sites free of redness, purulent drainage.

ONGOING ASSESSMENT

- Monitor temperature. *For the first 48 to 72 hours post-operatively, temperatures of up to 38.5° are expected as a normal stress response following major surgery. Beyond 72 hours, temperature should return to patient's baseline. Temperature spikes, usually occuring in the later afternoon or night, are often indications of infection.*
- ▲ Monitor WBC. *Elevated WBC is an indication of infection.*
- Assess incision, wound for redness, drainage, swelling, increased pain:
  Closed wounds/incisions: *Incisions which have been closed with sutures or staples should be free of redness, swelling, and drainage. Some incisional discomfort is expected. These incisions are usually kept covered by a dry dressing for 24 to 48 hours; beyond 48 hours, there is no need for a dressing.*
  Open wounds: *Wounds left open to heal by secondary intention should appear pink/ red, moist, and have minimal sero-sanguinous drainage. These wounds are usually*

Ongoing Assessment—cont'd

packed with sterile gauze moistened with sterile saline. Discomfort is expected upon packing.

- Assess all peripheral and central IV sites for redness, purulent drainage, and pain.
- Assess color, clarity and odor of urine. *Cloudy, foul smelling urine is an indication of urinary tract infection, which can occur as the result of an indwelling catheter.*
▲ Obtain culture of cloudy, foul-smelling urine *to determine pathogens present.*
- Assess stability of tubes/drains. *In-and-out motion of improperly secured tubes/drains allows access by pathogens through stab wounds where tubes/drains are placed.*
▲ Obtain culture of any unusual drainage from wound, incision, tubes, drains *to determine the presence of pathogens.*

Therapeutic Interventions

- Wash hands before contact with postoperative patient. *Handwashing remains the most effective method of infection control.*
- Use aseptic technique during dressing change, wound care, or handling or manipulating of tubes/drains.
- Ensure that closed drainage systems (urinary catheter, surgical tubes/drains) are not inadvertently interrupted (opened). Tape connectors, pin extension/drainage tubing securely to patient's gown *to minimize tension on tubes and connection. Opening of sterile systems allows access by pathogens and puts the patient at risk for infection.*
- Provide aseptic site care to all peripheral and central venous access devices per hospital policy.
- Provide meticulous meatal care daily *to reduce the number of pathogens around the urinary catheter entrance site.*
▲ Irrigate tubes/drains only with physician prescription. Use aseptic technique and sterile irrigant. *Intraabdominal infection can result from introduction of pathogens into interrupted systems.*
▲ Administer antibiotics and antipyretics as prescribed.

High Risk for Altered Tissue Integrity

Risk Factors

Delayed wound healing
Infection
Presence of seroma or hematoma
Increased intraabdominal pressure
Mechanical force

Expected Outcomes

Patient has an intact wound or has complications such as dehiscence, evisceration, or fistulalization recognized and treated promptly.

Ongoing Assessment

- Assess wound for hematoma (collection of bloody drainage beneath the skin) or seroma (collection of serous fluid beneath the skin); *presence of either predisposes the wound to separation and infection.*
- Assess wound for intactness *to detect wound dehiscence (separation of the suture line or wound).*
    Closed wound: *Wound edges should remain approximated, without tension, puckering, or open gaps between stitches/staples.*
    Open wounds: *Wounds left open to heal by secondary intention are open only as deep as the subcutaneous tissue is deep; the fascia, muscle, and peritoneum have usually been closed. The deepest portion of the wound will come together, with the presence of tissue beneath being visible.*
- Assess condition of stitches/staples and retention sutures, if present; report any closures that appear to have loosened or fallen out. *This is especially important during the first 48 hr, before wound strength begins to develop. Retention sutures (large sutures placed in addition to routine closures) are used when obesity, extreme abdominal distention, intraabdominal infection, poor nutritional status, and/or a history of wound evisceration is present.*
- Assess open wounds for evidence of evisceration (protrusion of abdominal contents).
- Assess wound/dressings for suspicious drainage. *The presence of yellow, green, or brown fluid or material with an acrid or fecal odor indicates the presence of a fistula, a communication between some portion of the bowel and the incision or open wound.*

Therapeutic Interventions

- Prevent strain on abdominal incision/wound:
    Keep head of bed elevated 30 degrees.
    Encourage patient to splint with pillow or hands before coughing.
    Ensure proper functioning of suction machine *to decrease nausea, which may lead to retching.*

Continued.

NURSING DIAGNOSES	EXPECTED OUTCOMES AND NURSING INTERVENTIONS / *RATIONALES* (■ = INDEPENDENT; ▲ = COLLABORATIVE)

	THERAPEUTIC INTERVENTIONS—cont'd
	▲ If dehiscence or evisceration occurs or is suspected:
	    Place patient in Fowler's position and keep patient quiet and still.
	    Use wide tape *to approximate wound edges as well as possible.*
	    Cover area with saline-solution-soaked gauze.
	    Notify physician; *this situation usually requires a return to surgery for repair.*
	▪ If fistula is suspected:
	    Save dressing with suspicious drainage to show physician.
	    Protect wound edges with petrolatum-based ointment or hydrocolloid.
	    See also Enterocutaneous fistula, p. 305.

High Risk for Altered Tissue Perfusion: Thrombophlebitis, Deep Vein Thrombosis **RISK FACTORS** Prolonged time in OR Position during OR Decreased postoperative activity Dehydration Decreased vascular tone	**EXPECTED OUTCOMES** Patient remains free of thrombophlebitis and deep vein thrombosis, as evidenced by bilaterally equal calves, absence of calf pain. **ONGOING ASSESSMENT** ▪ Assess legs for swelling; compare right leg to left leg. *Except for minor differences, calves should have the same approximate circumference. Unilateral swelling could indicate thrombophlebitis or deep vein thrombosis.* ▪ Assess for presence of distended leg veins, *which may indicate venous congestion and poor venous circulation.* ▪ Assess for bluish discoloration of legs, *which may also indicate venous congestion.* ▪ Assess for pain on compression of calf and calf pain upon dorsiflexion of foot. *Either is an indication of thrombophlebitis or deep vein thrombosis.* **THERAPEUTIC INTERVENTIONS** ▪ Reinforce/encourage leg exercises taught preoperatively; strive for 10 repetitions each hour until fully ambulatory. *Contracting the leg muscles decreases venous stasis and encourages good venous return; both decrease the opportunity for thromboembolic developments.* ▲ Use antiembolic stockings or sequential compression devices while the patient is in bed. *Both are useful in improving venous return.* ▪ Discourage gatching of bed at knee. *This contributes to venous pooling in the legs and decreased venous return.* ▲ Encourage ambulation by patient as soon as possible per physician's prescription. *Being fully upright is preferable to "dangling" or sitting in a chair, because contracted muscles push against the leg vessels and improve venous return most effectively when the patient is upright and legs are straight.* ▲ Administer prophylactic anticoagulant therapy as prescribed. ▲ Administer IV fluids/encourage ingestion of fluids as prescribed.

Knowledge Deficit
 	
RELATED FACTORS
Lack of previous experience with abdominal surgery
Need for home management
 	
DEFINING CHARACTERISTICS
Multiple questions
Lack of questions
Inability to provide self-care on discharge
	EXPECTED OUTCOMES
	Patient verbalizes understanding of and demonstrates ability to provide wound care, limit activities as appropriate.
	
	ONGOING ASSESSMENT
	▪ Assess patient's ability to perform wound care, verbalize appropriate activity, verbalize appropriate diet.
	▪ Assess patient's understanding of need for further therapy, if needed. *Patients who have had abdominal surgery for malignancies may require further therapy, such as chemotherapy, irradiation, or immunotherapy.*
	▪ Assess patient's understanding of need for close follow-up observation. *Patients who leave the hospital with sutures, staples, or drains in place need to return for their removal.*
	
	THERAPEUTIC INTERVENTIONS
	▪ Teach patient to perform appropriate wound care:
	    Closed abdominal incision: Staples/sutures and dressings have usually been removed by the time of discharge, and Steri-Strips have been placed *to maintain wound approximation. Steri-Strips should be left in place until they fall off.*
	    Open abdominal wounds: Wounds require twice daily wet-to-dry saline solution packings until wound has granulated in enough to close.

THERAPEUTIC INTERVENTIONS—cont'd

- Teach patient appropriate activity:
  No lifting heavier than 10 pounds for 6 wk.
  Mild exercise (e.g., walking) *to increase stamina.*
  Showering OK.
  Bathing OK except when there is an open wound, *which may take up to 8 wk to heal completely; hand-held shower head good way to clean this wound.*
  No driving until anterior abdominal wound has healed.
- Teach patient the following about diet: A well-balanced, high-calorie, high-protein diet is desirable for healing *that continues over a period of weeks. Patients who have undergone gastrectomy should be taught to eat small frequent meals, as they no longer have preoperative gastric capacity. Small, frequent meals are less likely to cause "dumping syndrome," which results from too large an osmotic load.*
- Teach patient the importance of any further cancer therapy planned (e.g., chemotherapy, radiation therapy, immunotherapy). *These therapies are typically offered if the pathology report indicates that the tumor was not confined to the bowel/bowel wall.*
- Teach patient that bowel function will return to preoperative baseline in 2-3 wk, *usually after the patient has returned to a normal schedule and diet.*
- Instruct patient to seek medical attention for any of the following: fever > 38° C, foul-smelling wound drainage, redness or unusual pain in any incision, absence of bowel movement.

By: Audrey Klopp, RN, PhD, ET

Acute abdomen

A condition characterized by abdominal pain, vomiting, anorexia, constipation or diarrhea, changes in bowel sounds, and fever. Accurate diagnosis depends on thorough physical assessment, appropriate testing, and observation. Treatment depends on cause. This care plan addresses conservative medical management; it does not include exploratory laparotomy for diagnosis or other surgical procedures that may follow definitive diagnosis. If a perforation is determined, surgery will be scheduled immediately.

NURSING DIAGNOSES	EXPECTED OUTCOMES AND NURSING INTERVENTIONS / *RATIONALE* (■ = INDEPENDENT; ▲ = COLLABORATIVE)

Pain

RELATED FACTORS

Pancreatitis, thrombosis, strangulating/infarcted bowel, renal/biliary colic, ruptured aneurysm, appendicitis, peritonitis, diverticulitis, obstruction, gastroenteritis, blunt/penetrating trauma, perforated GI malignancy, pelvic inflammatory disease (PID), inflammatory bowel disease (ulcerative colitis, Crohn's disease)

EXPECTED OUTCOMES

Patient verbalizes ability to tolerate pain.

ONGOING ASSESSMENT

- Assess pain: degree, location, sudden or gradual onset.
- Assess for precipitating and relieving factors, *such as position, application of heat or cold, intake of food or fluid.*
- Monitor for changes in type, degree, location of pain; notify physician of significant changes. *Changes in pain patterns are major diagnostic indicators in the patient with an acute abdomen. Significant change in pain may indicate perforation and need for immediate surgery.*
- Evaluate effectiveness of interventions.

THERAPEUTIC INTERVENTIONS

- Respond immediately to complaints of pain. *Pain is best relieved before it becomes severe, and although patients with an acute abdomen may go on to have severe pain, interventions such as positioning, massage are best used early.*

Continued.

Gastrointestinal and Digestive Care Plans

NURSING DIAGNOSES	EXPECTED OUTCOMES AND NURSING INTERVENTIONS / *RATIONALES* (■ = INDEPENDENT; ▲ = COLLABORATIVE)

DEFINING CHARACTERISTICS
Complaints of abdominal pain
Restlessness
Insomnia
Guarding behavior
Self-focusing
Moaning
Crying
Autonomic responses not seen in chronic stable pain (e.g., diaphoresis, changes in vital signs, pupillary dilatation)

THERAPEUTIC INTERVENTIONS—cont'd
- Place in semi-Fowler's position; use pillows for support. *This position facilitates relaxation of abdominal muscles which may help lessen sensation of pain.*
- ▲ Provide analgesics as prescribed. *Pain medications are typically withheld or given sparingly so as not to mask symptoms, which may help pinpoint diagnosis.*
- ▲ Administer antibiotics as prescribed. *Many causes of an acute abdomen include an inflammatory or infectious process, which antibiotics may improve; additionally, antibiotics are given to protect the patient from infection if bowel is ruptured.*

High Risk for Fluid Volume Deficit

RISK FACTORS
NPO status
Diaphoresis
Vomiting
Diarrhea
Fever
Ileus
Internal bleeding

EXPECTED OUTCOMES
Patient maintains normal fluid volume as evidenced by stable vital signs, urinary output > 30 ml/hr, moist mucous membranes.

ONGOING ASSESSMENT
- Monitor blood pressure, heart rate, and temperature.
- Assess skin turgor and condition of mucous membranes. *Both are sensitive indicators of fluid volume status.*
- Monitor urine output. *Urine output of at least 30 ml/hr indicates adequate fluid volume.*
- Assess urine specific gravity. *Concentration of urine (i.e., specific gravity > 1.020) may indicate dehydration.*
- ▲ Monitor hemoglobin and hematocrit *to determine significant blood loss from internal bleeding.*
- ▲ Monitor white blood count (WBC). *Elevated WBC indicates infection.*
- ▲ Monitor urine and serum amylase levels. *Patients with pancreatitis have high urine and serum amylase levels. This helps in ruling out other causes of an acute abdomen.*
- Assess for bowel sounds q4h. *Patients with paralytic ileus or bowel obstruction sequester large volumes of fluid in the lumen of the gut. This contributes to fluid volume deficit.*
- Assess for bowel elimination; note frequency, nature of stool, presence of blood.

THERAPEUTIC INTERVENTIONS
- ▲ Administer IV fluids as ordered.
- ▲ Insert NG tube and attach to low suction *to ease persistent vomiting and distention. If paralytic ileus or other type of bowel obstruction is present, fluid will continue to accumulate in the bowel, worsening fluid volume deficit.*
- ▲ Measure gastric output, and replace cubic centimeter per cubic centimeter with IV replacement fluid, usually 0.45 or 0.9 normal saline (NS) solution.
- ▲ Administer antiemetics as prescribed.

Knowledge Deficit

RELATED FACTORS
Acuity of illness
New diagnosis

DEFINING CHARACTERISTICS
Anxiety
Questioning
Anger/hostility
Withdrawal/depression
Noncompliance

EXPECTED OUTCOMES
Patient verbalizes understanding of illness and treatment plan.

ONGOING ASSESSMENT
- Assess knowledge of illness. *Conservative management and a "wait and see" approach may make the patient think nothing is being done.*
- Assess patient's understanding of treatment plan. *The patient needs to understand that careful observation in combination with fluid and medication administration helps to establish a clear diagnosis. The patient should also understand that surgery may occur, sometimes precipitously, depending on findings.*
- Assess patient's understanding of proposed diagnostic measures. *Frequent blood testing and x-ray procedures may be carried out to aid in diagnosis.*

THERAPEUTIC INTERVENTIONS
- Teach patient/significant other that symptoms of an acute abdomen may indicate a variety of disorders, including appendicitis, diverticulitis, pancreatitis, peritonitis, gastroenteritis, bowel obstruction, ruptured aneurysm, ectopic pregnancy, inflammatory bowel disease.

NURSING DIAGNOSES	EXPECTED OUTCOMES AND NURSING INTERVENTIONS / *RATIONALES* (■ = INDEPENDENT; ▲ = COLLABORATIVE)

THERAPEUTIC INTERVENTIONS—cont'd

- Teach patient/significant other that conservative medical management is appropriate therapy.
- Teach patient/significant other that surgery is a possible course of therapy.
- Explain the purpose of all diagnostic procedures.
- Answer questions honestly, sharing information as it is available.
- Teach the patient to report any change in pain immediately. *Sudden cessation of or worsening of pain may indicate a serious change (e.g., ruptured bowel, appendix, diverticulum) requiring immediate surgery to minimize the risks of peritonitis.*

See also:
Anxiety, p. 5.
Ineffective airway clearance, p. 3.

By: Kathleen Jaffry, RN

Cirrhosis

(LAËNNEC'S CIRRHOSIS; HEPATIC ENCEPHALOPATHY; ASCITES; LIVER FAILURE)

A chronic disease characterized by scarring of the liver. Although viral hepatitis, biliary obstruction, and severe right-sided heart failure may cause cirrhosis, alcohol is the most frequent cause. Cirrhosis is a major cause of death in the United States; its highest incidence is between ages 40 and 60. Cirrhosis has a 2:1 male/female ratio.

NURSING DIAGNOSES	EXPECTED OUTCOMES AND NURSING INTERVENTIONS / *RATIONALE* (■ = INDEPENDENT; ▲ = COLLABORATIVE)

Altered Nutrition: Less than Body Requirements

RELATED FACTORS

Poor eating habits
Excess alcohol intake
Lack of financial means
Altered hepatic metabolic function
Inadequate bile production
Nausea, vomiting, anorexia

DEFINING CHARACTERISTICS

Documented inadequate dietary intake
Weight loss
Muscle wasting, especially in extremities
Skin changes consistent with vitamin deficiency (flaking, loss of elasticity)
Coagulopathies

EXPECTED OUTCOMES

Patient achieves adequate nutrient intake, as evidenced by consumption of 3000 cal/day, weight stabilization.

ONGOING ASSESSMENT

- Obtain weight history.
- Assess for weight distribution. *Actual weight may remain steady while muscle mass deteriorates and ascitic fluid accumulates.*
- Document intake.
- ▲ Monitor serum electrolyte levels and albumin/protein levels. *Hypokalemia ($K^+ < 3.5$) is common in cirrhosis as a result of increased aldosterone levels, which increase K+ excretion. Serum protein levels are decreased secondary to decreased hepatic production of protein and loss of protein molecules to the peritoneal space.*
- ▲ Monitor glucose levels. *Patients with cirrhosis may be hypoglycemic as the liver fails to perform glycolysis (breakdown of stored glycogen) and gluconeogenesis (formation of glucose from amino acids).*
- ▲ Monitor coagulation profile. *Several coagulation factors are made by the liver. Patients with cirrhosis frequently have coagulopathy severe enough to precipitate bleeding.*

THERAPEUTIC INTERVENTIONS

- ▲ Provide diet high in calories from carbohydrate source. *Aberrant protein metabolism in failing liver can cause hepatic encephalopathy because ammonia, which is normally metabolized into urea (which can be excreted), passes through the damaged liver unchanged and goes on to become a cerebral toxin.*
- Schedule small frequent meals.
- Assist with meals as needed.
- ▲ Provide dietary/pharmacologic vitamin supplementation. *If bile production is impaired, absorption of fat soluble vitamins A, D, E, and K will be inadequate.*
- ▲ Provide enteral or parenteral nutritional support as ordered, using carbohydrates as calorie source.

Continued.

Gastrointestinal and Digestive Care Plans

NURSING DIAGNOSES	EXPECTED OUTCOMES AND NURSING INTERVENTIONS / *RATIONALES* (■ = INDEPENDENT; ▲ = COLLABORATIVE)

Fluid Volume Excess, Extravascular (Ascites)

RELATED FACTORS

Increased portal venous pressure
Hypoalbuminemia
Low serum oncotic pressure
Aldosterone imbalance

DEFINING CHARACTERISTICS

Increasing abdominal girth
Ballottement
Taut abdomen, dull to percussion

EXPECTED OUTCOMES

Patient experiences a decrease in ascites formation/accumulation, as evidenced by decreased abdominal girth.

ONGOING ASSESSMENT

- Assess for presence of ascites: *Ascites is the collection of protein-rich fluid in the peritoneal cavity. Its volume may be so severe as to impair respiratory and digestive functions, as well as mobility.*
  Measure abdominal girth daily, taking care to measure at same point consistently.
  Check abdomen for dullness on percussion.
  Check for ballottement. (Fluid wave on abdominal assessment).
- ▲ Monitor serum albumin and globulin levels. *Protein molecules act as fluid "magnets" that help maintain body fluid in correct compartments; low protein level allows shift of fluid to extravascular space.*
- Assess for signs of portal hypertension: history of upper GI bleeding, spider nevi.
- Monitor I & O.
- Assess for side effects of massive ascites: limited mobility, decreased appetite, inadequate lung expansion, altered body image, self-care deficit.

THERAPEUTIC INTERVENTIONS

- ▲ Restrict fluid and sodium intake as ordered. *Increased aldosterone levels contribute to aggressive sodium reabsorption.*
- ▲ Administer diuretics cautiously *as excess fluid is extravascular; aggressive diuresis can lead to dehydration and acute tubular necrosis or hepatorenal syndrome.*
- Assist with paracentesis as needed.
- For peritoneovenous shunt (LaVeen shunt, Denver shunt), facilitate shunt function. *Although paracentesis (removal of peritoneal fluid by needle) effectively removes ascitic fluid, it also wastes protein and is only a temporary measure. Peritoneovenous shunting returns ascitic fluid to the vascular space.*
  Apply abdominal binder.
  Encourage use of blow bottle or incentive spirometer. *Inspiring against resistance and the use of an abdominal binder increase intraperitoneal pressures, causing valve in shunt to open, allowing ascitic fluid to shunt into vascular space.*
- ▲ Administer spironolactone as prescribed. *Spironolactone, a diuretic, antagonizes aldosterone. It causes excretion of sodium and water but spares K^+.*

High Risk for Fluid Volume Deficit

RISK FACTORS

Overly aggressive diuresis
GI bleeding
Coagulopathies

EXPECTED OUTCOMES

Patient maintains normal fluid volume as evidenced by stable vital signs, urine specific gravity 1.010-1.020, moist mucous membranes.

ONGOING ASSESSMENT

- Monitor blood pressure and heart rate; check for orthostatic changes.
- Observe urine specific gravity, color.
- Check moisture of mucous membranes. *Dry mucous membranes indicate dehydration.*
- Monitor for hematemesis (vomited blood), hematochezia (bright red blood per rectum), melena (dark, tarry stool).
- Test any emesis, gastric aspirate, or stool for blood.

THERAPEUTIC INTERVENTIONS

- ▲ Administer IV fluids and/or blood products as prescribed.
- ▲ Hold diuretics, *which may deplete intravascular volume.*
- If GI bleeding occurs: increase IV fluids, *to expand intravascular fluid volume and prevent complications of hypovolemia (e.g., ATN, shock);* anticipate CVP or PAP line; prepare to administer volume expanders or blood products.
  See also GI bleeding, p. 311.

Sensory-Perceptual Alteration

RELATED FACTORS

Hepatic encephalopathy
Delirium tremens
Acute intoxication
Hepatic metabolic insufficiency

DEFINING CHARACTERISTICS

Altered attention span
Inability to give accurate history
Inability to follow commands
Disorientation to person, place, and/or time
Delusions
Inappropriate behavior
Self- or other-directed violence
Inappropriate affect
Evidence of hepatic encephalopathy

EXPECTED OUTCOMES

Patient remains arousable, oriented, able to follow directions.

ONGOING ASSESSMENT

▲ Monitor blood alcohol level on admission.
▲ Monitor blood ammonia levels. *Ammonia is a cerebral toxin that contributes to changed LOC.*
• Note time since last ingestion of alcohol. *Delirium tremens can occur up to 7 days after last alcohol intake.*
• Assess for signs/symptoms of hepatic encephalopathy; note stage:
  Stage I: minor mental aberrations, confusion.
  Stage II: asterixis, apraxia.
  Stage III: lethargy alternating with combativeness, stupor, EEG slowing.
  Stage IV: coma, further EEG slowing, fetor hepaticas, altered hepatic enzymes, altered liver function study findings.
• Document improvement/deterioration in level of encephalopathy.
• Monitor for evidence of violent, hallucinatory, and/or delusional thought.
• Evaluate factors that may increase cerebral sensitivity to ammonia (infections, acid-base imbalances).

THERAPEUTIC INTERVENTIONS

▲ Protect patient from physical harm:
  Pad side rails.
  Keep bed in low position.
  Restrain, if necessary.
  Administer sedatives *(nonhepatic metabolism)* as prescribed; document effectiveness; notify physician if dosage needs adjustment.
  Prevent oversedation *that may precipitate coma.*
• Orient patient to time, place, and person: place calendar and clock in room, provide environmental stimulation (television, radio, newspaper, visitors).
• Provide emotional support by reassuring patient of physiologic cause of confusion.
▲ Decrease intestinal bacteria content:
  Administer nonabsorbable antibiotics (neomycin, kanamycin) as prescribed.
  Administer lactulose as prescribed *to alter colonic pH and stimulate evacuation.*
▲ Decrease ammonigenic potential: order low-protein diet (0-40 g/day); check drugs for ammonia content; clean intestines of any old blood (lavage, suction, enemas).
• See also Thought process, altered, p. 65.

High Risk for Impaired Gas Exchange

RISK FACTORS

Decreased lung excursion related to ascites
Aspiration secondary to vomiting, retching
Altered LOC

EXPECTED OUTCOMES

Patient maintains adequate gas exchange as evidenced by ease of breathing, stable ABGs.

ONGOING ASSESSMENT

• Assess respirations; note quality, rate, depth, use of accessory muscles, position assumed for ease of breathing, and apparent impact of ascitic abdomen.
▲ Monitor ABGs. *Hypoventilation, secondary to decreased excursion, can lead to increased Pco_2 and decreased Po_2.*
• Assess for changes in orientation and/or behavior.

THERAPEUTIC INTERVENTIONS

▲ Administer O_2 as ordered.
• Assist patient to most effective position for breathing. *Elevating HOB to 30 degrees facilitates diaphragmatic excursion by displacing ascitic fluid from chest.*
• Assist patient in eating/drinking *to minimize risk of aspiration.*
• Withhold oral food/fluid from patient if LOC is altered.
• Suction if necessary.
• Encourage turning, coughing, and deep breathing.
• See also Gas exchange, impaired, p. 27.

Continued.

Gastrointestinal and Digestive Care Plans

NURSING DIAGNOSES	EXPECTED OUTCOMES AND NURSING INTERVENTIONS / *RATIONALES* (■ = INDEPENDENT; ▲ = COLLABORATIVE)

High Risk for Impaired Skin Integrity (Itching)

RISK FACTORS

Jaundice
Elevated bilirubin levels

EXPECTED OUTCOMES

Patient has intact skin.
Patient verbalizes decreased itching or ability to tolerate itching without scratching.

ONGOING ASSESSMENT

- Assess for jaundice *(yellow staining of skin by bilirubin).*
▲ Monitor findings of liver function tests, especially bilirubin levels. *Unexcreted bilirubin moves by diffusion into subcutaneous and cutaneous structures and irritates the tissue, causing histamine release and itching.*
- Assess itchiness and scratching.

THERAPEUTIC INTERVENTIONS

- Keep skin clean and well moisturized.
- Discourage scratching *(can introduce pathogens and cause localized infection).*
- Place mitts on patient if scratching cannot be discouraged by other means.
▲ Administer antihistamines as ordered.

Altered Health Maintenance

RELATED FACTORS

Lack of material resources
Ineffective coping
Perceptual/cognitive impairment
Inability to make thoughtful judgments

DEFINING CHARACTERISTICS

Demonstrated lack of knowledge regarding basic health practices
Observed inability to take responsibility for health
Reported lack of resources

EXPECTED OUTCOMES

Patient follows prescribed treatment regimen.
Patient identifies and uses available resources as appropriate.
Patient participates in alcohol treatment program as feasible/appropriate.

ONGOING ASSESSMENT

- Assess available support systems.
- Assess resources, ability to provide housing, food, medical care. *Alcoholic persons frequently have difficulty holding steady jobs or may use money to buy alcohol instead of food, medication, and so on. Also, many homeless individuals abuse alcohol.*
- Assess need for/readiness for alcohol rehabilitation. *Success in alcohol rehabilitation requires readiness of the patient.*

THERAPEUTIC INTERVENTIONS

- Teach the following: effects of alcohol intake/abstinence; need for high-calorie, low-protein diet *to facilitate regeneration of damaged liver cells.*
  Signs and symptoms of complications of cirrhosis: abdominal pain; vomiting, anorexia; loss of blood from GI tract; generalized bleeding (from gums, skin, GU tract); changes in level of consciousness.
- Teach dose, administration schedule, expected actions, and possible side effects of prescribed medications.
▲ Refer to alcohol rehabilitation program, if appropriate.

See also:
Body image disturbance, p. 7.
Impaired physical mobility, p. 47.
Impaired skin integrity, p. 59.

By: Audrey Klopp, RN, PhD, ET

Colon cancer

Colon cancer is the second most common cause of cancer death in the United States; it is second only to lung cancer in men, and breast cancer in women. Overall, men and women are equally affected. Cancers of the right colon are usually asymptomatic until very advanced, at which point the patient experiences weight loss and anemia. Cancers of the left colon typically present as changes in bowel elimination, rectal bleeding, and a feeling of incomplete evacuation. Colon cancers are staged by using Duke's classification; 5 year survival rate is about 50% and has not improved significantly. Surgery is the only definitive therapy for colon cancer, although irradiation may be used preoperatively. Chemotherapy, combinations of chemotherapy and irradiation, and immunotherapy are used, but with limited success. This care plan addresses the preoperative stage and the care of the patient who has undergone colon resection.

NURSING DIAGNOSES	EXPECTED OUTCOMES AND NURSING INTERVENTIONS / *RATIONALE* (■ = INDEPENDENT; ▲ = COLLABORATIVE)

Knowledge Deficit

RELATED FACTORS
New disease
Preoperative preparation

DEFINING CHARACTERISTICS
Questions
Lack of questions
Verbalized misconceptions
Inability to participate in making treatment decisions

EXPECTED OUTCOMES
Patient verbalizes understanding of proposed procedures.

ONGOING ASSESSMENT
- Assess patient's understanding of colon cancer. *Because many colon cancers are advanced by the time of diagnosis, patients may feel guilty about not having sought treatment sooner.*
- Assess patient's knowledge of proposed method of treatment and possible outcomes. *As with other cancers, patients may feel hopeless, that "nothing can be done."*
- Assess patient's knowledge of necessary diagnostic procedures. *The patient may have had multiple diagnostic examinations at this point and may not understand the importance of repeating procedures or making further diagnostic studies.*

THERAPEUTIC INTERVENTIONS
- Teach patient the following about colon cancer:
  Risk factors.
  > *The American diet (high-calorie, high-fat) is probably the greatest risk factor for cancer. Other risk factors include family history of colon cancer, history of inflammatory bowel disease, or history of other cancers, especially breast cancer in women.*

  Signs and symptoms.
  > *Because the right side of the colon is distensible, tumors on the right side are usually asymptomatic until the disease is widespread. Symptoms at that time include weight loss, anemia, weakness, and fatigue.*
  > *Tumors on the left side of the colon usually result in bleeding, constipation and/or diarrhea, a feeling of incomplete evacuation, and sometimes complete obstruction.*

  Method of spread/relationship to treatment.
  > *Colon cancer spreads by direct extension into surrounding tissue, by lymphatic channels, and by seeding into the peritoneal cavity. Excision of the tumor and surrounding tissue is the only curative treatment, although radiation therapy, chemotherapy, and immunotherapy may help to reduce the tumor and check the spread.*

  Types of surgical treatment.
  > *The type of surgery will be determined by the location of the tumor, and whether or not there is metasasis. Right or left hemicolectomy (removal of the right or left half of the colon or large intestine) is done to remove tumors of the ascending, transverse, descending, and sigmoid colon. Tumors that are too close to the anus are treated with abdominoperineal resection (resection of a portion of the colon, along with the rectum); this procedure results in a permanent colostomy because the rectum is gone. Tumors that are in the lower rectosigmoid colon or in the rectum may be treated with a low anterior resection, in which the tumor and surrounding colon are removed, and the colon is then anastomosed (no colostomy).*

Continued.

NURSING DIAGNOSES	EXPECTED OUTCOMES AND NURSING INTERVENTIONS / *RATIONALES* (■ = INDEPENDENT; ▲ = COLLABORATIVE)
	• Teach the patient about the following diagnostic procedures, as appropriate:

Colonoscopy.
> *Colonoscopy is a procedure that uses a flexible scope instrument to visualize the entire colon directly. Although a tumor may have been identified by digital examination, the entire colon should be examined before surgery; the presence of more than one tumor is possible.*

Carcinoembryonic antigen (CEA).
> *CEA is a blood test that gives an indication of ongoing cancer activity. Blood is drawn preoperatively so that progress can be monitored postoperatively.*

CT Scans.
> *CT scans are done to determine distant metastatic spread. This information helps the surgeon to decide how extensive a procedure is necessary.*

CBC.
> *Complete blood count is determined to assess for anemia. Colon tumors, particularly advanced colon tumors, bleed; bleeding may result in significant anemia, which is corrected before surgery.*

• Teach the patient about steps taken to prepare the bowel for surgery:
Clear liquid diet *to reduce the residue in the bowel.*
Antibiotics *to reduce the amount of bacteria normally present in the colon.*
CoLyte, GoLYTELY, osmotic agents *to induce diarrhea and clean bowel before surgery; may also be used before colonoscopy.*

• Prepare the patient for what to expect after surgery:
Incision(s), drains.
> *After colectomy, most patients have one midline incision. Patients who have had an abdominoperineal resection have an anterior midline incision, a perineal incision where the rectum was removed and a colostomy. Anterior incisions are typically sutured or stapled closed; perineal incisions may be closed or may be packed and left to heal by secondary intention. All patients have small drains in the lower abdomen to drain lymphatic fluid from the operative area.*

IVs.
> *Since patients resume oral feedings 72 to 96 hr postoperatively when peristalsis resumes; therefore administration of IV fluids is necessary and continues until the patient can tolerate oral fluids.*

Activity.
> *Patients should expect to get out of bed on the first postoperative day to prevent complications of immobility (deep vein thrombosis, atelectasis).*

Pain management.
> *Patients should be involved in choice of postoperative pain management. Options include traditional IM medications given prn, medications given under patient's control via PCA, or bolus or continuous-infusion epidural analgesics.*

Postoperative Pain

RELATED FACTORS

Surgical incision
Presence of tubes/drains

DEFINING CHARACTERISTICS

Report of incisional pain
Grimacing
Reluctance to move, cough, or take deep breaths
Protection of tubes/drains

EXPECTED OUTCOMES

Patient is free of pain or verbalizes ability to tolerate pain.

ONGOING ASSESSMENT

• Assess pain.
• Assess degree to which pain interferes with ability to turn, cough, and deep-breathe.
• Assess patient's use of chosen pain management method.
• Assess effectiveness of pain management.

THERAPEUTIC INTERVENTIONS

• Anticipate need for analgesia *to prevent peak pain periods.*
• Time administration of pain medication *to correspond with painful procedures (e.g., dressing changes, ambulation).*
• Teach patient to use hands or pillows *to splint incision when deep-breathing, coughing, or changing position.*
• Secure all tubes/drains *to minimize movement and subsequent pain.*
• See also Pain, p. 49.

NURSING DIAGNOSES	EXPECTED OUTCOMES AND NURSING INTERVENTIONS / *RATIONALES* (■ = INDEPENDENT; ▲ = COLLABORATIVE)

Altered Bowel Elimination: Postoperative Ileus

RELATED FACTORS
General anesthesia
Manipulation of bowel

DEFINING CHARACTERISTICS
Abdomen silent on auscultation
No stooling
Report of bloated feeling

EXPECTED OUTCOMES
Patient has bowel sounds within 96 hr postoperatively.

ONGOING ASSESSMENT
- Assess for bowel sounds every shift.
- Note passage of first flatus and stool. *Postoperative ileus usually resolves within 96 hr after surgery.*

THERAPEUTIC INTERVENTIONS
▲ Maintain NPO status until bowel sounds return.
- Ensure patency of NG tube *to keep stomach empty.*
- Encourage/assist with ambulation *to hasten resolution of ileus.*
- Document initial bowel movement.
- Assist patient with initial food/fluid selection *to minimize gaseous distention.*

Altered Nutrition: Less than Body Requirements

RELATED FACTORS
Increased metabolic demands (stress of surgery)
NPO
Primary diagnosis (cancer)
Fever

DEFINING CHARACTERISTICS
Weight loss
Poor wound healing
Low serum albumin (<3.5 gm/dl)

EXPECTED OUTCOMES
Patient maintains pre-operative weight.

ONGOING ASSESSMENT
- Assess postoperative weight; compare to preoperative weight.
- Remain cognizant of length of NPO status.
- Monitor vital signs, especially temperature. *Temperature of 38.5° C for 24-48 hr is a normal postop response.*
▲ Monitor serum albumin level. *< 3.5 gm/dl is an indication of inadequate visceral protein levels.*
- Monitor wound healing.

THERAPEUTIC INTERVENTIONS
▲ Administer IV fluids as ordered: *1 L of 5% dextrose provides approximately 200 cal, which may achieve protein sparing for short time.*
▲ If poor nutritional status and ileus have not resolved, consider peripheral or central hyperalimentation *to maintain anabolic state.*
▲ Administer antipyretics *to control fever; for each 1° C above normal body temperature, metabolic need for calories increases by 7%.*
- See also Nutrition, altered: less than body requirements, p. 44.

High Risk for Infection

RISK FACTORS
Length of procedure
Intraoperative leakage of bowel contents
Insertion of circular staple gun through rectum to abdominal cavity
Postoperative wound contamination

EXPECTED OUTCOMES
Patient remains free of infection as evidenced by temperature < 38.5° C; clean, dry wound.

ONGOING ASSESSMENT
- Assess wound for redness, drainage, pain, swelling, or dehiscence. *These are signs of wound infection.*
▲ Obtain culture of suspicious drainage. *Normal drainage is clear, yellow, odorless.*
- Monitor temperature. *Temperature above 38.5° C should arouse suspicion of infection.*
▲ Monitor WBC.

THERAPEUTIC INTERVENTIONS
- Wash hands on entering room. *Handwashing remains the most effective means of infection control.*
- Use aseptic technique for dressing changes.
▲ Administer antibiotics and antipyretics as prescribed.
- If stoma present, isolate fecal drainage by maintaining good skin seal.
- See also Infection, high risk for, p. 40.

Continued.

Colon cancer—cont'd

NURSING DIAGNOSES	EXPECTED OUTCOMES AND NURSING INTERVENTIONS / *RATIONALES* (■ = INDEPENDENT; ▲ = COLLABORATIVE)

Knowledge Deficit

RELATED FACTORS

Lack of previous experience
  with colon surgery
Need for home management
Need for long-term follow-up
  care

DEFINING CHARACTERISTICS

Multiple questions
Lack of questions
Inability to provide self-care
  on discharge

EXPECTED OUTCOMES

Patient/significant other verbalize knowledge and demonstrate ability to perform wound care, select appropriate diet, plan activity, report complications, get necessary follow-up care.

ONGOING ASSESSMENT

- Assess patient's ability to perform wound care, verbalize appropriate activity, verbalize appropriate diet.
- Assess patient's understanding of need for further cancer therapy (if needed).
- Assess patient's understanding of need for close follow-up care *to detect recurrence of cancer.*
- Assess patient's understanding of expected bowel function.

THERAPEUTIC INTERVENTIONS

- Teach patient to perform appropriate wound care:
    Anterior abdominal wound: *Staples/sutures and dressings have usually been removed by the time of discharge, and Steri-Strips have been placed to maintain wound approximation. Steri-Strips should be left in place until they fall off.*
    Perineal wound: *Sitz baths twice daily for cleansing and comfort, after which the wound is repacked with saline-solution-moistened gauze; usually clean technique (hands washed, clean but not sterile gloves) is used.*
- If patient has a colostomy, see also Fecal ostomy, p. 308.
- Teach patient appropriate activity:
    No lifting more than 10 lb for 6 wk
    Mild exercise (e.g., walking) desirable *to increase stamina*
    Showering OK.
    Bathing OK unless open perineal wound, *which may take up to 8 weeks to heal completely, hand-held shower head good way to clean this wound.*
    No driving until anterior abdominal wound has healed.
- Teach patient the following about diet:
    A well-balanced, high-calorie, high-protein diet is desirable for healing, *which continues over a period of weeks.*
    Fiber should be added to diet; *since patient has already had colon cancer, the risk for future tumors is high. Consumption of high-fiber diet is associated with more frequent bowel movements and less time for suspected carcinogenic food by-products to be in contact with the colonic mucosa. Foods high in fiber include grains, fruits, vegetables.*
- Teach patient the importance of any further cancer therapy planned (e.g., chemotherapy, radiation therapy, immunotherapy). *These therapies are typically offered if the pathology report indicates that the tumor was not confined to the bowel/bowel wall.*
- Teach patient the importance of follow-up colonoscopies *to allow early detection of any recurrent tumors. These are usually scheduled every 6 months for persons with history of colon cancer.*
- Discuss family risk with patients; *parents, siblings, and adult children beyond the age of 40 should be screened yearly for colon cancer.*
- Teach patient that bowel function may not return to preoperative baseline for several weeks. *The more colon resected, the longer the period of adaptation; during this time stool may be loose and stooling more frequent.*
- For patients who have had removal of rectum, teach that phantom rectum sensation and feeling of needing to have a normal bowel movement *(related to remaining nerve fibers in the perineum)* are normal and will subside over time.
- Instruct patient to seek medical attention for any of the following: fever > 38° C, foul-smelling wound drainage, redness or unusual pain in any incision, absence of bowel movement.

See also:
Anticipatory grieving, p. 28.

By: Audrey Klopp, RN, PhD, ET

Enteral tube feeding

(ENTERAL HYPERALIMENTATION; G-TUBE; JEJUNOSTOMY; DUODENOSTOMY)

A method of providing nutrition using a nasogastric tube, a gastrostomy tube, or a tube placed in the duodenum or jejunum. Feedings may be continuous or intermittent (bolus).

NURSING DIAGNOSES	EXPECTED OUTCOMES AND NURSING INTERVENTIONS / *RATIONALE* (■ = INDEPENDENT; ▲ = COLLABORATIVE)

Altered Nutrition: Less than Body Requirements

RELATED FACTORS

Mechanical problems during feedings, such as clogged tube, inaccurate flow rate, stiffening of tube, pump malfunction

DEFINING CHARACTERISTICS

Continued weight loss
Failure to gain weight
Weakness

EXPECTED OUTCOMES

Patient's nutritional status improves as evidenced by gradual weight gain, increased physical strength.

ONGOING ASSESSMENT

- Assess tubing for patency and free flow of enteral feeding.
- Assess equipment (pump) used for administration; assure that proper flow rate is indicated, and that pump is delivering enteral feeding at appropriate rate.
- Assess weight every other day, or as ordered. *Most commercially available tube feeding preparations contain 1 kcal/cc. The average size/weight adult requires 1800-2400 kcal/24h*
- Assess physical strength, daily; note improvement/deterioration.

THERAPEUTIC INTERVENTIONS

- Flush tubing with 20 cc of water *to reduce the risk of clotting.*
- Crush medications and dilute with water; use elixir form when possible.
- Keep pump alarms on.
- Attach to electrical outlet unless patient is traveling.
- ▲ Consult dietician *to assure that ongoing nutritional needs are being met as condition/situation changes.*
- If flow is interrupted for more than 1 hour, recalculate amount to be given over 8 hours and reset administration rate. *Rapid administration to "catch up" can precipitate a hyperglycemic crisis, because the pancreas may not be able to produce adequate insulin for the increased carbohydrate load. The risk of diarrhea also increases when rate is suddenly increased.*

High Risk for Aspiration

RISK FACTORS

Lack of gag reflex
Poor positioning
Overfeeding

EXPECTED OUTCOMES

Patient maintains a patent airway as evidenced by absence of coughing, no shortness of breath, no aspiration.

ONGOING ASSESSMENT

- Assess correct position of tube before initiation of feeding, by injecting air through tube and auscultating over stomach (a gurgling sound indicates correct tube placement). *This is especially important for gastrostomy tubes, because the potential for reflux is increased; duodenostomy and jejunostomy tubes carry somewhat less risk. Also, smaller-diameter, more flexible feeding tubes can easily enter the trachea during insertion.*
- Assess presence of gag reflex before each feeding.
- Assess LOC before administration of feeding. *High-risk patients are comatose, have decreased gag reflex, or cannot tolerate the HOB elevated. Nasoduodenal or gastroduodenal feeding tubes are preferred for high-risk patients.*
- Document patient's baseline respiratory status; monitor respiratory status throughout feeding. *Coughing, shortness of breath may indicate aspiration.*
- Assess for residual feeding before feeding. If patient is on continuous feedings, check residual q4h. *Feedings are held if residual is >110% of amount to be delivered in 1 hr.*
- Assess for coughing, shortness of breath during feedings.

THERAPEUTIC INTERVENTIONS

- Elevate HOB to 30 degrees during and for 30 min after each feeding, *to facilitate gravity flow of feeding past gastroduodenal sphincter; this reduces the risk of aspiration.*
- If patient has an endotracheal or tracheostomy tube, keep the cuff inflated during feedings. *This will protect the airway from inadvertent entry of feedings into the trachea.*
In case of aspiration:
- Stop the feeding.
- Notify the physician.
- Keep the HOB elevated.

Continued.

NURSING DIAGNOSES	EXPECTED OUTCOMES AND NURSING INTERVENTIONS / *RATIONALES* (■ = INDEPENDENT; ▲ = COLLABORATIVE)

THERAPEUTIC INTERVENTIONS—cont'd
- Suction airway as necessary.
- Document time feeding was stopped, patient's appearance, and change in respiratory status.
- See also Airway clearance, ineffective, p. 3.

High Risk for Diarrhea

RISK FACTORS

Intolerance to tube feeding caused by hyperosmolarity, temperature of feeding, rate of delivery, bacterial contamination of feeding, fiber content of feeding

EXPECTED OUTCOMES

Patient does not experience diarrhea during tube feedings.

ONGOING ASSESSMENT
- Assess bowel sounds.
- Assess number and character of stools. *Frequent, loose stools are an indication of intolerance to the tube feedings.*
- Note osmolarity and fiber content of the feeding. *Hyperosmolar or high-fiber feedings draw fluid into the bowel and can cause diarrhea.*
- Note history of lactose intolerance. *Milk-based feedings contain lactose, which is not tolerated by individuals with lactase deficiency.*

THERAPEUTIC INTERVENTIONS

Delivery of formula:
- Begin feedings slowly; consider dilute solution.
- ▲ Increase rate and strength to prescribed amount but not at same time. *High-rate feeding combined with high osmolality may precipitate diarrhea.*
- Administer feedings at room temperature. *Cold stimulates peristalsis.*
- Do not allow formula to hang longer than 8 hr at room temperature *to minimize risk of bacterial contamination.*
- Change setup daily.
- Encourage light activity after feeding *to facilitate digestion.*

High Risk for Fluid Volume Deficit

RISK FACTORS

Osmolarity of feedings
Glucose content of feedings

EXPECTED OUTCOMES

Patient maintains normal fluid volume, as evidenced by moist mucous membranes, good skin turgor, baseline mental status, normal blood glucose level.

ONGOING ASSESSMENT
- Monitor I & O.
- Assess for change in mental status. *Changes in mental status or LOC may be early signs of dehydration or hyperosmolar coma.*
- ▲ Monitor urine glucose and blood glucose levels by glucometer. *High glucose levels cause fluid shift resulting in dehydration. Patients who are unable to metabolize glucose are at risk.*

THERAPEUTIC INTERVENTIONS
- Keep pitcher of water at the bedside. *Availability of free water reduces the risk of fluid volume deficit, by allowing the patient to respond readily to thirst, an early sign of fluid volume deficit or hyperosmolarity.*
- ▲ Administer antihyperglycemic agents as prescribed.

See also:
Fluid volume deficit, p. 25.

Pain

RELATED FACTORS

Dry mucous membranes
Tape irritation
Presence of tube

DEFINING CHARACTERISTICS

Dry, cracked lips
Soiled tape
Reddened area where tube positioned
Swallowing difficulty
Verbalized discomfort

EXPECTED OUTCOMES

The patient remains comfortable as evidenced by moist mucous membranes, ease in swallowing.

ONGOING ASSESSMENT
- Assess mucous membranes. *The presence of a nasally inserted tube will cause mouth-breathing. This contributes to dry, cracked mouth and lips.*
- Assess tube insertion site for reddened areas.
- Assess pain on swallowing.

THERAPEUTIC INTERVENTIONS
- Provide skin/mucous membrane care: change position of tube at nares; retape q12h; apply water-soluble lubricant to nares.

NURSING DIAGNOSES	EXPECTED OUTCOMES AND NURSING INTERVENTIONS / *RATIONALES* (■ = INDEPENDENT; ▲ = COLLABORATIVE)

THERAPEUTIC INTERVENTIONS—cont'd

- Provide mouth care q4h. Avoid lemon-glycerin swabs, *which can lead to further drying.*
- Allow hard candy or gum if permissible *(stimulate salivary secretion).*
- ▲ Provide anesthetic mouthwash as ordered, *to numb throat and ease pain.*
- See also Pain, p. 49.

Knowledge Deficit: Need for Nutritional Support

RELATED FACTORS

New procedure and treatment

DEFINING CHARACTERISTICS

Verbalized inaccurate information

Inappropriate behavior

Questions

EXPECTED OUTCOMES

Patient verbalizes reasons for tube feedings and begins to participate in self-care.
Patient demonstrates independence in enteral feeding administration.

ONGOING ASSESSMENT

- Assess for prior experience with tube feeding.
- Assess knowledge of tube feeding: purpose, expected length of therapy, expected benefits.
- Assess patient's ability to administer own feedings. *Many patients require feedings well beyond hospitalization and can administer feedings to self.*
- Assess patient's ability to use equipment related to feeding: measuring devices, feeding pump, tubing.
- Assess patient's ability to minimize complications related to tube feedings: checking for residual, assuming sitting position, maintaining a bacteria-free feeding.

THERAPEUTIC INTERVENTIONS

- Demonstrate feedings and tube care. Allow return demonstration *so that necessary alteration in teaching plan can be undertaken.*
- Teach significant other or arrange for visiting nurse if patient is unable to feed self.

See also:
Body image disturbance, p. 7.

By: Frankie Harper, RN
   Audrey Klopp, RN, PhD, ET

Enterocutaneous fistula

Communication between any portion of the gastrointestinal tract and the skin. Fistulae may occur spontaneously or postoperatively and may be treated medically or surgically. Problems of greatest concern are nutritional status, fluid/electrolyte balance, and perifistulous skin integrity.

NURSING DIAGNOSES	EXPECTED OUTCOMES AND NURSING INTERVENTIONS / *RATIONALE* (■ = INDEPENDENT; ▲ = COLLABORATIVE)

Skin Integrity, Impaired

RELATED FACTOR

Continuous contact of bowel secretions with skin

DEFINING CHARACTERISTICS

Patient complains of burning, itching

Skin is red, tender

Skin is excoriated

EXPECTED OUTCOMES

Patient's skin is free of irritation caused by contact with drainage.

ONGOING ASSESSMENT

- Assess skin condition for redness, excoriation, tenderness.
- Assess secretion amount, quality, and pH. *The corrosiveness of the secretion will depend on where in the GI tract the fistula is located, because pH varies throughout the GI tract. Duodenal, gastric, and small intestinal fistulas will irritate the skin quickly.*

Continued.

Gastrointestinal and Digestive Care Plans

NURSING DIAGNOSES	EXPECTED OUTCOMES AND NURSING INTERVENTIONS / *RATIONALES* (■ = INDEPENDENT; ▲ = COLLABORATIVE)

THERAPEUTIC INTERVENTIONS

- Maintain intact perifistulous skin.
  Dressing method:
    Protect wound edges with hydrocolloid barriers.
    Change dressing as frequently as necessary *to keep wound edges dry.*
    Use alternate methods (net panties, Montgomery straps) *to hold dressing in place.*
    Adhesives can further compromise skin integrity. Note: If dressing changes are required more often than q2-3h, the dressing method is not appropriate.
  Pouch method:
    Choose appropriate pouch by evaluating skin condition *(pouch adhesives will not adhere to wet/moist skin)*; size and shape of abdomen; presence of current or recent sutures; fistula site; characteristics of fistula drainage.
- Clean and prepare perifistulous skin. *Skin preparation is the most important step in pouching the fistula.*
- Prepare pattern, as a guide to customize the fit of the pouch; apply hydrocolloid skin barrier.
- Fashion pouch; apply over skin barrier.
- Attach to gravity drainage if indicated. *Skin barrier is protected and pouch will last longer if drainage is channeled from skin seal.*
- Keep pouch emptied routinely if it is not connected to gravity.
- Change as necessary when leakage occurs.
    Suction method *(if neither pouch nor dressings maintain dryness):*
      Consult physician about placement of soft, fenestrated catheter near fistula site.
- Position and anchor catheter.
- ▲ Connect to low, intermittent suction device. *Note: Combining pouch and suction methods may increase wear time.*

High Risk for Fluid Volume Deficit

RISK FACTORS

Loss of intestinal fluids/electrolytes through fistula

EXPECTED OUTCOMES

Patient maintains normal fluid balance as evidenced by moist mucous membranes, urine output > 30 ml/hr, stable blood pressure and heart rate.

ONGOING ASSESSMENT

- Assess hydration status: skin turgor, mucous membranes, I & O, including fistula output, weight, vital signs, subjective indicators (thirst).
- ▲ Monitor serum and urine osmolality and specific gravity.
- ▲ Monitor K^+, Na^+, Mg^+ levels.
- Monitor changes in mental status. *Electrolyte imbalance can cause confusion, somnolence.*

THERAPEUTIC INTERVENTIONS

- ▲ Administer parenteral fluids as ordered.
- ▲ Offer ice chips and fluids as ordered/tolerated by patient. *Volume of oral intake should be kept to a minimum, because the amount of fluid passing through the gut may negatively influence spontaneous closure of a fistula.*
- ▲ Administer anticholinergic drugs as ordered. *Anticholinergic drugs decrease the amount of intestinal secretions by decreasing cholinergic (vagal) stimulation.*
- Report signs/symptoms of electrolyte imbalance and dehydration.

Altered Nutrition: Less than Body Requirements

RELATED FACTORS

Nutritional loss from fistula(s)
Decreased or bypassed absorptive surface
Prolonged therapeutic withholding of nutrients

EXPECTED OUTCOMES

Patient achieves nutritional status sufficient to support healing, as evidenced by stable weight, healing wounds.

ONGOING ASSESSMENT

- ▲ Assess nitrogen balance and serum albumin levels. *Nitrogen balance indicates total protein reserve; serum albumin level indicates visceral protein reserve.*
- If patient has hyperalimentation line, inspect insertion site for redness, swelling, oozing, and tenderness.
- Weigh patient daily.
- ▲ Check electrolytes daily.
- See also Nutrition, altered: less than body requirements, p. 44.

NURSING DIAGNOSES	EXPECTED OUTCOMES AND NURSING INTERVENTIONS / *RATIONALES* (■ = INDEPENDENT; ▲ = COLLABORATIVE)

DEFINING CHARACTERISTICS

Complaints of weakness
Weight loss
Negative nitrogen balance
Low serum albumin level
Low total iron-binding capacity
(TIBC)
Scaling skin

THERAPEUTIC INTERVENTIONS

- ▲ Administer hyperalimentation as prescribed.
- Maintain flow rate. *If administration is to be stopped or resumed for any reason, change flow rate to 50% of normal rate for at least 1 hr to allow appropriate pancreatic response. This allows for appropriate hormonal use of glucose.*
- Change occlusive dressing and tubing per policy.

Body Image Disturbance

RELATED FACTORS

Continuous fecal drainage
Fecal odor
Necessity of pouch, dressings,
and/or suction catheter

DEFINING CHARACTERISTICS

Verbalized concern of altered
pattern of excretion
Reluctance to look at or touch
pouch/dressing
Altered socialization

EXPECTED OUTCOMES

Patient maintains healthy, realistic body image as evidenced by ability to discuss/participate in own care.
Patient feels comfortable with collection device/technique, as evidenced by increased socialization, participation in own care.

ONGOING ASSESSMENT

- Note verbal indications of altered self-concept/body image.
- Note patient's willingness to socialize with family, friends, staff, other patients.
- Note patient's involvement in self-care.
- Note defensive behaviors about appearance.
- Note presence of odor and patient's reaction to it. *Small bowel fistulae have little odor, but large bowel (colonic) fistulae have a strong fecal odor.*

THERAPEUTIC INTERVENTIONS

- Encourage verbalization of feelings.
- Talk with patient empathetically.
- Provide adequate site care *so odor is minimized or eliminated.*
- Use pouch or room deodorants sparingly. *Overuse can call unnecessary attention to the problem.*
- Refer to support group as appropriate.

High Risk for Impaired Individual Coping

RISK FACTORS

Prolonged hospitalization
Painful uncomfortable pouch/
dressing changes
Prolonged nutritional support
Prolonged isolation from family, friends, and work
Possible need for surgery

EXPECTED OUTCOMES

Patient demonstrates positive coping methods as evidenced by relaxed appearance; ability to participate in care/activities; ability to rest

ONGOING ASSESSMENT

- Assess for signs of coping difficulty: Emotional tension, irritability, changes in eating pattern, sleeping difficulties, verbalized coping difficulties.
- Evaluate support systems available to patient while in hospital.

THERAPEUTIC INTERVENTIONS

- Discuss present status/anticipated therapy.
- Explain usual therapy course. *The usual course of treatment for an enterocutaneous fistula is bowel rest (complete NPO status) with aggressive nutritional support (parenteral hyperalimentation). If the fistula fails to close in 6-8 wk, surgery may be considered.*
- Provide simple explanations and reassurance. *Understanding how and why procedures are done may help decrease fear/anxiety and promote effective coping.*
- Point out progress being made, however slight (*e.g., decrease in drainage*).
- Assist patient in using usual coping behaviors.
- Express normalcy of such feelings about self under circumstances.
- Reinforce that once fistula is healed, elimination does return to normal.
- ▲ Initiate consultation with occupational/physical therapist *to provide opportunity for exercise and activity.*
- Encourage use of distractions (television, radio, newspapers).

By: Florencia Isidro-Sanchez, RN, BSN
Audrey Klopp, RN, PhD, ET

Fecal ostomy

(COLOSTOMY; ILEOSTOMY; FECAL DIVERSION; STOMA)

A surgical procedure that results in an opening into small or large intestine for the purpose of diverting the fecal stream past an area of obstruction or disease, protecting a distal surgical anastomosis, or providing an outlet for stool in the absence of a functioning intact rectum. Depending on the purpose of the surgery and the integrity and function of anatomical structures, stomas may be temporary or permanent. Peristomal irritation, adaptation, and learning are important nursing concerns.

NURSING DIAGNOSES	EXPECTED OUTCOMES AND NURSING INTERVENTIONS / *RATIONALE* (■ = INDEPENDENT; ▲ = COLLABORATIVE)

Preoperative Knowledge Deficit

RELATED FACTORS

Lack of previous similar experience
Need for additional information
Previous contact with poorly rehabilitated ostomate

DEFINING CHARACTERISTICS

Verbalized need for information
Verbalized misinformation/ misconceptions
Multiple questions
Lack of questions

EXPECTED OUTCOMES

Patient describes alteration in normal GI anatomy and physiology requiring surgical creation of the stoma.
Patient verbalizes that loss or bypass of anal sphincter will result in the need to wear a pouch.

ONGOING ASSESSMENT

- Assess previous surgical experience.
- Inquire as to information from surgeon about ostomy formation (i.e., purpose, site).
- Ascertain (from chart, physician) whether stoma will be permanent or temporary. *Learning readiness/adaptation is often delayed in patients with temporary stomas.*
- Explore previous contact patient has had with persons with stoma. *Expectations are frequently based on previous experience.*

THERAPEUTIC INTERVENTIONS

- Reinforce and reexplain proposed procedure. *Preoperative anxiety frequently makes necessary to repeat instructions/explanations several times in order for patients to comprehend.*
- Use diagrams, pictures, and AV equipment to explain anatomy, physiology of GI tract; pathophysiology necessitating ostomy; proposed location of stoma. *Ileostomy stomas are located in the right lower quadrant; colostomy stomas may be upper right quadrant, midabdomen at waistline, or left upper or lower quadrant.*
- Explain need for pouch in terms of loss of sphincter. *Patients should be told that preoperative bowel habits may return after surgery, but that control of defecation is lost, and that therefore, a pouch is necessary to collect/contain stool and gas.*
- Show patient actual pouch or one similar to the one that patient will wear after surgery.
- Allow patient to wear pouch preoperatively. *Stoma site selection is facilitated by observing adhesive faceplate in situ.*
- Offer visit from rehabilitated ostomate. *Often contact with another individual who has "been there" is more beneficial than factual information.*

High Risk for Self-care deficit: Toileting

RISK FACTORS

Presence of poorly placed stoma
Presence of pouch
Poor hand-eye coordination

EXPECTED OUTCOMES

Patient performs self-care independently (emptying pouch/changing pouch) as a result of preoperative stoma site selection.

ONGOING ASSESSMENT

- Assess for the following: presence of old abdominal scars, presence of bony prominences on anterior abdomen, presence of creases/skinfolds on abdomen, extreme obesity, scaphoid abdomen, pendulous breasts, ability to see and handle equipment. *Stoma placement is easier for a patient who has a flat abdomen that has no scars, bony prominences, or extremes of weight.*

THERAPEUTIC INTERVENTIONS

- ▲ Consult ET nurse or surgeon to mark proposed stoma site in area indelibly: patient can easily see; patient can easily reach; scars, bony prominences, skinfolds are avoided; hip flexion does not change contour; *Stoma location is a key factor in self-care. A poorly located stoma can delay/preclude self-care.*
- Note usual sites for stoma:
    Ileostomy: *lower right quadrant.*
    Ascending colostomy: *right upper or lower quadrant.*
    Transverse colostomy: *midwaist or just below midwaist.*
    Descending and sigmoid colostomies: *lower left quadrant.*
- If possible, have patient wear pouch over proposed site; evaluate effectiveness 12-24 hr after applying pouch.

NURSING DIAGNOSES	EXPECTED OUTCOMES AND NURSING INTERVENTIONS / *RATIONALES* (■ = INDEPENDENT; ▲ = COLLABORATIVE)

High Risk for Altered Stoma Tissue Perfusion

RISK FACTORS

Surgical manipulation of bowel
Postoperative edema
Tightly fitted faceplate
Pressure from rod or other support device

EXPECTED OUTCOMES

Patient's stoma remains pink and moist.

ONGOING ASSESSMENT

- Assess the following at least q4h: color of stoma (*stoma is a rerouted piece of intestine that should look pink/red and moist*), moist appearance of stoma, stomal edema, presence of rods/support devices. *Transverse or loop stomas are frequently supported by a rod or other support device, which usually is removed at the bedside on the 7th-10th postoperative day.*

THERAPEUTIC INTERVENTIONS

- Notify physician if stoma appears dusky or blue. *Stoma (a piece of intestine) should be pink, moist, indicating good perfusion and adequate venous drainage. Dusky or blue appearance may indicate venous congestion or poor blood supply, either of which could result in a necrotic stoma.*
- Anticipate/prepare patient for possible surgical stoma revision.

High Risk for Body Image Disturbance

RISK FACTORS

Presence of stoma
Loss of fecal continence
Presence of pouch
Primary disease (after cancer)
Fear of offensive odor
Fear of appearing "different"

EXPECTED OUTCOMES

Patient begins to verbalize feelings about stoma and body image.

ONGOING ASSESSMENT

- Assess perception of change in body structure and function.
- Assess perceived impact of change. *The patient's response to real or perceived changes in body structure and/or function is related to the importance the patient places on the structure or function (i.e., a very fastidious person may experience the visual presence of a stool-filled pouch on the anterior abdomen as intolerable).*
- Note verbal/nonverbal references to stoma. *Patients frequently "name" stomas as an attempt to separate the stoma from self. Others may look away or totally deny the presence of the stoma until able to cope.*
- Note patient's ability/readiness to look at, touch, care for stoma and ostomy equipment.

THERAPEUTIC INTERVENTIONS

- Acknowledge appropriateness of emotional response to perceived change in body structure and function. *Because control of elimination is skill/task of early childhood and socially private function, loss of control precipitates body image change and possible self-concept change.*
- Assist patient in looking at, touching, and caring for stoma when ready.
- Assist patient in identifying specific actions that could be helpful in managing perceived loss/problem related to stoma. *The most frequent concern is odor; helping patients to gain control over odor will facilitate an acceptable body image. (See Odor control in discharge planning section of this care plan.)*

Knowledge Deficit: Ostomy Self-Care

RELATED FACTORS

Presence of new stoma
Lack of similar experience

DEFINING CHARACTERISTICS

Demonstrated inability to empty and change pouch
Verbalized need for information about diet, odor, activity, hygiene, clothing, interpersonal relationships, equipment purchase, financial concerns

EXPECTED OUTCOMES

Patient is capable of partial ostomy self-care on discharge.

ONGOING ASSESSMENT

- Assess ability to empty and change pouch. *Most patients will be independent in emptying pouch by time of discharge; many will still need assistance with pouch change and may require outpatient follow-up care.*
- Assess ability to care for peristomal skin and identify problems.
- Assess appropriateness in seeking assistance.
- Assess knowledge of the following:
  Diet. (*Postoperatively patient should consume high-protein, high-carbohydrate diet to facilitate healing. Patient must understand that not eating in order to minimize fecal output is detrimental, and that the stoma will have output regardless.*)
  Activity. (*Patient should understand that activity should not be altered by the presence of the stoma/pouch.*)
  Hygiene.
  Clothing. (*No special clothing or alterations in existing clothing are necessitated by the presence of the stoma/pouch.*)

Continued.

Gastrointestinal and Digestive Care Plans

NURSING DIAGNOSES	EXPECTED OUTCOMES AND NURSING INTERVENTIONS / *RATIONALES* (■ = INDEPENDENT; ▲ = COLLABORATIVE)

THERAPEUTIC INTERVENTIONS

- Provide psychomotor teaching during first and subsequent applications of pouch. *Even before patients are able to participate actively, they can observe and discuss ostomy care.*
- Include one (or more) significant others as approved/desired by patient. *It is beneficial to teach others alongside the patient, so long as all realize that the goal is for the patient to become independent in self-ostomy care.*
- Gradually transfer responsibility for pouch emptying and changing to patient.
- Allow at least one opportunity for supervised return demonstration of pouch change before discharge. *Ostomy care requires both cognitive and psychomotor skills. Postoperatively, learning ability may be decreased, requiring repetition and opportunity for return demonstrations.*
- Instruct patient on the following regarding diet:
    For Ileostomy: *balanced diet: special care in chewing high-fiber foods (popcorn, peanuts, coconut, vegetables, string beans, olives): increased fluid intake during hot weather, vigorous exercise.*
    For colostomy: *balanced diet: no foods specifically contraindicated; certain foods (eggs, fish, green leafy vegetables, carbonated beverages) may increase flatus and fecal odor.*
- Discuss odor control and acknowledge that odor (or fear of odor) can impair social functioning. *Odor control is best achieved by eliminating odor-causing foods from diet; green leafy vegetables, eggs, fish, and onions are primary odor-causing foods. Oral deodorants and pouch deodorants may also help.*
- Discuss availability of ostomy support groups (United Ostomy Association, National Foundation for Ileitis and Colitis)
- Instruct patient to maintain contact with enterostomal therapy nurse *for follow-up and observation and problem solving.*

See also:
High risk for infection, p. 40.

By: Audrey Klopp, RN, PhD, ET

Gastrointestinal bleeding

(LOWER GASTROINTESTINAL BLEED; UPPER
GASTROINTESTINAL BLEED; ESOPHAGEAL VARICES;
ULCERS)

Loss of blood from the GI tract is most often the result of erosion or ulceration of the mucosa but may be the result of arteriovenous (AV) malformation, malignancies, increased pressure in the portal venous bed, or direct trauma to the gastrointestinal tract. Alcohol abuse is a major etiologic factor in GI bleeding. Varices, usually located in the distal third of the submucosal tissue of the esophagus and/or the fundus of the stomach, can also cause life-threatening GI hemorrhage. Treatment may be medical or surgical or may involve mechanical tamponade.

NURSING DIAGNOSES

EXPECTED OUTCOMES AND NURSING INTERVENTIONS / *RATIONALE*
(■ = INDEPENDENT; ▲ = COLLABORATIVE)

Fluid Volume Deficit

RELATED FACTORS

Upper GI bleeding (mouth, esophagus, stomach, duodenum) caused by gastric ulcer, duodenal ulcer, gastritis, esophageal varices, Mallory-Weiss tear, blunt or penetrating trauma, cancer

Lower GI bleeding (small or large intestine, rectum, anus) caused by tumors, inflammatory bowel disease (diverticular disease, Crohn's disease, ulcerative colitis), A-V malformations, blunt or penetrating trauma, hemorrhoids

Generalized GI bleeding: systemic coagulopathies, radiation therapy, chemotherapy, family history of GI bleeding, history of recent violent retching, history of alcohol abuse/use, altered coagulation profile, history of aspirin, steroid, nonsteroid, or ibuprofen use/abuse

DEFINING CHARACTERISTICS

Hematemesis (observed or reported)
Melena
Hematochezia (bright red blood per rectum)
Orthostatic changes
Tachycardia
Hypotension
Change in LOC
Thirst
Dry mucous membranes

EXPECTED OUTCOMES

Patient maintains normal fluid volume as evidenced by urine output of 30 ml/hr, stable blood pressure and heart rate, moist mucous membranes.

ONGOING ASSESSMENT

- Monitor color, consistency of hematemesis, melena, or rectal bleeding; encourage patient to describe unwitnessed blood loss accurately using common household measures (e.g., a cupful, a spoonful, a pint).
- Obtain history of use/abuse of substances known to predispose to GI bleeding: aspirin, aspirin-containing drugs, nonsteroidal antiinflammatory drugs, ibuprofen-containing drugs, alcohol, steroids.
- Monitor blood pressure for orthostatic changes (from patient lying prone to high Fowler's). Note orthostatic hypotension significance:
  >10 mm Hg drop: circulating blood volume is decreased by 20%.
  >20-30 mm Hg drop: circulating blood volume is decreased by 40%.
- Assess for tachycardia.
- ▲ Monitor coagulation profile, Hb, and Hct.
- Obtain diet history.
- Monitor urine output. *Urine output of at least 30 ml/hr is an indication of adequate renal perfusion.*

THERAPEUTIC INTERVENTIONS

- ▲ Start one or more large-bore IVs. *Rapid volume expansion is necessary to prevent/treat hypovolemia complications; IV medication and/or blood component administration is likely.*
- ▲ Insert NG tube *for stomach lavage, to monitor continuing blood loss closely, and for medication administration.*
- ▲ Lavage stomach until clots are no longer present, return is clear; use room temperature saline solution. *Iced saline solution may cause undesirable ischemic changes in gastric mucosa.*
- ▲ Provide volume resuscitation with crystalloids or blood products as ordered; monitor cardiopulmonary response to volume expansion. *Patients with history of alcohol abuse may have alcohol-related cardiomyopathies.*
- ▲ Assist with/coordinate diagnostic procedures performed to identify bleeding site:
  Endoscopy: *provides direct visualization of esophagus, stomach, and duodenum. Procedure must precede radiographs requiring barium ingestion to maximize visualization by endoscopist.*
  Sigmoidoscopy/proctoscopy/colonoscopy: *Provides direct visualization of rectum and colon.*
  Barium studies:
    Barium swallow: *indirect visualization of esophagus, stomach, and small intestine.*
    Barium enema: *indirect visualization of colon.*
    Small bowel follow-through: *indirect visualization of small intestine.*
  Angiography *(may be diagnostic or performed for arterial line placement to infuse vasoconstrictive medications locally; will be inconclusive diagnostically unless bleeding >0.5 cc/min).* After angiography: dress site with pressure dressing, connect arterial line to pressure/flush system.
- ▲ Administer vasopressin drip, *a potent vasoconstrictive agent.*
- ▲ Administer vitamin K as ordered *to allow coagulation factor production.*
- ▲ Administer antacids and H$_2$ receptor antagonists (i.e., Cimetadine, Zantac) *to suppress gastric/duodenal secretions.*

Continued.

Gastrointestinal bleeding—cont'd

NURSING DIAGNOSES	EXPECTED OUTCOMES AND NURSING INTERVENTIONS / *RATIONALES* (■ = INDEPENDENT; ▲ = COLLABORATIVE)

THERAPEUTIC INTERVENTIONS—cont'd

▲ Arrange/assist with transfer of patient to monitored area if hemodynamically unstable.

▪ Guard against inadvertent administration of drugs that may potentiate further bleeding.

If in critical care area:

▲ Prepare for insertion of Sengstaken-Blakemore tube for the patient bleeding from esophageal/gastric varices. *The Sengstaken-Blakemore tube has balloons that inflate in the esophagus and upper portion of the stomach to provide tamponade (pressure) against the vessels that are bleeding.*

High Risk Pain/Discomfort

RISK FACTORS

Invasive therapies
Diagnostic procedures
Vomiting
Diarrhea

EXPECTED OUTCOMES

Patient verbalizes absence of pain or tolerable levels of pain.
Patient appears comfortable.

ONGOING ASSESSMENT

▪ Assess for evidence of discomfort: verbalizing of pain/discomfort, facial grimacing, restlessness.

▪ Assess specific sources of discomfort.

▪ Ask patient what measure(s) he/she believes might provide comfort.

THERAPEUTIC INTERVENTIONS

▪ Tape/stabilize all tubes, drains, and catheters *to minimize movement causing discomfort.*

▪ Provide frequent oral hygiene *to remove blood/emesis and moisten mucous membranes.*

▪ For patient with traction helmet for stabilization of Sengstaken-Blakemore tube, pad parts contacting skin *to minimize occurrence of skin friction and/or ischemia.*

▪ Provide meticulous perineal care after all bowel movements.

▪ For patients with any indwelling nasogastric tube, moisten external nares with water-soluble lubricant at least once per shift *to reduce adherence of mucus (can dry and cause irritation).*

▪ Change linens as necessary *to minimize discomfort and reduce unpleasant melenic odor.*

▲ Use analgesics with caution *so LOC changes related to fluid volume deficit may be carefully evaluated.*

▪ See also Pain, p. 49.

High Risk for Altered Skin Integrity

RISK FACTORS

Bed rest
Frequent stooling
Hypovolemia leading to skin ischemia
Poor nutritional status

EXPECTED OUTCOMES

Skin remains intact.

ONGOING ASSESSMENT

▪ Assess condition of skin at least q2h for redness, irritation.

THERAPEUTIC INTERVENTIONS

▪ Turn patient side to side as hemodynamic status allows. *Hemodynamically unstable patients may have a drop in blood pressure when turned side to side.*

▪ Place pressure relief device(s) beneath patient.

▪ Do not allow patient to sit on bedpan for long periods.

▪ Clean perianal skin with soap and water after each bowel movement; dry well.

▪ Apply liquid film barrier to perianal area *so there is no direct skin contact with stool.*

▪ Minimize use of plastic linen protectors *(harbor moisture and enhance maceration).*

High Risk for Injury: Complications of Vasopressin (Pitressin) Therapy

RISK FACTORS

Vasoconstriction
Antidiuretic effect of vasopressin

EXPECTED OUTCOMES

Patient is free of complications related to vasopressin therapy, as evidenced by stable vital signs, normal sinus rhythm, no nausea/vomiting.

ONGOING ASSESSMENT

▪ Assess for side effects of vasopressin: anginal pain, ST-segment changes on ECG, sinus bradycardia, tremors, sweating, vertigo, pounding in head, abdominal cramps, circumoral pallor, nausea/vomiting, flatus, urticaria, fluid retention.

▪ Monitor blood pressure and heart rate.

▪ Assess peripheral pulses (rate, regularity) and capillary refill.

▪ Assess for abdominal distention; record abdominal girth.

NURSING DIAGNOSES	EXPECTED OUTCOMES AND NURSING INTERVENTIONS / *RATIONALES* (■ = INDEPENDENT; ▲ = COLLABORATIVE)

THERAPEUTIC INTERVENTIONS

▲ Administer vasopressin per order. *Vasopressin is a commercial preparation of antidiuretic hormone, which promotes vasoconstriction.*

If side effects occur:

▲ Stop infusion of vasopressin drip. *IV vasopressin preparation is short-acting; cessation of administration diminishes adverse effects rapidly.*

▲ Have atropine on hand for decreased heart rate.

▪ Provide patient comfort and assurance.

High Risk for Altered Level of Consciousness (LOC)

RISK FACTORS

Elevated cerebral toxin levels
Altered metabolic liver function
Increased cerebral sensitivity

EXPECTED OUTCOMES

Patient maintains normal level of consciousness.

ONGOING ASSESSMENT

▪ Assess for changes in level of consciousness: lethargy, confusion, somnolence.

▲ Monitor ammonia levels. *Ammonia is normally converted to urea by hepatic cells; when this does not occur, ammonia circulates and acts as a cerebral toxin.*

▲ Monitor acid base balance.

▪ Monitor temperature. *Both acid-base imbalance and fever increase cerebral sensitivity to circulating toxins.*

THERAPEUTIC INTERVENTIONS

▲ Reduce toxins available to the cerebral circulation by lavaging stomach *to remove blood,* giving enemas *to remove blood,* administering nonabsorbable antibiotics as prescribed *to reduce intestinal bacteria count (thus reducing ammonia production).*

▲ Administer antipyretics as ordered.

▲ Correct acid-base balance.

▪ See Consciousness, altered level of, p. 252.

Knowledge Deficit

RELATED FACTORS

First GI bleed
Unfamiliar environment

DEFINING CHARACTERISTICS

Multiple questions
Lack of questions
Verbalized misconceptions

EXPECTED OUTCOMES

Patient/significant other verbalizes understanding of cause(s) and management of GI bleeding.

ONGOING ASSESSMENT

▪ Assess understanding of the cause and treatment of GI bleeding.

▪ Assess understanding of the need for long-term follow-up, observation, and possible lifestyle changes.

THERAPEUTIC INTERVENTIONS

▪ Explain procedures necessary for diagnosis and/or treatment before they are performed. *Understanding the need for unpleasant procedures may help patient comply/participate and increase yield/effectiveness of treatment or procedure.*

▪ Encourage/stress importance of avoidance of substances containing aspirin, alcohol, nonsteroidal antiinflammatory drugs, ibuprofen, steroids.

▪ Teach patient the dose, administration schedule, expected actions, and possible adverse effects of medications that may be prescribed for long periods. *Drugs given to decrease gastric acid production may be prescribed indefinitely; patients must understand that cessation of bleeding or other symptoms does not mean need for medication has ended.*

▲ Refer patient to alcohol rehabilitation if indicated.

See also:
Fear, p. 23.
Ineffective management of
  therapeutic regimen, p. 39.

By: Lou Ann Ary, RN, BSN

Hemorrhoids/ hemorrhoidectomy

(RECTAL POLYPS; PILES)

Hemorrhoids are the vascular tumors formed in the rectal mucosa caused by the presence of dilated blood vessels. Treatment varies with condition, including banding, laser, and surgical ligation.

NURSING DIAGNOSES	EXPECTED OUTCOMES AND NURSING INTERVENTIONS / *RATIONALE* (■ = INDEPENDENT; ▲ = COLLABORATIVE)

Excess Fluid Volume, In Superior (Internal) and/or Inferior (External) Hemorrhoidal Plexus

RELATED FACTORS

Increased intravenous pressure in hemorrhoidal plexus

DEFINING CHARACTERISTICS

Large, firm lumps protruding from rectum
Presence of large, firm lumps on rectal examination
Anal itching
Painless, intermittent bleeding
Constant discomfort and bleeding
Rectal discomfort

EXPECTED OUTCOMES

Patient understands and controls factors that aggravate hemorrhoids.

ONGOING ASSESSMENT

- Solicit patient's history of signs/symptoms of hemorrhoids. *Severe bleeding and/or pain may indicate proctoscopy to diagnose internal hemorrhoids versus rectal polyps.*
- Examine rectal area for external hemorrhoids: *skin-covered, emerging from external anal tissue; protruding from anal canal, covered by rectal mucosa.*
- Check for rectal bleeding.
- Assess itching.

THERAPEUTIC INTERVENTIONS

- Encourage patient to avoid prolonged standing or sitting *(causes blood pooling and thrombosis).*
- ▲ Treat diarrhea/constipation (see also Diarrhea, p. 19, Constipation, p. 16).
- Discuss patient's life-style and predisposing factors to hemorrhoid development:
    Prolonged occupational standing or sitting, *which causes venous congestion.*
    Straining caused by diarrhea, constipation, vomiting, sneezing, and coughing.
    Loss of muscle tone (old age, rectal surgery, pregnancy, episiotomy, anal intercourse).
    Anorectal infections.
- Encourage patient to take corrective actions.
- Discuss self-care issues:
    Bowel elimination.
    Manual reduction of hemorrhoidal prolapse (gently pushing hemorrhoids into rectum).
    Dietary habits (provide dietary consultaion if necessary).

Pain

RELATED FACTORS

Thrombosis of external hemorrhoids or hemorrhoidal prolapse

DEFINING CHARACTERISTICS

Sudden rectal pain
Large, firm lumps protruding from rectum
Postoperative pain

EXPECTED OUTCOMES

Patient verbalizes relief of pain.

ONGOING ASSESSMENT

- Assess complaints of pain.
- Elicit comfort factors used in past.

THERAPEUTIC INTERVENTIONS

- ▲ Provide local anesthetic as ordered. *Analgesic and steroidal creams are useful in controlling hemorrhoidal pain.*
- Provide cold compresses.
- Encourage warm sitz baths.
- ▲ Administer analgesics as prescribed for intractable pain. *Pain will be present until thrombosis is resolved.*

High Risk for Fluid Volume Deficit

RISK FACTORS

Bleeding hemorrhoids
Preoperative or postoperative hemorrhoidal bleeding

EXPECTED OUTCOMES

Patient maintains normal fluid volume as evidenced by absence of bleeding, and stable vital signs.

ONGOING ASSESSMENT

Preoperative care
- Obtain history of past bleeding, frequency.
- Examine rectal area; assess amount of bleeding: small, moderate, or profuse; number of pads soaked.
- Assess blood pressure, heart rate.
- ▲ Assess Hct, Hb if anemia suspected in patient bleeding for a long time.
Postoperative care
- Examine rectal area for hematoma, swelling, drainage, and excessive bleeding.

THERAPEUTIC INTERVENTIONS

Preoperative care
- Provide gentle rectal hygiene and minimal manipulation *to prevent tearing thin rectal tissue.* Do *not* take rectal temperature.
- Notify physician of large blood loss, vital sign changes.
▲ Anticipate need for type and cross match. *Patients can loose significant amount of blood.*
- Prepare patient for surgery if indicated.

Postoperative care
▲ Administer medications as ordered. *(Metamucil to increase stool bulk).*
- Keep wound site clean by changing pads as needed and providing sitz baths if appropriate.

Knowledge Deficit

RELATED FACTORS

New condition
No previous surgical intervention

DEFINING CHARACTERISTICS

Requests for information
Repeated episodes of bleeding or thrombosis

EXPECTED OUTCOMES

Patient expresses understanding of treatment and prevention.

ONGOING ASSESSMENT

- Assess understanding of causes and treatment of hemorrhoids.

THERAPEUTIC INTERVENTIONS

- Instruct patient on importance of regular bowel habits. *Straining at stool is a common cause of exacerbation of hemorrhoids.*
- Discuss good anal hygiene:
  Suggest use of plain, nonscented white toilet paper. *Dyes and perfumes may irritate tissue and cause itching, bleeding.*
  Encourage use of medicated astringent pads for cleansing.
  Discuss avoidance of hand soaps and vigorous washing with hand towels. *Soap can irritate rectal mucosa. Vigorous washing can disrupt thin tissues and cause bleeding.*
▲ Provide dietary information/consultation. *High-fiber diets with ample fluids make defecation easier and reduce episodes of inflamed hemorrhoidal tissue.*
- Discuss other predisposing factors:
  Occupational: discourage prolonged sitting or standing.
  Sexual habits: discourage anal intercourse.
- If patient to have surgical or other intervention, provide accurate preoperative instruction; discuss postprocedural expectations.
- Upon discharge, provide patient with follow-up appointment and important telephone numbers.

By: Michele Knoll Puzas, RN,C, MHPE

Hepatitis

(SERUM HEPATITIS, INFECTIOUS HEPATITIS, HAV, HBV, HCV, NANB-PT, NANB-ET)

Inflammation of the liver caused by a virus. Type A (HAV) infectious hepatitis is commonly transmitted by fecal-oral route, poor sanitation, person-to-person contact, or contaminated food, water, or shellfish. Type B (HBV) serum hepatitis is commonly transmitted parenterally or by intimate contact with carriers; by blood, saliva, semen, and vaginal secretions; via contaminated needles and renal dialysis. Type non-A, non-B (sometimes called "C") is actually two distinct entities: non-A, non-B parenterally transmitted (PT), and non-A, non-B enterically transmitted (ET). Non-A, non-B ET is transmitted via the oral-fecal route; non-A, non-B PT is transmitted via parenteral routes, such as needle use/sharing, accidental sticks, and dialysis. Health care workers are at risk for all types.

NURSING DIAGNOSES	EXPECTED OUTCOMES AND NURSING INTERVENTIONS / *RATIONALE* (■ = INDEPENDENT; ▲ = COLLABORATIVE)

Knowledge Deficit

RELATED FACTORS

New condition
Unfamiliarity with disease
  course and treatment

DEFINING CHARACTERISTICS

Lack of questions
Many questions
Noncompliance with isolation
  procedures

EXPECTED OUTCOMES

Patient/significant other verbalize and demonstrate knowledge of and compliance with treatment regimen and isolation procedures.

ONGOING ASSESSMENT

- Determine understanding of disease process, disease transmission, complications, treatment, and signs of relapse.
- Observe compliance with treatment regimen.
- Observe compliance with isolation procedures. *Noncompliance may be related to incomplete understanding of disease transmission and/or treatment regimen.*

THERAPEUTIC INTERVENTIONS

- Teach patient/significant other about disease transmission:
  Hepatitis A: *fecal-oral transmission (crowded living conditions, poor personal hygiene, contaminated food, milk, raw shellfish).*
  Hepatitis B: *percutaneous and permucosal (needles, blood products, sex).*
  Hepatitis C: *percutaneous (blood products, needles).*
- Teach patient about treatment. *Adequate rest, nutrition, and prevention of complications are the mainstay of therapy for all types of hepatitis. Since the disease is viral, medications are not helpful.*
- Teach patients about isolation procedures, *which are related to preventing the transmission of disease.*
- Teach patients reasons that health care workers wear protective clothing: *to protect themselves and others from viral infection.*
- Discuss future need to avoid blood donation. *Even after patients with hepatitis are well, they may carry the virus and should refrain from blood donation to prevent risk of disease transmission.*
- Teach patient about possible complications/long-term sequelae of hepatitis. *Hepatitis can lead to chronic hepatitis and/or fulminant liver failure and death if it is untreated or treated unsuccessfully.*
- Teach patient that compliance with therapy improves prognosis and reduces the risk of serious complications.
- Teach patient that successful treatment and full recovery can take weeks to months; relapse is not uncommon.

Activity Intolerance

RELATED FACTORS

Decreased metabolism of nutrients
Increased basal metabolic rate
  caused by viral infection

EXPECTED OUTCOMES

Patient avoids fatigue/exhaustion by alternating activity with periods of rest.
Patient is able to perform required ADLs.

ONGOING ASSESSMENT

- Assess general energy levels and activity tolerance every shift; note specific trends. *Some patients have peak energy levels early in the day or after naps; nursing care should be scheduled accordingly to prevent exhaustion.*
- Assess vital signs before activity: respiratory rate, heart rate, blood pressure. *Baseline allows for recognition of significant changes.*
- Determine need for supplemental oxygen during activity.

NURSING DIAGNOSES	EXPECTED OUTCOMES AND NURSING INTERVENTIONS / *RATIONALE* (■ = INDEPENDENT; ▲ = COLLABORATIVE)

DEFINING CHARACTERISTICS

Fatigue
Weakness
Dyspnea associated with activity
Tachycardia and elevated BP associated with activity
Inability to initiate activity

ONGOING ASSESSMENT—cont'd

- Assess need for assistive devices, *which may decrease exertion.*
- ▲ Monitor liver enzyme levels. *Elevations in hepatic enzyme levels indicate damage or death of liver cells; new elevations or failure of enzyme levels to trend toward normal indicates continuing damage, which could result from premature activity or overexertion.*

THERAPEUTIC INTERVENTIONS

- ▲ Maintain bedrest until enzyme levels begin to normalize. *Healing damaged liver cells and generating new ones require metabolic expenditure; maintaining bedrest reduces the energy required for movement and increases the energy available for healing.*
- Allow bathroom use or provide a bedside commode when activity tolerance improves or if use of a bedpan requires more energy expenditure than getting up to use the bathroom or commode.
- Provide a quiet environment and promote rest using strategies that the patient identifies as helpful (music, reading, dim lights, etc.).
- Plan and pace nursing care *to provide for long, uninterrupted periods of rest and relaxation.*
- ▲ Administer sedatives or tranquilizers as prescribed *to facilitate rest; avoid medications that are metabolized by the liver.*
- Increase activity as tolerated.
- Provide information on energy conservation techniques.

High Risk for Diversional Activity Deficit

RISK FACTORS

Isolation
Lack of energy
Long-term hospitalization

EXPECTED OUTCOMES

Patient engages in meaningful activity within the limits of activity tolerance.

ONGOING ASSESSMENT

- Assess for evidence of diversional activity deficit: verbalized boredom, verbalized feelings of "being isolated" or "away from everyone and everything," daydreaming.
- Assess patient's desire for/ability to participate in diversional activities.
- Explore the usual diversional activities that the patients enjoys.

THERAPEUTIC INTERVENTIONS

- Assist patient in identifying realistic goals for engaging in diversional activity. *The patient may need assistance in balancing desire for diversional activities with the reality of need for rest and activity intolerance imposed by the disease process.*
- ▲ Consult specialists (occupational therapists, recreational therapists) *to provide diversional activities and resources to carry out activities.*
- Assist patient in planning day so that energy level will allow participation in diversional activities. *If the patient attempts diversional activities but is too exhausted to participate meaningfully, increased frustration about activity intolerance and diversional activity deficit may occur.*
- Encourage contact with significant others *to maintain involvement with significant home/work events.*

High Risk for Altered Nutrition: Less than Body Requirements

RISK FACTORS

Alteration in nutrient absorption
Alteration in nutrient metabolism
Decreased nutrient intake
Anorexia
Nausea/vomiting
Diarrhea

EXPECTED OUTCOMES

Patient maintains adequate nutritional status as evidenced by stable weight or weight gain.

ONGOING ASSESSMENT

- Document patient's actual weight.
- Obtain nutritional history *to ascertain weight loss history, food likes/dislikes, intolerances, and food allergies.*
- ▲ Monitor laboratory values indicative of nutritional status:
  Serum albumin level: *an indication of visceral protein reserve.*
  Hemoglobin level: *an important component of red blood cells; determines ability of blood to carry adequate amounts of oxygen.*
  Cellular immune response skin test: *an overall indicator of nutritional well-being; a patient who is anergic (has no response to the injection of intradermal antigens) is severely nutritionally compromised and cannot heal.*
- Determine patient's food preferences. *Anorexia is a major problem in hepatitis.*

Continued.

NURSING DIAGNOSES	EXPECTED OUTCOMES AND NURSING INTERVENTIONS / *RATIONALE* (■ = INDEPENDENT; ▲ = COLLABORATIVE)
	THERAPEUTIC INTERVENTIONS ▲ Administer antiemetics as prescribed before meals *to decrease nausea, increase food tolerance, and maximize intake.* ▲ Consult dietitian; diet should be high in calories *for energy,* high in carbohydrates *because carbohydrates are easily metabolized and stored by the liver,* and limited in fats, *which may trigger nausea.* ▪ Provide small meals with frequent snacks *to increase daily intake.* ▪ Provide largest meal at breakfast, *as anorexia tends to worsen later in the day.* ▪ Discourage alcoholic beverages. *Alcohol damages liver cells and provides "empty calories" (calories without nutritional value).* ▲ Administer vitamin supplements as prescribed. ▲ Administer total parenteral nutrition (see p. 324) as ordered *to nourish patients unable to maintain adequate oral intake of nutrients.*
High Risk for Fluid Volume Deficit **RISK FACTORS** Vomiting Diarrhea Decreased dietary intake	**EXPECTED OUTCOMES** Patient maintains normal fluid volume as evidenced by normal heart rate, moist mucous membranes, urine output ≥ 30 ml/hr. **ONGOING ASSESSMENT** ▪ Monitor I & O. ▪ Check weight daily. Note enteric losses of fluid (e.g., vomiting, diarrhea) *to determine fluid balance and plan for replacement.* ▲ Monitor serum sodium level and osmolarity *to determine hydration status,* total protein and serum albumin *levels to determine oncotic pressure.* ▪ Monitor for signs/symptoms of dehydration: tachycardia, concentrated urine, dry mucous membranes, decreased urine output < 30 ml/hr. **THERAPEUTIC INTERVENTIONS** ▪ Encourage oral intake of fluids. ▲ Administer enteral and parenteral fluids as prescribed *to supplement oral replacement and compensate for losses.*
High Risk for Impaired Skin Integrity **RISK FACTORS** Accumulation of bile salts in skin Prolonged bed rest Mechanical forces associated with bed rest (pressure, shearing) Frequent diarrhea Poor nutritional status	**EXPECTED OUTCOMES** Patient maintains intact skin. **ONGOING ASSESSMENT** ▪ Check skin for signs of breakdown or presence of lesions. ▪ Assess itchiness. *Patients with hepatitis often have jaundice (a buildup of bilirubin), which causes yellowish skin discoloration and itching produced by irritation of the skin.* **THERAPEUTIC INTERVENTIONS** ▪ Position patient at least q2h *to prevent pressure ulcers.* ▪ Use pressure-relieving devices as necessary. ▲ *For itching:* encourage cool shower or bath with baking soda, use calamine lotion, administer antihistamines as prescribed, keep fingernails short, provide patient with gloves *(prevent further injury from scratching).*

See also:
Constipation, p. 16.
Diarrhea, p. 19.
Total parenteral nutrition, p. 324.

By: Martha Dickerson, RN, MS, CCRN
   Audrey Klopp, RN, PhD, ET

Inflammatory bowel disease

(CROHN'S DISEASE; ULCERATIVE COLITIS, DIVERTICULITIS)

The term inflammatory bowel disease (IBD) refers to a cluster of specific bowel abnormalities whose symptoms are often so similar as to make diagnosis difficult and treatment empirical. Crohn's disease is associated with involvement of all four layers of the bowel and may occur anywhere in the GI tract, although it is most common in the small bowel. Ulcerative colitis involves the mucosa and submucosa only and occurs only in the colon. Cause is unknown for both diseases. Incidence is usually in the 15- to 30-yr-old age group. Diverticular disease occurs frequently in persons over age 40; seems to be etiologically related to high-fat, low-fiber diets; and occurs almost exclusively in the colon. IBD is treated medically. If medical management fails or complications occur, surgical resection and possible fecal diversion will be undertaken.

NURSING DIAGNOSES	EXPECTED OUTCOMES AND NURSING INTERVENTIONS / *RATIONALE* (■ = INDEPENDENT; ▲ = COLLABORATIVE)

Abdominal Pain, Joint Pain

RELATED FACTORS

Bowel inflammation and contractions of diseased bowel or colon

Systemic manifestations of IBD

DEFINING CHARACTERISTICS

Reports of intermittent colicky abdominal pain associated with diarrhea

Abdominal rebound tenderness

Chronic joint pain

Hyperactive bowel sounds

Abdominal distention

Pain and cramps associated with eating

EXPECTED OUTCOMES

Patient verbalizes freedom from pain or adequate relief from pain.

ONGOING ASSESSMENT

- Assess pain: intermittent, colicky abdominal pain, joint pain, pain and cramping associated with eating.
- Auscultate bowel sounds.
- Check abdomen for rebound tenderness.
- Evaluate patient's perception of dietary impact on abdominal pain. *Many IBD patients cannot tolerate dairy products, and may not tolerate many other foods.*
- Assess presence of changes in bowel habits, such as diarrhea.
- Determine measures patient has successfully used to control pain.

THERAPEUTIC INTERVENTIONS

- ▲ Administer medications as prescribed. *Sulfasalazine (Azulfadine), which contains aspirin, and corticosteroids, which decrease inflammation, are typically used to bring the disease to remission. Topical preparations of corticosteroids (enemas, rectal foam) may also relieve pain/discomfort. In the most severe cases, immunosuppressive drugs (e.g., Imuran) may be given.*
- Evaluate and document effectiveness; observe for signs of untoward effects.
- Institute use of diversional activities, hobbies, relaxation techniques, and psychosocial support systems *to facilitate comfort and relaxation.*
- Make necessary alterations in diet.

Altered Nutrition: Less than Body Requirements

RELATED FACTORS

Malabsorption/diarrhea

Increased nitrogen loss with diarrhea

Decreased intake

Poor appetite/nausea

DEFINING CHARACTERISTICS

Body weight > 10%-20% below ideal

Decreased/normal serum calcium, K^+, vitamins K and B_{12}, folic acid, and zinc

Muscle wasting

Pedal edema

Skin lesions

Poor wound healing

EXPECTED OUTCOMES

Patient's nutritional status improves as evidenced by weight gain or stabilization of weight, controlled diarrhea, normal serum electrolyte profile.

ONGOING ASSESSMENT

- Document patient's actual weight on admission (do not estimate).
- Obtain nutritional history.
- Assess for skin lesions, skin breaks, tears, decreased skin integrity, and edema of extremities.
- ▲ Assess serum electrolytes, Ca^+, vitamins K and B_{12}, folic acid, and zinc levels *to determine actual or potential deficiencies.*
- Assess patterns of elimination: color, amount, consistency, frequency, odor, and presence of steatorrhea.
- Monitor dietary intake.

THERAPEUTIC INTERVENTIONS

- ▲ Consult dietitian to review nutritional history, monitor calorie count, and assist in menu selection. *High-calorie, high-protein, low-residue diets are recommended to maximize calorie absorption.*
- Keep room as odor-free as possible. *A malodorous environment will adversely affect appetite/intake.*

Continued.

Inflammatory Bowel Disease—cont'd

NURSING DIAGNOSES	EXPECTED OUTCOMES AND NURSING INTERVENTIONS / *RATIONALE* (■ = INDEPENDENT; ▲ = COLLABORATIVE)
	THERAPEUTIC INTERVENTIONS—cont'd ▲ Administer vitamin/mineral supplements as ordered *to compensate for deficiencies.* ▪ Encourage family members to bring food patient enjoys and to stay during meals *to enhance the social nature of mealtime.* ▲ Administer total parenteral nutrition (TPN) as prescribed *for patients who cannot tolerate oral intake and/or require bowel rest.* ▲ Administer medications *to control diarrhea.*
High Risk for Fluid Volume Deficit: **RISK FACTORS** Presence of excessive diarrhea/nausea/vomiting Blood loss from inflamed bowel mucosa Poor oral intake	**EXPECTED OUTCOMES** Patient remains adequately hydrated as evidenced by good skin turgor, urine output > 30 ml/hr, moist mucous membranes. **ONGOING ASSESSMENT** ▪ Assess hydration status: skin turgor, mucous membranes, I & O, weight, and blood pressure, heart rate. ▪ Document hemoccult-positive stools or obvious presence of bloody diarrhea. *Blood loss is typically most severe in patients with ulcerative colitis, but patients with Crohn's disease also may have bloody diarrhea.* ▲ Monitor Hb and Hct *if patient is bleeding.* ▪ Monitor urine output and urine specific gravity. ▪ Measure all diarrhea. **THERAPEUTIC INTERVENTIONS** ▲ Administer medications as ordered, noting possible reactions. *Azulfidine affects inflammatory response; corticosteroids may be used for both antiinflammatory and immunosuppressive benefits.* ▲ Administer IV fluids *if patient unable to maintain adequate oral intake.*
High Risk for Infection **RISK FACTORS** Poor nutritional status Immunosuppression from steroid therapy **See also:** Granulocytopenia, p. 413	**EXPECTED OUTCOMES** Patient remains free of infection as evidenced by normal temperature, normal WBC. **ONGOING ASSESSMENT** ▪ Monitor temperature. ▲ Monitor WBC. *4000-12,000 cu/mm is normal.* ▪ Assess frequency of infectious episodes. ▪ Assess wounds for signs of healing. **THERAPEUTIC INTERVENTIONS** ▪ Maintain good handwashing and encourage patient to do some *to prevent nosocomial infection.* ▪ Discourage visits from individuals with colds, flu, sore throat, or fever. ▪ Instruct patient on good perianal hygiene (*wiping from front to back minimizes the risk of a urinary tract infection).*
Knowledge Deficit **RELATED FACTORS** Need for continuous and long-term management of chronic disease Change in health care needs related to remission/exacerbation of disease **DEFINING CHARACTERISTICS** Multiple questions by patient/significant others related to disease process and management Noncompliance with therapy **See also:** Skin integrity, impaired, p. 59 Total parenteral nutrition, p. 324	**EXPECTED OUTCOMES** Patient/significant other verbalize understanding of disease and management. **ONGOING ASSESSMENT** ▪ Assess understanding of IBD and necessary management. **THERAPEUTIC INTERVENTIONS** ▪ Discuss disease process and management. ▪ Explain that inflammatory bowel disease is characterized by remissions and exacerbations. ▪ Explain that careful medical management may eliminate/postpone the need for surgical intervention. ▪ Encourage patient to verbalize fears and feelings. ▲ Make appropriate referrals: dietary, psychiatric counseling, National Foundation for Colitis & Ileitis.

By: Vivian Jones, RN, and Audrey Klopp, RN, PhD, ET

Laparoscopic surgery

Laparoscopic surgery uses small abdominal incisions in combination with telescopic visualization of the abdominopelvic cavity to accomplish many surgeries that prior to 1988 required an open abdominal surgical approach. Surgeries now commonly using a laparoscopic approach include laparoscopic cholecystectomy, laparoscopic management of bile duct stones, laparoscopic appendectomy, and laparoscopic herniorraphy. Some surgeons are beginning to use laparoscopic approaches for small and large bowel resections. Nursing care interventions for patients undergoing laparoscopic procedures are similar for all types of procedures and will also be addressed in this care plan.

NURSING DIAGNOSES	EXPECTED OUTCOMES AND NURSING INTERVENTIONS / *RATIONALE* (■ = INDEPENDENT; ▲ = COLLABORATIVE)

Knowledge Deficit, Preoperative

RELATED FACTORS

Proposed surgical experience
Lack of previous similar surgical procedure

DEFINING CHARACTERISTICS

Questions
Lack of questions
Verbalized misconceptions

EXPECTED OUTCOMES

Patient verbalizes understanding of proposed surgical procedure and realistic expectations for the postoperative course.

ONGOING ASSESSMENT

- Assess patient's knowledge of proposed surgical procedure. *Patient should be aware of the nature of the surgical procedure, the reason it is being done, and whether the surgeon plans an open abdominal procedure or a laparoscopic procedure.*
- Assess patient's previous experience with surgery. *Patients who have had surgery in the past may have negative feelings related to side effects of anesthesia, postoperative pain, and lengthy recovery.*

THERAPEUTIC INTERVENTIONS

- Explain and reinforce surgeon's explanations regarding proposed surgical procedure.
- Prepare patients having laparoscopic procedures to expect to be discharged within 24 hours with:
    Two or three small incisions *(location will depend on nature of the surgical procedure)* covered with large bandages.
    Resumption of normal activity in 2-3 days. *Most patients are able to return to work on the third or fourth day after laparoscopic surgery.*
    Resumption of normal diet on the evening of surgery. *Patients having laparoscopic surgery do not experience a paralytic ileus and therefore are able to resume usual diet the day of surgery.*
    Minimal pain, managed with oral analgesic agents.

High Risk for Infection

RISK FACTORS

Abdominal incisions
Presences of tubes/drains

EXPECTED OUTCOMES

Patient remains free of infection, as evidenced by healing wound/incision free of redness, swelling, purulent discharge, pain; normal body temperature within 72 hr postoperatively.

ONGOING ASSESSMENT

- Monitor temperature. *For the first 48-72 hr postoperatively, temperatures of up to 38.5° C are expected as a normal stress response to major surgery. Beyond 72 hr, temperature should return to patient's baseline. Temperature spikes, usually occurring in the later afternoon or night, are often indications of infection.*
- Assess incisions for redness, drainage, swelling, increased pain. *Incisions that have been closed with sutures or staples should be free of redness, swelling, and drainage. Some incisional discomfort is expected. These incisions are usually kept covered by a dry dressing for 24-48 hr; beyond 48 hr, there is no need for a dressing.*
- Assess stability of tubes/drains. *In-and-out motion of improperly secured tubes/drains allows access by pathogens through stab wounds where tubes/drains are placed.*

THERAPEUTIC INTERVENTIONS

- Wash hands before contact with postoperative patient. *Handwashing remains the most effective method of infection control.*
- Use aseptic technique during dressing change, wound care, or handling or manipulating of tubes/drains.
- Ensure that surgical tubes/drains are not inadvertently interrupted (opened). Tape connectors, pin extension/drainage tubing securely to patient's gown *to minimize tension on tubes and connection. Opening sterile systems allows access by pathogens and puts the patient at risk for infection.*
- ▲ Administer antibiotics and antipyretics as prescribed.

Continued.

Laparoscopic surgery—cont'd

NURSING DIAGNOSES	EXPECTED OUTCOMES AND NURSING INTERVENTIONS / *RATIONALE* (■ = INDEPENDENT; ▲ = COLLABORATIVE)

Knowledge Deficit

RELATED FACTORS

Lack of previous experience
with laparoscopic surgery
Need for home management

DEFINING CHARACTERISTICS

Multiple questions
Lack of questions
Inability to provide self-care
on discharge

EXPECTED OUTCOMES

Patient verbalizes understanding of and ability to perform postoperative care after discharge.

ONGOING ASSESSMENT

- Assess patient's ability to perform wound care, verbalize appropriate activity, verbalize appropriate diet.
- Assess patient's understanding of need for close follow-up observation. *Patients who leave the hospital with sutures, staples, or drains in place need to return for removal.*

THERAPEUTIC INTERVENTIONS

- Teach patient to perform appropriate wound care:
  Abdominal incisions: *staples/sutures and dressings will be present at the time of discharge.*
  Dressings: *dressings are usually Band-Aids, which should be changed daily and after showering.*
- Provide patient with measuring receptacle and chart/flow sheet *for recording drain output. Drains are left in place until drainage is < 30 cc/24 hr; this usually occurs 3-7 days postoperatively.*
- Teach patient to empty drainage collection devices. *Patients should prepare a clean surface (e.g., clean paper towels) to work on and should wash hands under running water before emptying collection device. These measures reduce risk of infection.*
- Teach patient appropriate activity: no lifting heavier than 10 lb for 6 wk, return to work in 3 or 4 days, showering OK, bathing OK.
- Teach patient the following about diet: a well-balanced, high-calorie, high-protein diet promotes healing, *which continues over a period of weeks.*
- Teach patient that bowel function will return to preoperative baseline in 2-3 days.
- Instruct patient to seek medical attention for any of the following: fever > 38° C, foul-smelling wound drainage, redness or unusual pain in any incision, absence of bowel movement.
- Teach patient that minor abdominal pain and shoulder pain is normal after laparoscopic surgery and should be managed with oral analgesic agents. *During laparoscopic surgery, the peritoneal cavity is filled with CO_2; this facilitates visualization of structures by the surgeon. Until the gas is completely absorbed, some discomfort is typical.*

By: Audrey Klopp, RN, PhD, ET

Pancreatitis, acute

A nonbacterial inflammatory process of autodigestion of pancreatic tissue by pancreatic enzymes, resulting in edema, necrosis, and hemorrhage. The two most common causes are alcohol abuse and biliary obstruction. In severe cases, pancreatitis can be complicated by ARDS.

NURSING DIAGNOSES	EXPECTED OUTCOMES AND NURSING INTERVENTIONS / *RATIONALE* (■ = INDEPENDENT; ▲ = COLLABORATIVE)

Pain

RELATED FACTORS

Inflammation of pancreas and surrounding tissue
Biliary tract disease
Biliary obstruction
Excessive alcohol intake
Abdominal trauma/surgery
Infectious process

DEFINING CHARACTERISTICS

Epigastric pain or umbilical pain radiating to back/shoulders
Increasing pain in supine position
Pain aggravated by food
Abdominal distention with rebound tenderness
Extreme restlessness

EXPECTED OUTCOMES

Patient verbalizes relief of pain or adequate pain management.

ONGOING ASSESSMENT

- Assess pain characteristics.
- Assess history of previous attack.
- Assess precipitating factors. *Often a bout of pancreatitis is precipitated by an alcoholic binge or consumption of a large meal.*
- Observe for increased abdominal distention; auscultate abdomen for bowel sounds q2h; report decrease or absence of bowel sounds. *Extravasation of pancreatic enzymes causes paralytic ileus.*
- Observe sclera and skin for jaundice. *Patients with biliary obstruction will have jaundice because of inability to circulate and metabolize bilirubin normally. The bile pigment diffuses through tissue to skin and mucous membranes, staining them yellow.*
- Observe stool for fat, absence of bile, odor.

THERAPEUTIC INTERVENTIONS

▲ Reduce pancreatic stimulus by maintaining patient NPO or with nasogastric tube to low suction as ordered. *Oral intake causes vagally stimulated pancreatic secretion; the escape of pancreatic secretions into the pancreas causes damage by autodigestion and pain.*
- Anticipate need for pain medication. *Pain management is most effective when pain is treated before it becomes severe.*
▲ Administer medication, such as anticholinergic drugs *(mimic sympathetic stimulation and quiet pancreatic secretion);* avoid morphine derivatives *(may cause spasms of sphincter of Oddi, increasing pain).*
- Use repositioning and back rubs *to provide comfort.*

High Risk for Fluid Volume Deficit

RISK FACTORS

Vomiting
Decreased intake
Shifting of fluids to extravascular space
Hemorrhage
Ileus

EXPECTED OUTCOMES

Patient maintains normal fluid volume as evidenced by urine output > 30 ml/hr, good skin turgor, stable BP and heart rate.

ONGOING ASSESSMENT

- Monitor vital signs. *Fluid volume deficit occurs rapidly; subtle vital sign changes may indicate profound fluid volume deficit.*
- Assess hydration status, including skin turgor, daily weight, hemodynamic parameters (blood pressure decrease, heart rate increase).
- Observe for complications of dehydration. *Oliguria and impaired renal function can occur rapidly as a result of the severity of fluid volume deficit.*
▲ Monitor serum and urine amylase and renal-amylase creatinine clearance levels as prescribed.

THERAPEUTIC INTERVENTIONS

▲ Maintain circulatory volume; replace fluid and electrolyte losses:
▲ Administer IV fluid as prescribed.
▲ Administer volume expanders or blood transfusion as prescribed.
- See also Fluid volume deficit, p. 25.

Continued.

323

Pancreatitis, acute—cont'd

NURSING DIAGNOSES	EXPECTED OUTCOMES AND NURSING INTERVENTIONS / *RATIONALE* (■ = INDEPENDENT; ▲ = COLLABORATIVE)

Knowledge Deficit

RELATED FACTORS

Unfamiliarity with disease process

DEFINING CHARACTERISTICS

Multiple questions
Misconceptions
Repeat admissions to hospital
with recurrent bouts of pancreatitis

See also:
Ineffective breathing pattern,
p. 10.
Impaired skin integrity,
p. 59.
ARDS, p. 183.
Ineffective therapeutic management Regimen, p. 39.

EXPECTED OUTCOMES

Patient verbalizes understanding of causative factors for pancreatitis.

ONGOING ASSESSMENT

- Assess understanding of disease process, particularly potentially controllable behaviors that may trigger episodes of pancreatitis.

THERAPEUTIC INTERVENTIONS

- Teach about relationship of alcohol consumption to pancreatitis.
- Teach about the recurrent nature of pancreatitis.
- Teach patient that certain foods may precipitate a bout of pancreatitis. *These foods vary from person to person and are best identified by the patient.*

By: Susan Galanes, RN, MS, CCRN

Total parenteral nutrition (TPN)

(INTRAVENOUS HYPERALIMENTATION)

Total parenteral nutrition (TPN) is the administration of concentrated glucose and amino acid solutions via a central or large-diameter peripheral vein. TPN therapy is necessary when the gastrointestinal tract cannot be or is not used to meet the patient's nutritional needs. TPN solutions may contain 20% to 60% glucose and 3.5% to 10% protein (in the form of amino acids), in addition to various amounts of electrolytes, vitamins, minerals, and trace elements. These solutions can be modified, depending on the presence of organ system impairment and/or the specific nutritional needs of the patient. In order to provide necessary amounts of fat and the fat-soluble vitamins (A, D, E, and K), intralipids are often administered 2 to 3 times per week along with TPN.

NURSING DIAGNOSES	EXPECTED OUTCOMES AND NURSING INTERVENTIONS / *RATIONALE* (■ = INDEPENDENT; ▲ = COLLABORATIVE)

Altered Nutrition: Less than Body Requirements

RELATED FACTORS

Prolonged NPO status
Alterations in GI tract function
(e.g., GI surgery, fistulas,
bowel obstruction, esophageal injury/disease, dysphagia, stomatitis, nausea,
vomiting, or diarrhea)
Increased metabolic rate or
other conditions necessitating
increased intake (e.g., sepsis,
burns, or chemotherapy)
Psychological reasons for refusal to eat

EXPECTED OUTCOMES

Patient achieves an adequate nutritional status as evidenced by stable weight/weight gain, improved albumin levels.

ONGOING ASSESSMENT

- Perform a comprehensive nutritional assessment on admission and periodically thereafter and document findings.
- ▲ Assess response to nutritional support (e.g., daily weights, lab results: electrolyte, glucose, albumin levels; wound healing; skin condition).
- Obtain accurate calorie counts and I & O, including TPN.

THERAPEUTIC INTERVENTIONS

- Assist with insertion, maintenance of central or peripheral line.
- ▲ Administer prescribed TPN solution, preferably via infusion pump *(to assure constant infusion rate). Falling behind on TPN administration deprives the patient of needed nutrition; boluses (or too rapid administration) can precipitate a hyperglycemic crisis, because the hormonal response (i.e., insulin) may not be available to allow use of the increased glucose load.*

NURSING DIAGNOSES	EXPECTED OUTCOMES AND NURSING INTERVENTIONS / *RATIONALE* (■ = INDEPENDENT; ▲ = COLLABORATIVE)

DEFINING CHARACTERISTICS

Caloric intake less than body requirements

Weight loss (or weight 20% below ideal)

Poor skin turgor and wound healing

Decreased muscle mass

Decreased serum albumin, total protein, and transferrin levels

Electrolyte imbalances

THERPEUTIC INTERVENTIONS—cont'd

- Be familiar with additive content of TPN solution (glucose, amino acids, electrolytes, insulin, vitamins, and trace minerals).
- Assist with oral intake if indicated. *Unless complete bowel rest is indicated, patients may be fed orally in addition to TPN to maximize nutritional support.*
▲ Refer to/collaborate with appropriate resources: nutritional support team, dietitian, pharmacy.

High Risk for Fluid Volume Deficit

RISK FACTORS

Hyperglycemia

Inability to respond to thirst mechanisms because of NPO status

Low serum protein level

EXPECTED OUTCOMES

Patient maintains normal fluid volume as evidenced by good skin turgor, balanced I & O, urine output of at least 30 ml/hr.

ONGOING ASSESSMENT

- Assess for signs and symptoms of fluid volume deficit: decreased BP, increased HR, elevated body temperature, skin dryness, loss of turgor, high urine specific gravity.
- Monitor intake and output. *Output of at least 30 ml/hr indicates adequate fluid intake.*
▲ Monitor blood glucose levels. *Hyperglycemia can lead to hyperosmolar, nonketotic coma with subsequent dehydration secondary to osmotic diuresis.*
▲ Monitor serum protein levels per hospital policy, usually every 3-7 days. *Low serum protein level may lead to loss of fluids from intravascular spaces, secondary to low colloidal pressures.*
- Weigh patient daily and record.

THERAPEUTIC INTERVENTIONS

▲ Administer TPN at prescribed, constant rate; if infusion is interrupted, infuse 10% dextrose in water until TPN infusion is restarted. *This provides needed fluid in addition to protecting patient from sudden hypoglycemia.*
▲ Administer maintenance or bolus fluids as prescribed, in addition to TPN.
- Encourage oral intake of fluids, unless contraindicated.

High Risk for Fluid Volume Excess

RISK FACTORS

Overinfusion of TPN

Inability to tolerate increased vascular load

EXPECTED OUTCOMES

Patient maintains normal fluid volume as evidenced by balanced I & O, absence of edema.

ONGOING ASSESSMENT

- Assess for signs and symptoms of fluid volume excess: weight gain in excess of .5 kg/day, intake greater than output, shortness of breath and crackles *(caused by accumulation of fluid in the lungs),* edema *(caused by accumulation of fluid in the extravascular spaces),* elevated central venous pressures.
- Monitor intake and output.
- Weigh patient daily and record.
- Assess for edema. *Edema occurs when fluid accumulates in the extravascular spaces. Edema usually begins in the fingers, facial area, and the presacral area. Generalized edema, called anasarca, occurs later and involves the entire body.*
▲ Monitor serum sodium level. *Hypernatremia may cause/aggravate edema by holding fluid in the extravascular spaces.*

THERAPEUTIC INTERVENTIONS

▲ Administer diuretics as prescribed. *Diuretics aid in the excretion of excess body fluids.*
▲ Restrict fluid intake as prescribed.
▲ Restrict sodium intake, both TPN and in oral diet, as prescribed.
- Position patient to reduce risk of pulmonary complications related to fluid volume excess. *Elevating the head of the bed 30 degrees will allow for ease in breathing and prevent accumulation of fluid in the thoracic area.*
- Handle edematous extremities with caution *to prevent damage to taut skin.*

Continued.

Total parenteral nutrition (TPN)—cont'd

NURSING DIAGNOSES	EXPECTED OUTCOMES AND NURSING INTERVENTIONS / *RATIONALE* (■ = INDEPENDENT; ▲ = COLLABORATIVE)

High Risk for Injury

RISK FACTORS

Electrolyte imbalances:
  Hypokalemia (K^+ < 3.5 mEq/L)
  Hyponatremia (Na^+ < 115 mEq/L)
  Hypocalcemia (Ca^{++} < 6.8 mg/dl)
  Hypomagnesemia (Mg^+ < 1.5 mg/dl)
  Hypophosphatemia (PO_4 < 2.5 mg/dl)
Essential fatty acid deficiency (EFAD)
Hyperglycemia (glucose >200 mg/dl)
Hypoglycemia (glucose <60 mg/dl)

EXPECTED OUTCOMES

Patient maintains normal serum electrolyte levels as evidenced by K^+ > 3.5 mEq/L, Na^+ > 115 mEq/L, Ca^{++} > 6.8 mg/dl, Mg^+ > 1.5 mg/dl, PO_4 > 2.5 mg/dl.
Patient has normal serum triglyceride level (40-150 mg/dl).
Patient has blood glucose level of 70-200 mg/dl.

ONGOING ASSESSMENT

▲ Assess for signs and symptoms of electrolyte imbalance: *When patients are receiving TPN and no other nutrition, there is a risk, especially early in TPN therapy, that all electrolyte needs may not be met; as physiologic condition changes, patients may have altered needs for electrolytes, will require adjustment of the TPN solution.*
  Hypokalemia:
    Alteration in muscle function (e.g., weakness, cramping).
    ECG changes (e.g., ventricular dysrhythmias, ST-segment depression, or U-wave).
    Mental status changes (e.g., confusion, lethargy).
    Abdominal distention, loss of bowel sounds.
  Hyponatremia:
    Decreased skin turgor.
    Weakness.
    Tremors/seizures.
    Lethargy, confusion.
    Nausea, vomiting.
  Hypocalcemia:
    Paresthesias.
    Tetany.
    Seizures.
    Positive Chvostek's sign.
    Irregular heart rate.
  Hypomagnesemia:
    Muscle weakness, cramping, twitching.
    Tetany.
    Seizures.
    Irregular heart rate.
  Hypophosphatemia:
    Muscle weakness.
    Mental status changes.

▲ Assess for signs/symptoms of essential fatty acid deficiency (EFAD): *TPN solutions contain no fat; fat is a nutritional requirement that allows essential fat-soluble vitamins A, D, E, and K to be absorbed.*
    Alopecia.
    Tendency to bruise and thrombocytopenia *due to coagulopathy secondary to inadequate vitamin K levels.*
    Dry, scaly skin *related to vitamin D and E deficiencies.*
    Poor wound healing *related to vitamin A and E deficiencies.*

▲ Monitor serum triglyceride level twice weekly, if patient is receiving intralipids.

▪ For patients receiving intralipid therapy, monitor for signs and symptoms of adverse reactions: dyspnea, cyanosis, headache, flushing.

▲ Monitor serum glucose and urine fractionals.

▲ Assess for hyper- or hypoglycemia signs and symptoms; notify physician of presence of:
  Hypoglycemia:
    Glucose level <60 mg/dl.
    Weakness, agitation, clammy skin, tremors.
  Hyperglycemia:
    Glucose level >200 mg/dl.
    Glycosuria.
    Thirst, polyuria, confusion.

▪ Monitor vital signs and cardiac rhythm.

THERAPEUTIC INTERVENTIONS

▪ Be aware of TPN solution's electrolyte content. *For each gram of nitrogen infused (in the form of amino acids), electrolytes must be supplied in the following ratio: phosphorous 0.8 mg, sodium 3.9 mg, chloride 2.5 mEq, calcium 1.2 mEq.*

▲ Administer electrolyte replacement therapy as prescribed.

NURSING DIAGNOSES	EXPECTED OUTCOMES AND NURSING INTERVENTIONS / *RATIONALE* (■ = INDEPENDENT; ▲ = COLLABORATIVE)

THERAPEUTIC INTERVENTIONS—cont'd

▲ Administer 10% or 20% intralipids as ordered. *It is recommended that patients NPO and/or receiving only TPN >2 wk receive intravenous fat emulsions or intralipids. Intralipids can also be given in absence of EFAD to provide extra calories.*

• Piggyback intralipids into most proximal part of TPN tubing after preparing port aseptically. Do not infuse intralipids through filter. Secure tubing with tape *to prevent dislodgment.*

▲ If adverse reactions occur, stop the infusion immediately; notify physician.

• Maintain continuous flow of TPN solution (preferably via infusion pump). Do not "catch up" or "slow down" infusion rate if "off schedule."

• When discontinuing TPN therapy, taper rate over 2-4 hr *(to prevent hypoglycemic episode caused by abrupt TPN withdrawal).*

▲ Use corrective actions if TPN solution stops or must be stopped suddenly.

> For clotted catheter or if subsequent TPN bags not available: hang 10% dextrose and H_2O at rate of TPN infusion.
>
> For arrest situation: stop TPN infusion; administer bolus doses of 50% dextrose.
>
> For hyperglycemia, administer insulin as prescribed.

High Risk for Infection

RISK FACTORS

Central venous line used for TPN (provides access for bacterial entry)

High glucose concentration of TPN solution (provides excellent microbial growth medium)

Preexisting susceptibility to infection secondary to poor nutritional status

EXPECTED OUTCOMES

Patient remains free of infection as evidenced by normal temperature, WBC 4000-11,000; clean, dry central line insertion site that is free of redness and purulent drainage.

ONGOING ASSESSMENT

• Monitor for signs/symptoms of infection.

• Monitor temperature. Notify physician of temperature >38.6° C.

▲ Monitor WBC count.

▲ If line-related infections are suspected, assist with obtaining specimens for culture and sensitivity.

THERAPEUTIC INTERVENTIONS

▲ Assist with central line placement for TPN under sterile conditions.

• Use sterile technique when caring for central line during dressing tubing and solution changes.

• Change TPN tubing and filter q24h or according to institutional policy.

• Maintain sterile, occlusive TPN dressing. Perform dressing changes under sterile technique q48h or according to policy.

▲ Change individual TPN bag after 24 hr or more often, as prescribed. *(High glucose concentration of TPN provides excellent microbial growth medium.)*

• Keep TPN solutions refrigerated until needed.

• Never use TPN line for medications, blood draws, or CVP readings *(to lessen risk of contamination of line).*

• Do not place additives in prepared TPN solution. Return TPN solution to pharmacy if additives are needed. *TPN is prepared in the pharmacy under a laminar air flow hood to decrease risk of microbial contamination of fluid.*

• Do not infuse TPN into preexisting central lines or Swan-Ganz catheters.

▲ If line-related infections are suspected, assist physician with reinsertion of central line at new site. Use new TPN solution, tubing, and filter.

▲ If infection is present, administer antibiotics as prescribed.

High Risk for Injury: Air Embolism

RISK FACTORS

Entry of air into vascular system via central TPN catheter

EXPECTED OUTCOMES

Patient is free of dyspnea, tachypnea, pain or ABG deterioration.

ONGOING ASSESSMENT

• Obtain vital signs, including respiratory rate, q4h. Observe for dyspnea and tachypnea.

• Assess breath sounds every shift.

▲ Monitor arterial blood gases as prescribed.

• Monitor TPN infusion rate q1h. *Do not let infusion run dry, as air can be pumped into patient.*

• Monitor for changes in mental status.

THERAPEUTIC INTERVENTIONS

• Use Luer-Lock tubings on TPN line and tape all connections securely.

• Use infusion device that will detect presence of air in line. *Air will then be detected before reaching patient.*

Continued.

NURSING DIAGNOSES	EXPECTED OUTCOMES AND NURSING INTERVENTIONS / *RATIONALE* (■ = INDEPENDENT; ▲ = COLLABORATIVE)

	TEHERAPEUTIC INTERVENTIONS—cont'd
	• If TPN infusion runs dry, clamp tubing, aspirate air from line, and remove all air from line before continuing infusion with new bag.
	• Have patient perform Valsalva's maneuver during tubing changes *(prevents patient from taking breath, which would cause air to be sucked into an "open" central line).*
	▲ Use air elimination filter according to hospital policy.
	   If air embolus is suspected:
	      Immediately turn patient on left side, in Trendelenburg's position. *If air has already traveled into heart, it will then stay on right side of RA or RV and away from pulmonic valve.*
	      Call physician stat. *This is a life-threatening emergency.*
	      Assist physician with aspiration of air through central line while patient performs Valsalva's maneuver.

High Risk for Injury: Pneumothorax
 	
RISK FACTORS
 	
Placement of central line for TPN
	EXPECTED OUTCOMES
	Patient remains free of pneumothorax as evidenced by normal, bilateral breath sounds after insertion of central line, radiographic evidence of correct central line placement.
	
	ONGOING ASSESSMENT
	• Assess breath sounds before and after central line placement. *This allows comparison of breath sounds from baseline to postprocedure status. Pneumothorax (air in the pleural space) will result in diminished breath sounds; occasionally the opposite side will be more diminished as the side with the pneumothorax pushes the normal lung over and inhibits expansion.*
	• Assess for subcutaneous emphysema and asymmetrical chest movement.
	▲ Obtain chest radiograph after line placement *to determine correct placement of the line and to rule out pneumothorax.*
	
	THERAPEUTIC INTERVENTIONS
	• Properly position patient for placement of central line. *The proximity of the apex of the lung and local vasculature creates risk at the time of line insertion. This risk is minimized by correct positioning of the patient during central line placement.*
	   Place head of bed flat.
	   Place towel roll between shoulder blades *to allow shoulders to drop back, revealing correct anatomic placement of subclavian vein.*
	▲ After central line is placed, infuse 5% dextrose in water *until radiograph report confirms proper placement of the line.*

By: Debbie Lazzara, RN, MS, CCRN

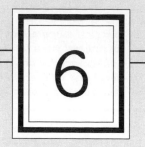

Musculoskeletal Care Plans

Amputation of a lower extremity, surgical

Surgical amputations may be required as a result of extensive peripheral vascular disease, infection, trauma, thermal injury, malignancy, or congenital deformity. The most distal amputation level that will facilitate wound healing, maintain joint mobility, and create a stump appropriate for later prosthesis is selected.

NURSING DIAGNOSES	EXPECTED OUTCOMES AND NURSING INTERVENTIONS / *RATIONALE* (■ = INDEPENDENT; ▲ = COLLABORATIVE)

Knowledge Deficit: Preoperative

RELATED FACTORS

Unfamiliarity with hospital routines, medical or surgical procedures

DEFINING CHARACTERISTICS

Increased anxiety level
Questioning
Verbalized misconceptions
Fears about level of independence

EXPECTED OUTCOMES

Patient verbalizes understanding of postoperative routines, exercises, and activity regimen.

ONGOING ASSESSMENT

- Assess understanding of type of procedure to be performed (above vs. below knee amputation) and type of prosthesis (if any) planned (immediate postsurgical fitting vs. delayed fitting).
- Assess knowledge of rehabilitation program involved in amputation.

THERAPEUTIC INTERVENTIONS

- Instruct patient of the following *to prepare for smooth transition through recovery:*
  Postoperative care of residual limb
  Preparation for prosthesis: ROM exercises, positioning, stump bandaging.
  Muscle strengthening exercises *to facilitate crutch walking*
  Phantom pain phenomena (sensations "felt" in amputated leg, which may persist for several weeks, months)
  Appropriate use of assistive devices (e.g., walker, crutches, cane, trapeze).
  Practice walking preoperatively can aid in subsequent rehabilitation process.
- Prepare patient to experience emotional withdrawal and depression during adjustment period. *Rehabilitation period can be long and difficult. Avoid unrealistic goal setting.*

Impaired Skin Integrity

RELATED FACTORS

Surgical incision
Skin breakdown caused by immobility
Abnormal wound healing

DEFINING CHARACTERISTICS

Redness
Pain
Edema
Drainage/discharge

EXPECTED OUTCOMES

Patient manifests signs of optimal wound healing, as evidenced by intact skin, absence of skin breakdown, well-fitting prosthesis.

ONGOING ASSESSMENT

- Assess wound for normal healing, bleeding/hemorrhage, proper fit of cast or pressure dressing, prolonged pressure on tissues associated with immobility.
- Assess nutritional status. *Adequate calories/protein are needed for healing and energy for ambulation/transfer techniques.*

THERAPEUTIC INTERVENTIONS

- Reinforce dressing as needed; use aseptic technique; note drainage.
- Instruct patient to report slippage of cast, rigid dressing, or compression dressing. *These appliances help prevent edema, minimize pain with movement, and facilitate shaping of stump for later prosthesis.*
- Assist with stump wrapping; use elastic bandage when indicated (stump shrinker is sometimes preferred).
- Check stump for signs of impaired circulation (i.e., edema, pain).
- Rewrap stump q3-4hr or as needed for bunching or slippage. *Correct wrapping reduces swelling, promotes shaping of stump for prosthesis.*
- Discuss weight-bearing limitations and their importance *to prevent skin breakdown and facilitate proper wound healing.*

Impaired Physical Mobility

RELATED FACTORS

Change in center of gravity creating balance problems
Activity limitations caused by loss of body part
Difficulty in using assistive devices
Pain upon mobility
Fatigue
Postoperative protocol

EXPECTED OUTCOMES

Patient achieves optimal level of mobility (walking with prosthesis, crutches; use of wheel chair).
Patient maintains functional alignment of all extremities and avoids contractures.

ONGOING ASSESSMENT

- Assess proper positioning techniques; individualize to patient.
- Assess activity tolerance.
- Assess understanding of mobility and restrictions.
- Assess understanding of postoperative activity and exercise program.
- ▲ Assess whether patient is candidate for a prosthesis (type, time for application). *Elderly or debilitated patients may not be able to handle a prosthesis; a wheel chair may be more appropriate. Prosthesis can be fitted when wound healing is satisfactory.*

NURSING DIAGNOSES	EXPECTED OUTCOMES AND NURSING INTERVENTIONS / *RATIONALE* (■ = INDEPENDENT; ▲ = COLLABORATIVE)

DEFINING CHARACTERISTICS

Inability to move purposefully within environment

Reluctance to attempt movement

Limited range of motion

THERAPEUTIC INTERVENTIONS

- Reinforce teaching of muscle strengthening and balancing exercises *to strengthen muscles and increase sense of balance.*
- Reinforce proper positioning and need for exercise:
  Have patient lie on back, keeping pelvis level and hip joint extended *to prevent contractions.*
  Maintain neutral rotation.
  Have patient lie prone with lower extremity in extension 30 min three or four times a day *to prevent deformities (flexion contraction).*
  Instruct patient to perform ROM exercises.
- Encourage early ambulation (patient should be able to stand within 48 hr) *to promote confidence about regaining independence.*
- Encourage use of assistive devices. *Patient may use walker, crutches, wheelchair as appropriate.*
- Encourage patient to ask for needed assistance.
- Assist patient with transfers and ambulation until able to perform safely.
- Teach prevention of postoperative complications (flexion abduction and external rotation of hip): avoid sitting for long periods; avoid use of pillows under residual limb; maintain proper alignment; avoid flexing residual limb while sitting or lying.
- If patient is not a candidate for prosthesis, instruct in self-care activities from amputee wheelchair.

Body Image Disturbance

RELATED FACTORS

Loss of body part

Loss of independence

Inability to maintain prior lifestyle

DEFINING CHARACTERISTICS

Verbal preoccupation with changed body part

Refusal to discuss change

Actual change in function

Change in social behavior

EXPECTED OUTCOMES

Patient demonstrates enhanced body image, as evidenced by ability to look at and talk about amputated leg, ability to provide self-care to stump (as appropriate).

ONGOING ASSESSMENT

- Assess ability to adjust to loss of body part. *The acute (vs. chronic) nature of the causative factor requiring amputation, the patient's prior health and age, and significant other all impact on adjustment to amputation.*
- Assess ability to use coping mechanisms.
- Assess perceived impact of change on ADL, social behavior, personal relationships, occupational activities.
- Assess need for support group.

THERAPEUTIC INTERVENTIONS

- Encourage verbalization of feelings. *Loss of a limb requires significant psychological adjustment. Allow patient time to work through grief stages.*
- Listen and support verbalized feelings about body and life-style changes.
- Encourage participation in care of residual limb when able *to promote independence.*
- Explore successful past coping techniques.
- Encourage use of clothing *to enhance appearance.*
- Encourage patient to participate fully in therapy regimen *(fosters sense of control).*
- Encourage family members to support patient and allow independence.
- Discuss use of prosthesis for cosmetic as well as ambulatory purposes.
- ▲ Consult social services for support groups. *Lay persons in similar situations offer a unique type of support that is perceived as helpful.*

Pain

RELATED FACTORS

Phantom pain

Surgical procedure

Decreased mobility

DEFINING CHARACTERISTICS

Verbal complaints

Facial expressions of discomfort

Protection of stump

Crying, moaning

Restlessness

Withdrawal/Irritability

EXPECTED OUTCOMES

Patient verbalizes relief of postoperative discomfort.

Patient verbalizes understanding of phantom limb pain.

ONGOING ASSESSMENT

- Assess description of pain.
- Assess for nonverbal signs of pain.
- Assess previous pain experience and successful relief measures.
- Assess understanding of occurrence/management of phantom limb sensations. *Phantom limb sensations are due to nerve stimulation proximal to the level of amputation but perceived as coming from the amputated limb. Phantom limb sensations are normal and can last for months.*

Continued.

NURSING DIAGNOSES	EXPECTED OUTCOMES AND NURSING INTERVENTIONS / *RATIONALE* (■ = INDEPENDENT; ▲ = COLLABORATIVE)
	THERAPEUTIC INTERVENTIONS ▲ Provide medications as prescribed for surgical pain relief; evaluate effectiveness. ▲ Use additional comfort measures as appropriate to relieve phantom sensations: diversional activities; relaxation techniques; position change, exercise; ROM of stump; application of pressure to residual limb; transcutaneous electrical nerve stimulation (TENS). *Analgesics are less appropriate/effective than these measures.*
Knowledge Deficit: Discharge Instructions **RELATED FACTORS** New condition New role/life-style **DEFINING CHARACTERISTICS** Expressed concerns about home management Questions about medications/treatment	**EXPECTED OUTCOMES** Patient verbalizes understanding of limb, prosthetic, and follow-up care. **ONGOING ASSESSMENT** ▪ Assess knowledge of the following *to facilitate smooth transition from hospital to home:* care of residual limb, phantom limb pain management, signs/symptoms of circulatory problems, prosthetic care, follow-up appointments, community resources. **THERAPEUTIC INTERVENTIONS** ▪ Reinforce teaching for care of residual limb (e.g., stump wrapping, skin care, and weight-bearing limitations) *to promote optimal rehabilitation.* ▪ Provide information for phantom limb pain/sensation management. ▪ Discuss signs/symptoms of circulatory problems. ▪ Reinforce teaching about care of prosthesis if applicable. ▪ Inform of discharge medications, exercises, and follow-up appointments. ▲ Coordinate social services, physical therapy, and occupational therapy *to provide adequate discharge planning and home treatments after discharge.* ▲ Contact social services for information about community resources and support groups (i.e., visiting nurses, homemakers, outpatient therapy).

See also:
Anxiety/Fear, p. 523.
Impaired Individual Coping, p. 18.
Activity Intolerance, p. 2.

By: Sherry Weber, RN
Carol Clark, RN

Arthritis, rheumatoid

A chronic, systemic, inflammatory disease that usually presents as symmetric synovitis primarily of the small joints of the body. Extraarticular manifestations may include rheumatoid nodules, pericarditis, scleritis, arteritis. Rheumatoid arthritis is characterized by periods of remission and exacerbation of the disease. The specific cause of rheumatoid arthritis is unknown, but it may occur secondary to autoimmunity, infection, or genetic factors. It affects women more than men.

NURSING DIAGNOSES	EXPECTED OUTCOMES AND NURSING INTERVENTIONS / *RATIONALE* (■ = INDEPENDENT; ▲ = COLLABORATIVE)

Joint Pain

RELATED FACTORS

Inflammation associated with increased disease activity
Degenerative changes secondary to long-standing inflammation

DEFINING CHARACTERISTICS

Patient's/significant other's report of pain
Guarding on motion of affected joints
Facial mask of pain
Moaning or other sounds associated with pain

EXPECTED OUTCOMES

The patient verbalizes a decrease in pain and is able to participate in self-care activities.

ONGOING ASSESSMENT

- Assess for signs of joint inflammation (redness, warmth, swelling, decreased motion).
- Evaluate location and description of pain. *Pain occurs primarily in small joints, such as hands, wrists, fingers, ankles.*
- Assess interference with life-style.

THERAPEUTIC INTERVENTIONS

▲ Administer antiinflammatory medication as prescribed. Give first dose of day as early as possible, with small snack. *Antiinflammatory drugs should not be given on an empty stomach (can be very irritating to stomach lining and lead to ulcer disease).*
▲ Use nonnarcotic analgesic as necessary. *Narcotic analgesia appears to work better on mechanical than on inflammatory types of pain. Narcotics can be habit-forming.*
■ Encourage patient to assume anatomically correct position. Do not use knee gatch or pillows to prop knees. Use small flat pillow under head.
▲ Encourage patient to wear splints as prescribed. *Splints provide rest to inflamed joint, may reduce muscle spasm.*
▲ Consult occupational therapist for proper splinting of affected joints.
▲ Use hot (e.g., heating pad) or cold packs on painful, inflamed joints. Consult clinical specialist or physical/occupational therapist for suggestions. *Some individuals prefer heat to cold or vice versa. Patient may need to alternate. Try what works best at the time.*
■ Encourage use of ambulation aid(s) when pain is related to weight bearing.
■ Apply bed cradle *to keep pressure of bed covers off inflamed lower extremities.*
■ Encourage use of alternative methods of pain control such as relaxation, guided imagery, or distraction.

Joint Stiffness

RELATED FACTORS

Inflammation associated with increased disease activity
Degenerative changes secondary to long-standing inflammation

DEFINING CHARACTERISTICS

Patient's/significant other's complaint of joint stiffness
Guarding on motion of affected joints
Refusal to participate in usual self-care activities
Decreased functional ability

EXPECTED OUTCOMES

The patient verbalizes decrease in stiffness and is able to participate in self-care activities.

ONGOING ASSESSMENT

- Solicit patient's description of stiffness: location (generalized or localized), timing: (morning, night, all day). *Stiffness characteristically occurs upon awakening in morning.*
  Length of stiffness. Ask patient, "How long do you take to loosen up after you get out of bed?" Record in hours or fraction of hour. *Usually 30 min, may last longer as disease progresses.*
  Relationship to activities (aggravate/alleviate stiffness). *Usually aggravated by prolonged inactivity, may be precipitated by joint motion.*
- Determine past measures to alleviate stiffness.
- Assess interference with life-style. *Rheumatoid arthritis is a chronic disease with periods of remission and exacerbations.*

THERAPEUTIC INTERVENTIONS

- Encourage patient to take 15-min warm shower or bath upon rising. Localized heat (hand soaking) is also useful. *Reduces stiffness; relieves pain and muscle spasms.*
- Encourage patient to perform ROM exercises after shower or bath, two repetitions per joint.
- Allow patient sufficient time for activities.
- Avoid scheduling tests or treatments when stiffness present.
▲ Administer antiinflammatory medications as prescribed. Give first dose of day as early in morning as possible, with a small snack.

Continued.

NURSING DIAGNOSES	EXPECTED OUTCOMES AND NURSING INTERVENTIONS / *RATIONALE* (■ = INDEPENDENT; ▲ = COLLABORATIVE)

THERAPEUTIC INTERVENTIONS—cont'd

- Ask patient about normal home medication schedule; try to continue it. *The sooner patient takes the medication, the sooner stiffness will abate. Many patients prefer to take these medications as early as 6 or 7 A.M. Antiinflammatory drugs should not be given on empty stomach.*
- Suggest use of elastic gloves (e.g., Isotoner) at night *to decrease hand stiffness.*
- Remind patient to avoid prolonged periods of inactivity.

Fatigue

RELATED FACTORS

Increased disease activity
Anemia of chronic disease

DEFINING CHARACTERISTICS

Patient's/significant other's description of lack of energy, exhaustion, listlessness
Excessive sleeping
Decreased attention span
Facial expressions: yawning, sadness
Decreased functional capacity

EXPECTED OUTCOMES

The patient verbalizes a higher level of energy and appears rested.

ONGOING ASSESSMENT

- Solicit patient's description of fatigue: timing (afternoon or all day), relationship to activities, aggravating and alleviating factors.
- Determine nighttime sleep pattern. *Pain may interfere with achieving a restful sleep.*
- Determine whether fatigue is related to psychologic factors (stress, depression).

THERAPEUTIC INTERVENTIONS

- Provide periods of uninterrupted rest throughout day (30 min 3-4 times/day). *Patients often have limited energy reserve. Fatigue may cause flare-up of disease.*
- Reinforce principles of energy conservation:
    Pacing activities (alternating activity with rest). *Patient often uses more energy than others to complete same tasks.*
    Adequate rest periods (throughout day and at night).
    Organization of activities and environment.
    Proper use of assistive/adaptive devices.
  If fatigue is related to interrupted sleep:
- Encourage warm shower or bath immediately before bedtime. *Warm water relaxes muscles, facilitating total body relaxation.*
- Encourage gentle ROM exercises (after shower/bath) *to maximize effects of heat.*
- Encourage patient to sleep in anatomically correct position (do not prop knees or head). Should change positions frequently during night.
- Avoid stimulating foods (caffeine) and activities before bedtime.
- Encourage use of progressive muscle relaxation techniques.
▲ Administer nighttime analgesic/long-acting antiinflammatory drug as prescribed.

Impaired Physical Mobility

RELATED FACTORS

Pain
Stiffness
Fatigue
Psychosocial factors
Altered joint function
Muscle weakness

DEFINING CHARACTERISTICS

Patient's/significant other's description of difficulty with purposeful movement
Decreased ability to transfer and ambulate
Reluctance to attempt movement
Decreased muscle strength
Decreased ROM

EXPECTED OUTCOMES

The patient verbalizes/demonstrates increased ability to move purposefully.

ONGOING ASSESSMENT

- Solicit patient's description of aggravating and alleviating factors, joint pain and stiffness, interference with life-style. *Symptoms will change as the disease progresses.*
- Observe patient's ability to ambulate, move all joints functionally. *Pain may cause progressive loss of function.*
- Assess need for analgesics before activity. *Pain may be dealt with effectively by preventing/reducing it.*

THERAPEUTIC INTERVENTIONS

- Allow patient adequate time for all activities. *Patient may need more time than others to complete same tasks.*
- Provide adaptive equipment (e.g., cane, walker) as necessary or ask significant other to bring them from home.
▲ Reinforce proper use of ambulation devices as taught by physical therapist. *Reduces load on joints and may promote safety.*
- Encourage patient to wear proper footwear (well-fitting, with good support and nonskid bottoms) when ambulating and avoid house slippers.
- Assist with ambulation as necessary.
▲ Reinforce techniques of therapeutic exercise taught by physical therapist. *ROM, muscle strengthening, and endurance exercise promote joint function and increase physical stamina.*

NURSING DIAGNOSES	EXPECTED OUTCOMES AND NURSING INTERVENTIONS / *RATIONALE* (■ = INDEPENDENT; ▲ = COLLABORATIVE)

THERAPEUTIC INTERVENTIONS—cont'd

- Instruct patient to avoid excessive exercise during acute inflammatory flare-up.
- ▲ Reinforce principles of joint protection taught by occupational therapist.
- Reinforce proper body alignment when sitting, standing, walking, and lying down. *Improper body alignment can lead to unnecessary pain and contracture.*

Self-Care Deficit

RELATED FACTORS

Pain
Stiffness
Fatigue
Psychosocial factors
Altered joint functions
Muscle weakness

DEFINING CHARACTERISTICS

Patient's/significant other's description of difficulty with self-care activities

EXPECTED OUTCOMES

The patient participates in self-care activities.

ONGOING ASSESSMENT

- Observe patient's ability to bathe, carry out personal hygiene, dress, toilet, eat. *Joint pain and stiffness interfere with performing ADLs.*
- Assess impact of self-care deficit on life-style. *Some patients may have successfully adjusted their routines and complete required tasks. Other patients may be unable to care for themselves.*
- Determine assistive/adaptive devices used in self-care activities. *The patient may not have knowledge of newly available devices.*
- Assess need for home health care after discharge.

THERAPEUTIC INTERVENTIONS

- Encourage independence: assist only as necessary; provide necessary adaptive equipment (raised toilet seat, dressing aids, eating aids) or ask significant other to bring them from home. *Such aids promote independence and may enhance safety.*
- ▲ Refer specialized needs to occupational therapy. *Patients' self-image improves when they can perform personal care independently.*
- Allow patient adequate time for self-care activities. *Standing/soaking in warm water may relieve joint stiffness.*
- Encourage a shower or bath rather than bed bath.
- Do not schedule tests/activities during self-care time. *Patients need to conserve energy.*
- Offer patient guidance in pacing activities.
- ▲ Reinforce self-care techniques taught by occupational therapist.

Knowledge Deficit

RELATED FACTORS

New disease/procedures
Unfamiliarity with treatment regimen
Lack of interest

DEFINING CHARACTERISTICS

Multiple questions
Lack of questions
Verbalized misconceptions
Verbalized lack of knowledge
Inaccurate follow-through of previous instructions

EXPECTED OUTCOMES

Patient verbalizes understanding of the disease and treatment.

ONGOING ASSESSMENT

- Assess patient's level of knowledge of rheumatoid arthritis and its treatment.

THERAPEUTIC INTERVENTIONS

- Introduce/reinforce disease process information: unknown cause, chronicity of rheumatoid arthritis, process of inflammation, joint and other organ involvement, remissions and exacerbations, control vs. cure.
- Introduce/reinforce information on drug therapy. *Patients may be taking many drugs and need to understand the different methods of administration and the potential side effects to watch for.*
  Side effects of long-term prednisone: facial puffiness, buffalo hump, diabetes mellitus, osteoporosis, avascular necrosis, increased appetite, increased risk of infection/glaucoma.
  Side effects of immunosuppressants: increased risk of infection *caused by bone marrow suppression,* nausea/vomiting, sterility, hemorrhagic cystitis, cancer.
  Importance of wearing Medic-Alert tag stating use of prednisone/immunosuppressants.
  Importance of never altering prednisone dose unless prescribed.
- Introduce/reinforce self-management techniques: ROM exercises, muscle strengthening exercises, pain management, joint protection, pacing activities, adequate rest, splinting, use of assistive devices.
- Introduce/reinforce nutritionally sound diet. Explain need for salt restriction if on steroid therapy.
- Stress importance of long-term follow-up observation. *Patient is living with a chronic illness and requires ongoing help.*
- Encourage patient to discuss new or over-the-counter treatments with health care worker. *Patient may be vulnerable to fads/ads claiming curative effects of high-dose vitamins, special health foods, copper bracelets.*

Continued.

NURSING DIAGNOSES	EXPECTED OUTCOMES AND NURSING INTERVENTIONS / *RATIONALE* (■ = INDEPENDENT; ▲ = COLLABORATIVE)
	THERAPEUTIC INTERVENTIONS—cont'd
	▪ Inform of resources such as the Arthritis Foundation.
	▪ Suggest referral to arthritis specialist for optimal treatment and emotional support. *This may be necessary for dealing/coping with chronic disease.*

See also:
Impaired coping, p. 18.
Altered nutrition: more than
  body requirements, p. 45.
Altered nutrition: less than
  body requirements, p. 44.
Body image disturbance,
  p. 7.
Powerlessness, p. 52.

By: Sue A. Connaughton, RN, MSN, Psy D Candidate
    Linda Ehrlich, RN, MSN

Extremity fracture

(CLOSED REDUCTION; OPEN REDUCTION;
INTERNAL FIXATION; EXTERNAL FIXATION)

A fracture is a break or disruption in the continuity of a bone. Fractures occur when a bone is subjected to more stress than it can absorb. Fractures are treated by one or a combination of the following: closed reduction—alignment of bone fragments by manual manipulation without surgery; open reduction—alignment of bone fragments by surgery; internal fixation—immobilization of fracture site during surgery with rods, pins, plates, screws, wires, or other hardware; immobilization through use of casts, splints, traction, posterior molds, etc.; external fixation—immobilization of bone fragments with the use of rods/pins that extend from the incision externally and are fixed.

NURSING DIAGNOSES	EXPECTED OUTCOMES AND NURSING INTERVENTIONS / *RATIONALE* (■ = INDEPENDENT; ▲ = COLLABORATIVE)
Pain	**EXPECTED OUTCOMES**
	Patient verbalizes relief or reduction in pain.
RELATED FACTORS	Patient appears comfortable.
Fracture	
Soft tissue injury	**ONGOING ASSESSMENT**
	▪ Assess for pain or discomfort.
DEFINING CHARACTERISTICS	▪ Determine past experience with pain and pain relief measures.
Complaints of pain or discomfort	**THERAPEUTIC INTERVENTIONS**
Guarding behavior	▪ Maintain immobilization and support of affected part. *Immobility prevents further tissue damage and muscle spasm.*
Muscle spasm	▪ Reposition and support unaffected parts as permitted *to promote general comfort.*
Increased pulse rate	▪ Elevate affected part *to decrease vasocongestion.*
Increased blood pressure	▪ Apply cold *to decrease swelling* (first 24-48 hr). Apply for 20-30 min q1-2hr.
Crying, moaning	▲ Respond immediately to request for analgesia. Consider round-the-clock or continuous patient-controlled anesthesia (PCA).
Grimacing	▪ Medicate 30 min before wound/pin care or physical therapy *to decrease pain from movement.*
Anxiety	
Restlessness	▪ Teach relaxation techniques.
Withdrawal	▲ Administer muscle relaxants as necessary.
Irritability	

NURSING DIAGNOSES	EXPECTED OUTCOMES AND NURSING INTERVENTIONS / *RATIONALE* (■ = INDEPENDENT; ▲ = COLLABORATIVE)

High Risk for Infection

RISK FACTORS

Open fracture
External fixation or traction
  pins
Surgical intervention

EXPECTED OUTCOMES

Patient is free of infection, as evidenced by normal temperature, absence of drainage or odors around fracture site.

ONGOING ASSESSMENT

- Assess wound and/or pin site for local signs of infection, skin tension around pins, signs of developing gangrene (*vesicles filled with red watery fluid and gas bubbles coming from tissue*).
- Assess for systemic infection signs.
- Monitor vital signs.
- Assess for odors or drainage through immobilization devices that are not removed (i.e., casts, splints).

THERAPEUTIC INTERVENTIONS

- Maintain adequate hydration and nutritional status *to promote wound healing.*
- Use sterile technique when changing wound dressings. *This is necessary in absence of intact first line of defense.*
- ▲ Keep dressing dry and intact. Give wound care as ordered.
- Initiate wound precautions if purulent drainage is present *to prevent cross-contamination of other patients.*
- ▲ Administer antibiotics as prescribed.
- ▲ Administer tetanus toxoid and/or hypertet as indicated.
- ▲ Perform appropriate pin site care:
    Provide care to all pin sites every 8-24 hr.
    Provide pin care as prescribed or use standard protocol (e.g., cleanse each pin site with hydrogen peroxide with sterile applicator and rinse with normal saline solution to remove crusting from pin site). *Removal of crusting from pin sites allows free drainage of fluids, which prevents infection along pin tract.*
    Apply sterile dressing and/or ointment as prescribed. Wipe off fixator with alcohol.

Impaired Physical Mobility

RELATED FACTORS

Cast
Fixation device
Pain
Surgical procedure
Immobilizer device

DEFINING CHARACTERISTICS

Reluctance to attempt movement
Limited ROM
Mechanical restriction of movement
Decreased muscle strength and/or control
Impaired coordination
Inability to move purposefully within physical environment (bed, mobility, transfer, ambulation)

EXPECTED OUTCOMES

Patient maintains maximum mobility within prescribed restrictions.

ONGOING ASSESSMENT

- Assess ROM of unaffected parts proximal and distal to immobilization device.
- Assess ability to perform basic ADLs.
- Assess ability to ambulate.
- Assess present and preinjury mobility level.
- Assess muscle strength in all extremities.

THERAPEUTIC INTERVENTIONS

- Encourage isometric, active, and resistive ROM exercises to all unaffected joints qid and as tolerated *to prevent muscle atrophy and maintain adequate muscle strength required in mobility.*
- ▲ Apply splint to support foot in neutral position (applied to LE frames and traction) *to prevent foot drop.*
- Perform flexion and extension exercises to proximal and distal joints of affected extremity when indicated.
- Assist up to chair when ordered; teach transfer technique.
- Lift extremity by external fixation frame if stable; avoid handling of injured soft tissue.
- ▲ Reinforce crutch ambulation taught by physical therapist; use appropriate weight-bearing techniques. Assist with gait belt until gait is stable.
- ▲ Obtain occupational therapy consultation as indicated.

High Risk for Impaired Skin Integrity

RISK FACTORS

Presence of immobilization device
Improper immobilization device
Bed rest

EXPECTED OUTCOMES

Patient maintains intact skin.

ONGOING ASSESSMENT

- Assess immobilized extremity for redness/breakdown.
- If casted, check edges of cast for roughness.
- Assess bony prominences for redness/breakdown.

Continued.

NURSING DIAGNOSES	EXPECTED OUTCOMES AND NURSING INTERVENTIONS / *RATIONALE* (■ = INDEPENDENT; ▲ = COLLABORATIVE)
	THERAPEUTIC INTERVENTIONS · Use antipressure devices (i.e., flotation devices, eggcrate mattress, air mattress), as appropriate. · Maintain adequate hydration and nutritional status. *Good nutrition is necessary for tissue growth and repair.* · Reposition q2hr. · Prevent pressure on toes from sheets; use bed cradle if necessary. · Trim and petal tape rough edges of a cast *to prevent irritation.* · Massage skin around cast with alcohol *to toughen skin.* · Pad pin edges *to protect injury to other areas.* · Turn and provide skin care q2-4hr.
High Risk for Injury **RISK FACTOR** Loss of continuity of cast	**EXPECTED OUTCOMES** Patient maintains intact cast. **ONGOING ASSESSMENT** · Assess cast for cracks, weakened areas, indentations, softened or wet areas. **THERAPEUTIC INTERVENTIONS** · Leave cast open to air until completely dry. *Drying of plaster cast takes 24-48 hr. Air drying promotes drying from inside out to ensure a stable cast. A fiberglass cast will dry in just a few hours.* · Prevent indenting cast by moving it with palms of hands and supporting it on nonplastic pillows until dry. *Plastic traps heat released during application.* · Reposition patient and cast q2hr *to allow for drying of cast on all sides.* · Keep cast clean and dry. Prevent soiling from urine/feces.
High Risk for Altered Tissue Perfusion **RISK FACTORS** Trauma Surgery Compartment syndrome Neurovascular compromise	**EXPECTED OUTCOMES** Patient maintains adequate tissue perfusion, as evidenced by warm skin, bilateral pulses, absence of pain and edema. **ONGOING ASSESSMENT** · Assess distal to fracture site for cool, cyanotic skin; diminished or absent pulse; slow/absent capillary refill; edema; hematoma; numbness, tingling; pain (progressive and disproportional to injury); pain on passive stretching of muscle; tightness of muscle compartment. · Compare to opposite extremity. **THERAPEUTIC INTERVENTIONS** · Remove restrictive clothing and/or jewelry from affected part. · Elevate affected part above level of heart on pillows or by suspension traction if prescribed *to promote venous return and decrease edema.* Do not elevate *above* level of heart if compartment syndrome is suspected; arterial pressure should be maintained by keeping limb at heart level. *This will promote arterial blood flow.* ▲ Encourage exercise of unaffected parts distal to site as allowed *to promote circulation.* ▲ Report any neurovascular compromise to physician immediately. · Have cast cutter available *for splitting, bivalving, or removal of cast if necessary.* · Prepare patient for surgical intervention (i.e., fasciotomy) if compartment syndrome is probable. *Severe tissue swelling that decreases blood flow causes ischemia and may result in permanent motor and/or sensory damage.*
High Risk for Fluid Volume Deficit **RISK FACTORS** Multiple fractures Long bone fractures Blood vessel damage with bleeding Third spacing of fluids caused by trauma	**EXPECTED OUTCOMES** Patient maintains adequate fluid volume, as evidenced by normal heart rate, urine output >30 ml/hr, normal blood pressure, alert mentation. **ONGOING ASSESSMENT** · Assess for symptoms of hypovolemia: weak, rapid pulse; cool, clammy skin; rapid, shallow respirations; decreased blood pressure; slow capillary refill; decreased urinary output; anxiety; altered level of consciousness. · Assess amount of bleeding from external wounds. · Assess for third spacing or bleeding around fracture site.

NURSING DIAGNOSES	EXPECTED OUTCOMES AND NURSING INTERVENTIONS / *RATIONALE* (■ = INDEPENDENT; ▲ = COLLABORATIVE)

ONGOING ASSESSMENT—cont'd

- Obtain a circumference measurement of injured area q8hr *to assess for further bleeding/ third spacing fluid.*
- Note amount of bleeding on cast.

THERAPEUTIC INTERVENTIONS

- ▲ Administer IV fluids and blood products as prescribed.
- Maintain alignment and immobility of fracture site *to prevent disruption of the bone healing process.*
- ▲ Administer humidified oxygen as prescribed.

High Risk for Self-Esteem Disturbance

RISK FACTORS

Loss of body function
Inability to meet role responsibilities
Loss of control

EXPECTED OUTCOMES

Patient verbalizes positive expressions, feelings and reactions about self and situation.

ONGOING ASSESSMENT

- Assess prior/current coping mechanisms used by patient.
- Assess effect of injury on self-esteem.

THERAPEUTIC INTERVENTIONS

- Identify and reinforce patient's strengths.
- Support continued significant roles with family/friends; provide for visits, phone calls, written work, etc., as tolerated.
- Encourage patient to plan, participate in care activities. Adapt care to patient's routines and needs.
- Provide opportunities for independent activities. *Independence facilitates coping.*
- Arrange environment to promote independent use of materials needed for ADLs. *To develop self-esteem, patient/significant others must participate actively in rehabilitation.*
- Continually teach and inform patient/family about physical status, treatment plan, etc.
- See also Diversional activity deficit, p. 21.
- ▲ Make social service referral early in hospitalization for financial and resource counseling as needed.

Knowledge Deficit: Home Management

RELATED FACTORS

New procedures/treatment
New condition
Home care needs

DEFINING CHARACTERISTICS

Verbalizes inadequate knowledge of care/use of immobilization device, mobility limitations, complications, and follow-up care
Confusion; asking multiple questions
Lack of questions
Inaccurate follow-through of instruction
Improper performance
Inappropriate or exaggerated behaviors (i.e., hostile, agitated, hysterical, apathetic)

EXPECTED OUTCOMES

- Patient/significant other verbalize understanding of treatment, possible complications, and follow-up care.

ONGOING ASSESSMENT

- Solicit current understanding of diagnosis, treatment, follow-up care, etc.
- Assess patient's/family's readiness and ability to assume care responsibility.

THERAPEUTIC INTERVENTIONS

- Instruct patient to:
  Elevate extremity above level of heart with pillows during reclining position *to prevent swelling;* prop affected leg on footstool or chair during sitting.
  Do prescribed exercises several times a day *to maintain muscle tone.*
  Use appropriate assistive device (walker, crutches) and maintain prescribed weight-bearing status.
  Identify and report to physician signs of neurovascular compromise of extremity: pain, numbness, tingling, burning, swelling, or discoloration.
  Use pain relief measures safely.
  Obtain proper nutrition *to promote bone/wound healing and prevent constipation.*
  Arrange for follow-up care.
- Instruct patient in cast to:
  Notify physician if cast cracks or breaks, of foul odor under cast, of fresh drainage through cast, if anything gets inside cast, of areas of skin breakdown around cast, of pain or burning inside cast, of warm areas on cast.
  Keep cast clean and dry; tub bath only if cast is protected, not immersed.
  Inspect skin around cast edges for irritation.
  Do *not* put anything under cast, poke under cast, or put powder or lotion under cast. *This may abrade skin and cause infection.*
- Instruct patient with surgical incision to observe incision for infection signs and notify physician if they develop.

Continued.

NURSING DIAGNOSES	EXPECTED OUTCOMES AND NURSING INTERVENTIONS / *RATIONALE* (■ = INDEPENDENT; ▲ = COLLABORATIVE)

THERAPEUTIC INTERVENTIONS—cont'd

- Instruct patient with external fixation device to perform pin care, perform wound care, observe for loosening of pins, cleanse device.
- Involve patient/significant others in procedure.
- Supervise those performing procedures.
- Provide patient with own supplies as needed.

See also:
Body Image Disturbance, p. 7.
Diversional Activity Deficit, p. 21.
Impaired Ineffective Coping, p. 18.
Ineffective Breathing Pattern, p. 10.
Altered Nutrition: Less than Body Requirements, p. 44.

By: Michele Knoll Puzas, RNC, MHPE
Marilyn R. Magafas, RN, MBA.

Low back pain; lumbar laminectomy

(DISK HERNIATION; SPINAL STENOSIS; BACK TRAUMA)

A syndrome characterized by pain and tenderness in the muscles or their attachments in the lower lumbar, lumbosacral, or sacroiliac regions. Pain may be referred to one or both legs if nerve root compression occurs. This phenomenon is called radiculopathy. The most common cause is intervertebral disk herniation. Other causes of low back pain include uterine or prostatic disorders, infection, arthritis, and metastatic cancer. Low back pain is usually successfully treated with conservative measures (e.g., bedrest, analgesics). Surgery is indicated when conservative measures fail: severe, incapacitating recurrent pain; progressive nervous system involvement (weakness, increased sensory loss). Laminectomy is the excision of a small part of the lamina, the posterior arch of the vertebrae. This allows the surgeon access to the foramen, through which nerve roots pass to the disk in the lower back.

NURSING DIAGNOSES	EXPECTED OUTCOMES AND NURSING INTERVENTIONS / *RATIONALE* (■ = INDEPENDENT; ▲ = COLLABORATIVE)

Motor-Sensory Deficit

RELATED FACTORS

Disk herniation (herniated nucleus pulposus)
Spinal stenosis
Osteoarthritis
Mechanical instability
Back trauma
Infection
Metastatic cancer
Postoperative difficulties

EXPECTED OUTCOMES

Patient maintains optimal neurologic functioning, as evidenced by movement in lower legs, adequate strength, normal reflexes.

ONGOING ASSESSMENT

- Evaluate history/onset: injury/spontaneous, work-related, postoperative, unknown.
- Assess neurologic status: movement and strength of lower extremeties, sensation, equality of foot strength, reflexes (knee, ankle, Babinski). *If laminectomy was performed, preassessments need to be compared to postoperative condition; some sensations such as tingling/numbness may temporarily persist during early recovery.*
- Assess vascular status of lower extremities: pulses, temperature.

NURSING DIAGNOSES	EXPECTED OUTCOMES AND NURSING INTERVENTIONS / *RATIONALE* (■ = INDEPENDENT; ▲ = COLLABORATIVE)

DEFINING CHARACTERISTICS

Low back pain
Radiating pain into lower extremities
Paresthesia
Weakness in lower extremity
Bladder/bowel difficulties
Decreased/absent deep tendon reflex
Limited straight leg raising
Urinary retention

ONGOING ASSESSMENT—cont'd

- Evaluate for specific lumbar nerve root syndromes:
  L3-4: quadriceps (difficulty climbing stairs); patella reflex (knee jerk)
  L4-5: weakness, dorsiflextion of foot/large toe; sensory loss in large toe and medial side of foot
  L5-S1: Inability to stand on tiptoe, sensory loss on lateral aspect of foot; decreased/absent ankle jerk.
  Cauda equina: Compression may result in paraparesis and sphincteric disturbances. *Early surgical decompression is warranted.*
- Assess bladder/bowel functioning: I & O, dribbling, incontinence, rectal sphincter tone, retention. *May occur secondary to disk herniation or be complication of surgery.*
- Inquire about previous episodes of back pain and related hospitalization and treatment: bed rest, pelvic traction, transcutaneous nerve stimulation, heat/massage, exercise program, medications.
- Inquire about previous tests, dates, and results, if known:
  Myelogram
  CT scan: Injection of contrast into lumbar subarachnoid space followed by CT scan *to delineate disk protrusion, obliteration/displacement of nerve root(s), and presence of osteoarthritis causing nerve root compression/distortion at one or more levels.*
  Electromyogram: *May be useful in differentiating root compression from peripheral neuropathy.*
  Lumbosacral radiographic studies
  Sedimentation rate: *May be elevated in the presence of infection (e.g., disk space infection).*
  Magnetic resonance imaging (MRI) scan: *Especially helpful to evaluate abnormality such as lesions in the brain stem or spinal cord, possible related vascular anomalies.*
- Inquire about previous surgery for low back pain: lumbar laminectomy, fusion, chemonucleolysis: injection of a bulging disk with chymopapain to decrease disk size (not currently used).
- Inquire about location of pain/radiation, aggravating factors, alleviating factors.

THERAPEUTIC INTERVENTIONS

- Reinforce need for bed rest as indicated.
- Provide bedside commode or assist patient to bathroom as needed.
- Provide raised toilet seat if appropriate.
▲ Apply pelvic traction: 15-20 lb 4 times/day as ordered.
- Elevate knees about 10-20 degrees *to relieve sciatic stretch and promote comfort.*
- Assist patient with application of lumbosacral corset, if appropriate, *to promote proper body alignment.*
- Evaluate motor strength, reflexes, sensory status q4-6hr *for improvement or deterioration of neurologic status.*
- Prior to discharge teach and encourage isometric abdominal and gluteal muscle tightening.
▲ Coordinate therapy with physical therapist.
- Postlaminectomy: maintain proper body alignment; maintain bedrest as ordered; log roll for position change.

Pain

RELATED FACTORS

Low back pain
Disk herniation
Muscle spasm, strain
Postoperative laminectomy

DEFINING CHARACTERISTICS

Complaints of discomfort
Decreased physical activity
Slow, guarded movement
Irritability, restlessness, altered sleep pattern
Palpable muscle spasm

EXPECTED OUTCOMES

- Patient verbalizes relief from/reduction in pain
- Patient appears comfortable.

ONGOING ASSESSMENT

- Evaluate for signs of discomfort.
- Assess location and intensity of pain.
- Inquire about previous episodes, hospitalization, and treatment.

THERAPEUTIC INTERVENTIONS

▲ Anticipate need for pain medication/muscle relaxant as prescribed. *Attention to pain relief promotes trust, increases confidence, and facilitates patient independence.*
▲ Apply heating pad with setting on low heat as ordered.
- Use ice packs. *May be more helpful for easement of muscle spasms.*

Continued.

341

Low back pain; lumbar laminectomy—cont'd

NURSING DIAGNOSES	EXPECTED OUTCOMES AND NURSING INTERVENTIONS / *RATIONALE* (■ = INDEPENDENT; ▲ = COLLABORATIVE)

	THERAPEUTIC INTERVENTIONS—cont'd
	• Raise knee gatch 10-20 degrees (or place pillow under knees) *to reduce stretch on sciatic nerve and to promote comfort.*
	• Instruct patient to exhale when turning in bed. *This reduces muscle tightening and may ease muscle spasm.*
	• Instruct patient in how to get out of bed with minimum of discomfort:
	    Roll onto the side.
	    Elevate head of bed.
	    Lower legs over side.
	    Use arms to prop self upright
	    Sit over side of bed with feet firmly on the floor for several minutes before standing.
	    Use leg muscles to progress from sitting to standing position.
	• Instruct patient in how to get back into bed by reversing order.
	• Instruct patient to avoid bending at the waist. Rather instruct to squat or use an arm extender device to pick up an object on the floor.
	• Postlaminectomy: instruct in log rolling for comfort; provide reassurance that movement is okay.

High Risk for Impaired Physical Mobility
 	
RISK FACTORS
Pain
Muscle weakness
Imposed bed rest
Postoperative laminectomy pain
	EXPECTED OUTCOMES
	• Patient maintains mobility within limits of disease.
	• Patient performs ADLs independently.
	
	ONGOING ASSESSMENT
	• Evaluate for signs of alteration in mobility:
	Difficulty with movement and position changes:
	    Inability to move
	    Reluctance to attempt movement
	    Limited ROM
	    Decreased muscle strength
	• Assess for potential complications of immobility (e.g., phlebitis, pulmonary embolism, altered skin integrity).
	
	THERAPEUTIC INTERVENTIONS
	• Encourage slow deep breathing exercises about 10 times/hr while awake.
	• Instruct in foot-ankle exercises (plantar and dorsiflexion of foot with rotation at ankle) about 10 times/hr while awake.
	• Assist with repositioning as needed at least q2hr.
	▲ Anticipate use of support hose (e.g., TED hose) and sequential compression devices until patient is ambulating in the hall. *Protect against clot formation.*
	▲ Postlaminectomy, encourage early ambulation as ordered. *Protocols vary among surgeons.*
	• Discuss need for/role of physical therapist.
	• If signs of altered mobility are present, see also Impaired Physical Mobility, p. 47.

Knowledge Deficit **RELATED FACTORS** New onset of low back pain and rehabilitation of back with or without surgery **DEFINING CHARACTERISTICS** Multiple questions Misconceptions Fear of spinal complications	**EXPECTED OUTCOMES** Patient/significant others verbalize cause of low back pain and discuss recommended ADL modifications. **ONGOING ASSESSMENT** • Evaluate patient's knowledge of body mechanics (bending from waist, lifting objects, rotating spine), cause of low back pain (if known), ADLs, surgical recovery, discharge instructions. **THERAPEUTIC INTERVENTIONS** • Discuss causes of low back pain (e.g., *repeated stress on lower back, poor body mechanics*). • Define disk herniation. • Discuss symptoms of disk herniation (e.g., *lower back pain, radiation of pain, weakness, changes in sensation*).

| NURSING DIAGNOSES | EXPECTED OUTCOMES AND NURSING INTERVENTIONS / *RATIONALE*
(■ = INDEPENDENT; ▲ = COLLABORATIVE) |

THERAPEUTIC INTERVENTIONS—cont'd

- Discuss recommended alterations in life-style:
  - When to return to work:
  - When to resume driving (usually not for 2 wks after surgery)
  - Date and time of follow-up appointment
  - Name and telephone number of physician
  - Recreational restrictions
- Discuss exercises for muscle strengthening. *Strong muscles help support back; proper muscle tone can improve posture and reduce chances of recurring muscle strain:*
  - Isometric abdominal and gluteal muscle exercises begin 7-10 days after surgery
  - Flexion-extension exercises initiated as prescribed.
- Discuss ADL guidelines with patient:
  - Sleeping: Recommend a firm mattress. *Sleeping on the side with knees and hips flexed is preferable to sleeping on the back or abdomen.*
  - Bathing: Showers are preferable to tub baths. If tub baths are important to patient, instruct in avoiding flexing lower back when getting into and out of tub.
  - Bending: Instruct patient to squat rather than bend at waist.
  - Lifting: When physician allows resumption of lifting (recommend not more than 20 lb) instruct patient to squat, hold object close to body, straighten knees, and *never* lift anything heavy above waist.
  - Reaching: Instruct patient not to reach or strain to pick up object, to rise to level required; to avoid movements such as bending backward, twisting to reach telephone, or crouching over desk.
  - Sexual activities: Recommend abstinence for 1-2 wk. Then for about 8-12 wk, the patient should assume underlying position with pillow under buttocks. Alternative: woman lies on side with knees bent, man lying behind and facing back.
  - If lower back pain occurs, instruct patient to go to bed and rest back.

See also:
Constipation, p. 16.
Impaired Individual Coping, p. 18.

By: Linda Arsenault, RN, MSN, CNRN

Osteoarthritis

(DEGENERATIVE JOINT DISEASE [DJD])

Osteoarthritis is a common progressive degenerative joint disease that affects articular cartilage and subchondral bone. Clinical manifestations vary from annoying symptoms to progressively disabling disease. Treatment is aimed at relieving pain, maintaining optimal joint function, and preventing progressive disability.

| NURSING DIAGNOSES | EXPECTED OUTCOMES AND NURSING INTERVENTIONS / *RATIONALE*
(■ = INDEPENDENT; ▲ = COLLABORATIVE) |

Pain

RELATED FACTORS

Joint degeneration
Muscle spasm
Physical activity

EXPECTED OUTCOMES

The patient verbalizes reduction in or relief of pain.
The patient verbalizes ability to cope with chronic pain.

ONGOING ASSESSMENT

- Assess description of pain. *Usually provoked by activity and relieved by rest. May occur in fingers, hips, knees, lower lumbar, and cervical vertebrae.*
- Assess previous experiences with pain and pain relief.
- Determine patient's emotional reaction to chronic pain. *Patient may find coping with progressive disease difficult.*

Continued.

Musculoskeletal Care Plans

NURSING DIAGNOSES	EXPECTED OUTCOMES AND NURSING INTERVENTIONS / *RATIONALE* (■ = INDEPENDENT; ▲ = COLLABORATIVE)

DEFINING CHARACTERISTICS

Patient's/significant other's report of pain
Facial grimaces
Moaning, crying
Protective, guarded behavior
Restlessness
Withdrawal
Irritability

THERAPEUTIC INTERVENTIONS

- Develop pain relief regimen based on patient's identified aggravating and relieving factors.
- Change patient's position while maintaining functional alignment (e.g., turning, adjusting pillows).
▲ Administer analgesics and/or antiinflammatory medication:
  Aspirin/nonsteroidal antiinflammatory drugs (NSAIDS): *Commonly used to relieve pain and any secondary inflammation. Patients need to be evaluated for hypertension, renal disease, and heart disease because of the salt retention properties of these medications. These medications are excreted by the kidneys.*
  Analgesics (such as Tylenol): *To relieve pain.*
- Apply hot or cold packs *to provide comfort. Some patients have preference for hot vs. cold therapy.*
- Encourage adequate rest periods. *Fatigue impairs ability to cope with discomfort.*
- Provide adaptive equipment (i.e., cane, walker) as necessary *to assist ambulation and reduce joint stress.*
- Eliminate additional stressors.
▲ Medicate for pain before activity and exercise therapy.
- See also Pain, p. 49.

Impaired Physical Mobility

RELATED FACTORS

Pain
Stiffness
Fatigue
Restricted joint movement
Muscle weakness

DEFINING CHARACTERISTICS

Reluctance to move
Limited ROM
Decreased muscle strength
Decreased ability to transfer and ambulate

EXPECTED OUTCOMES

The patient verbalizes and demonstrates ability to move purposefully.

ONGOING ASSESSMENT

- Assess ROM. *Pain on motion may cause progressive loss of function.*
- Assess ability to perform ADLs.
- Assess previous use of assistive ambulatory devices.

THERAPEUTIC INTERVENTIONS

- Assist patient with isometric, active, and passive ROM exercises to all extremities. *Muscular exertion through exercise promotes circulation and free joint mobility, strengthens muscle tone, develops coordination, and prevents nonfunctional contracture.*
- Increase activity as indicated. Consult physical therapy (PT) staff. *Home exercise can be effective in maintaining joint function and independence.*
- Encourage patient to ambulate with assistive devices (i.e., crutches, walker, cane, raised toilet seat). *Reduces the load on the joint and promotes safety.*
- Encourage sitting in a chair with a raised seat and firm support. *Facilitates getting in and out of chair.*
- Provide adequate rest periods.
- Allow patient adequate time for activities.
- Discuss environmental barriers to mobility.

NURSING DIAGNOSES	EXPECTED OUTCOMES AND NURSING INTERVENTIONS / *RATIONALE* (▪ = INDEPENDENT; ▲ = COLLABORATIVE)

Knowledge Deficit

RELATED FACTORS

New disease/procedures
Unfamiliarity with treatment
 regimen

DEFINING CHARACTERISTICS

Multiple questions
Lack of questions
Verbalized misconceptions
Verbalized lack of knowledge

EXPECTED OUTCOMES

Patient verbalizes understanding of disease and treatment.

ONGOING ASSESSMENT

▪ Assess knowledge of ostoearthritis and its treatment.

THERAPEUTIC INTERVENTIONS

▪ Introduce/reinforce disease process information. *Adequate health knowledge increases person's ability to understand health problem, prevent harm to self, and participate in care.*
   Cause; mechanical factors contributing to disease process (injury to the joint, trauma, congenital problems)
   Sites of involvement
▪ Introduce/reinforce information on drug therapy. *Some potential side effects of NSAIDs include stomach irritation and salt retention.*
▪ Provide information on needed adaptive equipment.
▪ Discuss weight loss if patient is overweight. *The excess body weight puts added strain on already compromised joints and can increase pain.*
▪ Discuss need for relaxation techniques. *Many different approaches may be indicated for dealing with the chronic disease.*
▪ Discuss need for exercise. *Water exercise is ideal because the buoyancy of the water reduces stress on the joints. The aerobic program should be designed by a health professional.*
▪ Stress importance of long term follow-up care. *Patients with progressive loss of function and habitual pain may require surgical intervention (i.e., arthroscopy, total joint replacement).*
▪ Suggest referral to community resources such as the Arthritis Foundation

See also:
Skin Integrity, p. 59.
Self-care Deficit, p. 53.
Body Image Disturbance,
 p. 7.

By: Linda Ehrlich, RN, MSN

Osteomyelitis

Escherichia coli infection of the bone, caused by a pathogenic organism, usually Staphylococcus, Streptococcus or Salmonella and introduced via soft tissue trauma, open wounds, or infections at other sites. Osteomyelitis may be acute (less than 1 month duration) or chronic (more than 1 month).

NURSING DIAGNOSES	EXPECTED OUTCOMES AND NURSING INTERVENTIONS / *RATIONALE* (▪ = INDEPENDENT; ▲ = COLLABORATIVE)

Bone Infection

RELATED FACTORS

Infection that has migrated to
 bone tissue

DEFINING CHARACTERISTICS

Local inflammation of involved
 bone characterized by pain/
 guarding, edema, warmth,
 redness

EXPECTED OUTCOMES

Patient responds to antibiotic therapy, as evidenced by normal WBC, negative wound culture findings.

ONGOING ASSESSMENT

▪ Assess affected area for signs/symptoms of infection.
▲ Assess lab values, especially WBC and sedimentation rate.
▲ Assess bone scan findings. *Aid in establishing diagnosis.*
▲ Obtain appropriate cultures and sensitivities: blood; aspirate from bone abscess if present. *Wound cultures are necessary to identify causative organism.*

Continued.

Musculoskeletal Care Plans

NURSING DIAGNOSES	EXPECTED OUTCOMES AND NURSING INTERVENTIONS / *RATIONALE* (■ = INDEPENDENT; ▲ = COLLABORATIVE)
	THERAPEUTIC INTERVENTIONS—cont'd
	▲ Administer IV antibiotics as ordered. *Aggressive antibiotic treatment is the primary therapy.*
	▲ Administer antipyretics.
	■ Provide fluids *to prevent dehydration in febrile state.*
	■ Immobilize affected site.
	■ Ensure sterile technique during dressing changes. Prevent cross-contamination.
	For chronic osteomyelitis:
	▲ Prepare for surgical débridement. *May be necessary for removal of infected tissue.*
	▲ Anticipate constant wound irrigation with antibiotics. *Sepsis and unsuccessful antibiotic therapy are major complications.*
Pain	**EXPECTED OUTCOMES**
RELATED FACTORS	Patient verbalizes relief or reduction in pain and appears comfortable.
Infection	
Inflammation	**ONGOING ASSESSMENT**
	■ Assess affected area for pain with movement.
DEFINING CHARACTERISTICS	■ Assess verbal and nonverbal signs of pain.
Verbalized bone pain with/ without movement	■ Assess analgesic effectiveness.
Nonverbal signs (i.e., moans, restlessness, and grimaces)	■ Monitor vital signs for signs/symptoms of pain.
Physical signs (e.g., increased heart rate, increased blood pressure, and diaphoresis)	**THERAPEUTIC INTERVENTIONS**
	▲ Administer analgesics as prescribed.
	■ Immobilize limb. Use care and support when moving affected extremity. *Motion can aggravate pain.*
	■ Maintain good functional alignment.
	■ Provide diversional activities.
High Risk for Injury	**EXPECTED OUTCOMES**
RISK FACTORS	Patient avoids fracture/injury to healing bone.
Necrosis of bone	
Fragile bone	**ONGOING ASSESSMENT**
	■ Assess for guarded movement of affected limb, pain in affected bone with movement or ROM, bone scan findings of bone destruction.
	THERAPEUTIC INTERVENTIONS
	■ Immobilize affected area. *Extensive manipulation and movement can result in pathologic fractures.*
	■ Provide passive ROM as indicated.
	▲ Obtain PT consultation.

NURSING DIAGNOSES	EXPECTED OUTCOMES AND NURSING INTERVENTIONS / *RATIONALE* (■ = INDEPENDENT; ▲ = COLLABORATIVE)

Knowledge Deficit

RELATED FACTORS

Hospitalization and treatment
Lack of experience

DEFINING CHARACTERISTICS

Verbalized lack of understanding
Questioning

EXPECTED OUTCOMES

- Patient verbalizes understanding of diagnostic process, antibiotic therapy, wound care, and follow-up care.

ONGOING ASSESSMENT

- Assess understanding of disease process, treatment, follow-up care.

THERAPEUTIC INTERVENTIONS

- Provide explanation of the development of osteomyelitis.
- Explain necessity for tests (e.g., aspirations, blood culture and sensitivity, x-ray films, and scans).
- Explain importance of long-term IV therapy. *Compliance with prolonged therapy is essential for adequate treatment of osteomyelitis. Chronic osteomyelitis results from failed initial therapy.*
- Stress importance of continuing oral antibiotic after discharge.
- Instruct in wound care.
- Provide follow-up appointments, prescriptions, and home health services if home treatment is possible.

See also:
Impaired Physical Mobility, p. 47.
Impaired Individual Coping, p. 18.
Self-care Deficit, p. 53.
Diversional Activity Deficit, p. 21.

By: Susan Geoghegan, RN, BSN

Osteoporosis

A metabolic bone disease characterized by a decrease in bone mass resulting in porosity/brittleness. This leads to a greater risk of bone fractures and deformities. It is more common in women after menopause.

NURSING DIAGNOSES	EXPECTED OUTCOMES AND NURSING INTERVENTIONS / *RATIONALE* (■ = INDEPENDENT; ▲ = COLLABORATIVE)

High Risk for Ineffective Calcium Utilization

RISK FACTORS

Insufficient dietary intake of calcium
Hormonal changes
Postmenopausal patient not having estrogen replacement therapy

EXPECTED OUTCOMES

Patient identifies high-calcium foods.
Patient maintains balanced, calcium-rich diet.

ONGOING ASSESSMENT

- Obtain history of calcium intake: *1000 mg/day is usually required; 1500 mg/day needed for postmenopausal women not taking estrogen supplement.*
- Assess whether patient is postmenopausal or has had hysterectomy with bilateral oophorectomy. *Reabsorption of bone is accelerated with natural or surgically induced menopause.*
- Assess tobacco, alcohol, and exercise history. *Smoking, drinking alcohol, and having only minimal weight-bearing exercise are risk factors for development of osteoporosis.*
- Assess for calcium supplementation. *Necessary if dietary intake is inadequate.*
- Assess whether patient is taking medications that decrease calcium absorption: cortisone, antacids, tetracycline, laxatives.
- ▲ Monitor calcium levels. *Elevated calcium levels indicate calcium malabsorption (may indicate need for vitamin D supplement to aid calcium absorption).*

Continued.

NURSING DIAGNOSES	EXPECTED OUTCOMES AND NURSING INTERVENTIONS / *RATIONALE* (■ = INDEPENDENT; ▲ = COLLABORATIVE)

	THERAPEUTIC INTERVENTIONS
	• Encourage increased intake of calcium-rich foods: skim milk/cheeses/yogurt/ice cream; whole-grain cereals; green leafy vegetables; almonds/hazelnuts. *Natural sources of calcium may provide more elemental or useful forms.*
	▲ Consult dietician when appropriate. Reinforce meal planning taught by dietitian.
	▲ Administer calcium supplementation therapy as ordered *to reduce bone resorption.*
	    Calcitonin: *Given by injection or nasal spray to women who cannot take estrogen.*
	    Bisphosphonate therapy: oral.
	    Dironel: Not FDA approved yet.
	▲ Administer estrogen therapy as indicated.

Pain **RELATED FACTORS** Fracture Deformities **DEFINING CHARACTERISTICS** Patient's/significant other's report of pain Guarding on motion of affected area Facial mask of pain Moaning or other pain-associated sounds	**EXPECTED OUTCOMES** The patient verbalizes a decrease in pain. **ONGOING ASSESSMENT** • Solicit patient's description of pain. *Although osteoporosis occurs throughout the skeletal body, fractures/problems are more evident in the spine, hips, and wrists.* • Assess patient's response to pain medication or therapeutics aimed at abolishing/relieving pain. **THERAPEUTIC INTERVENTIONS** ▲ Administer pain medications as necessary as prescribed. *Newer treatment includes calcitonin.* • Encourage use of ambulation aid(s) for pain related to weight bearing. *Assistive devices can help support body weight that otherwise could add to pain in fractures of weight-bearing joints/bones.* • See also Pain, p. 49.
Impaired Mobility **RELATED FACTORS** Deformities Fractures Pain **DEFINING CHARACTERISTICS** Patient's/significant other's report of difficulty of purposeful movement Decreased ability to transfer and ambulate Reluctance to attempt movement Decreased muscle strength Decreased ROM	**EXPECTED OUTCOMES** Patient verbalizes/demonstrates increased ability to move purposefully. Patient is free of falls. Patient identifies/implements safe environment practices at home. **ONGOING ASSESSMENT** • Solicit patient's description of aggravating and alleviating factors, joint/bone pain and stiffness, interference with life-style. • Observe patient's ability to ambulate, to move all body parts functionally. • Assess environment for safety. *Osteoporosis is the leading cause of fractures in postmenopausal women.* **THERAPEUTIC INTERVENTIONS** ▲ Promote mobility through physical therapy and exercise. Suggest moderate weight-bearing exercise (e.g., walking, bicycling, or dancing) for 30 min 3 times/wk. *Weight bearing stimulates osteoblastic activity and new bone growth.* ▲ Reinforce techniques of therapeutic exercise (ROM and muscle strengthening) taught by physical therapist. • Assist with ambulation as necessary. • Recommend low, comfortable shoes for walking. *Pathologic fractures are a complication of falls.* • Provide adaptive equipment (e.g., cane, walker) as necessary to assist with ambulation. • Provide safe hospital environment: bed rails up, bed in down position, necessary items (e.g., telephone, call light, walker, cane) within reach, adequate lighting, grab bars in bathroom (if available). • Teach patient to create safe environment at home: remove or tack down throw rugs; wear firm-soled shoes; install grab bars in bathroom; do not carry heavy objects. *Safe home environment is necessary to prevent falls and potential fractures.*

| NURSING DIAGNOSES | EXPECTED OUTCOMES AND NURSING INTERVENTIONS / *RATIONALE*
(■ = INDEPENDENT; ▲ = COLLABORATIVE) |

Body Image Disturbance

RELATED FACTORS

Deformities
Fractures
Use of assistive devices

DEFINING CHARACTERISTICS

Verbalization of feelings about altered structure/function of body part or use of assistive devices
Preoccupation with altered body part or function
Refusal to use assistive devices

EXPECTED OUTCOMES

Patient verbalizes positive aspects of body and self.
Patient identifies supportive person as appropriate.

ONGOING ASSESSMENT

- Assess perception of change in body part structure/function. *Bone loss causes loss of height and appearance of humped back (dowager's hump).*
- Assess perceived impact of change on ADL, social behavior, personal relationships, occupational activities. *Patient may isolate self for fear of falling, difficulty in getting around, or self-consciousness about changed appearance.*

THERAPEUTIC INTERVENTIONS

- Acknowledge normality of emotional response to actual or perceived change in body structure/function.
- Assist patient in incorporating actual changes in ADL, social life, interpersonal relationships, occupational activities.
- Allow patient adequate time for self-care activities. Assist as necessary. *Patient's self-image improves when he or she can perform personal care independently.*
- ▲ Reinforce self-care techniques taught by occupational therapist.
- Encourage participation in support groups. *Allows for open, nonthreatening discussion of feelings with others with similar experiences. Groups can give realistic picture of the condition and suggestions for problem solving and coping.*
- See also Body image disturbance, p. 7.

Knowledge Deficit

RELATED FACTORS

New disease
Unfamiliarity with treatment regimen

DEFINING CHARACTERISTICS

Patient's/significant other's multiple questions, verbalized misconceptions, verbalized lack of knowledge
Lack of questions

See also:
Self-care deficit, p. 53.
Impaired individual coping, p. 18.

EXPECTED OUTCOMES

Patient verbalizes understanding of the disease and treatment.

ONGOING ASSESSMENT

- Assess patient's knowledge of osteoporosis and treatment.

THERAPEUTIC INTERVENTIONS

- Schedule educational sessions when patient is most comfortable. *Pain will distract patient and may lead to inability to absorb new information.*
- Introduce/reinforce disease process information:
  Causes: Estrogen deficiency in postmenopausal women, early menopause, premenopausal estrogen deficiency.
  Risk factors: Besides above, inadequate calcium intake, Caucasian and Asian race, female gender, inactivity, cigarette and alcohol abuse, increasing age, some endocrine diseases
  Process: Though osteoporosis occurs throughout the body, the process is more evident in the spine, hips, and wrists.
- Describe diagnostic tests available:
  Bone density measurement. *Provides information on fracture risk.*
  Biochemical assessment. *Tests such as serum osteocalcin provide information on osteoblastic activity.*
- Introduce/reinforce information on medications: calcium/vitamin D supplements, estrogen therapy, calcitonin injection, bisphosphonate.
- Introduce/reinforce self-management techniques:
  Physical activity. *Weight bearing along with calcium intake stimulates development and maintenance of bone mass.*
  Use of assistive devices.
  Protection from injury/falls
- Reinforce dietary teaching about increased calcium intake.

By: Linda Ehrlich, RN, MSN
Meg Gulanick, RN, PhD

Partial anterior acromiectomy with or without rotator cuff repair

(BANKART REPAIR; PUTTI-PLATT OPERATION; BRISTOW REPAIR)

Decompression of the subacromial space by osteotomy of the anterior/inferior margin of the acromion and transsection of the coracoacromial ligament, with examination of rotator cuff muscles and repair of defect if indicated.

NURSING DIAGNOSES	EXPECTED OUTCOMES AND NURSING INTERVENTIONS / RATIONALE (■ = INDEPENDENT; ▲ = COLLABORATIVE)

Knowledge Deficit

RELATED FACTORS

New surgical procedures
Unfamiliarity with surgical routines

DEFINING CHARACTERISTICS

Many questions
Lack of questions
Increased anxiety level
Verbalized misconceptions

EXPECTED OUTCOMES

Patient verbalizes understanding of preoperative instructions and postoperative care.

ONGOING ASSESSMENT

- Assess knowledge of present problem and recommended treatment.

THERAPEUTIC INTERVENTIONS

- Verbally review operative protocol.
- Instruct patients about:
    Hospital educational television with general pre-, intra- and postoperative information
    Preoperative routines
    Preoperative strength testing (Cybex testing) if necessary
    Immediate postoperative routines (e.g., closed wound suction, drains, IV, diet, pain management)
    Coughing and deep breathing exercises
    Mobility limitations and postoperative exercises
    Knowledge increases patient's ability to understand health problem, reduces postoperative complications, and may reduce postoperative pain.

Pain

RELATED FACTORS

Surgical procedure

DEFINING CHARACTERISTICS

Patient's/significant other's report of pain
Facial grimaces
Moaning, crying
Protective, guarded behavior
Restlessness
Withdrawal
Irritability

EXPECTED OUTCOMES

Patient verbalizes reduction or relief of pain.
Patient appears relaxed and comfortable.

ONGOING ASSESSMENT

- Assess description of pain.
- Assess previous experiences with pain and pain relief.
- Assess pain relief measure effectiveness.

THERAPEUTIC INTERVENTIONS

▲ Give analgesics as prescribed.
- Alter patient's position (turn to nonoperative side, adjust pillows to support affected shoulder, seat in chair or bed).
- Encourage appropriate rest periods. *Rest conserves energy necessary for cellular metabolism needed for tissue healing.*
- Eliminate additional stressors; encourage diversional activity.
- Instruct patient to report pain *so relief measures can be implemented.*
▲ Consider use of patient-controlled anesthesia as appropriate.

High Risk for Altered Peripheral Tissue Perfusion to Affected Extremity

RISK FACTORS

Surgical procedure
Restricted movement
Swelling

EXPECTED OUTCOMES

Patient maintains optimal tissue perfusion, as evidenced by warm skin, good capillary refill, absence of edema and pain.

ONGOING ASSESSMENT

- Use preoperative neurovascular assessment to establish baseline status for postoperative comparison.
- Assess upper extremities; compare temperature, color, sensation, movement, edema, pulse, and capillary refill. *Coldness, pallor, pain, sluggish or absent capillary refill, pressure within muscle compartment, edema are all signs of compromised circulation.*
- Assess for increasing pain in affected extremity.

THERAPEUTIC INTERVENTIONS

▲ Notify physician of neurovascular status changes. *Diminished tissue oxygenation results from impaired circulation, which increases potential for tissue necrosis.*

NURSING DIAGNOSES	EXPECTED OUTCOMES AND NURSING INTERVENTIONS / *RATIONALE* (■ = INDEPENDENT; ▲ = COLLABORATIVE)

High Risk for Self-Care Deficit

RISK FACTORS
Restricted movement of extremity

EXPECTED OUTCOMES
Patient performs self-care activities independently (using assistive devices as needed).

ONGOING ASSESSMENT
- Assess ability to perform ADLs independently. *Presence of immobilizer, sling, or shoulder spica cast can significantly impair purposeful movement.*
- Assess available home support systems.
- Assess hand dominance.

THERAPEUTIC INTERVENTIONS
▲ Refer to occupational therapy for needed ADL training. *Immobilization of upper extremity demands alternative methods of performing ADLs.*
- Assist in ADL training, using one-handed technique.
▲ Reinforce use of assistive devices if prescribed.
▲ Request social service consultation for home needs
- Instruct on wearing large clothing that fits over arm. *Arm must remain immobilized to allow for healing.*

Knowledge Deficit: Home Management

RELATED FACTORS
Unfamiliarity with postoperative activity

DEFINING CHARACTERISTICS
Many questions
Increased anxiety about impending discharge

EXPECTED OUTCOMES
Patient verbalizes understanding of home management.

ONGOING ASSESSMENT
- Assess knowledge of postoperative activity.

THERAPEUTIC INTERVENTIONS
- Emphasize importance of maintaining position in shoulder immobilizer, sling, or cast for 3-6 wk.
- Educate patient to put nothing under cast or immobilizer.
- Instruct on positions to avoid (abduction, lifting, etc.), need to keep incision dry and clean, need to inspect skin around immobilizer or cast for irritation.
- Instruct patient to notify physician of:
  Pain, numbness, tingling, edema, or discoloration of fingers. *May signify compromised circulation.*
  Pain, redness, drainage from incision. *Signifies possible infection.*
  Persistent fever
  Cracking or softened areas in cast
  Pain, numbness, drainage, foul odors, or warm areas under cast
  Anything inside cast. *Causes pressure and injury to skin*
  Areas of skin breakdown around cast or immobilizer
- Discuss courses of rehabilitation: Review instructions for follow-up visit.

See also:
High Risk for Infection, p. 40.
Ineffective Airway Clearance, p. 3.
Impaired Individual Coping, p. 18.

By: Sandra Eungard, RN, MS
Marilyn Magafas, RN, MBA

Pelvic fracture

(STABLE PELVIC FRACTURE; UNSTABLE PELVIC FRACTURE)

Traumatic interruption of the pelvic ring by osseous injury, ligamentous injury, or a combination of both. Pelvic fractures are classified by location and the resulting effect on the stability of the pelvis. Type I fractures are stable without a break in the pelvic ring. Type II fractures include single breaks in the pelvic ring with little or no displacement of the fracture fragment and therefore are stable. Type III fractures involve double breaks in the pelvic ring and are always unstable. Type IV fractures are unstable with acetabular fractures. Motor vehicle accidents, crush injuries and falls generating forces of 400 to 2600 pounds account for most pelvic fractures.

NURSING DIAGNOSES	EXPECTED OUTCOMES AND NURSING INTERVENTIONS / *RATIONALE* (■ = INDEPENDENT; ▲ = COLLABORATIVE)

Pain

RELATED FACTORS

Trauma
Surgical procedure
Rehabilitation program

DEFINING CHARACTERISTICS

Verbalization of pain
Crying, moaning, grimacing
Increased pulse, BP
Irritability, impatience
Restlessness
Guarded or limited movement
 of body and extremities

EXPECTED OUTCOMES

Patient expresses relief or reduction of pain.
Patient appears comfortable.

ONGOING ASSESSMENT

- Assess pain characteristics.
- Assess the degree of pelvic fracture.
- Assess for proper body and traction alignment.
- Assess effectiveness of pain relief measures.

THERAPEUTIC INTERVENTIONS

- Maintain immobilization and support of affected part. *Immobility prevents further tissue damage and muscle spasm.*
- Reposition and support unaffected parts as permitted *to promote general comfort.*
- ▲ Administer pain medication as prescribed.
- Encourage use of analgesic 30 min before physical therapy if indicated or any activity that might intensify pain. *Adequate pain management is essential to allow active participation in the physical therapy regimen.*

Impaired Physical Mobility

RELATED FACTORS

Imposed bedrest caused by
 injury and immobilization
 device—pelvic sling, skeletal
 traction, external fixator, hip
 spica cast, or brace
Surgical procedure—internal
 fixation

DEFINING CHARACTERISTICS

Mechanical restriction of
 movement
Decreased muscle strength,
 control, coordination, and
 range of motion
Reluctance to move

EXPECTED OUTCOMES

Patient achieves maximal independence within activity restrictions.
Patient maintains muscle strength/tone.

ONGOING ASSESSMENT

- Assess degree of pelvic stability/instability and extent of activities and movement allowed.
- Assess ability to carry out ADLs and tolerance of activities.
- Assess muscle strength and ROM.

THERAPEUTIC INTERVENTIONS

- ▲ Maintain bedrest as indicated, approximately 6-8 wk for *unstable* pelvic fracture.
- Assist with repositioning and turning as appropriate.
- Encourage independence within patient's activity limitations.
- Assist and encourage to perform quad sets, gluteal sets, and ROM exercises if appropriate *to prevent muscle atrophy and maintain adequate muscle strength required in mobility.*
- ▲ For stable pelvic fractures, assist with ambulation and appropriate use of assistive walking devices—walker or crutches as indicated. *There is an inherent tendency to overprotect the area of injury/surgery, thus the need for encouragement and emotional support when ambulating.*

High Risk for Altered Peripheral Tissue Perfusion

RISK FACTORS

Restricted movement
Swelling
Surgical procedure

EXPECTED OUTCOMES

Patient maintains adequate tissue perfusion, as evidenced by warm extremities, strong bilateral pulses, good capillary refill, absence of pain or edema.

ONGOING ASSESSMENT

- Monitor neurovascular status for any signs or symptoms of neurovascular insufficiency: coldness, pallor, edema, pain, pulselessness, sluggish or absent capillary refill, numbness, tingling sensation, cyanosis, hematoma.
- Assess for increased pain in affected extremity/ies.
- Assess for presence of positive Homan's sign.

THERAPEUTIC INTERVENTIONS

- Elevate extremity/ies if indicated.
- Maintain functional alignment.
- ▲ Apply sequential compression devices and/or antiembolic stockings as prescribed.
- Instruct to perform ROM exercises *to increase venous return and decrease probability of deep vein thrombosis.*
- ▲ Notify physician of signs of altered tissue perfusion.

High Risk for Fluid Volume Deficit

RISK FACTORS

Blood vessel damage
Multiple fractures
Soft tissue swelling and bruising

EXPECTED OUTCOMES

Patient maintains adequate blood/fluid volume, as evidenced by normal heart rate; warm, dry skin; good capillary refill; normal blood pressure.

ONGOING ASSESSMENT

- Assess amount of any blood loss.
- Assess degree of pelvic fracture. *Because pelvic fractures are generally associated with high energy forces, multiple injuries should be anticipated and systematically evaluated. Hemorrhage continues to be the primary cause of early mortality after an unstable pelvic fracture.*
- Assess for signs of hypovolemia: weak, rapid pulse; decreased BP; rapid, shallow respiration; cold, clammy skin; sluggish capillary refill; cyanosis; decreased urinary output; change in level of consciousness.
- Monitor intake and output.
- ▲ Monitor laboratory values—CBC, Hb, Hct. Determine baseline values.

THERAPEUTIC INTERVENTIONS

- Apply pressure to bleeding areas.
- ▲ Administer intravenous fluids and blood products as prescribed.
- Encourage fluid intake if not contraindicated.

High Risk for Impaired Skin Integrity

RISK FACTORS

Physical immobility
Presence and contact with immobilization device

EXPECTED OUTCOMES

Patient maintains intact skin.
Risk of further breakdown is reduced through ongoing assessment and early intervention.

ONGOING ASSESSMENT

- Assess skin for color, texture, moisture, and general appearance.
- Assess immobilized part of body for redness or breakdown.
- Assess actual wound appearance if present.
- Remove antiembolic devices every shift for inspection of skin integrity.

THERAPEUTIC INTERVENTIONS

- ▲ Turn and position q2hr if not contraindicated. *Shifting body weight off bony prominences is necessary to prevent pressure areas from developing and prevent tissue from breaking down.*
- Apply pressure relief device to bed (flotation devices, air mattress, foam or eggcrate mattress) as appropriate.
- Maintain padding under immobilization device *to prevent rubbing.*
- Keep as clean and dry as possible if patient is unable to control bowel or bladder function.
- Keep bed linens free of wrinkles and foreign matter.
- Clean, dry, and moisturize skin as necessary, especially over bony prominences.
- Lift patient as necessary. Do not allow friction of skin when placing or removing bedpan. Do not drag or pull patient to position.
- Apply overhead frame and trapeze if patient is able to assist self to move in bed.
- Keep heels off bed at all times. Apply heel/elbow protectors as needed.
- Maintain adequate nutritional status. *Ischemia and progressive tissue deterioration are more likely to appear in malnourished persons who are in negative nitrogen balance.*
- Administer pressure sore care as needed.

Continued.

Pelvic fracture—cont'd

NURSING DIAGNOSES	EXPECTED OUTCOMES AND NURSING INTERVENTIONS / *RATIONALE* (■ = INDEPENDENT; ▲ = COLLABORATIVE)

High Risk for Infection at Pin Sites and/or Open Wounds

RISK FACTORS

External fixation device applied to stabilize sacral fracture

Use of pelvic slings in conjunction with longitudinal skeletal traction to facilitate reduction of pelvic fracture

Interrupted first line of defense

EXPECTED OUTCOMES

Patient avoids infection at wound/pin site, as evidenced by normal WBC, afebrile state, no drainage/odor at wound site.

ONGOING ASSESSMENT

- Assess pin sites or open wounds for signs of infection.
- Monitor vital signs, especially temperature.
▲ Monitor WBC.
- Assess for skin tension at pin sites.

THERAPEUTIC INTERVENTIONS

▲ Perform sterile pin site care/wound care with betadine, hydrogen peroxide, normal saline solution, or as prescribed q8hr.
▲ Administer antibiotics as ordered.
- Maintain adequate nutrition and hydration *to promote wound healing*
- Teach patient/family purpose of pin/wound care, signs and symptoms of infection, and pin site care/wound care.

High Risk for Altered Urinary Elimination

RISK FACTORS

Urinary tract injuries (e.g., urethral tear secondary to high-velocity trauma)

Bladder rupture secondary to punctures from bony fragments

Immobility

Presence of catheter

Infection

EXPECTED OUTCOMES

Patient maintains adequate urine output (>30 ml/hr) without complications.

ONGOING ASSESSMENT

- Assess frequency, amount, and character of urine.
- Observe for gross hematuria, pelvic hematoma, edematous and ecchymotic scrotum.
- Record intake and output accurately.
- Monitor for incontinence.
- Assess for poor emptying *secondary to neuropathic bladder. Pelvic injuries frequently cause internal injury to the urinary tract; IVP, cystogram, and KUB may be required for diagnosis.*
- Monitor for urine retention: decreased urine output, bladder distention, suprapubic pain.
▲ Assess for signs and symptoms of urinary tract infection: frequency, burning on urination, elevated temperature, elevated WBC.

THERAPEUTIC INTERVENTIONS

- Encourage fluids and juices. *If the urine is kept dilute, calcium particles are less likely to precipitate and stasis with resultant infection is less likely.*
- Provide privacy during void.
▲ Insert Foley catheter or institute intermittent catheterization using aseptic technique as prescribed.
▲ Administer antibiotics as prescribed.
▲ Notify physician immediately of any abnormalities in urine and the process of voiding.

High Risk for Injury

RISK FACTORS

Improper positioning of immobilization device—sling, traction, external fixator

If cast in place, loss of continuity of cast

EXPECTED OUTCOMES

Patient maintains correct body position and alignment.
Patient's cast dries correctly.

ONGOING ASSESSMENT

- Assess immobilization device periodically for weights, knots, and ropes.
- Assess patient's position in the immobilization apparatus.
- Assess that bed linens are not interfering with the immobilization device.
- Assess cast for cracks; weakened, softened, or wet areas; or indentations.

THERAPEUTIC INTERVENTIONS

Traction:
- Maintain proper alignment of pelvis area and/or affected extremity in the desired position *that reduces the fracture.*
▲ Maintain continuous traction at all times.
- Maintain mechanics of traction at all times. Maintain adequate countertraction by avoiding elevation of head of bed more than 30 degrees, except during mealtimes.
- Tighten all traction equipment and check that weights hang freely.

NURSING DIAGNOSES	EXPECTED OUTCOMES AND NURSING INTERVENTIONS / *RATIONALE* (■ = INDEPENDENT; ▲ = COLLABORATIVE)

THERAPEUTIC INTERVENTIONS—cont'd

- Maintain the foot of bed in gatch position *to enhance circulation and relieve back strain while in pelvic sling if not contraindicated.*
- ▲ Verify from physician how much lifting and turning the patient is allowed.

Cast:

- Leave cast open to air until completely dry.
- Prevent indenting cast by moving and supporting it with palms of hands.
- Reposition patient and cast q2hr *to allow for drying.*
- Keep cast clean and dry; avoid soiling from urine/feces.

High Risk for Altered Nutrition: Less than Body Requirements

RISK FACTORS

Trauma to the viscera and abdominal organs
Nausea/vomiting
Abdominal distention
Absent bowel sounds
Abdominal pain

EXPECTED OUTCOMES

Patient maintains optimal nutritional status, as evidenced by stable weight, progression to solid food.

ONGOING ASSESSMENT

- Auscultate for bowel sounds in all abdominal quadrants. *Abdominal trauma should always be suspected in cases of major pelvic fractures until proved otherwise. The proximity of the abdominal cavity accounts for a large number of associated injuries to abdominal organs.*
- Measure abdominal girth every morning if distention is present.
- Monitor intake and output.
- Monitor patient's tolerance of fluids or food.
- Assess for abdominal pain/discomfort or cramps.

THERAPEUTIC INTERVENTIONS

- ▲ If absent bowel sounds, infuse IV fluids as ordered.
- ▲ If nasogastric tube is present: keep patient NPO; irrigate NGT as needed.
- Provide supplemental nourishment as indicated.
- ▲ Notify physician of nausea, vomiting, abdominal distention, absence of flatulence, abdominal pain/discomfort, or cramps.

High Risk for Ineffective Coping

RISK FACTORS

Posttraumatic response
Restricted activity
Dependence
Self-care deficit

EXPECTED OUTCOMES

Patient begins to verbalize positive expressions, feelings, and reactions about self and situation.
Patient identifies available resources/support staff.

ONGOING ASSESSMENT

- Assess psychosocial status before hospitalization—life-style, physical capabilities, body image, attitudes.
- Assess degree of dependence.
- Assess for signs of behavior change and level of acceptance of injury and treatment.

THERAPEUTIC INTERVENTIONS

- Provide time for listening to patient's concerns. *Consider that because the accidents that cause unstable pelvic fractures are major ones, signs of posttraumatic stress disorder may be exhibited.*
- Provide diversionary activities as allowed by his/her condition.
- Explain procedures and treatment *to alleviate anxiety.* Avoid false assurances.
- Identify and reinforce patient's strengths and assist with weaknesses.
- Encourage patient to plan, participate in care activities. Adapt care to patient's routines and needs.
- Provide opportunities for independent activities. *Independence facilitates coping.*
- Arrange environment to promote independent use of materials needed for ADLs. *To develop self-esteem, patient/significant others must participate actively in rehabilitation.*
- Continually teach and inform patient/family of physical status, treatment plan, etc.
- ▲ Initiate social service and/or psychiatry referrals as needed.

Continued.

NURSING DIAGNOSES	EXPECTED OUTCOMES AND NURSING INTERVENTIONS / *RATIONALE* (■ = INDEPENDENT; ▲ = COLLABORATIVE)

Knowledge Deficit

RELATED FACTORS
New condition
New procedure/treatment

DEFINING CHARACTERISTICS
Verbalized lack of knowledge
  of care of pelvic fracture
Multitude of questions
Lack of questions

EXPECTED OUTCOMES
Patient/significant other verbalize understanding of treatment, possible complications, and
  follow-up care.

ONGOING ASSESSMENT
- Solicit understanding of diagnosis, treatment, follow-up, care, etc.
- Assess patient's/family's readiness and ability to assume care responsibility.

THERAPEUTIC INTERVENTIONS
- Instruct patient/family/significant other about:
    Signs of possible complications and appropriate actions to take if they occur
    Mobility restrictions
    Exercises *to maintain muscle tone*
    Pain relief measures
    Nutritional needs
    Proper use of ambulatory devices if applicable
    Pin care if external fixator is present
    Cast care if cast is present
    Follow-up care after discharge
▲ Refer to social worker to arrange for home physical therapy and homemaker if needed.

See also:
Body Image Disturbance, p.
  7.
Diversional Activity Deficit, p.
  21.
Ineffective Breathing Pattern,
  p. 10.
Extremity Fracture, p. 336.
Traction, p. 371.

By: Rachel Ongsansoy, RN, BSN
    Marilyn Magafas, RN, MBA

Systemic lupus erythematosus

(SLE; LUPUS)

A chronic, systemic inflammatory disease characterized by multi-system involvement. Mild disease can affect joints and skin. More severe disease can affect kidneys, heart, lung, blood vessels, and central nervous system as well as joints and skin. Women are affected six times more often than men.

NURSING DIAGNOSES	EXPECTED OUTCOMES AND NURSING INTERVENTIONS / *RATIONALE* (■ = INDEPENDENT; ▲ = COLLABORATIVE)

Altered Skin Integrity

RELATED FACTORS

Inflammation
Vasoconstriction

DEFINING CHARACTERISTICS

Redness
Pain/tenderness
Itching
Skin breakdown
Oral/nasal ulcers
Skin rash

EXPECTED OUTCOMES

The patient maintains optimal skin integrity as evidenced by absence of rashes and skin lesions.

ONGOING ASSESSMENT

- Assess skin integrity: note size of lesions, including oral, nasal, fingertip, and leg ulcers.
- Solicit patient's description of pain.

THERAPEUTIC INTERVENTIONS

- Clean, dry, and moisturize intact skin; use warm (not hot) water, especially over bony prominences, using unscented lotion (Eucerin or Lubriderm). *Scented lotions may contain alcohol, which dries skin.*
- Encourage adequate nutrition and hydration.
- Provide prophylactic pressure-relieving devices (e.g., special mattress, elbow pads).
- Instruct to avoid contact with harsh chemicals (e.g., household cleaners, detergents), and to wear cotton-lined latex gloves as needed.

For skin rash:
- Instruct patient to avoid ultraviolet light: *Sun can exacerbate skin rash.*
  Wear maximum protection sunscreen (SPF 15 or above) in sun.
  Wear wide-brim hat and carry umbrella.
  Wear protective eyewear.
  Sunbathing is contraindicated.
- ▲ Introduce/reinforce information about use of hydroxychloroquine sulfate (Plaquenil Sulfate). *It is a slow-acting medicine used to relieve or reduce rash. It may take 8-12 wk for effect. A potential side effect is retinal toxicity. Patient must be followed by ophthalmologist q6 mo.*
- Inform patient of availability of special makeup (at large department stores) to cover rash, especially facial rash: Covermark (Lydia O'Leary), Dermablend, Marilyn Miglin.

For oral ulcers:
- Instruct to rinse mouth with half-strength hydrogen peroxide tid. *Hydrogen peroxide helps keep oral ulcers clean.*
- Instruct to avoid irritating foods (e.g., spicy or citric).
- Instruct to keep ulcerated skin clean and dry. Apply topical ointments as prescribed.

Altered Skin Integrity: Alopecia (Scalp Hair Loss)

RELATED FACTORS

Inflammation
Exacerbation of disease process
High-dose corticosteroid use
Use of immunosuppressant drugs

DEFINING CHARACTERISTICS

Diffuse hair loss areas
Loss of discrete scalp hair patches
Scalp hair loss may or may not be accompanied by scarring

EXPECTED OUTCOMES

The patient verbalizes ability to cope with hair loss.
The patient identifies ways to conceal scalp loss as appropriate.

ONGOING ASSESSMENT

- Assess amount and distribution of scalp hair loss. Note scarring in areas of scalp hair loss. *Patient may experience total or patchy hair loss.*
- Assess degree to which symptom interferes with patient's life-style.

THERAPEUTIC INTERVENTIONS

- Instruct patient to avoid scalp contact with harsh chemicals (e.g., hair dye, permanent, curl relaxers). *These aggravate condition.*
  Use mild shampoo (e.g., P & S).
  Decrease frequency of shampooing.
- Instruct patient that scalp hair loss occurs during exacerbation of disease activity. *Scalp hair loss may be first sign of impending disease exacerbation.* Scalp hair loss may not be permanent; *as disease activity subsides, scalp hair begins to regrow.*
- Suggest short haircut during times of scalp hair loss.

Continued.

Systemic lupus erythematosus—cont'd

NURSING DIAGNOSES	EXPECTED OUTCOMES AND NURSING INTERVENTIONS / *RATIONALE* (■ = INDEPENDENT; ▲ = COLLABORATIVE)

THERAPEUTIC INTERVENTIONS—cont'd

- Explain that regrown hair may have different texture, often finer; hair will not regrow in areas of scarring.
- Instruct patient that scalp hair loss may be caused by high-dose corticosteroids (prednisone) and/or immunosuppressant drugs. *(Hair will regrow as dose decreases).*
- Encourage patient to investigate ways *(scarfs, hats, wigs)* to conceal scalp hair loss, if interfering with life-style.

Fever

RELATED FACTORS

Inflammation

DEFINING CHARACTERISTICS

Temperature greater than 101° F (38.4° C)
Chills
Shaking chills (rigor)
Diaphoresis
Dehydration

EXPECTED OUTCOMES

The patient maintains optimal body temperature.

ONGOING ASSESSMENT

- Assess for elevated temperature. *Fever is a common disease manifestation seen during active disease.*
- Assess for chills, shaking, and diaphoresis.
- Assess for signs of dehydration: decreased skin turgor, dry mucous membranes, decreased urine output.

THERAPEUTIC INTERVENTIONS

- ▲ Administer antipyretics as ordered. If aspirin used, monitor patient for elevated liver enzyme level. *Aspirin use by febrile lupus patients is documented to cause transient liver toxicity.*
- ▲ Administer steroids in divided dose.
- Encourage hydration.
- ▲ If temperature remains above 103° F (39.5° C), apply cooling mattress.
- See also Hyperthermia, p. 37.

Altered Peripheral Tissue Perfusion

RELATED FACTORS

Raynaud's phenomenon: vasospasm, structural changes

DEFINING CHARACTERISTICS

Pain, numbness, cold sensation
Triphasic color changes: white, blue, red

EXPECTED OUTCOMES

The patient maintains optimal tissue perfusion as evidenced by normal color of fingers and toes.

ONGOING ASSESSMENT

- Assess hands and feet for color, temperature, and skin integrity. *Raynaud's phenomenon is a common manifestation of lupus.*
- Solicit description of pain, numbness, and cold sensations.
- Assess interference with ADLs and life-style.

THERAPEUTIC INTERVENTIONS

- Keep extremities warm (socks, blankets, gloves, mittens).
- Remove vasoconstricting factors when possible.
- ▲ Administer vasodilating medications (e.g., Nifedipine) as ordered.
- Instruct patient to avoid undue cold exposure:
    Wear oven mitts for refrigerator or freezer.
    Wear multiple clothing layers (hat/cap, ear muffs, nose protector, mittens/gloves, socks) in cold environment.
    Suggest wearing items made of wool, cotton, down, or thinsulate *(provide most protection from cold exposure).*
- Instruct patient to avoid caffeine and nicotine *(cause vasoconstriction).*
- Instruct patient in stress management *(stress can precipitate vasospasm).*
- ▲ Refer to specialized stress reduction program as needed.

NURSING DIAGNOSES	EXPECTED OUTCOMES AND NURSING INTERVENTIONS / *RATIONALE* (■ = INDEPENDENT; ▲ = COLLABORATIVE)

Joint Pain

RELATED FACTORS

Inflammation

DEFINING CHARACTERISTICS

Pain
Guarding on motion of affected joints
Facial mask of pain
Moaning or other pain-associated sounds

EXPECTED OUTCOMES

Patient verbalizes a reduction in pain.

ONGOING ASSESSMENT

- Assess for signs of joint inflammation (redness, warmth, swelling, decreased motion).
- Solicit description of pain.
- Determine past measures used to alleviate pain. *Patient may not know of or have tried all currently available treatments.*
- Assess interference with life-style.

THERAPEUTIC INTERVENTIONS

▲ Administer antiinflammatory medication as prescribed. Give first dose of day as early in morning as possible, with small snack. *Antiinflammatory drugs should not be given on an empty stomach (can be very irritating to stomach lining and lead to ulcer disease).*
▲ Use nonnarcotic analgesic as necessary. *Narcotic analgesia appears to work better on mechanical than on inflammatory types of pain. Narcotics can be habit-forming.*
- Encourage patient to assume anatomically correct position of joint. Do not use knee gatch or pillow to prop knees; use small flat pillow under head.
- Encourage use of ambulation aid(s) when pain is related to weight bearing.
- Apply bed cradle *to keep pressure of bed covers off inflamed lower extremities.*
▲ Consult occupational therapist for proper splinting of affected joints.
▲ Encourage patient to wear splints as ordered. *Provides rest to inflamed joint.*
- Encourage use of alternative methods of pain control, such as relaxation, guided imagery, or distraction.
- See also Pain, p. 49.

Joint Stiffness

RELATED FACTOR

Inflammation

DEFINING CHARACTERISTICS

Verbalized complaint of joint stiffness

EXPECTED OUTCOMES

Patient verbalizes reduction in stiffness.
Patient demonstrates ability to perform required ADLs.

ONGOING ASSESSMENT

- Solicit description of stiffness:
  Location. generalized or localized
  Timing: morning, night, all day
  Length of stiffness. Ask patient, "How long do you take to loosen up after you get out of bed?" Record in hours or fraction of hour.
  Relationship to activities
  Aggravating/alleviating factors
- Assess interference with life-style. *Usually lupus does not result in deformity as in rheumatoid arthritis.*

THERAPEUTIC INTERVENTIONS

- Encourage patient to take 15-min warm shower/bath on rising. *Warmth reduces stiffness, relieves pain. Water should be warm. Excessive heat may promote skin breakdown.*
- Encourage patient to perform ROM exercises after shower/bath, two repetitions per joint.
- Allow sufficient time for all activities.
- Avoid scheduling tests or treatments when stiffness is present.
▲ Administer antiinflammatory medication as prescribed. First dose of day should be as early in morning as possible, with small snack. Ask about normal home medication schedule and try to continue it. *The sooner patient takes medication, the sooner stiffness will abate.* Many patients prefer to take medications as early as 6 or 7 A.M. *Antiinflammatory drugs should not be given on empty stomach.*
- Remind patient to avoid prolonged periods of inactivity.

Continued.

Systemic lupus erythematosus—cont'd

NURSING DIAGNOSES	EXPECTED OUTCOMES AND NURSING INTERVENTIONS / *RATIONALE* (■ = INDEPENDENT; ▲ = COLLABORATIVE)

High Risk for Injury

RISK FACTORS

Altered renal function
Inflammation and sclerosis of glomeruli
Side effects of connective tissue disease

EXPECTED OUTCOMES

The patient will maintain optimal renal function within limits of disease as evidenced by normal BUN and creatinine levels, and minimal edema.

ONGOING ASSESSMENT

- Assess urinary output at least q2hr.
- Monitor fluid intake.
- Obtain nutritional history.
▲ Monitor electrolyte levels for elevated BUN and creatinine levels.
- Monitor urine specific gravity.
- Assess for edema, especially of lower extremities.
- Assess for elevated blood pressure.
- Assess for LOC changes.
- Weigh daily.

THERAPEUTIC INTERVENTIONS

▲ Obtain dietary consultation as needed.
▲ Administer immunosuppressant medications as ordered: methylprednisolone, cyclophosphamide.
- Instruct patient of potential immunosuppressant medication side effects. See also Potential for injury: side effects related to prednisone and immunosuppressant medication, p. 362; Renal failure, acute, p. 436; Hypertension, p. 122; Cardiac output, decreased, p. 12.

High Risk for Injury

RISK FACTORS

Inflammation
Severe, active SLE (usually occurs early in disease course, often combined with increased disease activity in other organ systems)
CNS altered by organic psychosis, organic brain syndrome

EXPECTED OUTCOMES

The patient maintains optimal CNS function as evidenced by normal mentation and ability to perform normal daily activities.

ONGOING ASSESSMENT

- Assess for presence of headaches. *Headaches, often severe and throbbing, are usually accompanied by seizures or organic brain syndrome.*
- Assess for presence of seizure activity: *Seizures are most often grand mal.*
- Assess for presence of organic psychosis: impaired judgment, inappropriate speech, disorganized behavior, disorientation, decreased attention, hallucinations. *Organic psychosis may be caused by high-dose corticosteroids.*
- Assess for the presence of organic brain syndrome: impaired memory, disorientation, impaired judgment, increased or decreased psychomotor activity, loss of higher cortical functions (e.g., asphasia [language disorder], apraxis [motor disorder], agnosia [failure to recognize objects]), personality changes.

THERAPEUTIC INTERVENTIONS

For headaches:
- Provide quiet, restful environment during headaches.
▲ Administer analgesics.
▲ Give corticosteroids as prescribed. *These reduce the active inflammatory process of CNS lupus.*
For seizures:
- Maintain seizure precautions
- Provide quiet, safe environment during seizures.
▲ Administer neuroleptics, corticosteroids, and immunosuppressants as prescribed. *Underlying disease process must also be treated with steroids and immunosuppressants.*

NURSING DIAGNOSES	EXPECTED OUTCOMES AND NURSING INTERVENTIONS / *RATIONALE* (■ = INDEPENDENT; ▲ = COLLABORATIVE)

THERAPEUTIC INTERVENTIONS—cont'd

For organic psychosis or organic brain syndrome:
- Provide safe, structured, predictable environment when organic psychosis or organic brain syndrome is present:
    - Maintain consistent staff for daily care; one-to-one care may be necessary.
    - Decrease environmental stimuli. Keep patient in private room if necessary.
    - Remove potentially dangerous objects from room.
    - Orient patient to person, place, and time as necessary. Keep clock and calendar in room.
    - Provide clear, concise instructions.
    - Decrease ambiguity and confusion by offering limited choices.
- ▲ Administer antipsychotic, corticosteroid, and immunosuppressant drugs as prescribed. *Corticosteroids may also cause psychosis. It is difficult to differentiate CNS lupus from corticosteroid psychosis.*

Fatigue

RELATED FACTORS

Increased disease activity
Anemia of chronic disease

DEFINING CHARACTERISTICS

Lack of energy, exhaustion, listlessness
Excessive sleeping
Decreased attention span
Facial expressions: yawning, sadness
Decreased functional capacity

EXPECTED OUTCOMES

The patient verbalizes reduction in fatigue level.
The patient demonstrates use of energy conservation principles.

ONGOING ASSESSMENT

- Solicit patient's description of fatigue: timing (afternoon or all day), relationship to activities, aggravating and alleviating factors.
- Determine night sleep pattern.
- Determine whether fatigue is related to psychologic factors (stress, depression).

THERAPEUTIC INTERVENTIONS

- Provide periods of uninterrupted rest throughout day (30 min 3 to 4 times/day). *Patients often have limited energy supply.*
- Reinforce energy conservation principles:
    - Pacing activities (alternating activity with rest). *Patient often needs more energy than others to complete same tasks.*
    - Adequate rest periods (throughout day/night)
    - Organization of activities and environment
    - Proper use of assistive/adaptive devices

If fatigue is related to interrupted sleep:
- Encourage warm shower/bath immediately before bedtime. *Warm water relaxes muscles, facilitating total body relaxation, excessive heat may promote skin breakdown.*
- Encourage gentle ROM exercises (after shower/bath) *to maximize warm bath/shower benefits.*
- Encourage patient to sleep in anatomically correct position. Do not prop up affected joints. Change position frequently during night.
- Avoid stimulating foods (caffeine), activities before bedtime.
- Encourage use of progressive muscle relaxation techniques.
- ▲ Administer nighttime analgesic and/or long-acting antiinflammatory drug as ordered.

Continued.

NURSING DIAGNOSES	EXPECTED OUTCOMES AND NURSING INTERVENTIONS / *RATIONALE* (■ = INDEPENDENT; ▲ = COLLABORATIVE)

Knowledge Deficit

RELATED FACTORS:

New disease/procedures
Unfamiliarity with treatment regime
Lack of interest

DEFINING CHARACTERISTICS

Multiple questions
Lack of questions
Verbalized misconceptions
Verbalized lack of knowledge
Inaccurate follow-through on previous instructions

See also:
Impaired Gas Exchange, p. 27.
Self-Care Deficit, p. 53.
Altered Nutrition: Less than Body Requirements, p. 44.
Altered Nutrition: More than Body Requirements, p. 45.
Ineffective Individual Coping, p. 18.
Altered Sexuality Patterns, p. 58.
Anticipatory Grieving, p. 28.
Sleep Pattern Disturbance, p. 61.

EXPECTED OUTCOMES

Patient verbalizes increased awareness of disease and treatment.

ONGOING ASSESSMENT

▪ Assess knowledge of lupus and its treatment.

THERAPEUTIC INTERVENTIONS

▪ Schedule educational sessions when patient is most comfortable. *Pain will distract patient and may lead to inability to absorb new information.*
▪ Introduce/reinforce disease process information: unknown cause, chronicity of lupus, processes of inflammation and fibrosis, skin and other organ involvement, remissions and exacerbations, control versus cure.
▪ Introduce/reinforce information on drug therapy. Instruct patient on potential effects of prednisone/immunosuppressant medication. *Potential effects are related to long-term use or high dosage.*

    Prednisone: facial puffiness, buffalo hump, diabetes mellitus, osteoporosis, avascular necrosis, increased appetite, increased infection risk, glaucoma

    Immunosuppressants: increased infection risk *caused by bone marrow suppression,* nausea/vomiting, sterility, hemorrhagic cystitis, cancer

    Importance of wearing Medic Alert tag at all times stating use of prednisone/immunosuppressants

    Importance of not altering prednisone dose. *Steroids must be tapered slowly after high-dose or long-term use. Body produces the hormone cortisol in adrenal glands. After high-dose/long-term use of extraneous forms of steroids, body no longer produces adequate cortisol level. Increased cortisol levels are needed in times of stress. Without supplementation, steroid-dependent person will enter Addisonian crisis.*

By: Linda Ehrlich, RN, MSN
    Sue A. Connaughton, RN, MSN, Psy D Candidate

Total hip arthroplasty/replacement

(HIP HEMIARTHROPLASTY; TOTAL HIP SURFACE
ARTHROPLASTY; CUP/MOLD ARTHROPLASTY)

Total hip arthroplasty (THA)/replacement: *a total joint replacement by surgical removal of the diseased hip joint, including the femoral neck and head, as well as the acetabulum. The femoral canal is reamed to accept a metal component placed into the femoral shaft, replacing the femoral head and neck. A polyethylene cup replaces the reamed acetabulum.*

Hip hemiarthroplasty *(e.g., Austin Moore, Bateman, bipolar, or Leinbach hemiarthroplasty): surgical removal of the femoral head and neck and replacement with metal component.*

Total hip surface arthroplasty: *reaming out of the acetabulum and implantation of an acetabular cup while the femoral head is only reamed down to accept a metal femoral head.*

Cup/mold arthroplasty: *the acetabulum and head of the femur are reamed down to an untraumatized surface, and an appropriate-sized metal cup is fitted over the head of the femur.*

NURSING DIAGNOSES	EXPECTED OUTCOMES AND NURSING INTERVENTIONS / *RATIONALE* (■ = INDEPENDENT; ▲ = COLLABORATIVE)

High Risk for Injury: Hip Dislocation

RISK FACTORS

Improper hip joint positioning

EXPECTED OUTCOMES

Patient maintains hip in anatomically correct position, as evidenced by normal hip contour, both legs the same length, legs/hip in abduction.

ONGOING ASSESSMENT

- Assess knowledge of proper position after total hip arthroplasty (THA). *Proper positioning is paramount in preventing dislocation. Improper movement increases the potential for injury.*
- Assess leg position in bed, in chair, and during ambulation.
- Assess transfer techniques during position changes.
- Assess for signs of dislocation after position changes and transfer: increased pain in affected hip joint, misalignment (position of legs in internal rotation or adduction), change in hip joint contour (dislocated hip may be palpated), change in length of affected extremity (leg may appear shortened).
- If possibility of dislocation is suspected, review radiographs.

THERAPEUTIC INTERVENTIONS

- Frequently instruct/reinforce hip positions: abduction of legs, flexion of hip <90 degrees, neutral or external rotation of affected leg. *Constant practice of precautions is essential to prevent dislocation of new hip joint.*
- Maintain abduction of legs and abduction device (in and out of bed). *Abduction device between patient's legs prevents adduction of legs.*
- ▲ Turn patient side to side in bed with abduction device between legs (may turn on to affected hip unless contraindicated by physician). *Prevents adduction.*
- Use raised toilet seat and high firm chair. *Prevents hip flexion >90 degrees.*

Pain

RELATED FACTORS

Bone and soft tissue trauma
caused by surgery
Intense physical therapy/
rehabilitation program
Restricted mobility

DEFINING CHARACTERISTICS

Complaint of pain
Facial grimaces, guarding behavior, crying
Withdrawal, restlessness, irritability
Altered vital signs

EXPECTED OUTCOMES

Patient verbalizes relief or reduction in pain.
Patient appears comfortable.

ONGOING ASSESSMENT

- Assess description of pain. *First step in alleviating pain is assessing location, severity, and degree of both physical and emotional pain.*
- Assess mental and physical ability to use patient-controlled analgesia (PCA) vs. IM/PO analgesics. *Successful use of PCA requires patient to have knowledge of its use and the manual dexterity to operate it.*
- Assess effectiveness of pain-relieving interventions.

Continued.

Total hip arthroplasty/replacement—cont'd

NURSING DIAGNOSES	EXPECTED OUTCOMES AND NURSING INTERVENTIONS / *RATIONALE* (■ = INDEPENDENT; ▲ = COLLABORATIVE)
	THERAPEUTIC INTERVENTIONS • Explain analgesic therapy, including medication and schedule. If patient is a PCA candidate, explain concept and routine. ▲ Administer analgesics as prescribed. Instruct patient to request analgesic before pain becomes severe. *Cycle of pain must be broken to be relieved. If pain is too severe before analgesics/therapy are instituted, relief takes longer.* • Encourage use of analgesics 30 to 45 min before therapy. *Unrelieved pain hinders rehabilitation progress.* • Change position (within hip precautions) q2hr. *Inability to move freely and independently causes pressure and pain on bony prominences.*
Impaired Physical Mobility **RELATED FACTORS** Surgical procedure Discomfort **DEFINING CHARACTERISTICS** Limited ability to ambulate or move in bed	**EXPECTED OUTCOMES** Patient maintains optimal mobility within limitations (sitting, transferring, ambulation). Patient adheres to prescribed mobility restrictions/guidelines. **ONGOING ASSESSMENT** • Assess fear/anxiety of transferring/ambulating. *Allaying anxiety/fear will allow patient to concentrate on correct techniques.* • Assess level of understanding of THA precautions. *Precautions must be maintained at all times to prevent dislocation.* **THERAPEUTIC INTERVENTIONS** • Encourage ROM in bed with all unaffected extremities. *Bedrest causes loss of muscle tone and pooling of venous blood.* • Encourage quadriceps, gluteal sets, and straight leg raise exercises *to increase muscle strength/tone.* • Encourage use of analgesic before position changes. *Decreased or controlled pain allows better performance during therapy.* ▲ Keep abduction pillow between legs while turning patient in bed *to prevent adduction, which can cause dislocation.* May turn onto operative side unless otherwise specified. • Use trapeze in bed *to assist in mobility.* ▲ Instruct patient on maintaining THA precautions during position changes *to prevent hip dislocation.* • Dangle patient at bedside several minutes before changing positions *to prevent orthostatic hypotension.* ▲ Reinforce physical therapist's instructions for exercises, ambulation techniques and devices. Maintain weight-bearing status on affected extremity as prescribed. *Consistent instructions from interdisciplinary team members promote safe, secure rehabilitation environment.*

NURSING DIAGNOSES	EXPECTED OUTCOMES AND NURSING INTERVENTIONS / *RATIONALE* (■ = INDEPENDENT; ▲ = COLLABORATIVE)
High Risk for Altered Tissue Perfusion to Lower Extremities (Neurovascular) **RISK FACTORS** Surgical procedure Immobility	**EXPECTED OUTCOMES** Patient maintains adequate tissue perfusion, as evidenced by warm extremities, good color; good capillary refill; absence of pain/numbness; bilaterally equal pulses. **ONGOING ASSESSMENT** • Assess and compare neurovascular status of both lower extremities preoperatively and postoperatively. *Assessment must include unaffected and affected extremity to monitor for change in neurovascular status.* • Assess lower extremities for signs of neurovascular compromise/damage: pain, coolness; pallor; cyanosis; decreased pulse; paresthesia; edema; sluggish/absent capillary refill noted in one or both lower extremities; foot drop. ▲ Check sequential compression device/TED stocking for extreme tightness *(produces tourniquet effect on extremity).* **THERAPEUTIC INTERVENTIONS** ▲ Notify physician immediately if signs of altered circulation are noted.
High Risk for Injury **RISK FACTORS** Surgery Immobility	**EXPECTED OUTCOMES** Patient is free of signs/symptoms of DVT/pulmonary embolus/fat embolism, as evidenced by negative Homan's sign, normal respiratory status, stable vital signs, normal ABGs. **ONGOING ASSESSMENT** • Assess for signs/symptoms of deep vein thrombosis (DVT): positive Homan's sign; swelling, tenderness, redness in calf; palpable cords; abnormal blood flow study findings (if prescribed). *Deep vein thrombosis is a* serious complication after joint replacement surgery. ▲ Assess for signs/symptoms of pulmonary embolus: abnormal ABGs, abnormal ventilation-perfusion scan result, tachypnea, DVT signs/symptoms, chest pain, dyspnea, tachycardia, hemoptysis, cyanosis, anxiety. • Assess for signs/symptoms of fat embolism: *pulmonary:* dyspnea, tachypnea, cyanosis; *cerebral:* headache, irritability, delirium, coma; *cardiac:* tachycardia, decreased blood pressure, petechial hemorrhage of upper chest, axillae, conjunctiva; fat globules in urine. *(fat embolism is usually seen the second day after surgery).* **THERAPEUTIC INTERVENTIONS** • Encourage leg exercises, including quad sets, gluteal sets, active ankle ROM. ▲ Encourage patient to be out of bed as soon as prescribed. Maintain THA precautions and weight-bearing status. • Encourage incentive spirometry q1hr while awake *to increase lung expansion and prevent atelectasis, hypoxemia, pneumonia.* ▲ Institute antiembolic devices as prescribed (sequential compression device or TED hose). *Antiembolic devices increase venous blood flow to heart and decrease risk of DVT, PE.*

Continued.

Musculoskeletal Care Plans

NURSING DIAGNOSES	EXPECTED OUTCOMES AND NURSING INTERVENTIONS / *RATIONALE* (■ = INDEPENDENT; ▲ = COLLABORATIVE)

**Knowledge Deficit:
Discharge**

RELATED FACTORS
New condition

DEFINING CHARACTERISTICS
Lack of/multitude of questions
Confusion about THA precautions

EXPECTED OUTCOMES
Patient verbalizes understanding of discharge instructions.

ONGOING ASSESSMENT
- Assess understanding of discharge instructions.
- Assess home support systems.

THERAPEUTIC INTERVENTIONS
Review THA precautions:
▲ Maintain abduction with ABD device.
- Always keep legs externally or neutrally rotated.
- Avoid hip flexion >90 degrees.
- Avoid bending. Kneel or use a reacher. *Bending causes hip flexion >90 degrees.*
- Lie flat in bed at least 1-2 hr/day *to prevent hip flexion contracture.*
- Do not cross legs. *Causes adduction, which can lead to dislocation.*
▲ Ambulate (weight bearing as instructed) with assistive device (walker/crutches). *Protected ambulation promotes healing of the affected hip.*
- Do not shower/tub bathe until all Steri-Strips on incision are off (usually 4-5 days after application). *Steri-Strips ensure approximation of the wound, to allow for primary closure of incision.*
▲ Resume sexual activity as long as THA precautions are observed (best positions are supine and side-lying). *Hip precautions must be incorporated into all aspects of normal activities.*
- Instruct to use raised toilet seat. *Prevents hip flexion >90 degrees.*
▲ Use ABD device at home, especially at night, until next physician appointment. *During sleep there is an increased risk of improper positioning that can cause dislocation.*
- Build up low chairs with firm pillow *to prevent hip flexion >90 degrees.*
▲ Continue exercise program of physical therapist. Home physical therapist will visit 3 times/wk for 1 mon to continue rehabilitation. *Successful rehabilitation requires 6-8 wk of extensive physical therapy.*
- Call physician immediately if sharp pain, "popping" of affected extremity, hip feeling "out of socket." *This can be a sign of "dislocation" that requires emergency medical attention.*
- Inform physicians/dentists of prosthetic devices when undergoing procedures. *Bacteremia can cause infection and failure of prosthesis.*
- Notify physician of signs of infection or other complications.
- Assist patient to understand the limitations (if any) of the surgery. *Full resumption of all desired activities may not be realistic.*
- Ask social worker to arrange home physical therapy and homemaker (if needed).

See also:
High Risk for Infection, p. 40.
Impaired Skin Integrity, p. 59.
Self-care Deficit, p. 53.
Activity Intolerance, p. 2.
Altered Health Maintenance, p. 31.
Impaired Individual Coping, p. 18.
Constipation, p. 16.
Ineffective Airway Clearance, p. 3.

By: Hope Tolitano, RN
    Catherine Dunning, RN, BSN
    Marilyn Magafas, RN, MBA

Total knee arthroplasty/replacement

(KNEE HEMIARTHROPLASTY)

Replacement of deteriorated femoral, tibial, and patellar articular surfaces with prosthetic metal and plastic components.

NURSING DIAGNOSES	EXPECTED OUTCOMES AND NURSING INTERVENTIONS / *RATIONALE* (■ = INDEPENDENT; ▲ = COLLABORATIVE)

Impaired Physical Mobility

RELATED FACTORS

Movement restricted by postoperative protocol
Surgical procedure

DEFINING CHARACTERISTICS

Decreased muscle strength, control, and coordination
Reluctance to move

EXPECTED OUTCOMES

Patient achieves independence in ambulation and ADLs.

ONGOING ASSESSMENT

- Assess ROM.
- Assess ability to carry out ADLs.
- Assess knowledge of early ambulation and physical therapy.
- Assess experience with use of crutches or walker.

THERAPEUTIC INTERVENTIONS

▲ If prescribed, apply continuous passive motion machine (CPM) to affected leg at prescribed degrees. *CPM facilitates joint ROM, promotes wound healing, and prevents formation of adhesions to operative knee.*

▲ Maintain proper position in CPM: maintain leg in neutral position; adjust CPM so knee joint corresponds to bend in CPM machine; adjust foot plate so foot is in neutral position in boot; instruct patient to keep opposite leg away from machine *to prevent injury by moving parts.*

■ Assist and encourage to perform quad sets, gluteal sets, and ROM to both legs *to increase muscle strength/tone.*

▲ Reinforce ROM (extension/flexion) and muscle strengthening exercises taught by physical therapist *to optimize return of full knee extension.*

■ Elevate leg on pillow when not in CPM. Place pillow under calf *to promote full leg extension.*

▲ Encourage and assist patient to sit in chair on first and second postoperative days. Instruct to sit with legs dependent several times a day *to promote flexion of knee.*

▲ Initiate weight bearing as prescribed. Weight-bearing status:
For cemented prosthesis: as tolerated.
For partially or fully uncemented prothesis: toe-touch to partial weight bearing.
Protective weight bearing is required for 6 wk with uncemented prosthesis to allow bony ingrowth into prosthesis

▲ Encourage ambulation with walker or canes after initiated by PT.

■ Encourage use of assistive devices provided by OT to carry out ADLs (reacher, sock aid, long-handled sponge, long-handled shoehorn).

▲ At discharge, instruct in need to continue progressive exercises *to improve ROM and strengthen muscles.*

High Risk for Altered Peripheral Tissue Perfusion

RISK FACTORS

Surgical procedure
Restricted movement
Swelling

EXPECTED OUTCOMES

Patient maintains optimal perfusion to extremities, as evidenced by warm legs, strong bilateral pulses, good capillary refill, absence of pain.

ONGOING ASSESSMENT

- Use preoperative neurovascular assessment to establish baseline status for postoperative comparison of lower extremities.
- Assess lower extremities; compare temperature, color, sensation, movement, pulses, edema, and capillary refill. *Coldness, pallor, pain, decreased pulse, edema, sluggish or absent capillary refill are signs of compromised circulation.*
- Remove antiembolic devices every shift *to inspect skin.*
- Assess for increased pain to affected extremity.

THERAPEUTIC INTERVENTIONS

- Maintain functional alignment.
- Instruct to perform ROM exercises *to increase venous return and decrease probability of DVT.*
▲ Apply TED hose and/or sequential compression devices as prescribed.
▲ If signs of altered tissue perfusion are noted, notify physician immediately.

Continued.

Musculoskeletal Care Plans

NURSING DIAGNOSES	EXPECTED OUTCOMES AND NURSING INTERVENTIONS / *RATIONALE* (■ = INDEPENDENT; ▲ = COLLABORATIVE)
Pain **RELATED FACTORS** Surgical procedure Rehabilitation program **DEFINING CHARACTERISTICS** Verbal report of pain Facial grimaces Moaning, crying Protective, guarding behavior Restlessness Withdrawal Irritability	**EXPECTED OUTCOMES** Patient verbalizes relief or reduction in pain. Patient appears comfortable. **ONGOING ASSESSMENT** · Obtain description of pain. · Assess behavior and facial expressions. · Assess pain relief measure effectiveness. **THERAPEUTIC INTERVENTIONS** ▲ Give analgesics as prescribed; evaluate effectiveness. · Alter patient's position (turning, adjusting pillows, etc.). ▲ Encourage use of analgesic 30 min before PT *to facilitate patient's participation in exercise session.* · Encourage appropriate rest periods. · Eliminate additional stressors; encourage diversional activity. · Instruct patient to report pain *so relief measures can be started.* ▲ Apply ice to knee 20-30 min, q2hr and after exercising *to decrease edema.* ▲ Consider use of PCA as appropriate.
Knowledge Deficit: Home Care **RELATED FACTOR** New condition **DEFINING CHARACTERISTICS** Lack of/multitude of questions Confusion about precautions	**EXPECTED OUTCOMES** Patient verbalizes understanding of discharge instructions. **ONGOING ASSESSMENT** · Assess understanding of discharge instructions. · Assess home support systems. **THERAPEUTIC INTERVENTIONS** ▲ Review position/activity restrictions/precautions as described in "Impaired Physical Mobility" above. ▲ Reinforce the need to continue prescribed ROM exercises. *May require home physical therapy.* · Demonstrate/reinforce proper use of assistive devices. · Instruct in signs/symptoms of infection or other leg complication to report immediately. ▲ Refer to social service/OT/PT as indicated *to provide adequate discharge planning.* · Reinforce need for follow-up appointments. · Emphasize importance of removing environmental hazards (throw rugs, low tables, pets, electrical cords, toys, etc.) *to prevent falls/injury.*

See also:
Self-Care Deficit, p. 53.
High Risk for Infection, p. 40.
Impaired Skin Integrity, p. 59.
Ineffective Breathing Pattern, p. 10.
Constipation, p. 16.

By: Sandra Eungard, RN, MS

Total shoulder arthroplasty/replacement

(SHOULDER HEMIARTHROPLASTY)

Total shoulder arthroplasty *is the surgical removal of the head of the humerus and the glenoid cavity of the scapula, with replacement by an articulating prosthesis.*
Shoulder hemiarthroplasty *is the surgical removal of the head of the humerus with replacement by a prosthesis.*

NURSING DIAGNOSES	EXPECTED OUTCOMES AND NURSING INTERVENTIONS / *RATIONALE* (■ = INDEPENDENT; ▲ = COLLABORATIVE)

Impaired Physical Mobility

RELATED FACTOR

Pain
Spasm

DEFINING CHARACTERISTICS

Limited ROM of affected extremity

EXPECTED OUTCOMES

Patient maintains optimal ROM.

ONGOING ASSESSMENT

- Assess preoperative full ROM of affected extremity.
- Assess postoperative ROM; document improvement/failure to progress.
- Assess performance of ADL.

THERAPEUTIC INTERVENTIONS

▲ Maintain arm in shoulder immobilizer 1-2 days or as prescribed.
▲ After immobilizer is removed (with physician's prescription), apply sling.
▲ Begin ROM exercises (extension, abduction, flexion) of hand, elbow, and wrist in conjunction with PT personnel. *Passive ROM helps prevent development of adhesions yet does not strain tissues. Achieving increasing mobility is prime goal of surgery, along with elimination of pain.*
- Reinforce/assist with shoulder exercises after initiation/demonstration in PT department.
▲ Encourage and assist patient in performing basic ADL: self-feeding, brushing teeth, combing hair.

High Risk for Injury: Altered Neurovascular Status

RISK FACTORS

Surgical procedures
Edema with compression

EXPECTED OUTCOMES

Patient maintains optimal neurovascular status as evidenced by warm skin; bilateral pulses; absence of edema, numbness, pain; good capillary refill.

ONGOING ASSESSMENT

- Assess color, peripheral pulses, sensation (including numbness and paresthesia), and motor function postoperatively; compare to preoperative status.
- Monitor and document neurovascular assessment (*allows early detection of compromised perfusion of arm/nerve compressions within arm*).
- Measure extremity *to detect increased circumference or presence of edema.*
▲ Notify physician if circumference increase is noted.

THERAPEUTIC INTERVENTIONS

▲ Report change in neurovascular status to physician immediately. *Important findings include: cool, cyanotic, or pulseless extremity; altered sensation or movement of extremity; sluggish/absent capillary refill; edema.*

Pain

RELATED FACTORS

Surgical procedure
Physical therapy

DEFINING CHARACTERISTICS

Patient's/significant others' complaint of pain or discomfort
Withdrawal, guarding behavior, moaning, grimacing, anxiety, rigidity, tachycardia, diaphoresis

EXPECTED OUTCOMES

Patient verbalizes relief or reduction of pain.
Patient appears comfortable.

ONGOING ASSESSMENT

- Assess for complaints of pain or discomfort.
- Assess effectiveness of intervention(s) in relieving pain/discomfort.

THERAPEUTIC INTERVENTIONS

▲ Give analgesics as prescribed and as needed. Encourage patient to take medications before pain becomes severe or, if patient has PCA device, operate according to policy/procedures and physician prescription. *Pain management is very important to prevent vicious cycle of pain-tension-anxiety that breeds more pain and, equally important, prevents participation in PT and self-care activities. Many patients are unprepared for the level of immediate postoperative pain experienced.*
▲ Offer analgesia 30-45 min before PT.
- Try other measures to relieve pain/discomfort:
  Heat or ice pack to shoulder after exercise as needed (with physician's prescription).
  Reposition patient q1-2hr. Avoid positioning on operative side.
  Elevate HOB to 45-60 degrees or as tolerated.
  Place pillow under affected elbow.

Continued.

NURSING DIAGNOSES	EXPECTED OUTCOMES AND NURSING INTERVENTIONS / *RATIONALE* (■ = INDEPENDENT; ▲ = COLLABORATIVE)

Knowledge Deficit

RELATED FACTORS

Unfamiliarity with postdis-
charge activity and self-care

DEFINING CHARACTERISTICS

Multiple questions
Lack of questions
Confusion about instructions

EXPECTED OUTCOMES

Patient verbalizes activities that may cause dislocation of the affected extremity or disruption of the surgical repair and demonstrates ability to perform usual ADLs.

ONGOING ASSESSMENT

- Ask patient to verbalize questions related to activities/limitations after shoulder arthroplasty *so better able to adapt to stress of gradual progress (as long as 1 yr before full power, strength, and function are restored).*
- Assess ability to perform usual ADLs (dressing, transferring, positioning, eating, bathing).

THERAPEUTIC INTERVENTIONS

Explain activity restrictions:
- Perform only passive ROM exercises for first 25 days. Thereafter, active exercises may be started.
- Avoid activities such as heavy lifting, pulling, pushing.
- Avoid activities that involve exaggerated external rotation and abduction (e.g., push-ups, golf, volleyball).
- Avoid activities in which affected extremity is required to support body weight, or if collisions or falls are likely (contact sports and skiing).

Follow-up care:
- Instruct to inform physician of infection signs (increased edema, tenderness, warmth along incision line, temperature above 38.3° C (101° F), increased pain, pus, bulging, dehiscence. *Early detection may prevent spread to prosthesis and surrounding structures and prevent osteomyelitis (all are serious and difficult to treat).*
- Reinforce need for follow-up appointments.
- ▲ Refer to social service/PT/OT as indicated *to provide adequate discharge planning.*

See also:

Self-care Deficit, p. 53.
High Risk for Infection, p. 40.
Impaired Skin Integrity, p. 59.
Ineffective Breathing Pattern, p. 10.

By: Cynthia Gordon, RN, BSN
 Marilyn Magafas, RN, MBA

Traction

Traction is the application of a pulling force to an area of the body or to an extremity. Skeletal traction is applied directly through the bone via Steinmann pins or Kirschner wires. It is commonly used for cervical spine, femur, tibia, and humerus fractures. Traction can also be applied through the use of balanced suspension or skin traction. Skin traction is often used to relieve muscle spasms and pain.

NURSING DIAGNOSES	EXPECTED OUTCOMES AND NURSING INTERVENTIONS / *RATIONALE* (■ = INDEPENDENT; ▲ = COLLABORATIVE)

Knowledge Deficit

RELATED FACTORS

Lack of experience with traction

DEFINING CHARACTERISTICS

High anxiety level
Multitude of questions
Lack of questions
Patient/family verbalized lack of knowledge of traction

EXPECTED OUTCOMES

Patient verbalizes understanding of purpose and application of traction.

ONGOING ASSESSMENT

- Assess knowledge of traction.

THERAPEUTIC INTERVENTIONS

- Explain purpose of traction as related to injury/illness and healing process. *Providing information helps alleviate anxiety, enables patient to absorb and retain further information and instructions.*
- Explain traction apparatus.
- Teach prevention of possible injury- and traction-related complications (e.g., pain, malalignment).
- For skeletal traction, explain pin insertion procedure, pin and traction removal procedure, and application of cast/brace as appropriate.

Pain

RELATED FACTORS

Fractured limb
Skeletal pins (pain at insertion site)
Muscle spasms

DEFINING CHARACTERISTICS

Verbalized pain
Irritability
Restlessness
Crying/moaning
Facial grimaces
Altered vital signs: increased pulse, increased blood pressure, increased respirations
Withdrawal
Unwilling to change position
Inability to sleep

EXPECTED OUTCOMES

Patient expresses relief of or reduction in pain.
Patient appears comfortable.

ONGOING ASSESSMENT

- Assess for signs and symptoms of pain.
- Assess types of activity that increase pain.
- Assess past experience with pain and pain relief measures.
- Assess effectiveness of present pain relief measures.
- Assess for correct positioning of traction and alignment of affected extremity. *Incorrect positioning and malalignment can be sources of pain.*

THERAPEUTIC INTERVENTIONS

- ▲ Give analgesics as prescribed and evaluate effectiveness *to determine whether comfort has been provided or another relief approach is needed. Dosage, drug, or route may also need to be revised.*
- Eliminate additional stressors or sources of pain/discomfort by providing comfort measures: relaxation techniques; diversionary activity (books, games, television, sewing, radio) heat or cold application; position changes; touch (backrubs). *Directing attention away from pain or to other body areas decreases perception of pain.*
- Explain that traction decreases muscle spasms and will gradually help lessen pain.

Impaired Physical Mobility

RELATED FACTORS

Fractured limb
Imposed restrictions related to traction and injury

DEFINING CHARACTERISTICS

Reluctance to move
Inability to move
Limited ROM and muscle strength

EXPECTED OUTCOMES

Patient maintains optimal mobility within restrictions.
Patient maintains muscle strength.

ONGOING ASSESSMENT

- Assess ability to perform ADLs.
- Assess present and preinjury level of mobility.
- Assess ROM of unaffected extremity.
- Assess muscle strength.

THERAPEUTIC INTERVENTIONS

- Encourage independence within limitation. *Patient may have full use of other extremities.*
- Instruct in use of assistive devices (overhead trapeze and side rails).
- Teach isometric exercises to affected extremity as appropriate.

Continued.

NURSING DIAGNOSES	EXPECTED OUTCOMES AND NURSING INTERVENTIONS / *RATIONALE* (■ = INDEPENDENT; ▲ = COLLABORATIVE)
	THERAPEUTIC INTERVENTIONS—cont'd • Teach strengthening exercises to affected extremities as appropriate. *Quad sets, ankle pumps, straight leg raises, gluteal sets, push ups, heel slides, and abductor sets help prevent development of stiff joints and muscle atrophy.* • Assist with repositioning. Maintain body in functional alignment. ▲ Initiate consultation for exercise program. • Instruct on complications of immobility and measures to decrease occurrence.
High Risk for Infection: Pin Sites/Open Wounds **RISK FACTORS** Interrupted first line of defense Interruption of bone structure	**EXPECTED OUTCOMES** Patient manifests no signs of infection, as evidenced by afebrile state, normal WBC, no redness/drainage at pin site/wound. **ONGOING ASSESSMENT** • Assess pin sites/open wounds for signs of infection. • Assess for skin tension at pin sites. • Assess vital signs (especially temperature). ▲ Monitor lab values (WBC). **THERAPEUTIC INTERVENTIONS** ▲ Perform pin care q8hr as prescribed. • Use aseptic technique to perform pin care, change dressings. ▲ Administer antibiotics as prescribed. • Instruct on purpose of pin care and infection signs/symptoms. • Encourage foods high in protein and vitamin C. *Vitamin C facilitates wound healing.*
High Risk for Impaired Skin Integrity **RISK FACTORS** Immobility Prolonged bed rest Contact with traction apparatus Countertraction (patient's body weight)	**EXPECTED OUTCOMES** Patient maintains intact skin. **ONGOING ASSESSMENT** • Examine skin for preexisting breakdown or potential problem areas. • Assess for preexisting risk factors for skin breakdown. *Factors such as physical health, increasing age, altered mental state, and immobility increase potential for breakdown.* • Inspect skin at least q8hr (especially of the affected extremity maintained in traction). **THERAPEUTIC INTERVENTIONS** • Clean, dry, and moisturize skin daily. Remove traction boot if possible. • Massage bony prominences. (Never massage reddened areas). • Maintain correct padding for affected extremity in traction. *Pressure areas and skin irritation can develop under or at edge of traction device and/or other equipment.* • Keep bed linen wrinkle free and dry. • Apply prophylactic pressure-relieving mattress to bed if needed. • Encourage adequate hydration and teach importance of balanced diet. • For actual skin breakdown, see also Impaired skin integrity, p. 59.
High Risk for Injury **RISK FACTORS** Improper positioning of traction Malalignment of bone ends Pin migration Edema with neurovascular compromise Compartment syndrome	**EXPECTED OUTCOMES** Patient is free of complications, as evidenced by proper body alignment, intact pins, optimal neurovascular status. **ONGOING ASSESSMENT** *Traction device:* • Assess traction apparatus every shift: weight, knots, ropes. • Assess patient's position in traction. • Assess that ropes are not frayed or stretched. • Assess that spreader bars, foot plate, or splints do not touch foot of bed. • Assess that bed linens do not interfere with traction. • Assess whole body alignment. *Weight of traction is often enough to pull body out of alignment.*

ONGOING ASSESSMENT—cont'd

Pin sites:
- Assess pin sites every shift for migration.
- Assess skin around pin for tears.
- Assess for pain at pin sites.

Tissue Perfusion/Compartment Syndrome:
- Assess affected extremity for signs/symptoms of altered perfusion or compartment syndrome. *Compartment syndrome results from severe tissue swelling that decreases blood flow, causes ischemia, and may cause permanent motor/sensory damage.*
- Assess for pain upon passive stretch of involved muscles, progressive pain disproportionate to expectations, pallor or cyanosis distal to injury site, edema of limb distal to injury, decreased active and passive muscle movement to injury site, numbness/tingling, tightness of compartment.
- Assess for positive Homan's sign.
- Compare affected extremity to unaffected and to previous assessments.
- Perform assessments of muscular strength with neurovascular checks.

THERAPEUTIC INTERVENTIONS

Traction:
- ▲ Maintain affected extremity in functional traction.
- Tighten all traction equipment; secure all knots with tape.
- Keep weights hanging freely. *Deviations alter amount of traction applied, as well as therapeutic effect.*
- ▲ Maintain continuous traction if prescribed.
- Maintain rope in center of pulley.
- Maintain adequate countertraction. (Avoid elevating head of bed >30 degrees except during meals.) *Countertraction is necessary for effective traction.*
- Anchor upper body to the bed as needed *to prevent sliding toward traction.*
- ▲ Provide foot plate or wrist splint *to maintain proper position of affected extremity.*

Pin sites:
- Report signs of pin migration to physician.
- Cover pin with cork or adhesive tape *to protect from accidental injuries.*

Tissue Perfusion/Compartment Syndrome:
- Instruct, encourage exercises for affected and unaffected extremities as allowed.
- ▲ Apply antiembolic stockings or sequential compression devices as prescribed; remove regularly for skin inspection.
- Report neurovascular compromise to physician.
- Inform patient/family of complications/warning signs of impaired circulation, methods to prevent complications.

See also:
High Risk for Constipation,
  p. 16.
High Risk for Ineffective
  Breathing Patterns, p. 10.
High Risk for Altered Urinary
  Elimination, p. 74.
Impaired Individual Coping,
  p. 18.
Diversional Activity Deficit,
  p. 21.

By: Catherine Dunning, RN, BSN
   Michele Knoll Puzas, RNC, MHPE

Hematolymphatic and Oncologic Care Plans

Acquired immunodeficiency syndrome (AIDS)

(HUMAN IMMUNODEFICIENCY VIRUS [HIV]; OPPORTUNISTIC INFECTIONS)

Human immunodeficiency virus (HIV), either alone or in combination with other viral or idiopathic cofactors, causes acquired immunodeficiency syndrome (AIDS). The virus is spread in three ways: across the placenta, during sexual activity (heterosexual and homosexual), and by sharing of intravenous drug equipment. Early in the epidemic, blood products spread the virus, but measures to screen donors greatly improved the safety of blood products. Most of the early victims of the syndrome were gay men; however, in many cities today, infected IV drug users, their sexual partners, and their children outnumber infected gay men. Between 4 and 24 weeks after infection, an antibody to HIV appears in the adult patient's blood. Between 1 and 30 years later (8 years on average), the adult patient's immune system weakens enough to allow an opportunistic infection to develop. Patients present at various stages of the disease. Treatment regimens are changing rapidly.

NURSING DIAGNOSES	EXPECTED OUTCOMES AND NURSING INTERVENTIONS / *RATIONALE* (■ = INDEPENDENT; ▲ = COLLABORATIVE)

Knowledge Deficit: Disease and Transmission

RELATED FACTORS
New condition
Fear of AIDS

DEFINING CHARACTERISTICS
Multiple questions
Lack of questions
Confusion about disease, complications

EXPECTED OUTCOMES
Patient verbalizes understanding of disease process, transmission, complications, and treatment modalities.

ONGOING ASSESSMENT
- Assess patient's knowledge of disease process, routes of transmission, complications, and treatment modalities.
- Determine patient/significant other's concerns about AIDS.
- Determine sexual orientation; number, kinds of sexual partners; recent, usual sexual activities.
- Elicit patient's feelings about changed sexual behavior.

THERAPEUTIC INTERVENTIONS
- Instruct patient in dose, schedule, and side effects of antiviral, fungalstatic, and prophylactic medication.
- Instruct patient about schedule of outpatient appointments and treatments.
- Instruct patient in signs/symptoms of disease, opportunistic infections, and neoplasms and the person to whom information should be reported.
- Instruct patient in routes of HIV transmission.
- Instruct patient in methods of preventing HIV transmission:
  Safe sex: kissing, touching, mutual masturbation
  Probably safe: vaginal or anal intercourse with latex condom and spermicidal lubricant. *Nonoxyl-9 spermicide inactivates HIV in vitro; efficacy and side effects in vivo are untested. Properly used, latex condom reduces HIV transmission risk for both partners.*
  Unsafe: vaginal or anal intercourse without condom; sexual activities that cause bleeding.
  Uncertain: oral intercourse between man and woman, two men, two women. *Although early studies indicated less risk during oral intercourse than vaginal or anal without condom, risk difficult to measure and unknown.*
- Explore ways to express physical intimacy that do not lead to infection.
- Explore patient's sexual partner's perception of personal risk of HIV infection.
- Role play to practice new behaviors in situations that may lead to transmission (e.g., saying no or negotiating condom use).
- Explore possible benefits/drawbacks of sexual or needle-sharing partner's being tested for HIV. *Benefits include initiation of antiviral therapy if CD4 counts are low. Drawbacks include possible discrimination and emotional depression.*
- Instruct patient/partners to prevent pregnancy. Instruct in birth control methods, including condom use. *Approximately 25%-50% of infants of HIV-infected mothers are infected.*
- Encourage use of clean IV equipment with recreational drugs. *HIV is quickly killed by 10% hypochlorite solution. Flush syringe and needles with household bleach diluted ninefold with water; rinse with tap water. Refer to drug rehabilitation program as appropriate.*
- Explain importance of:
  Refraining from donating blood, semen, or organs.

Continued.

NURSING DIAGNOSES	EXPECTED OUTCOMES AND NURSING INTERVENTIONS / *RATIONALE* (■ = INDEPENDENT; ▲ = COLLABORATIVE)

THERAPEUTIC INTERVENTIONS—cont'd

Not sharing razors, toothbrushes.

Cleaning blood or excreta containing blood with 10% hypochlorite solution. *Not necessary to use bleach to wash patient's dishes, clothes, or personal items.*

■ Instruct patient to avoid exposure to infectious diseases:

Avoid contact with people who have infectious diseases.

Avoid sexual practices that lead to sexually transmitted diseases (STDs). *Used properly, condoms can help prevent STD spread during vaginal or anal intercourse. Immunocompromised people are especially vulnerable to viral infections (e.g., herpes or genital warts). Syphilis is more difficult to diagnose and treat in HIV-infected persons and progresses more rapidly. Normally nonpathogenic intestinal flora may cause disease in HIV-infected persons; therefore, they should refrain from anal-oral sexual activities.*

Avoid changing cat's litter box. *Toxoplasmosis gondii may be transmitted from stool of infected cat.*

Avoid raw vegetables, fish, milk, and meat (*harbor bacteria and protozoa that may cause infection in immunocompromized person*).

■ Instruct patient to observe for signs of lactose intolerance; if present, change diet.

Infection

RELATED FACTOR

HIV infection

DEFINING CHARACTERISTICS

Decreased number of CD4 cells
Altered CD4 cell function
Reversed CD4/CD8 ratio
Altered cellular immune response
Altered humoral immune response
Decreased response to antigens in skin testing
Positive HIV antibody with confirmatory Westin blot
Positive P-24 antigen
Increased B-2 microglobulin

EXPECTED OUTCOMES

Patient does not experience opportunistic infections.
The number of CD4 cells stabilizes or declines more gradually.
The number of B-2 microglobulins decreases.
P-24 antigen becomes negative.

ONGOING ASSESSMENT:

■ Assess for presence of Defining Characteristics.

THERAPEUTIC INTERVENTIONS

▲ Administer antiretrovirals as ordered. *Antiretrovirals interfere with one of the HIV enzymes (reverse transcriptase) required for replication.*

▲ Administer Zidovudine (also called AZT or ZDV) as ordered. *Usually prescribed for asymptomatic patients with fewer than 500 CD4 cells and taken as long as tolerated. May be combined with other antiretrovirals.* Advise patient to take with food *to mitigate upset stomach and nausea. May also cause headaches, depression, insomnia, fatigue, or muscle inflammation. Minor side effects are worse during the first few months of therapy.* Monitor CBC for neutropenia and especially anemia. *Some patients require blood transfusions to correct anemia.*

▲ Administer dideoxyinosine (also called Videx or ddI) as ordered. *Usually prescribed if patient is intolerant to ZDV or in combination with ZDV for more advanced HIV disease (fewer than 300 CD4 cells.)* Advise patient to take on an empty stomach *to increase absorption. May cause diarrhea, peripheral neuropathy, or pancreatitis (pancreatitis is more likely with a history of alcohol abuse, or while the patient is receiving IV pentamidine or IV ganciclovir). Decreases the absorption of dapsone, ketoconaole, or quinolones and tetracyclines if given simultaneously.* Advise patient to abstain from drinking alcohol. Monitor for signs of peripheral neuropathy, such as pain, tingling, or weakness in hands or feet. Monitor for signs of pancreatitis, such as abdominal pain, nausea, vomitting, and increased serum amylase level.

▲ Administer dideoxycytidine (also known as HIVID or ddC) as ordered. *Usually prescribed in combination with ZDV for more advanced HIV disease (fewer than 300 CD4 cells). May cause neutropenia, pancreatitis, or peripheral neuropathy.* Monitor CBC. Monitor for signs of peripheral neuropathy, such as pain, tingling, or weakness in hands or feet. Monitor for signs of pancreatitis, such as abdominal pain, nausea, vomiting, and increased serum amylase level.

▲ Administer therapeutic vaccines as ordered. *Therapeutic vaccines are started while the patient still has a high number of CD4 cells. They stimulate the production of antibodies that keep HIV in check.*

▲ Follow local regulations for obtaining a separate consent to be tested for HIV and for reporting results to the health department.

NURSING DIAGNOSES	EXPECTED OUTCOMES AND NURSING INTERVENTIONS / *RATIONALE* (■ = INDEPENDENT; ▲ = COLLABORATIVE)

Impaired Individual Coping

RELATED FACTORS

Change in or loss of body part
Diagnosis of serious illness
Recent change in health status
Unsatisfactory support system
Inadequate psychological re-
  sources (poor self-esteem;
  lack of motivation)
Personal vulnerability
Inadequate coping method
Situational crises
Maturational crises

DEFINING CHARACTERISTICS

Verbalization of inability to
  cope
Inability to make decisions
Inability to ask for help
Destructive behavior toward
  self
Inappropriate use of defense
  mechanisms
Physical symptoms such as:
  Overeating; lack of appetite
  Overuse of tranquilizers
  Excessive smoking/drinking
  Chronic fatigue
  Headaches
  Irritable bowel
Chronic depression
Emotional tension
High illness rate
Insomnia
General irritability

EXPECTED OUTCOMES

Patient identifies adaptive/maladaptive behaviors.
Patient identifies and uses appropriate resources.
Patient verbalizes ability to cope.

ONGOING ASSESSMENT

- Determine patient's previous coping patterns. *Accurate appraisal can facilitate development of appropriate coping strategies.*
- Assess patient's perception of current situation. *Patients under stress may fail to recognize the "normalness" of having difficulty coping with a stressful situation. They may have unrealistic expectations of themselves without being aware of it.*
- Assess patient's support network.
- Observe and document expressions of grief, anger, hostility, and powerlessness.
- Determine suicide potential. *Patients at risk for self-directed harm or violence require immediate intervention.*

THERAPEUTIC INTERVENTIONS

- Maintain nonjudgmental attitude when giving care.
- Encourage patient to participate in own care.
- Provide patient opportunity to express feelings. *Unexpressed feelings can increase stress. Patients need to be able to talk of fears, such as dying.*
- Provide outlets that foster feelings of personal achievement and self-esteem.
- Provide information patient wants and needs. Do not provide more than patient can handle. *Patients who are coping ineffectively have a reduced ability to assimilate information.*
- Assist patient to grieve and work through the losses of chronic illness if appropriate.
- Support patient's effective coping strategies.
- Support patient's social network. *Lovers/nontraditional extended family may offer more support than traditional family.*
- Provide opportunities for patient/family/significant other interaction. *Without intervention, hospitalizations may isolate patient and decrease ability to cope.*
▲ Refer to psychiatric liaison or social worker as needed.
- After discharge, refer to an AIDS support group. *Support groups can offer a realistic picture of dealing with the physical and emotional aspects of AIDS.*

High Risk for Fluid Volume Deficit

RISK FACTORS

Altered nutritional status
Cryptoporidiosis
Enteric CMV disease
Intestinal parasites/diarrhea

EXPECTED OUTCOMES

Patient maintains adequate fluid volume, as evidenced by absence of weight loss, normal serum/urine osmolarity, normal urine specific gravity, good skin turgor.

ONGOING ASSESSMENT

- Assess hydration status. *Reduced skin turgor and dry mucous membranes are signs of fluid deficit.*
- Monitor I and O. Assess for presence/history of diarrhea.
- Record changes in weight.
▲ Monitor laboratory test results for increased serum sodium level, serum and urine osmolarity, and increased urine specific gravity.
▲ Culture stools for ova and parasites.
- Monitor for tachycardia and hypotension. *Are signs of reduced fluid volume and cardiac output.*
- Monitor for side effects of antibiotics given. *Many of the treatment drugs for fluid deficit have other multisystemic side effects.*

THERAPEUTIC INTERVENTIONS

- Encourage oral fluid intake.
▲ Administer parenteral fluids as ordered. *Tachypnea, pain, nausea, and esophageal candidiasis may prevent oral intake. Vomiting, diarrhea, and night sweats may increase output.*
▲ Administer antidiarrheal medication as prescribed.
▲ Administer antiparasitic medication as prescribed.
▲ If due to enteric CMV, administer prescribed medications. *Ganciclovir (also called DHP6 or Cytovene) is commonly given bid for 2 wk, then daily indefinitely. It is usually administered through a central line. Side effects include profound neutropenia, thrombocytopenia, and renal toxicity.*

Continued.

Acquired immunodeficiency syndrome (AIDS)—cont'd

NURSING DIAGNOSES	EXPECTED OUTCOMES AND NURSING INTERVENTIONS / *RATIONALE* (■ = INDEPENDENT; ▲ = COLLABORATIVE)

High Risk for Impairment of Skin Integrity

RISK FACTORS

Altered nutritional status
Diarrhea
Herpes infection
Perianal *Candida* infection
Seborrheic dermatitis
Ulcerated cutaneous Karposi sarcoma
Dermatologic staphylococcal infections
Immobility from fatigue
Prolonged unrelieved pressure

EXPECTED OUTCOMES

Patient maintains intact skin, as evidenced by absence of reddened, ulcerated areas.

ONGOING ASSESSMENT

- Check skin color, moisture, texture, and temperature.
- Assess for signs of ischemia, redness, pain.
- Assess nutritional status.
- Assess for pruritis.

THERAPEUTIC INTERVENTIONS

- Turn patient according to established schedule.
- Provide prophylactic pressure-relieving devices: alternating pressure mattress, Stryker boots, and elbow pads.
- Maintain functional body alignment.
- *Increase tissue perfusion* by massaging around affected pressure area.
- Keep skin clean and dry. *Night sweats and diarrhea macerate and damage skin.*
- Maintain adequate hydration and nutrition.
- See also Skin integrity, impaired, p. 59.
- ▲ Administer antiviral/antimonilial medication as ordered.
- ▲ If skin impairment due to herpes, administer acyclovir (Zovirax). *Side effects include nephrotoxicity.*
- ▲ If skin impairment due to seborrheic dermatitis, wash affected areas with coal tar shampoo and apply 1% hydrocortisone cream as prescribed.
- ▲ If skin impairment due to dermatologic staph infections, obtain culture of lesions and administer antibiotics as prescribed. *Common infections include bellous impetigo, ecthyma, folliculitis, or cellulitis. Staphylococcal infections are very common in HIV disease.*

Altered Nutrition: Less than Body Requirements

RELATED FACTORS

Loss of appetite
Fatigue
Oral or esophageal candidiasis
Cryptospondiosis
Enteric CMV disease
MAI (cultured from blood, bone marrow, or lymph node biopsy)
Increased nutritional needs
Nausea/vomiting

DEFINING CHARACTERISTICS

Weight loss
Caloric intake inadequate to meet metabolic requirements

EXPECTED OUTCOMES

Patient regains weight or does not lose additional weight.
Patient verbalizes understanding of necessary caloric intake.

ONGOING ASSESSMENT

- Assess changes in weight
- Obtain nutritional history: intake, difficulty in swallowing, weight loss.
- Inspect mouth for Candida infection. *Causes difficulty in swallowing.*
- Evaluate for possible adverse reactions to medications. *Many drugs used to treat AIDS can cause anorexia, nausea/vomiting, weight loss.*
- ▲ If patient receives TPN, monitor serum glucose and electrolyte levels.

THERAPEUTIC INTERVENTIONS

- Provide dietary planning to encourage intake of high-calorie, high-protein foods.
- ▲ Provide antiemetics before meals.
- Assist with meals as needed. *Fatigue/weakness may prevent patient from eating.*
- Encourage exercise as tolerated.
- ▲ Administer dietary supplements/total parenteral nutrition (TPN) as ordered. *Despite supplements, HIV may cause wasting syndrome.*
- Administer antimonilial medication as prescribed. *Oral and esophageal candidiasis can cause sore throat, may cause lack of appetite.*
- ▲ Administer megestrol acetate (Megace) as prescribed. *Dose will be individualized to degree of wasting and patient's response. It increases body weight by increasing appetite. Side effects include carpal tunnel syndrome, thrombophlebitis, alopecia, reduced sex drive, and impotence.*
- ▲ If Megace is ineffective, anticipate/administer Merinol as prescribed. *Side effects may also include clouded sensorium or euphoria.*
- ▲ Administer medications for opportunistic pathogens affecting the GI tract. *Bowel inflammation from opportunistic infections causes malabsorption of nutrients.*
- ▲ If wasting is caused by MAI medications, anticipate readjustment of medication. *Therapy will be lifelong; therefore, the optimal drug regimen must be determined.*

High Risk for Altered Thought Process

RISK FACTORS

HIV infection
CNS infections: *Toxoplasmosis gondii* encephalitis, cryptococcal meningitis
Intracranial lesions:
  Progressive multifocal leukoencephalopathy (PML)
  CNS lymphoma
  AIDS dementia complex (ADC)
  Neurosyphilis (terminal phase of disease)
Organic mental disorders associated with other physical disorders.

EXPECTED OUTCOMES

Patient can interact with others appropriately.
Patient follows prescribed treatment plan.

ONGOING ASSESSMENT

- Assess for mental status changes, such as loss of short-term memory, impaired ability to perform ADLs, decreased cognitive functioning, altered behavior, disorientation, altered or labile mood, poor judgment, short attention span/confusion.
- Assess for neurological status changes, such as seizures, headaches, abnormal gait.
▲ Review results of diagnostic tests. *Cause guides appropriate therapy. Nurses' understanding promotes optimal patient education. Common tests include serum antibody positive to Toxoplasma gondii, MRI or CT scan with lesions characteristic of toxoplasma infection, or PML, lumbar puncture results consistent with neurosyphilis.*

THERAPEUTIC INTERVENTIONS

▲ Administer antiviral agents as prescribed. *Dementia may herald acute CNS infection or chronic HIV infection. Anti-HIV treatment improves dementia caused by chronic HIV infection.*
- Supervise patient; remove potentially dangerous items from environment *to ensure safety.*
- See also Thought Processes, altered, p. 65.
▲ If caused by crytococcal meningitis, give prescribed medications (usually amphotericin B). *May be followed by fluconazole, which may be prescribed for lifelong maintenance.*
▲ If caused by toxoplasmic encephalitis (TE), anticipate treatment with pyremthamine-sulfadiazine. *This medication has many significant side effects. Folinic acid (Leucovorin) may be prescribed to reduce the hemotologic toxicity. Dexamethasone may also be prescribed to reduce cerebral edema. Antiseizure medications are frequently prescribed.*
- If PML is diagnosed, anticipate nursing home, or hospice care. *As yet there is no effective medication available for treatment. Although patients may experience progressively decreasing levels of consciousness, they usually do not become agitated or combative.*
▲ If CNS lymphoma is diagnosed, administer chemotherapy as prescribed.
▲ If neurosyphilis is diagnosed, anticipate antibiotic treatment, such as IV penicillin. *Important to assess for allergy and observe for signs of hypersensitivity.*
▲ If the patient has problems with motor function, determine whether caregiver can assist with ADLs at discharge. Initiate social service/physical therapy consultations as needed.
▲ If the patient becomes agitated in relation to the *pain* of the terminal phase of HIV disease, administer narcotics such as morphine drip as prescribed. Use patient-controlled analgesia regulating pump as appropriate.

High Risk for Ineffective Breathing Pattern

RISK FACTORS

Pneumocystis carinii Pneumonia (PCP)
Pulmonary Tuberculosis (TB)
Pulmonary Karposi Sarcoma
Pulmonary *Mycobacterium avium* Complex (MAC)
Pulmonary CMV

EXPECTED OUTCOMES

Patient is afebrile, has clear breath sounds, no cough, ABGs within normal limits, no infiltrates on chest radiograph, usual skin color without cyanosis, normal respiratory rate and rhythm, no SOB or dyspnea.

ONGOING ASSESSMENT

- Assess for signs of respiratory difficulty: dyspnea/shortness of breath, tachypnea, cough, cyanosis, crackles/rhonchi, use of accessory muscles.
▲ Monitor ABGs; note changes.
▲ Monitor chest radiograph results.
▲ Monitor LDH. *May be increased with PCP.*
▲ Evaluate PPD skin test results. *Area of induration > 5 mm is considered TB-positive for HIV-infected patients. Additional skin tests such as those for Candida, mumps, or tetanus antigens, may be administered to determine the patient's ability to mount a delayed-hypersensitivity-type reaction. Many patients with fewer than 200 CD4 cells are no longer able to respond to skin tests.*
▲ Monitor sputum culture results for PCP, MAC, and TB. *Respiratory therapist may be needed to collect specimen by induced sputum. Specimen must be delivered immediately to lab for PCP staining.*

Continued.

Acquired Immunodeficiency Syndrome (AIDS)

Hematolymphatic and Oncologic Care Plans

NURSING DIAGNOSES	EXPECTED OUTCOMES AND NURSING INTERVENTIONS / *RATIONALE* (■ = INDEPENDENT; ▲ = COLLABORATIVE)
	THERAPEUTIC INTERVENTIONS

- Position with proper body alignment for optimal breathing pattern. *Sitting position improves lung excursion and chest expansion.*
- Explain to patient the need for bronchoscopy if required for diagnosis. *Aids in diagnosis of PCP and KS. Tissue cultures are used for CMV.*
- See also Breathing pattern, ineffective, p. 10.
▲ If respiratory problems are due to PCP, administer IV pentamidine as prescribed (usually 14-21 days):
  Monitor closely for hypotension.
  Instruct patient to lie down during administration and ambulate only with assistance.
  Infuse over 1 hr *to reduce hypotension. Side effects include hypoglycemia, renal failure, pancreatitis.*
▲ If PCP is diagnosed and patient is intolerant to pentamadine, anticipate treatment with trimethoprim-sulfa methoxazole (TMP-SMX [Bactrim, Septra]). Determine any allergies to sulfa.
▲ If patient is unresponsive to PCP therapies, anticipate use of an experimental drug such as BW556C80 as prescribed. *This drug is currently available for compassionate use.*
▲ After acute PCP is resolved, continue antiinfective therapy as prescribed for secondary prophylaxis. *Patients with fewer than 200 CD4 cells usually begin prophylaxis even without a history of PCP.*
▲ Anticipate pentamidine aerosol treatment as needed. *May be given on monthly basis.*
▲ If pulmonary TB is diagnosed, administer isoniazid (INH), vitamin B6, ethambutol (Myambutol), rifampin (Rifadin, Rifamate), or pycizinade (PZA) as ordered. *The specific combination therapy is determined by resistance information obtained from culture results. Treatment is long and requires patient cooperation in order to prevent resistant strains from emerging.*
▲ For TB, maintain respiratory isolation until treatment has begun and coughing subsides; use skin testing to screen household contacts.
▲ If sputum is positive for *Mycobacterim avium* and there is no response to PCP treatment, anticipate treatment for MAI.
▲ If CMV is recovered from a bronchoscopy and other causes of respiratory distress have been eliminated, administer ganciclovir (DHP6 or Cytoven) as prescribed.

High Risk for Visual Impairment

EXPECTED OUTCOMES

Patient's vision is improved or maintained.

RISK FACTOR
CMV retinitis

ONGOING ASSESSMENT

- Determine whether patient has any visual floaters, blurred vision, or loss of peripheral or field vision.

THERAPEUTIC INTERVENTIONS

▲ Refer to ophthamologist as indicated. *A positive fundoscopic examination result indicates CMV.*
- *To ensure safety,* supervise patient. Remove potentially dangerous items from environment.
▲ Administer ganciclovir (DHP6 or Cytovene) as prescribed, usually for 2 weeks, then daily indefinitely.
▲ Make referral for home-health nurse to administer ganciclovir at home after patient discharge.

| NURSING DIAGNOSES | EXPECTED OUTCOMES AND NURSING INTERVENTIONS / *RATIONALE* (■ = INDEPENDENT; ▲ = COLLABORATIVE) |

High Risk for Infection

Risk Factors

Accidental contact with HIV by health care worker
Accidental contact with HBV
Contact with TB

Expected Outcomes

Health care worker is not infected with HIV through patient exposure.
Health care worker verbalizes universal precautions to be followed.

Ongoing Assessment

- Assess for exposure to HBV- or HIV-positive blood, semen, vaginal excretion, breast milk, amniotic fluid, wound drainages, blood-tinged body fluids, or fluids derived from blood
- Assess for exposure to untreated patient with pulmonary TB.
- ▲ Screen for HBV antibody.
- ▲ Skin test for TB q6mo.
- Monitor CDC guidelines for prevention of spread/protection.

Therapeutic Interventions

Use universal precautions *to prevent HIV spread:*
- Avoid unprotected contact with blood, semen, vaginal secretions, blood-tinged body fluids, wound drainage, breast milk, and fluids derived from blood (e.g., amniotic fluid, pericardial effusion). *These body fluids harbor HIV in quantities that may cause infection.*
- Wear gloves when exposed to potentially infectious fluids. *Latex gloves provide effective barrier against HIV.*
- Wear gloves when handling specimens.
- Label specimens with blood/body fluids precautions label; place specimen in plastic bag.
- Wear gown when soiling is anticipated.
- Wear mask and goggles when potentially infectious body fluids may spray.
- Keep disposable Ambu bag and mask at bedside.
- Immediately clean spills of potentially infectious fluids with sodium hypochlorite (bleach) solution. *Bleach, cleaning solutions labeled tuberculocidal will kill HIV.*
- Prevent injury with needles or other sharp instruments. *Although most needle-stick injuries do not result in infection, risk exists.* A month-long course of ZVD starting within hours of exposure may reduce the chance of infection.
- Do not recap needles, resheath instruments. *Recapping needles is the most common cause of needle-stick injuries.*
- Dispose of sharps in rigid plastic container.
- Keep needle disposal container in patient's room.
- Obtain assistance to restrain confused or uncooperative patient during venipuncture or other invasive procedure.
- Take care to prevent needle-stick injuries during arrests/other emergencies.
- If accidental needle-stick injury occurs, complete incident report; notify employee health service.
- Receive series of HBV vaccine.
- Receive hyperimmune HBV globulin if acutely exposed to HBV and not previously vaccinated.
- ▲ Maintain respiratory isolation for patients with pulmonary MTB.
- ▲ If TB skin test result becomes positive, examine chest radiograph or sputum culture result to rule out active disease and consider prophylactic course of isoniazid and vitamin B_6.

See also:
Altered Sexual Patterns, p. 58.
Spiritual Distress, p. 62.
Hopelessness, p. 36.
Self-care Deficit, p. 53.
Anticipatory Grieving, p. 28.

By: Jeff Zurlinden, RN, MS

Aplastic anemia

Aplastic anemia is a disease of diverse causes characterized by a decrease in precursor cells in the bone marrow and replacement of the marrow with fat. The underlying cause of aplastic anemia remains unknown. Possible pathophysiologic mechanisms include certain infections, toxic dosages of chemicals and drugs, radiation damage, and impairment of cellular interactions necessary to sustain hematopoiesis.

NURSING DIAGNOSES	EXPECTED OUTCOMES AND NURSING INTERVENTIONS / *RATIONALE* (■ = INDEPENDENT; ▲ = COLLABORATIVE)

Knowledge Deficit

RELATED FACTORS

Unfamiliarity with disease
Lack of resources

DEFINING CHARACTERISTICS

Many questions
Verbalized misconceptions
Lack of questions

EXPECTED OUTCOMES

Patient describes known facts about own disease and treatment plan.

ONGOING ASSESSMENT

- Assess understanding of new medical vocabulary. *Most persons have little exposure to hematologic diseases and therefore have not heard/do not understand terms commonly used by health professionals.*
- Assess understanding of possible causative factors.

THERAPEUTIC INTERVENTIONS

- Explain hematologic vocabulary and functions of blood elements, such as white blood cells and platelets.
- Instruct patient to avoid causative factor if known (i.e., certain chemicals.)
- Explain necessity for bone marrow aspiration and biopsy for definitive diagnosis.
- Explain the need for patient transfer to a major treatment center. *Advanced treatments such as bone marrow transplantation may be indicated.*
- Explain the need for rapid human leukocyte antigen (HLA) typing. *Performed to identify possible marrow donors.*
- Explain that allogeneic bone marrow transplant is the recommended treatment for patients less than 40 yr old and who have HLA-identical related donors.
- Explain that blood transfusions from prospective marrow donors should be avoided because of histocompatibility antigens that could lead to rejection of donor marrow.
- Explain that immunosuppressive therapy is the treatment of choice in patients without HLA-matched donors and/or over age 40.
- Describe the major therapies and potential complications:
    Immunosuppressive therapy: antihuman thymacyte globulin (ATG) and antihuman lymphocyte globulin (ALG). *These have become standard therapy for patients who do not have an HLA-identical donor.*
      Drug administration requires continuous monitoring of heart rate and blood pressure.
      Emergency resuscitation equipment must be immediately available because of risk of severe anaphylaxis. Some centers admit patients to the critical care unit for drug administration.
    Allogeneic bone marrow transplantation. *Autologous transplantation is not an option because the patient's own marrow is defective. Marrow must be transferred from an identically matched donor who is healthy (i.e., allogeneic transplantation with identical HLA-matched donor).*
    Complications:
      Rejection of donor marrow. *Results from sensitization to histocompatibility antigens acquired during previous blood transfusions and carries a high mortality rate. Conditioning regimens using cytoxin and total lymphoid irradiation show a reduction in the risk of graft failure.*
      Acute graft versus host disease (GVHD). *A red maculopapular rash 7-14 days post transplantation signals acute GVHD and carries a 20%-40% mortality rate.*
      Chronic graft versus host disease. *Can be manifested by many symptoms. Mucosal degeneration leading to guaiac-positive diarrhea, vomiting, and malnutrition is one manifestation.*
- See also Bone Marrow Transplantation, p. 386.

NURSING DIAGNOSES	EXPECTED OUTCOMES AND NURSING INTERVENTIONS / *RATIONALE* (■ = INDEPENDENT; ▲ = COLLABORATIVE)

High Risk for Infection

RISK FACTORS

Bone marrow malfunction
Replacement with factor

EXPECTED OUTCOMES

Patient has reduced risk of infection as evidenced by normal WBC, absence of fever, implementation of preventive measures.

ONGOING ASSESSMENT

▲ Monitor WBC and differential.
■ Assess for local or systemic signs of infection, such as fever, chills, malaise, swelling, pain.

THERAPEUTIC INTERVENTIONS

▲ Provide a private room for protective isolation. *Necessary if absolute neutrophil count is less than 500 mm³.*
■ Practice vigilant handwashing.
■ Assist with daily hygiene and mouth care.
▲ Anticipate need for antibiotic, antifungal, and antiviral IV agents *to counteract opportunistic infections.*

High Risk for Injury: Bleeding

RISK FACTORS

Thrombocytopenia caused by bone marrow malfunction
Replacement with factor

EXPECTED OUTCOMES

Patient has reduced risk of bleeding as evidenced by normal/adequate platelet levels, absence of bruises/petechiae.

ONGOING ASSESSMENT

▲ Monitor platelet count daily.
■ Assess skin for evidence of petechiae or bruising.
■ Observe for frank bleeding from nose, gums, urinary or GI tract.
■ Monitor stools and urine for occult blood.

THERAPEUTIC INTERVENTIONS

■ Institute bleeding precautions. *Necessary when platelet count falls below 50,000/mm³.*
■ Avoid rectal procedures such as enemas and rectal temperature taking. *Can stimulate bleeding.*
■ Avoid shaving with straight razors.
■ Consolidate laboratory blood sampling tests
▲ If platelet counts are low, anticipate need for platelet transfusions and premedication with antipyretics and antihistamines.

Activity Intolerance

RELATED FACTOR

Fatigue caused by reduced number of red blood cells (RBCs)

DEFINING CHARACTERISTICS

Report of weakness or fatigue
Exertional discomfort or dyspnea
Abnormal heart rate or blood pressure response to activity

EXPECTED OUTCOMES

Patient achieves adequate activity tolerance, as evidenced by ability to perform ADLs, verbalization of return to normal/near-normal activity levels.

ONGOING ASSESSMENT

■ Assess activity level before hospitalization.
■ Assess specific cause of fatigue. *Besides anemia, patient may have associated depression or related medical problem that can compromise activity tolerance.*
▲ Assess Hb and Hct counts 3 times/wk.

THERAPEUTIC INTERVENTIONS

■ Plan ADLs with patient. Prioritize activities for the day *to reduce fatigue.*
■ Use energy conservation principles.
▲ Anticipate need for transfusion of packed red blood cells *to increase O₂ supply to organ systems.*
▲ Administer medications that may stimulate RBC production in the bone marrow.

High Risk for Anticipatory Grieving

RISK FACTOR

Poor prognosis associated with this life-threatening disease

EXPECTED OUTCOMES

Patient verbalizes feelings about condition.
Patient maintains support system for self.

ONGOING ASSESSMENT

■ Monitor patient's response to immunotherapy or bone marrow transplantation. *Failure of therapy makes death more imminent.*
■ Assess patient's family and social resources.

Continued.

NURSING DIAGNOSES	EXPECTED OUTCOMES AND NURSING INTERVENTIONS / *RATIONALE* (■ = INDEPENDENT; ▲ = COLLABORATIVE)

THERAPEUTIC INTERVENTIONS

- Answer questions about treatment carefully yet honestly. *Major therapies for this disease are complex and often require critical care interventions.*
- Be prepared to explain and interpret lab values and diagnostic test results for the patient.
- Allow patient to express feelings, as in crying.
- Encourage patient to speak about individual concerns.
- Help significant others to understand hospital environment and patient's condition.
- See also Anticipatory grieving, p. 28.

By: Mary T. McCarthy, RN, MSN, CS

Blood and blood product transfusion therapy

Homologous donated blood, autologous blood, or blood components infused to achieve hemodynamic equilibrium.

(WHOLE BLOOD; PACKED RBCS; RANDOM DONOR; PLATELET PHERESIS PACKS; PLATELETS; FRESH FROZEN PLASMA; ALBUMIN; COAGULATION FACTORS [VIII, AUTOPLEX])

NURSING DIAGNOSES	EXPECTED OUTCOMES AND NURSING INTERVENTIONS / *RATIONALE* (■ = INDEPENDENT; ▲ = COLLABORATIVE)

Knowledge Deficit

RELATED FACTORS
Unfamiliarity with transfusion process
Misinformation about risks of transfusion

DEFINING CHARACTERISTICS
Questioning
Verbalized misconceptions
Refusal to permit transfusion

EXPECTED OUTCOMES

Patient/family verbalize understanding of the need for a transfusion and the screening process performed before the transfusion begins.

ONGOING ASSESSMENT

- Assess knowledge of transfusion process.
- Assess patient's moral, ethical, and religious background as it relates to administration of blood. *Some religions prohibit the transfusion of blood products. If a critical need for blood products arises in a patient with such prohibitions, there is a need for sensitive discussion, decision making, and possible legal action, depending on individual clinical circumstances.*

THERAPEUTIC INTERVENTIONS

- Offer explanation of precautionary measures employed by blood bank (*blood tested for hepatitis B, non A-, non-B; syphilis; HIV antibody*).
- Explain the specific type of blood product to be transfused and reason for infusion. *Patients should understand the specific clinical conditions they are being treated for and the results/improvements to be anticipated. They should also understand that transfusion administration time frames differ for individual blood components.*
- Acknowledge concerns.
- Explain procedure for administering blood *so patient is not concerned when vital signs are taken frequently.*

High Risk for Injury

RISK FACTORS
Hemolytic reaction
Allergic reaction
Febrile transfusion reaction
Circulatory overload

EXPECTED OUTCOMES

Patient receives blood without reaction.
Risk of transfusion reaction is reduced through accurate assessment and early intervention.

ONGOING ASSESSMENT

- Assess medical history for recent trauma, clotting disorders, chemotherapy, bone marrow suppression, fluid shifts/imbalances. *These contribute to a critical decrease in essential blood components and necessitate replacement for homeostasis.*

ONGOING ASSESSMENT—cont'd

- Assess for previous transfusions or reactions. *Patient may require premedication.*
- Check for signed consent for blood transfusion. *Infusion of blood product should begin within 30 min of receipt of blood on unit.*
- Check that component order is appropriate, that volume order is within safe range, and that rate of transfusion is appropriate. *Patient's cardiopulmonary status must be considered when determining rate of infusion.*
- Assess adequacy and patency of venous access.
- Check blood product and patient ID along with blood type and expiration date. *Discrepancies must be resolved before product is administered.*
- Take vital signs before therapy begins, then q15min for next hour, and q1hr thereafter.
- Assess for signs and symptoms of reaction to blood product:

    Hemolytic reaction: chills, fever, low back pain, tachycardia, tachypnea, hypotension, bleeding, oppressive feeling, and acute renal failure. *Hemolytic reaction is the most serious reaction and potentially life threatening. It is caused by infusion of incompatible blood products.*

    Allergic reaction: flushing, itching, hives, wheezing, laryngeal edema, and anaphylaxis. *These reactions are caused by sensitivity to plasma protein or donor antibody that reacts with recipient antigen.*

    Febrile nonhemolytic reaction: sudden chills and fever, headache, flushing, and anxiety. *Common transfusion reaction caused by hypersensitivity to donor white cells, platelets, or plasma proteins. Use of a leukocyte-poor filter when transfusing blood products to a person requiring frequent transfusions may reduce or prevent febrile nonhemolytic reactions.*

    Circulatory overload: dyspnea, cough, distended neck veins, increased blood pressure, and crackles heard on pulmonary auscultation. *Occurs when fluid is administered at a rate or volume greater than the circulatory system can manage.*

THERAPEUTIC INTERVENTIONS

- ▲ Follow hospital policy for obtaining blood product from blood bank.
- Prime blood tubing with normal saline solution and connect to patient's IV access. *Used as standby for infusion when blood completed or should reaction occur.*
- ▲ Premedicate with prescribed antipyretics, antihistamines, and/or steroids for those patients who have received frequent previous transfusions. *These patients have been sensitized to donor's white blood cell antigens and may experience febrile transfusion reactions if not premedicated.*
- If any type of reaction occurs, stop the transfusion immediately. Keep the IV access open with 0.9% normal saline (NS) solution and notify physician.
- If no reaction occurs:

    Infuse total ordered blood product; flush IV line with normal saline solution and reconnect maintenance solution.

    Obtain posttransfusion vital signs.

    Complete documentation of transfusion per hospital policy.

- ▲ For hemolytic reaction:

    Be prepared to treat shock. *This is a potentially life-threatening reaction.*

    Maintain blood pressure with IV colloids.

    Insert Foley catheter and monitor hourly urine output.

    Draw testing blood samples and collect urine sample. *Urine is tested for presence of red blood cells. Blood sample permits repeat typing and crossmatch to examine compatibility.*

    Anticipate possible transfer to ICU and initiation of dialysis if renal failure develops.

    Return blood product to Blood Bank. *Testing will be done to reexamine compatibility between product and recipient.*

- ▲ For allergic reaction:

    Give antihistamines as prescribed.

    Anticipate need for intubation to maintain airway.

    Anticipate need for epinephrine and pressor medications. *Emergency treatment may be needed if severe respiratory distress, hypotension, or shock is present.*

- ▲ For febrile, nonhemolytic reaction:

    Give antihistamines as prescribed; check vital signs as soon as rigor is controlled; give antipyretics as prescribed; send blood sample, blood bag, and urine sample to lab to reexamine compatibility.

- ▲ For circulatory overload: keep patient in high Fowler's (upright) position; administer diuretics, oxygen, and morphine as prescribed; insert Foley catheter; anticipate transfer to ICU if pulmonary edema is severe.

By: Mary T. McCarthy, RN, MSN, CS
and Nedra Skale, RN, MS, CNA

Blood and Blood Product Transfusion Therapy

Bone marrow/peripheral blood stem cell transplantation

Bone marrow transplantation is both a standard curative and an investigational treatment for malignant and nonmalignant diseases. Bone marrow transplantation is used to prevent potentially lethal marrow toxicities resulting from treatment with high-dose chemotherapy alone or in combination with radiation therapy. The three major types of bone marrow transplantations are so named to indicate the source of the donor marrow that is transplanted into the recipient: (1) In autologous transplantation, the recipient receives his or her own marrow that was harvested during remission or before treatment. (2) In allogeneic transplantation, the recipient receives marrow donated by another person (can be matched, partially matched, related, or unrelated person). (3) In syngeneic marrow transplantation, the recipient receives marrow donated by a genetically identical twin. In peripheral blood stem cell (PBSC) transplantation, the recipient receives stem cells collected from own peripheral blood via a cell separator (apheresis) machine. Peripheral blood stem cells are capable of reproducing themselves and reconstituting the bone marrow. The patient is managed as in autologous bone marrow transplantation.

NURSING DIAGNOSES	EXPECTED OUTCOMES AND NURSING INTERVENTIONS / *RATIONALE* (■ = INDEPENDENT; ■ = COLLABORATIVE)

Knowledge Deficit

RELATED FACTORS

Unfamiliarity with procedures and treatments in bone marrow transplantation
Unfamiliarity with overall schedule of events
Unfamiliarity with discharge/follow-up care

DEFINING CHARACTERISTICS

Verbalized lack of knowledge
Expressed need for information
Multiple questions
Lack of questions
Verbalized misconceptions

EXPECTED OUTCOMES

Patient/significant other verbalize understanding of procedures, treatments, possible complications, follow-up care.

ONGOING ASSESSMENT

- Solicit patient's/significant others' understanding of procedure(s), treatment protocol, potential side effects/complications, schedule of overall treatment plan, anticipated length of hospitalization, follow-up care after discharge.

THERAPEUTIC INTERVENTIONS

- Share with patient written calendar/schedule of overall treatment plan.
- Instruct patient (significant other as needed) about central venous catheter insertion if not already in place. See also Central venous catheter, p. 408.
- Explain bone marrow/peripheral stem cell harvest (if not already collected): preoperative/postoperative care, collection/storage of bone marrow, potential complications. See also Bone marrow harvest, p. 396.
- Discuss high-dose chemotherapy/radiation therapy administration: potential short- and long-term side effects/toxicities, preventive measures to minimize/alleviate toxicities (antiemetic, oral/skin care regimens, pain control, etc.).
- Discuss bone marrow transplantation: procedure for bone marrow/peripheral stem cell infusion, potential complications, preventive measures to minimize/alleviate potential complications, time frame for marrow engraftment.
- Discuss protective environment (private room, laminar air flow room, etc.) *to protect patient from environmental contagions during myelosuppression period.* Provide information about isolation techniques/procedures.
- Discuss blood component transfusions (i.e., packed red cells, white cells, and platelets) *that constitute adjunct management of anemia, infections, and thrombocytopenia.* Encourage patient/significant other to participate in blood component donor accrual to fulfill frequent, often prolonged transfusion requirements.
- Assist patient/significant other in formulating visiting schedule in accordance with isolation precautions, visitor policy, and patient care needs.
- Discuss antibacterial, antiprotozoal, antifungal, and antiviral therapy *to prevent/treat infections. Oral nonabsorbable antibiotics (Gentamicin/Vancomycin/Nystatin/Polymyxin) may be administered prophylactically to suppress patient's own GI flora, which, during myelosuppression, potentially become pathogenic and eventually are source of infection/sepsis. Efficacy of oral nonabsorbable antibiotics is controversial; patient compliance/tolerance generally is poor.*

NURSING DIAGNOSES	EXPECTED OUTCOMES AND NURSING INTERVENTIONS / *RATIONALE* (■ = INDEPENDENT; ▲ = COLLABORATIVE)

THERAPEUTIC INTERVENTIONS—cont'd

- Discuss dietary modifications that may include low-bacterial diet (no fresh fruits/vegetables, "well cooked" food items) *to decrease bacterial contamination of alimentary tract. Total parenteral nutrition (TPN) initiated when patient's oral intake no longer meets daily nutritional requirements.*
- Explain need for frequent blood sampling *to assess for electrolyte and metabolic changes, cardiac/pulmonary/renal alterations, bone marrow function, need for blood component transfusion(s), and presence of infection.*
- Explain need for frequent inspection/culturing of all orifices/potential infection sites *for surveillance of opportunistic microorganisms, early detection, and prompt treatment of infection.*
- Discuss discharge planning/teaching. *Depends on course of postengraftment period, but usually begins about 2 wk after transplantation. Discharge criteria include absolute granulocyte count >1000/mm³, oral intake 1000 cal/day, and no evidence of infection:*
  ADLs
  Medications after discharge
  Importance of balanced diet, adequate fluid intake. Outpatient follow-up care after discharge
  Central venous catheter care (Hickman, Permcath)
  Measures to prevent infection (*patient's immune function not fully restored until about 6-9 mo after transplantation; many patients are fearful of leaving hospital's "protective isolation" environment*)
  Recognition/report of signs/symptoms of bleeding, low red blood cell count, and infection
  Sexual relations/contraception
  Return to work or school

Impaired Physical Mobility

RELATED FACTORS

Treatment-related side effects
Disease process
Pain and discomfort
Depression/severe anxiety
Generalized weakness/deconditioning
Physical restrictions on movement (i.e., protective isolation)

DEFINING CHARACTERISTICS

Pain/discomfort on movement
Weakness/lethargy
Decreased attempt to move
In bed most of time

EXPECTED OUTCOMES

Patient maintains optimal level of physical mobility and independence as evidenced by ROM within normal limits, participation in self-care activities.

ONGOING ASSESSMENT

- Assess for presence of Defining Characteristics.

THERAPEUTIC INTERVENTIONS

- Teach importance of activity and possible hazards of immobility. *Thorough explanation of purpose, goal, and importance of activity often increases patient compliance.*
- ▲ Notify physical therapist of patient's admission *for assessment and formalization of individualized activity regimen.*
- Facilitate procurement of stationary bicycle *to assist patient in maintaining muscle strength.*
- Encourage daily use of exercise bicycle as appropriate.
- Encourage patient involvement/participation in care activities.
- See also Mobility, impaired physical, p. 47.

High Risk for Altered Nutrition: Less than Body Requirements

RISK FACTORS

Side effects of chemotherapy/radiation therapy (inability to taste and smell foods, loss of appetite, nausea/vomiting, mucositis, mouth lesions, xerostomia, diarrhea)
Intestinal graft versus host disease: abdominal cramping, diarrhea, malabsorption of nutrients
Increased metabolic rate secondary to fever/infection

EXPECTED OUTCOMES

Patient demonstrates normal elimination pattern as evidenced by stools of normal frequency, consistency, and amount; absence of abdominal cramping/pain.

ONGOING ASSESSMENT

- Obtain history of side effects of previous chemotherapy/radiation therapy and treatment measures effective in past.
- Solicit patient's description of nausea/vomiting pattern.
- Evaluate effectiveness of antiemetic regimen.
- Obtain diet history, including dietary habits and sociocultural influences.
- Monitor daily calorie counts *to determine whether patient's oral intake meets daily nutritional requirements.*
- ▲ Monitor lab values: CBC/differential; electrolytes; serum iron, TIBC, total protein, albumin. *These provide information on nutritional, fluid, and electrolyte status.*
- Weigh daily on same scale *to assure accuracy of weight.*
- Monitor closely for tolerance to TPN solution and for any potential adverse complications. *Common problems include hyper/hypoglycemia, hypophosphatemia, electrolyte disorders, hyperosmolarity, dislodgment of catheter/infiltration, catheter sepsis.*
- Monitor intake and output.

Continued.

NURSING DIAGNOSES	EXPECTED OUTCOMES AND NURSING INTERVENTIONS / *RATIONALE* (■ = INDEPENDENT; ▲ = COLLABORATIVE)

THERAPEUTIC INTERVENTIONS

▲ Administer antiemetic on timed rather than prn schedule before, during, and after chemotherapy/radiation therapy *to maintain adequate blood levels.*
■ Teach methods to minimize/prevent nausea/vomiting:
  Small dietary intake before treatments
  Foods with low potential for nausea (e.g., dry toast, crackers, ginger ale, cola, popsicles, gelatin, baked/boiled potatoes)
  Avoidance of spices, gravy, greasy foods
  Modification of food consistency/type as needed
  Small, frequent nutritious meals
  Attractive servings
  Sufficient time for meals
  Rest periods before and after meals
  Quiet, restful environment
  Comfortable position
  Oral hygiene measures before, after, and between meals
  Avoidance of coaxing, bribing, or threatening in relation to intake
  Antiemetic half-hour before meals as prescribed
■ Identify and provide favorite foods; avoid serving them during periods of nausea/vomiting *as patient may develop aversion.*
▲ Administer supplemental feedings/fluids as prescribed.
■ Implement appropriate graft versus host disease diet or NPO status ("Gut rest") in the presence of abdominal cramps, pain, diarrhea. *These generally indicate injury to intestinal mucosal surfaces, resulting in nutrient malabsorption, making TPN support necessary.*
▲ Administer TPN solution at prescribed rate via infusion control device *to assure accurate flow rate.*
■ Exercise meticulus care in maintaining aseptic technique when handling TPN solutions/delivery *to reduce infection.*
■ See also Total parenteral nutrition, p. 324.

Diarrhea

RELATED FACTORS

Side effects of high-dose chemotherapy/radiation therapy
Antiemetic therapy
Oral magnesium
Antacids
Antibiotic therapy
Infection
Intestinal graft versus host disease

DEFINING CHARACTERISTICS

Abdominal pain
Cramping
Frequency of stools
Loose/liquid stools
Urgency
Hyperactive bowel sounds/sensations

ONGOING ASSESSMENT

■ Check bowel sounds; observe for abdominal distention/rigidity.
■ Observe stool pattern; record frequency, character, and volume. *Diarrhea can be the first manifestation of GVHD; it is usually high-volume (500-1500 cc/day), watery green, containing mucus strands, protein, and cellular debris.*
▲ Obtain stool specimen for culture and sensitivity as prescribed.
■ Hematest all watery stools. *Aids in detecting possible GI mucosal sloughing caused by chemotherapy/radiation therapy, or GVHD-related mucosal injury.*

THERAPEUTIC INTERVENTIONS

▲ Administer antidiarrheal, antispasmodic medication as prescribed; document effectiveness.
▲ Administer IV analgesics *to relieve abdominal pain/cramping.*
■ Implement meticulous perianal care regimen *to prevent mucosal irritation/breakdown.*
▲ Administer parenteral nutrition as prescribed *to maintain optimal nutritional support in view of inadequate PO intake/decreased absorption secondary to diarrhea/intestinal GVHD.*
■ See also Diarrhea, p. 19.

High Risk for Injury: Bleeding

RISK FACTORS

Invasion of bone marrow by malignant cells

Bone marrow suppression secondary to chemotherapy/ radiation therapy

Prolonged bone marrow re- generation

Decrease in total circulating platelets <50,000/mm^3

Failure of bone marrow graft

DIC

Tumor erosion ulcerations (i.e. stress ulcer, gastrointestinal mucosal sloughing secondary to chemotherapy/radiation therapy)

Hemorrhagic cystitis second- ary to high-dose Cytoxan therapy

EXPECTED OUTCOMES

Patient maintains reduced risk of bleeding, as evidenced by normal platelet count, absence of signs of bleeding, early report of any signs of bleeding.

ONGOING ASSESSMENT

- Assess for any signs of bleeding: *Signs may be obvious (e.g., epistaxis, bleeding gums, hematemesis, hemoptysis, retinal hemorrhages, melena, hematuria, vaginal bleeding) or occult (e.g., neurologic changes, dizziness).*
- Monitor vital signs as needed. *Increased heart rate and orthostatic changes accompany bleeding.*
- ▲ Monitor platelets, Hb/Hct daily *to detect changes early.*

THERAPEUTIC INTERVENTIONS

- ▲ Implement bleeding precautions for platelet count <50,000/mm^3 *(level at which spon- taneous bleeding can occur).*
- ▲ Communicate anticipated need for platelet support to transfusion center *to assure avail- ability and readiness of platelets.*
- ▲ Transfuse single or random donor platelet as prescribed. *Note: Orders to irradiate all blood products before administration (except bone marrow, peripheral stem cells, buffy coat) may be written to prevent graft-versus-host disease (GVHD), which, in autologus bone marrow transplantation patient, may be caused by imbalance in T_4/T_8 ratio, as well as presence of component donor's white blood cells. Irradiation of blood compo- nents continues 6-12 mo after patient discharge.*
- ▲ Maintain a current blood sample for "type and screen" in transfusion center *to ensure availability and readiness of packed red blood cells.*
- ▲ If significant drop in Hb and Hct is noted, transfuse packed red cells as prescribed *to restore Hb/Hct to levels where patient experiences minimal symptoms.* (Check whether blood components were irradiated before transfusion.)
- See also Aplastic Anemia, p. 382; Leukemia, acute, p. 420.

High Risk for Injury: Liver Dysfunction

RISK FACTORS

Venoocclusive disease (VOD)

Graft versus host disease

Hepatitis

Infection

Fatty liver (from parenteral nutrition)

Drug injury (chemotherapy/ antimicrobial therapy)

Hepatic malignancy

Liver failure

EXPECTED OUTCOMES

Patient maintains optimal liver function, as evidenced by serum and urine lab values within normal limits, absence of ascites, balanced intake and output, normal weight for patient.

ONGOING ASSESSMENT

- Assess for signs of liver dysfunction: sudden weight gain, enlarged liver, right upper quadrant pain, ascites, jaundice, tea-colored urine, labored and shallow respirations, dys- pnea, confusion, and lethargy/fatigue. *Typically, symptoms develop 1-3 wk after trans- plantation. Patients usually present with some but not all of these symptoms.*
- ▲ Monitor lab values daily for:
    Increased alkaline phosphatase, bilirubin, serum glutamic oxaloacetic transaminase (SGOT)/serum glutamic pyruvic transaminase (SGPT)/lactic dehydrogenase (LDH), ammonia levels.
    Decreased serum albumin level
    Electrolyte imbalance
    Abnormal coagulation profile
- Monitor weight bid.
- Measure abdominal girth. *Begin day 8 post transplantation to detect/monitor for ascites.*
- Assess risk factors predisposing to development of VOD:
    Age (under 15)
    Liver abnormalities before transplantation
    TBI (single dose versus fractionated)
    Intense toxic conditioning regimen (i.e., high-dose combination versus single high- dose chemotherapy)
    Diagnosis other than acute lymphocytic leukemia (ALL)
    Allogeneic bone marrow transplantation
    Second bone marrow transplantation

Continued.

Bone marrow/peripheral blood stem cell transplantation—cont'd

NURSING DIAGNOSES	EXPECTED OUTCOMES AND NURSING INTERVENTIONS / *RATIONALE* (■ = INDEPENDENT; ▲ = COLLABORATIVE)

THERAPEUTIC INTERVENTIONS

▲ Maintain sodium restriction as indicated.

▲ Restrict fluids as prescribed.

▲ Administer IV medications with minimal amount of solution. Consult pharmacist.

▲ Administer 25% normal serum albumin (human) as prescribed *to keep serum levels within normal range and maintain plasma oncotic pressure.*

▲ Administer diuretics as prescribed *to decrease amount of ascites and maintain adequate renal perfusion.*

▲ Transfuse packed RBCs as prescribed *to maintain intravascular fluid volume. The goal of hypertransfusion of PRBCs is to attain a HCT ≥40, which helps maintain high osmotic pressure within the vascular space. This in turn draws extravascular interstitial fluid back into the vessels.*

▲ Administer analgesics as prescribed for patient comfort. *Narcotics/sedatives with shorter half-lives and fewer metabolites (i.e., morphine/hydromorphine) given in reduced doses should be considered to prevent compounding of hepatic encephalopathy.*

▲ Consult dietician about dietary modifications in enteral/parenteral nutrition. *Oral protein may need to be restricted; TPN solutions may need to be concentrated.*

High Risk for Impaired Renal Function

RISK FACTORS

High-dose chemotherapy
Nephrotoxic drugs (i.e., aminoglycosides, amphotericin B, cyclosporine, methotrexate, acyclovir, DMSO)
Dehydration
Hemolysis
Venoocclusive disease
Ascites
Septic shock
Tumor lysis
Cardiotoxic effects
Congestive heart failure

EXPECTED OUTCOMES

Patient maintains optimal renal function as evidenced by balanced I & O, weight within normal limits, normal vital signs, alert mentation.

ONGOING ASSESSMENT

▪ Monitor urine output. Measure urine volume for a single shift and compare with volume for previous shift. *Decreased urine volume and increased serum creatinine suggest renal insufficiency.*

▲ Monitor lab data: Na, K, blood urea nitrogen (BUN), creatinine, Mg, CO_2, Hb, Hct, osmolality. *These reflect fluid and electrolyte balance, level of vital organ function, and acid-base balance.*

▪ Monitor fluid balance (I&O, weight) bid. *Determines the compartmental distribution of fluid in the body.*

▪ Observe for presence of peripheral and/or dependent edema.

▪ Measure abdominal girth bid *to detect/monitor ascites. An increase in girth without concomitant increase in weight usually indicates a decrease in intravascular volume.*

▪ Monitor vital signs for orthostatic changes in blood pressure and increased heart rate. *Caused by depletion of intravascular volume (hypovolemia).*

▪ Monitor for changes in mental status. *BUN and other waste products can build up in the blood and cause uremic encephalopathy.*

▪ Monitor drug profile for medications potentially contributing to renal insufficiency and/or mental status changes. *Drug dosage adjustment/discontinuation may be necessary to prevent toxic side effects of poorly excreted drugs.*

▲ Collect urine specimens for renal function tests.

▪ Monitor urine for specific gravity; dipstick for pH, protein, blood.

THERAPEUTIC INTERVENTIONS

▲ Administer IV fluids/diuretics as prescribed *to correct vascular volume disequilibrium.*

▲ Administer electrolytes in intravenous fluids *to match calculated loss and correct deficit or excess.*

▲ Administer low-dose ("renal dose") dopamine *to maintain urine flow.*

▲ Consult dietician about dietary modifications in enteral/parenteral nutrition.

▪ See also: Nephrotic syndrome, p. 447, and Acute renal failure, p. 436.

NURSING DIAGNOSES	EXPECTED OUTCOMES AND NURSING INTERVENTIONS / *RATIONALE* (■ = INDEPENDENT; ▲ = COLLABORATIVE)

High Risk for Infection

RISK FACTORS

Altered immunologic responses related to immunosuppression secondary to high-dose chemotherapy/radiation therapy

Bone marrow suppression

Antimicrobial therapy (i.e., superimposed infection)

Prolonged bone marrow regeneration

Failure of bone marrow graft

Cytomegalovirus (CMV)/herpes simplex virus (HSV) seropositivity

EXPECTED OUTCOMES

Patient is at reduced risk of local/systemic infection, as evidenced by negative blood/surveillance culture findings, compliance with preventive measures, normal chest radiograph, intact mucous membranes/skin, prompt reporting of early signs of infection.

ONGOING ASSESSMENT

▲ Monitor WBC/differential daily for evidence of rising/falling counts. *Gradually rising blood counts signal successful bone marrow engraftment/function (generally occurs 14-20 days after transplantation).*

▪ Monitor vital signs as needed for decreased blood pressure, increased heart rate and respiration.

▪ Auscultate lung fields.

▪ Note presence/type of cough.

▪ Observe for changes in color/character of sputum, urine, stool.

▪ Inspect body sites with high potential for infection (mouth, throat, axilla, perineum, rectum).

▪ Inspect peripheral IV/central catheter site(s) for redness/tenderness.

▪ Assess for fever; flushed appearance; diaphoresis; rigors/shaking chills; fatigue/malaise; changes in mental status; pleuritic pain; conjunctivitis; vaginal discharge.

▪ Assess risk factors predisposing to CMV infection: allogeneic bone marrow transplantation, CMV seropositivity, total body irradiation (TBI), acute graft versus host disease (GVHD).

▲ Obtain appropriate cultures (surveillance cultures) *to determine microorganism(s) causing the infection and antibiotic drug sensitivity.*

THERAPEUTIC INTERVENTIONS

▲ Place patient in protective isolation per transplant protocol.

▪ Ensure thorough handwashing (using vigorous friction) by staff/visitors before physical contact with patient *to remove transient/resident bacteria from hands, thus minimizing/preventing transmission to patient.*

▪ Provide care for neutropenic patients before other patients, taking strict precautions to prevent transferring infectious agent(s) to neutropenic patients in accordance with institutional isolation policy/procedure.

▪ Teach/provide meticulous total body hygiene with special attention to high-risk areas *(often sites of infection).*

▪ Use aseptic/sterile technique in patient care/treatments per isolation protocol/procedure.

▪ Use separate towel/washcloth for area of infection *to prevent cross contamination.*

▲ Institute low-bacterial or sterile diet *to protect patient from exposure to pathogens from foods at a time of greatly compromised host defenses.*

▪ Implement meticulous oral hygiene regimen.

▲ Administer antibacterial/antifungal/antiviral/antiprotozoal drugs as prescribed on time *to maintain therapeutic drug levels.*

▪ Describe to patient/significant other WBC role in infection prevention: normal range of WBC, function of leukocytes and neutrophils, meaning/importance of "absolute" neutrophil count, risk of bacterial infection associated with "absolute" neutrophil count ($<500/mm^3$: severe risk, $500/mm^3$: moderate risk, $>1000/mm^3$: minimal risk, $1500-2000/mm^3$: no significant risk).

▪ Explain effects of chemotherapy/radiation therapy on immune system.

▪ Teach patient/significant other measures to prevent infection after discharge until immune function fully restored (about 9-12 mo after transplantation):

    Avoid crowds or contact with persons with known infections.

    Avoid cleaning cat-litter boxes, fish tanks, or bird cages.

    Avoid contact with dog/human excreta.

    Avoid contact with barnyard animals.

    Avoid swimming in private/public pools.

    Practice meticulous oral/body hygiene, including frequent handwashing.

    Use aseptic technique when caring for central venous catheter.

    Maintain balanced diet with sufficient protein, calories, vitamins, minerals, and fluids.

    Limit number of sexual partners; practice "gentle" sex; use adequate lubrication; avoid rectal intercourse/douching; use contraceptive method(s) approved by physician.

▪ See also Leukemia, acute, p. 420; Granulocytopenia, p. 413.

Continued.

NURSING DIAGNOSES	EXPECTED OUTCOMES AND NURSING INTERVENTIONS / *RATIONALE* (■ = INDEPENDENT; ▲ = COLLABORATIVE)

High Risk for Fluid Volume Overload

RISK FACTORS

Aggressive IV hydration with high-dose Cytoxan-based preparatory regimen
Antidiuretic effect of Cytoxan
Bone marrow/peripheral stem cell reinfusion
Multiple IV drug therapy (oral route unsuitable secondary to nausea, vomiting, mucositis, etc.)
Parenteral nutrition
Blood component transfusions

EXPECTED OUTCOMES

Patient maintains optimal fluid balance, as evidenced by balanced intake and output, normal weight, normal breath sounds.

ONGOING ASSESSMENT

- Monitor vital signs.
- Auscultate chest as needed for rales, rhonchi, wheezes, increased respiratory effort.
- Weigh patient daily at same time with same scale *to assure accuracy.*
- Record accurate I & O.
- Monitor for signs of fluid overload: shortness of breath, dyspnea, edema, distended neck veins, restlessness.

THERAPEUTIC INTERVENTIONS

▲ Administer diuretics as prescribed; evaluate effectiveness and look for side effects; document. *Hypokalemia and hypovolemia are common side effects.*
▲ Administer IV medications with minimal amount of solution.
▲ Infuse IV solutions as prescribed via infusion control device *to assure accurate flow rate and prevent unintentional fluid overload.*
- Plan activities with minimum energy expenditure.
- Maintain physical/emotional rest *to reduce associated dyspnea.*
▲ Administer O_2 as prescribed.
- See also Fluid Volume Excess, p. 26.

High Risk for Decreased Cardiac Output

RISK FACTORS

Cardiac damage secondary to high-dose Cytoxan therapy or radiation therapy

EXPECTED OUTCOMES

Patient maintains optimal cardiac output, as evidenced by normal breath sounds, strong pulses, heart rate and blood pressure within normal limits.

ONGOING ASSESSMENT

- Assess for significant alterations in:
  Radial/apical/peripheral pulses, cardiac rhythm, blood pressure, pulsus paradoxus
  Heart sounds
  Lung sounds/respiratory pattern
  Jugular venous distention. *Sign of right-sided ventricular dysfunction.*
  Skin color, temperature. *Cool clammy skin is sign of compromised output.*
  Fluid balance: I & O, weight, presence of peripheral/dependent edema
  ABGs, chest radiograph
- Monitor ECG rate, rhythm, and change in ST segments during high-dose Cytoxan therapy. *Note that nonspecific ST changes are not uncommon with high-dose Cytoxan therapy.* Continue to monitor 48 hr after administration of last Cytoxan dose *to assess for potential myocardial damage.*
▲ Monitor serum electrolyte levels. *(Diuretic therapy may produce electrolyte depletion, i.e., hypokalemia.)*

THERAPEUTIC INTERVENTIONS

If signs of compromised cardiac output are noted:
▲ Administer O_2 as indicated.
▲ Administer medications as ordered: diuretics *to reduce volume overload,* digitalis *to slow and strengthen heart beat,* morphine *to reduce pulmonary vascular congestion and anxiety associated with dyspnea.*
- See also Cardiac output, decreased, p. 12.

High Risk for Injury (Drug/Blood Component Reaction)

Risk Factors

Chemotherapy
Radiation therapy
Antiemetic drugs
Antifungal drugs
Colony stimulating factors
Immunoglobulins
Immunosuppressive therapy (i.e., cyclosporine, methotrexate, steroids, antithymocyte globulins)
Bone marrow reinfusion
Blood component transfusion(s)

Expected Outcomes

Patient is free of injury from drug/radiation/blood therapy as evidenced by normal vital signs, absence of pain, absence of nausea/vomiting, normal cardiopulmonary status.

Ongoing Assessment

- Check for history of drug allergies.
- Monitor vital signs.
- Assess for reaction from *chemotherapeutic drugs*: restlessness, facial edema/flushing, wheezing, skin rash, tachycardia, hypotension, hematuria (Cytoxan), increased uric acid levels.
- Assess for reactions from *radiation therapy*: nausea/vomiting, fever, diarrhea, flushing, swelling of parotid glands, pancreatitis.
- Assess for reactions from *antiemetic drugs*: agitation, hypotension, irritability, spasm of neck muscles, dystonias.
- Assess for reactions from *antifungal drugs*: fever, chills, rigors, hypotension, headache, nausea/vomiting, hypokalemia.
- Assess for reactions from *colony-stimulating factors* (G-CSF/GM/CSF): headache, myalgia/arthralgia, skeletal bone pain, facial edema, erthyemia/fever, hypotension, fatigue, nausea/vomiting, capillary leak syndrome, rash, and chills/rigors.
- Assess for reactions from *immunoglobulins*: urticaria, pain (local erythema), headache, muscle stiffness, fever/malaise, nephrotic syndrome, angioedema, and anaphylaxis.
- Assess for reactions to *immunosuppressive therapy*: mucositis, nausea/vomiting, bone marrow suppression, fluid retention, hypertension, headache, hypomagnesemia, renal toxicity, tingling in extremities, tremors, and anaphylaxislike reactions.
- Assess for reactions to *bone marrow reinfusion*: chills/rigors, fever, rash/hives, hyper/hypotension, nausea/vomiting, dyspnea/shortness of breath, pulmonary emboli/fat emboli, volume overload, chest pain, sensation of tightness or fullness in throat, renal failure.
- Assess for reactions to *packed red cell/platelet transfusion*: fever, chills/rigors, and hives.
- Check urine pH as prescribed until 48 hr after administration of last Cytoxan dose.
- Test urine for blood *to check for hematuria caused by irritation of bladder lining secondary to metabolites from Cytoxan therapy. High urine flow, alkalinization of urine, and frequent voiding help prevent concentration of Cytoxan metabolites in bladder, thus reducing risk of hemorrhagic cystitis.*
- Perform pretransplantation assessment before bone marrow/peripheral stem cell infusion: take baseline vital signs; auscultate chest and heart; check patency of central venous catheter (24-72 hr after completion of chemotherapy depending on biologic clearance rates of drugs given). *In autologous transplantation, frozen bone marrow/peripheral stem cells are taken to patient's bedside, thawed in water bath, and administered intravenously via central venous catheter. In allogeneic or syngeneic transplant, freshly harvested donor marrow is taken from the operating room to patient's bedside and infused (much like a blood transfusion) via central catheter.*

Therapeutic Interventions

- ▲ Administer premedications as prescribed; monitor for effectiveness.
- Keep emergency drugs (IV Benadryl, hydrocortisone, Epinephrine 1:1000) readily available.
- ▲ Administer IV fluids and diuretics before, during, and after Cytoxan therapy as prescribed *to maintain good urine output and counteract antidiuretic effect of Cytoxan. As chemotherapy destroys tumor cells, uric acid is liberated and accumulates in blood. High urine flow prevents uric acid deposits in kidneys. See also Tumor lysis syndrome, p. 429.*
- ▲ Administer supplemental sodium bicarbonate as prescribed to maintain urine pH above 7, *thus increasing solubility of uric acid in urine and diminishing changes of crystalline deposits in kidneys, which could potentially cause uric acid nephropathy. Allopurinol may be added.*
- Instruct patient to void q1-2hr until 24 hr after completion of last Cytoxan dose.
- ▲ Administer analgesics as needed; apply topical ice packs to swollen parotid gland(s) *(helps reduce pain of parotitis). Symptomatic parotitis may occur 4-24 hr after single-dose 1000-rad total body irradiation (TBI); generally resolves in 1-4 days. Side effect less frequent when TBI administered in divided (fractionated) doses.*
- Have patient void before bone marrow reinfusion and assist in assuming position of optimal comfort *(prevents/minimizes interruptions to transplantation procedure).*

Bone Marrow/Peripheral Blood Stem Cell Transplantation

Continued

Bone marrow/peripheral blood stem cell transplantation—cont'd

NURSING DIAGNOSES	EXPECTED OUTCOMES AND NURSING INTERVENTIONS / *RATIONALE* (■ = INDEPENDENT; ▲ = COLLABORATIVE)

THERAPEUTIC INTERVENTIONS—cont'd

▲ Premedicate patient with antiemetic and antihistamine as prescribed before reinfusion *to reduce incidence of nausea/vomiting and allergic reactions. Nausea/vomiting caused by garliclike odor of dimethyl sulfoxide (DMSO) chemical used to preserve autologous bone marrow/peripheral stem cells. Allergic reactions, including shortness of breath (SOB), possibly result of liberation of histamines from broken marrow cells.*

■ Provide warm blankets if chills occur during reinfusion. *Chills usually secondary to cool temperature of thawed marrow/peripheral stem cell concentrate.*

■ Inform patient that urine will be pink or red for several hours after infusion *because of red color of tissue culture medium contained in reinfused components.*

▲ Do the following when drug/transfusion reaction suspected: stop infusion; notify physician; administer emergency drugs as prescribed; reassure patient.

See also:
Blood and blood product transfusion therapy, p. 384
Pulmonary thromboembolism, p. 216
Anaphylactic shock, p. 156, if allergic reactions during or after procedure

---

High Risk for Impaired Skin Integrity

RISK FACTORS:

Side effects of chemotherapy/radiation therapy
Malignant skin lesions
Impaired physical mobility secondary to treatment-related side effects
Allergic reaction secondary to drug/blood component therapy
Infection
Graft versus host disease (GVHD)

EXPECTED OUTCOMES

Patient maintains intact skin.
Patient is at reduced risk of altered skin integrity, as evidenced by compliance with preventive measures, prompt reporting of early signs of impairment.

ONGOING ASSESSMENT

■ Assess skin integrity daily; note color, moisture, texture, and temperature.

■ Inspect "high-risk" areas daily for skin breakdown: bony prominences, skin folds (e.g., axillae, breast folds, buttocks, perineum, groin), radiation port and exit site(s).

■ Assess movement/positioning ability.

■ Assess risk factors predisposing to development of GVHD: age above 30 years, sex-mismatched donor, HLA-mismatched donor, total body irradiation (TBI).

■ Assess for signs of acute skin GVHD:
Stage 1: presence of rubellalike rash on face, trunk, palms of hands, and/or soles of feet. *This maculopapular rash is the most common initial presentation.*
Stage 2: Progression of rash to general erythroderma, dryness, scaling of skin.
Stage 3: Generalized erythroderma.
Stage 4: Generalized erythroderma with progression to blisters and desquamation of skin.

■ Observe skin/mucosal biopsy sites for potential bleeding/infection.

■ Promote comfort: bed cradle to keep linen off body; egg crate mattress, low airless bed; nonadherent disposable sheets; body positioning and supports; systemic analgesics.

■ Maintain dressing placement with wrap (Kerlix or Surgiflex) *to prevent use of tape on sensitive skin.*

■ Implement measures to prevent dryness of nonirradiated skin: include Alpha Keri Oil in bath water; apply Eucerin lotion or Aloe cream liberally.

■ Implement measures *to prevent irritation to irradiated skin:* avoid constricting clothing (i.e., belts, girdles, brassieres); avoid irritating substances (e.g., perfumed soap, perfume, ointments, lotions, cosmetics, talcum, deodorants).
Avoid use of oil-based creams, ointments, and lotions during radiation treatment (*may contain heavy metals and leave coating on skin that may interfere with radiation therapy*).
Use only topical ointments, creams, powders, etc., as prescribed by radiologist *for skin tenderness, dryness, and itching.*
Avoid hot or cold applications (e.g., heating pad, ice compress) as well as sun exposure (*may increase irritation*).
Avoid vigorous scrubbing of skin.
Avoid scratching/peeling skin.
Wear soft cotton clothing.

ONGOING ASSESSMENT —cont'd

- Inform patient that skin discoloration is temporary; skin will return to normal color though texture may continue to be dry.
- Inform patient of early signs/symptoms of skin changes to report.
- Implement the following once signs of GVHD (stages 1-3) are present:
  Use AVEENO soap and AVEENO oatmeal bath preparation bid *to soothe dry, flaky irritated skin.*
  Administer antipruritic medications (i.e., antihistamines).
  Trim nails and discourage patient from scratching; consider use of mittens.
  Lubricate skin well with frequent applications of a mixture of half and half mineral oil and ointment (A&D) (or any other lubricant as prescribed).
- Implement the following comfort measures if bullae and desquamation are present:
  Use of low air loss or silicone bead bed.
  Use of burn sheets (Soft-Kare) on bed. *These sheets are nonirritating and fluid-absorbing, thereby minimizing further tissue damage.*
  Bathe patient with sterile warm saline solution or water. *This aids in débridement. Use sterile "burn pack."*
  Cover all open areas after bathing with a mixture of Silvadene and Mycostatin (or topical treatment as prescribed). Apply with sterile gloved hand *to prevent infection.*
  Provide warmth to maintain body temperature.
- Administer immunosuppressive drugs as prescribed *to prevent or treat acute GVHD (i.e., cyclosporine, methotrexate, steroids). GVHD results when the T lymphocytes in the transplanted donor bone marrow recognize the marrow recipient as "foreign" and mount an immunologic "attack" against the "host." GVHD presents clinically in two forms: acute and chronic.*
  Acute GVHD may present 7-100 days post transplantation; chronic GVHD may present 100-360 days post transplantation (usually after discharge).
  Acute GVHD involves the skin, liver, and GI tract; chronic GVHD involves the skin, eyes, GI tract, lungs, vagina, neuromuscular and immune systems. GVHD generally is seen in patients receiving allogeneic bone marrow transplantations. The incidence of GVHD is about 50%; it remains one of the major causes of transplantation-related mortality rates.

See also:
Anxiety/Fear, p. 5, 23.
Body Image Disturbance, p. 7.
Ineffective Individual Coping, p. 18.
Chemotherapy, p. 403.
Activity Intolerance, p. 2.

By: Christa M. Schroeder, RN, MSN
Victoria Frazier-Jones, RN, BSN

Bone marrow harvest: care of the bone marrow donor

The collection of bone marrow via multiple needle aspirations from the posterior iliac crest under general or spinal anesthesia. The anterior iliac crest and sternum may also be used. Bone marrow needles are placed through the skin into the inner cavity of the bone; marrow, along with some blood, is withdrawn. Approximately 200 aspirations are required to collect the desired amount of bone marrow, which is usually 1 to 1½ quarts or about 10% of the patient's total marrow volume.

NURSING DIAGNOSES

EXPECTED OUTCOMES AND NURSING INTERVENTIONS / *RATIONALE*
(■ = INDEPENDENT; ▲ = COLLABORATIVE)

Knowledge Deficit

RELATED FACTORS

Unfamiliarity with procedure, postoperative care, recovery
Unfamiliarity with discharge activity

DEFINING CHARACTERISTICS

Verbalized lack of knowledge or misconceptions
Expressed need for information
Multiple questions
Increased anxiety

EXPECTED OUTCOMES

Patient/significant others verbalize understanding of the bone marrow harvest procedure and recovery.

ONGOING ASSESSMENT

- Solicit patient's description and understanding of procedure, postoperative care, self-care of bone marrow aspiration sites, potential complications, marrow recovery.

THERAPEUTIC INTERVENTIONS

- Instruct patient on the following:
  Preoperative care
  Data base: labs, ECG, chest radiograph.
  Determination of type of anesthesia (spinal or general).
  Self-donation of blood. *Used as replacement transfusion during bone marrow harvest to prevent risk of transfusion-related complications (hepatitis, HIV)*
  Bone marrow aspirations:
  Anatomic location/distribution/function of marrow.
  Aspiration sites: posterior and/or anterior iliac crests.
  Procedure for aspiration. *Is performed in operating room by inserting special needles into the center of the pelvis bones and aspirating the liquid marrow into syringes. Several needle insertions/aspirations are required to collect the desired amount of marrow stem cells. The procedure lasts 1-2 hr.*
  Amount of bone marrow to be harvested. *About 500-1000 cc, depending on the number of marrow stem cells needed for engraftment. This is determined by the recipient's body size (usually 10 cc/kg body weight.) The aspirated marrow volume is replenished by the donor in about 2-3 wk.*
  Processing of bone marrow:
  Filtering of aspirated marrow to remove fat and bone particles.
  Collection of marrow stem cells into standard blood administration bag(s) *for further processing or intravenous infusion into recipient.*
  Postoperative care:
  Transfer from operating room to recovery room until patient recovers from anesthesia.
  Same day discharge or transfer to nursing unit if further observation indicated.
  Potential complications:
  Anesthesia-related complications.
  Fluid volume deficit (bonemarrow/peripheral blood volume loss).
  Bleeding from aspiration sites.
  Pain at aspiration site.
  Paresthesia (tingling/sharp pain radiating from posterior iliac crest to thigh and/or calf). *Caused by needle irritation or injury to sacral nerve plexus during aspirations.*
  Site care:
  Importance of keeping puncture sites clean, dry, and dressed for 72 hr after harvest or until healed.
  Signs and symptoms of infection to report.
  Pain Management:
  Use of analgesics before pain becomes severe.
  Avoidance of pressure against iliac crest; wearing of loose, nonrestrictive clothing.
  Use of shoes with low heels (sandals, tennis shoes) *to prevent "foot shock" (sensation of dull or sharp "ache" radiating from heel to pelvic bone).*
  Activity:
  Return to all activities as tolerated.

Fear

RELATED FACTORS

Impending surgery
Threat of anesthesia
Anticipated pain
Threat to or change in health status
Threat of death
Feelings about bone marrow recipient
Responsibility of being donor
Fear of unknown

DEFINING CHARACTERISTICS

Increased questioning
Restlessness
Tense appearance
Uncertainty
Jitteriness
Apprehension

EXPECTED OUTCOMES

Patient verbalizes reduction in fear.
Patient verbalizes ability to cope.
Patient expresses willingness, commitment, and positive feelings about being a donor.

ONGOING ASSESSMENT

- Assess level of fear and normal coping patterns.
- Assess patient's relationship with bone marrow recipient if appropriate. *Patient may feel "obligated" or "pressured" to donate marrow especially when it is the only tissue "match" suitable for transplantation.*

THERAPEUTIC INTERVENTIONS

- Reassure patient that fear is normal.
- Encourage verbalization of feelings, especially about donor role, if appropriate.
- Explore potential economic hardships (e.g., loss of work time, cost of travel and hospitalization).
- ▲ Involve other staff (social work, psychiatric liaison, etc.) as indicated.
- Assist patient in use of previously successful coping measures.
- Provide environment of confidence and reassurance.
- See also Fear, p. 23.

High Risk for Fluid Volume Deficit

RISK FACTORS

Restricted intake before procedure
Bone marrow volume loss
Peripheral blood volume loss
Bleeding from bone marrow aspiration sites
Postanesthesia vomiting

EXPECTED OUTCOMES

Patient maintains normal fluid volume, as evidenced by balanced I & O, normal skin turgor, normal blood pressure.

ONGOING ASSESSMENT

- Assess for signs of fluid volume deficit: dizziness, tachycardia, hypotension, decreased skin turgor, hemoconcentration, decreased urine output.
- Review operating room (OR) records to determine total volume of bone marrow collected.
- Assess I & O from IV infusions, packed RBC transfusions (intra- and postoperative), vomitus, urine as appropriate.
- ▲ Monitor lab (e.g., serum electrolytes, Hct) values as prescribed.
- Inspect pressure dressings over bone marrow aspiration site(s) frequently *to detect signs of undue oozing or hemorrhage. Dressings may have small areas of blood (normal). May be caused by residual effects of preoperative heparin bolus administered to facilitate marrow aspiration.*
- ▲ Monitor PT/PTT as prescribed.

THERAPEUTIC INTERVENTIONS

- ▲ Initiate IV therapy with lactated Ringer's solution or normal saline solution as prescribed.
- ▲ Reinfuse patient's own red cells as soon as available (if patient is own donor, i.e., autologous marrow).
- If patient is nauseous, give clear liquid diet and advance as tolerated.
- ▲ Administer antiemetics as prescribed *to minimize/prevent postanesthesia vomiting.*
- Reinforce pressure dressings as needed.
- ▲ If bleeding persists, administer protamine sulfate as prescribed *(to neutralize heparin).*
- Instruct patient to move slowly and bed *to prevent dizziness/hypotension*
- See also Fluid volume deficit, p. 25.

Continued.

Bone Marrow Harvest: Care of the Bone Marrow Donor

NURSING DIAGNOSES	EXPECTED OUTCOMES AND NURSING INTERVENTIONS / *RATIONALE* (■ = INDEPENDENT; ▲ = COLLABORATIVE)

Pain/Discomfort

RELATED FACTORS

Multiple puncture wounds in skin and bone
Endotracheal intubation (if procedure performed under general anesthesia)
Injection site of local anesthetic (if procedure performed under spinal anesthesia)

DEFINING CHARACTERISTICS

Facial grimacing
Moaning
Verbal complaints of discomfort and pain
Restlessness
Autonomic responses seen in acute pain (diaphoresis, changes in BP, pulse rate, increased or decreased respiratory rate)
Sore throat
Headache

EXPECTED OUTCOMES

Patient verbalizes relief of pain.
Patient appears comfortable.

ONGOING ASSESSMENT

- Assess patient for signs/symptoms of discomfort (see Defining Characteristics).
- Evaluate effectiveness of pain medication and nonmedication measures to relieve pain.

THERAPEUTIC INTERVENTIONS

- Encourage patient to request analgesic at early sign of discomfort *to prevent severe pain.*
- ▲ Administer analgesics as prescribed; evaluate effectiveness, observe for any signs/symptoms of adverse effects.
- Offer throat lozenges, popsicles/cold beverages as needed. *These are soothing to throat and mucous membranes irritated by endotracheal intubation.*
- Reposition as needed; use pillows for support.
- Handle patient gently and carefully.
- Avoid use of rolling board *to prevent exacerbation of discomfort/pain.*
- See also Pain, p. 49.

High Risk for Infection

RISK FACTORS

Interruption of skin and bone integrity secondary to bone marrow aspirations

EXPECTED OUTCOMES

Patient is free of infection, as evidenced by normal temperature, no drainage from puncture sites.

ONGOING ASSESSMENT

- Observe puncture sites at time of dressing change for evidence of infection: skin puncture sites red, tender, warm, swollen; drainage from skin puncture sites; persisting or increasing pain at operative site or near surrounding area; elevated body temperature.
- ▲ Obtain culture if ordered before wound cleansed *to obtain true sample of microorganisms present.*

THERAPEUTIC INTERVENTIONS

- Change postoperative pressure dressing day after harvest.
- Use aseptic technique when performing daily dressing changes: wipe over *each* skin puncture site with *new* Betadine wipe; let dry; apply small amount of Betadine ointment to each puncture site; cover with sterile adhesive bandage; keep dressings dry and intact.
- Report first signs of infection.

See also:
Impaired Mobility, p. 47
Ineffective Breathing Pattern, p. 10

By: Christa M. Schroeder, RN, MSN
Victoria Frazier-Jones, RN, BSN

Breast cancer/mastectomy

Breast cancer is the most common cancer in American women, occuring in one out of nine. It is the second leading cause of death in women between the ages of 35 and 54 years. With the use of breast self-examination and early mammography, breast cancer is being diagnosed at an earlier stage. In reality, breast cancer is many diseases depending on the type of tissue involved, the age of the patient, and whether the patient is estrogen-dependent. Treatment is dictated by the staging of the tumor. It may include surgery, irradiation, and chemotherapy. Prognosis is related to the type of tumor and the number of nodes involved. The use of adjuvant chemohormonal therapy has decreased recurrence and improved survival rate in most subgroups of patients. However, metastatic breast cancer is still considered incurable with standard therapies.

Mastectomy: segmented and modified radical

A segmented mastectomy involves removal of a quadrant of the breast or of only a tumor. A modified radical mastectomy involves removal of the breast and axillary contents, leaving the pectoral muscles intact to facilitate reconstruction. These procedures are currently done in the presence of malignant breast tumors. Breast-sparing lumpectomies are also performed. There is considerable controversy about the type of surgery and combination of therapies (i.e., radiation therapy, chemotherapy, and surgical intervention) that ensure no recurrence of malignant disease. This care plan addresses the care of a patient post mastectomy. See also Cancer Chemotherapy, p. 403.

NURSING DIAGNOSES	EXPECTED OUTCOMES AND NURSING INTERVENTIONS / *RATIONALE* (■ = INDEPENDENT; ▲ = COLLABORATIVE)

Knowledge Deficit

RELATED FACTORS

Unfamiliarity with proposed treatment plan and procedures

Uncertainty about treatment options

Misinterpretation of information

Decisional conflict

DEFINING CHARACTERISTICS

Expressed need for information

Verbalized confusion over treatment options

Verbalized misconceptions

Multiple questions

EXPECTED OUTCOMES

Patient verbalizes understanding of breast cancer, its diagnosis, various treatment options, and prognosis.

ONGOING ASSESSMENT

- Solicit understanding of diagnostic/metastatic testing.
- Assess understanding of relationship of stage of disease to prognosis and treatment.
- Assess understanding of treatment strategies: surgery, irradiation, chemotherapy, hormonal therapy, autologous bone marrow transplantation.

THERAPEUTIC INTERVENTIONS

- Describe rationale for diagnostic/metastatic testing procedures:

  Physical examination of breasts: *Lesion usually occurs in upper outer quadrant of the breast. It is usually hard, irregularly shaped, nonmobile, and poorly delineated.*

  Complete physical with pelvic examination, evaluation for signs of cancer in other locations (e.g., lymph nodes, liver)

  Blood tests to determine:

  Organ function and detect metastases (e.g., liver function tests (SGOT, LDH, alkaline phosphatase)

  Tumor markers (e.g., serum carcinoembryonic antigen (CEA) and CA 15-3) *to help determine prognosis and monitor course of disease.*

  Tumor tissue test, including hormone receptor assays, DNA, and other protein markers with potential diagnostic and prognostic value. *Estrogen and progesterone are the female hormones that affect breast cancer tissue. The amount of estrogen and progesterone receptors present in a tumor signifies that tumor's dependence on these hormones. Tumors are classified as estrogen or progesterone (ER/PR) positive or negative on the basis of the amount of receptor protein present. This classification determines tumor behavior and treatment. Tumors with positive receptors (usually more prevalent in postmenopausal women) are associated with better prognosis and longer survival.*

  Mammography. *To locate position/extent of known tumor and to screen for presence of other masses not detected on physical examination. Not all cancers are detected by this technique.*

Continued.

NURSING DIAGNOSES	EXPECTED OUTCOMES AND NURSING INTERVENTIONS / *RATIONALE* (■ = INDEPENDENT; ▲ = COLLABORATIVE)

THERAPEUTIC INTERVENTIONS— cont'd

Bone scan. *To rule out bone metastasis.*

CT scan. *To evaluate dense breasts and abdomen.*

Breast biopsies. *Usually performed by fine needle aspiration, needle core biopsy, open biopsy, or needle localization for microscopic examination to confirm benign or malignant tissue diagnosis and for surgical removal of lump or tumor.*

- Discuss rationale for selected treatment based on site, type, and stage of tumor.

The TNM classification system. *This system is used to stage breast cancer according to extent of primary tumor (T), absence or presence of regional lymph node metastasis (N), and absence or presence of distant metastasis (M).*

Clinical stages. *The clinical stages range from stage 0 to IV. Stage 0 implies in situ (localized) cancer; stage IV implies extensive metastasis.*

Stage 0: Usually treated by segmental mastectomy with or without radiation.

Stages I-II: Treated by lumpectomy, segmental mastectomy with radiation therapy/ modified radical or total mastectomy with adjuvant chemotherapy/radiation therapy.

Stages III-IV: Modified radical or radical mastectomy; chemotherapy/radiation/ hormonal therapy/autologous bone marrow transplantation.

Chemoprevention. *Is a new research area. Involves the prophylactic use of Tamoxifen in women at high risk for development of breast cancer.*

- Provide information and clarify misconceptions about newer treatment approaches:

Autologous bone marrow transplantation (ABMT). *Efficacy of treatment for metastatic/ high-risk early stage breast cancer is under clinical investigation. Studies suggest that ABMT offers a chance for long-term disease control rather than cure.*

Hormonal therapy. *Goal is to increase survival time in women with metastatic disease. ER/PR receptor-positive tumors respond well to hormonal treatment with the antiestrogen Tamoxifen, which blocks the action of estrogen in tumor cells.*

- Provide appropriate teaching materials (videotape, slide presentation, booklet) as adjunct to individualized education. Contact the National Cancer Institute in Bethesda, Maryland (1-800-4-CANCER) for additional patient teaching materials.

High Risk for Pain

RISK FACTORS

Contraction of tissue resulting from surgery and healing process

Intraoperative arm position

Possible injury to brachial plexus

Lymphedema

EXPECTED OUTCOMES

Patient verbalizes reduced pain/discomfort.

Patient appears comfortable.

Patient performs ROM with minimal discomfort.

ONGOING ASSESSMENT

- Note subjective reports of pain/discomfort.
- Assess neurovascular status of affected arm immediately after surgery and at regular intervals *for early detection of potential brachial plexus injury.*
- Measure biceps 2 in above elbow of affected arm immediately after surgery and every shift *to detect increase in circumference.*
- Evaluate ROM of affected arm.
- Report signs of infections/phlebitis in affected arm (pain, redness, warmth, swelling).

THERAPEUTIC INTERVENTIONS

- Prevent constriction of affected arm *to prevent impaired circulation.*
- Keep arm elevated on two pillows while patient in bed *to decrease edema and promote lymph drainage.*
- Protect affected arm from injury. *Mastectomy procedures remove the lymph nodes and lymphatic vessels draining the arm on the involved side of the body, thus increasing the risk of injury/infection in the involved arm.*
- Post notice at head of bed: no BP reading, no blood drawing, no IV, no injections.
- Instruct, encourage patient in straight extension and abduction exercises (straight elbow raises and wall climbing) on first postoperative day *to increase ROM progressively:*

Perform exercises 5-10 times/hr as tolerated *to prevent abduction and stiffness of shoulder and to promote lymphatic drainage and reduce swelling of the arm.*

Continue for 1 mo after surgery.

▲ Obtain elastic sleeve for affected arm with severe lymphedema (as prescribed) *to stimulate circulation.*

▲ Administer analgesics for pain.

NURSING DIAGNOSES	EXPECTED OUTCOMES AND NURSING INTERVENTIONS / *RATIONALE* (■ = INDEPENDENT; ▲ = COLLABORATIVE)

High Risk for Injury: Seroma

RISK FACTORS
Altered lymph drainage
Drain malfunction

EXPECTED OUTCOMES
Patient is at reduced risk for injury, as evidenced by absence of postoperative complications such as drain malfunction, lymphatic stasis.

ONGOING ASSESSMENT
- Immediately after surgery and at regular intervals, check drain for vacuum, clots, air leaks, diminished/absent drain output. *Seroma formation is the most common complication post surgery.*
- Document amount of output from drain.
- Assess for presence of fluid accumulation beneath flap.
- Assess for flap tenderness.

THERAPEUTIC INTERVENTIONS
- ▲ Milk/strip drain tubing q1hr *to maintain patency.*
- ▲ Notify physician of drain malfunctions, fluid accumulation beneath flap.

High Risk for Self-Esteem Disturbance/Body Image Disturbance

RISK FACTORS
Excision of breast and adjacent tissue
Beginning scar tissue
Asymmetric breasts caused by implant or prosthesis fit
Diagnosis of cancer

EXPECTED OUTCOMES
Patient adjusts to changes in body image, as evidenced by use of positive coping strategies, use of available resources, decreased/absent number of self-deprecating remarks.

ONGOING ASSESSMENT
- Assess for impact of change in patient's self-perceptions after surgery, such as behavior focused on altered body part, concerns about loss of femininity/sexual identity, negative feelings about body image. *The disfiguring surgery may be devastating to self-esteem.*

THERAPEUTIC INTERVENTIONS
- Encourage patient to verbalize feelings about effects of surgery on ability to perform roles, such as woman, sexual partner, worker.
- Assist patient in wearing temporary, nonweighted prosthetic insert at time of discharge. *Weighted prosthesis can be worn after healing.*
- Provide information on shops specializing in prostheses.
- Encourage family (especially husband) to provide positive input (e.g., feelings of being loved and needed). *The patient may have difficulty if social supports are limited or impaired.*
- Contact Reach-to-Recovery volunteer, facilitate visit. *Contact with women who have successfully dealt with mastectomy can help patients before surgery and afterward when they are struggling to adjust to its impact on life.*
- Help patient get information about reconstruction. *Disfigurement caused by amputation need not be permanent; reconstruction techniques are effective.*
- See also Body Image Disturbance, p. 7.

High Risk for Anxiety/Fear

RISK FACTORS
Breast loss
Diagnosis of cancer
Uncertain prognosis

EXPECTED OUTCOMES
Patient/family demonstrate reduced levels of anxiety, as evidenced by use of positive coping strategies, decreased/absent number of verbalized fearful, helpless, or other self-defeating statements.

ONGOING ASSESSMENT
- Assess for signs of anxiety/fear such as withdrawal, crying, restlessness, inability to focus. *The threat to health, life, and role resulting from cancer can predispose one to anxiety.*
- Assess previous successful coping strategies. *These may be useful in dealing with current crisis.*

THERAPEUTIC INTERVENTIONS
- Encourage patient to verbalize feelings; allow her to grieve for her loss and to express her anger, fears, and anxiety.
- Reassure patient that these feelings are normal.
- Assist in use of previously successful coping measures *(may need to be modified for this crisis).*
- ▲ Involve other departments (psychiatry, social services) as indicated for supportive care.
- Support realistic assessment; avoid false reassurance.
- See also Fear, p. 23; Anxiety, p. 5.

Continued.

NURSING DIAGNOSES	EXPECTED OUTCOMES AND NURSING INTERVENTIONS / *RATIONALE* (■ = INDEPENDENT; ▲ = COLLABORATIVE)

Knowledge Deficit

RELATED FACTORS

Lack of similar experience
Unfamiliarity with information resources
Information misinterpretation

DEFINING CHARACTERISTICS

Verbalized knowledge deficit
Demonstrated inability to grasp information
Questioning

EXPECTED OUTCOMES

Patient verbalizes importance of follow-up care and proper wound/arm care.

ONGOING ASSESSMENT

- Assess knowledge of home care and health maintenance.

THERAPEUTIC INTERVENTIONS

- Teach about wound/arm care:
    Arm will be stiff and sore; stiffness will cease but armpit numbness will remain for a long time if nodes were dissected.
    Continue exercises at least 1 mo *to ease tension in arm/shoulder and maintain muscle tone.*
    Protect arm from injury and infection.
    Use electric razor when shaving, gloves when gardening or doing dishes, and mitts when handling hot dishes.
    Avoid blood draws, IVs/injections during subsequent hospitalizations.
    Avoid tight-fitting sleeves, watches, jewelry.
    Carry heavy packages or handbags in other arm.
    Use of deodorant is safe.
    Massage incision site gently with cocoa butter or vitamin E cream *to promote healing and skin softness.*
    Wear temporary prosthesis or brassiere from time of discharge *to help adjust to recent loss of breast.*
- Explain activity guidelines: return to all activities as tolerated, resumption of sexual activity as tolerated, swimming permitted after prosthesis obtained, driving resumed as tolerated.
- Instruct regarding follow-up care:
    Importance of monthly breast self examination (BSE),
    Annual mammogram of remaining breast. *Increased risk of cancer: 15% develop breast cancer in the opposite breast. Mammography is a valuable complement to BSE; it offers the advantage of identifying breast malignancies before they become palpable.*
    Reconstructive surgery (if desired) usually done within 3 mo of surgery. *It is contraindicated in locally advanced, progressively metastatic, or inflammatory breast cancer.*
    Importance for large breasted women to be fitted for weighted prosthesis as soon as wound heals *to provide balance for proper posture.*
- Inform regarding family needs:
    May be familial breast cancer tendency *as risk is increased 2-3 times in daughters or sisters of women with breast cancer, and 7-8 times in daughters or sisters of women with premenopausal bilateral breast cancer.*
    All women in family over age 20 should examine breasts monthly.
    Women over age 35 should have annual mammogram.
- Instruct on follow-up consultation with medical and radiation specialist depending on nodal status.
- Provide appropriate educational materials from the American Cancer Society/National Cancer Institute/WYCA's ENCORE program *to enhance learning compliance.*

See also:
Chemotherapy, p. 403.
Bone Marrow Transplant, p. 386.
Impaired Individual Coping, p. 18.
Anticipatory Grieving, p. 28.
Potential for Infection, p. 40.
Potential for Impaired Skin Integrity, p. 59.

By: Christa M. Schroeder, RN, MSN

Cancer chemotherapy

Cancer chemotherapy is the administration of cytotoxic drugs by various routes (topical, oral, intramuscular, subcutaneous [SQ], intravenous, intraarterial, intracavitary, intrathecal, and intravesicular), for the purpose of destroying malignant cells. The goal of chemotherapy may be cure, palliation, or symptom relief.

NURSING DIAGNOSES	EXPECTED OUTCOMES AND NURSING INTERVENTIONS / *RATIONALE* (■ = INDEPENDENT; ▲ = COLLABORATIVE)

Knowledge Deficit

RELATED FACTORS

Unfamiliarity with proposed treatment plan/procedures
Misinterpretations of information
Unfamiliarity with discharge/follow-up care

DEFINING CHARACTERISTICS

Verbalized lack of knowledge
Expressed need for information
Multiple questions
Lack of questions
Verbalized misconceptions
Verbalized confusion over events

EXPECTED OUTCOMES

Patient/significant other verbalize understanding of chemotherapy treatment, including rationale for treatment, self-management of interventions to prevent or control side effects, follow up care.

ONGOING ASSESSMENT

■ Solicit understanding of diagnosis, rationale for chemotherapy, goal of treatment, chemotherapeutic agents to be used, rationale for occurrence of side effects, strategies (including interventions for self-management) aimed at prevention or control of adverse side effects, method of chemotherapy administration, potential problems experienced during chemotherapy administration, schedule of overall treatment plan, anticipated length and number of hospitalizations, and clinic/office visits, follow-up care.

THERAPEUTIC INTERVENTIONS

■ Instruct patient/significant others as needed:
Treatment plan:
  Schedule and need for laboratory tests before and during treatment *to assess for electrolyte and metabolic changes, cardiac/pulmonary/renal alterations, bone marrow function, need for blood component transfusion(s), and presence of infection*
  Chemotherapy agents to be used
  Method of administration
  Schedule of administration
Chemotherapy:
  Potential short- and long-term side effects/toxicities
  Period of anticipated side effects/toxicities
  Preventive measures to minimize/alleviate potential side effects/toxicities
Discharge planning/teaching:
  ADLs
  Return to work or school
  Sexual relations/contraception
  Catheter care (central venous, arterial, intraperitoneal catheters/devices)
  Signs/symptoms to report to health care professionals (e.g., bleeding, fever, shortness of breath, intractable nausea/vomiting, inability to eat/drink, diarrhea)
  Measures to prevent infection (*patient's immune function impaired by chemotherapy-induced bone marrow suppression*)
  Importance of balanced diet and adequate fluid intake
  Dietary/medications restrictions if indicated
  Medication(s) after discharge
  Outpatient follow-up care after discharge
  Community resources/support systems

Body Image Disturbance

RELATED FACTORS

Loss of hair (scalp, eyebrows, eyelashes, pubic/body hair)
Discoloration of fingernails, veins
Breakage/loss of fingernails
Changes in skin color/texture
Generalized "wasting"

EXPECTED OUTCOMES

Patient verbalizes understanding of temporary nature of side effects.
Patient verbalizes positive remarks about self.

ONGOING ASSESSMENT

■ Assess for presence of Defining Characteristics.
■ Observe for verbal/nonverbal cues to note image alteration.

THERAPEUTIC INTERVENTIONS

■ Acknowledge normality of emotional response to actual/perceived changes in physical appearance. *For some patients the fear of treatment side effects can feel worse than the disease.*

Continued.

403

NURSING DIAGNOSES	EXPECTED OUTCOMES AND NURSING INTERVENTIONS / *RATIONALE* (■ = INDEPENDENT; ▲ = COLLABORATIVE)

DEFINING CHARACTERISTICS

Self-deprecating remarks
Refusal to look at self in mirror
Crying
Anger
Decreased attention to grooming
Verbalized ambivalence
Compensatory use of makeup, concealing makeup, clothing, devices
Decreased social interaction

THERAPEUTIC INTERVENTIONS—cont'd

- Encourage verbalization of feelings; listen to concerns *to alleviate anxiety.*
- Convey feelings of acceptance and understanding.
- Provide anticipatory guidance on hair alternatives, makeup, skin care, and clothing by supplying/recommending appropriate teaching materials.
- Offer realistic assurance of temporary nature of some physical changes. *Important that patient understand that hair/nails will regrow; external/implanted access devices will eventually be removed, etc.*
- Refer to support group. *Groups that get together for mutual support and information can be a valuable resource.*
- See also Body image disturbance, p. 7.

Altered Nutrition: Less than Body Requirements

RELATED TO

Treatment effects:
Side effects of chemotherapy (inability to taste and smell foods, loss of appetite, nausea, vomiting, mucositis, dry mouth, diarrhea)
Medications (e.g., narcotics, antibiotics, vitamins, iron, digitalis)
Disease effects:
Primary malignancy/metastasis to CNS
Increased intracranial pressure resulting from tumor, intracranial bleeding
Obstruction of GI tract by tumor
Tumor waste products
Renal dysfunction
Electrolyte imbalances (e.g., hypercalcemia, hyponatremia)
Pain
Psychogenic effects:
Conditioning to adversive stimuli (e.g., anticipatory nausea/vomiting; tension, anxiety, stress)
Depression

DEFINING CHARACTERISTICS

Weight loss
Documented inadequate caloric intake
Weakness; fatigue
Poor skin turgor
Dry, shiny oral mucous membranes
Thick, scanty saliva
Muscle wasting

EXPECTED OUTCOMES

Patient maintains optimal nutritional status as evidenced by caloric intake adequate to meet body requirements, balanced intake and output, weight gain or reduced loss, absence of nausea/vomiting, good skin turgor.

ONGOING ASSESSMENT

- Obtain history of previous patterns of nausea/vomiting, treatment measures effective in past.
- Solicit patient's description of nausea/vomiting pattern.
- Evaluate effectiveness of antiemetic/comfort measure regimens.
- Observe patient for potential complications of prolonged nausea/vomiting: fluid/electrolyte imbalance (e.g., dehydration, hypokalemia, decreased Na and Cl), weight loss, decreased activity level, weakness, lethargy, apathy, anxiety, aspiration pneumonia, esophageal trauma, and tenderness/pain in abdomen and chest.
- Weigh patient daily at same time with same scale *to assure accuracy.*
- Monitor calorie counts daily *to determine whether oral intake meets daily nutritional requirement.*
- ▲ Monitor appropriate lab values (e.g., CBC/differential, electrolytes, serum iron, TIBC, total protein, albumin). *These reflect nutritional/fluid status.*

THERAPEUTIC INTERVENTIONS

- ▲ Administer antiemetics around the clock rather than "prn" during periods of high incidence of nausea/vomiting. *They maintain adequate plasma levels and thus increase effectiveness of antiemetic therapy.*
- Institute/teach measures to minimize/prevent nausea/vomiting:
  Small dietary intake before treatment(s)
  Foods with low potential to cause nausea/vomiting (e.g., dry toast, crackers, ginger ale, cola, Popsicles, gelatin, baked/boiled potatoes, fresh/canned fruit)
  Avoidance of spices, gravy, or greasy foods
  Modifications in diet (e.g., choice of bland foods)
  Small, frequent nutritious meals
  Attractive servings
  Avoidance of coaxing, bribing, or threatening in relation to intake. (Help family to avoid being "food pushers.")
  Sufficient time for meals
  Rest periods before and after meals
  Sucking on hard candy while receiving chemotherapeutic drugs with "metallic taste" (e.g., Cytoxan, Dacarbazine (DTIC), Cisplatinum, Actinomycin D, Mustargen, Methotrexate)
  Minimal physical activity and no sudden rapid movement during times of increased nausea (*may actually potentiate nausea/vomiting*)
  Quiet, restful, cool, well-ventilated environment
  Comfortable position
  Diversional activities
  Relaxation/distraction techniques
  Antiemetic half hour before meals as prescribed

NURSING DIAGNOSES	EXPECTED OUTCOMES AND NURSING INTERVENTIONS / *RATIONALE* (■ = INDEPENDENT; ▲ = COLLABORATIVE)

THERAPEUTIC INTERVENTIONS—cont'd

- Identify and provide favorite foods; avoid serving during nausea/vomiting. *Patient may develop aversion.*
- Explain rationale and measures to increase sensitivity of taste buds: perform mouth care before and after meals; change seasonings to compensate for altered sweet/sour threshold; increase use of sweeteners/flavorings in foods; warm foods to increase aroma.
- Serve foods cold if odors cause aversions.
- Offer meat dishes in morning. *Aversions tend to increase during day: chicken, cheese, eggs, fish usually well-tolerated protein sources.*
- Serve supplements between meals; have patient sip slowly *to prevent bloating/nausea/vomiting/diarrhea.*
- Explain rationale and measures to provide moisture in oral cavity if indicated:
    Frequent intake of nonirritating fluids (e.g., grape or apple juice)
    Sucking on smooth, flat substances (e.g., lozenges; tart, sugar-free candy; hot tea with lemon) *to increase saliva flow*
    Use of artificial saliva
    Liquids sipped with meals
    Foods moistened with sauces/liquids
    Strict oral hygiene before and after meals; avoidance of alcohol-containing commercial mouthwashes or lemon-glycerin swabs *(drying to oral mucosa)*
    Lips moistened with balm, water-soluble lubricating jelly, lanolin, or cocoa butter
    Humid environment air via vaporizer or pan of water near heat *(except when patient is luekopenic because of risk of Pseudomonas infection).*
- ▲ Titrate dosage/frequency of antiemetic(s)/analgesic(s) within prescribed parameters as needed until effective therapeutic levels are achieved.
- Position patient during vomiting episode *to decrease aspiration risk.*

High Risk for Infection

RISK FACTORS

Treatment effects:
Granulocytopenia/leukopenia secondary to bone marrow toxicity of chemotherapy
Side effect of radiation therapy with bone marrow producing sites in treatment field (e.g., skull, sternum, ribs, vertebrae, pelvis, ends of long bones)
Disease effects:
Invasion or "crowding" of bone marrow by malignant cells (especially secondary to hematologic malignancies, e.g., leukemia, lymphoma, multiple myeloma)
Anergy (absence of immune response)

EXPECTED OUTCOMES

Patient has reduced risk of local/systemic infection as evidenced by afebrile state, absence of sore throat/cough, normal CBC.

ONGOING ASSESSMENT

- Assess for signs of infection: fever, sore throat, tachycardia, urinary frequency/burning, redness/tenderness over peripheral IV/central line sites.
- ▲ Monitor WBC, differential, and absolute granulocyte count daily. *Absolute granulocyte count (AGC) calculated by multiplying white blood cell (WBC) count by percentage of granulocytes in differential (e.g., AGC = WBC × % granulocytes).*

THERAPEUTIC INTERVENTIONS

- Determine anticipated nadir and recovery of bone marrow after chemotherapy administration *to plan for appropriate nursing care measures. Nadir: time of greatest bone marrow suppression (e.g., when RBCs, WBCs, and platelets at lowest points). Each chemotherapeutic agent causes nadir at different time for each blood element; however, most drugs demonstrate nadir 7-14 days after start of chemotherapy with bone marrow recovery over another 5-10 days.*
- See also Granulocytopenia, p. 413; Leukemia, acute, p. 420.

High Risk for Injury: Bleeding

RISK FACTORS

Treatment effects:
Thrombocytopenia secondary to bone marrow toxicity of chemotherapy/radiation therapy
Mucosal soughing
Anticoagulants

EXPECTED OUTCOMES

Patient has reduced risk of bleeding as evidenced by platelets within acceptable limits, coagulation/fibrinogen within acceptable limits, absence of overt and occult bleeding.

ONGOING ASSESSMENT

- ▲ Monitor platelets daily *to detect changes early;* anticipate platelet count nadir.
- ▲ Monitor coagulation parameters (fibrinogen, thrombin time, bleeding time, fibrin degradation products) if indicated. *Changes in coagulation profile may be marked by ecchymoses, hematomas, petechia, blood in body excretions, bleeding from body orifices, change in neurologic status.*
- Monitor vital signs for increased heart rate, decreased blood pressure.

Continued.

NURSING DIAGNOSES	EXPECTED OUTCOMES AND NURSING INTERVENTIONS / *RATIONALE* (■ = INDEPENDENT; ▲ = COLLABORATIVE)

RISK FACTORS—cont'd

Disease effects:
Invasion of bone marrow by malignant cells
Disease of bone marrow
Genetically transmitted platelet deficiency coagulopathies (tumor-related or other)
Abnormal hepatic/renal function
Fever
Infection/sepsis
DIC
Pharmacologic effects:
Aspirin/indocin

ONGOING ASSESSMENT—cont'd
- Inspect patient regularly for evidence of:
  Spontaneous petechiae (all skin surfaces, including oral mucosa)
  Prolonged bleeding or new areas of ecchymoses or hematoma from invasive procedures (venipuncture, injection, and bone marrow sites)
  Oozing of blood from nose/gums

THERAPEUTIC INTERVENTIONS
- Inform patient/significant other of relationship between platelets and bleeding:
  Platelet function
  Normal platelet count
  Effects of chemotherapy on bone marrow function, platelet count
  Risk of bleeding associated with decreased platelet count:
    <20,000/mm^3: severe risk
    20,000-50,000/mm^3: moderately severe risk
    50,000-100,000/mm^3: mild risk
    >100,000/mm^3: no significant risk
- ▲ Implement bleeding precautions for platelet count <50,000/mm^3. *At this level spontaneous bleeding can occur.*
- See also Leukemia, acute, p. 420, for bleeding precautions/nursing interventions.
- Emphasize to patient/significant other the importance of consistent practice of measures to prevent bleeding and of prompt reporting of all signs/symptoms of suspected or actual bleeding.
- ▲ Communicate anticipated need for platelet support to transfusion center *to assure availability, readiness of platelets when needed (e.g., platelets <20,000/mm^3 or in presence of active bleeding).*
- ▲ Transfuse single or random donor platelets as ordered.
- ▲ Administer fresh frozen plasma or coagulation factors as prescribed *to replace needed clotting factors.*

High Risk for Injury: Anemia

RISK FACTORS

Treatment effects:
Anemia secondary to bone marrow toxicity of chemotherapy/radiation therapy
Disease effects:
Primary disease bone marrow (e.g., leukemia, aplastic anemia)
Infiltration of bone marrow by malignant cells
Autoimmune disorders
Renal disease
Exposure to toxic substances (e.g., benzene, antibiotics)
Nutritional deficiencies (e.g., decreased vitamin K, folic acid, B$_{12}$, iron intake absorption/use)

EXPECTED OUTCOMES

Patient is free of anemia, as evidenced by heart rate, blood pressure within normal limits, Hb/Hct within normal limits, ability to perform ADLs.

ONGOING ASSESSMENT
- Assess for signs of anemia: tiredness, weakness, lethargy, fatigue; pallor (skin, nailbeds, conjunctiva, circumoral); dyspnea on exertion, palpitations/chest pain on exertion; dizziness/syncope; hypersensitivity to cold, increased pulse, decreased blood pressure.
- ▲ Monitor Hb/Hct daily *to detect changes early;* anticipate nadir.
- Determine nadir, anticipated recovery of bone marrow after chemotherapy administration.

THERAPEUTIC INTERVENTIONS
- Estimate energy expenditures of ADLs; prioritize activities accordingly.
- Plan/promote rest periods *to lower body's oxygen requirement and decrease cardiopulmonary strain.*
- Provide warm clothing/blankets, comfortable environment; avoid drafts.
- ▲ Maintain current blood sample for "type and screen" in transfusion center *to assure availability, readiness of packed red blood cells when needed.*
- ▲ Transfuse packed red cells as ordered *to restore Hb/Hct to levels where patient experiences minimal symptoms.*
- See also Blood and blood product transfusion therapy, p. 384; Aplastic anemia, p. 382.

NURSING DIAGNOSES	EXPECTED OUTCOMES AND NURSING INTERVENTIONS / *RATIONALE* (■ = INDEPENDENT; ▲ = COLLABORATIVE)

High Risk for Injury

RISK FACTORS

Hypersensitivity to drug(s)
Potential side effects/toxicities
of drug(s)

EXPECTED OUTCOMES

Patient has reduced risk of injury from drug therapy, as evidenced by normal vital signs, absence of reaction, prompt reporting of adverse signs/symptoms.

ONGOING ASSESSMENT

- Note allergy history.
- Monitor for potential hypersensitivity/side effects/toxicities to chemotherapeutic drugs: restlessness, facial edema/flushing, wheezes, bronchospasms, tachycardia, hypotension/ hypertension, diaphoresis, fever, increased uric acid levels, runny nose, skin rash, temporal-mandibular joint pain, frontal sinusitis, ileus, diarrhea.
- Monitor for hypersensitivity/side effects/toxicities to common antiemetic drugs: agitation/ restlessness, hypotension/tachycardia, irritability, facial flushing, extrapyramidal reactions, dry mouth, sedation, blurred vision, drowsiness/dizziness, headache, diarrhea/urine retention.
- ▲ Monitor relevant lab data. *CBC, differential, platelets, ECG provide baseline and response data.*
- See also Tumor lysis syndrome, p. 429.

THERAPEUTIC INTERVENTIONS

- Verify written order for specific drug name, dose, route, time, and frequency of antiemetic/chemotherapy drugs to be administered.
- Know immediate and delayed side effects of drug(s) to be administered.
- Inform patient/significant other to report adverse effects. Delineate which changes indicate emergencies that must be reported immediately (*changes patient perceives as "minor" may be highly significant*).
- Maintain/restore adequate fluid balance *to reduce potential drug toxicity as fluids help clear body of accumulated metabolic by-products.*
- ▲ Keep emergency drugs (IV Benadryl, hydrocortisone, Epinephrine 1:1000) readily available when administering chemotherapeutic drugs with higher than usual risk for anaphylaxis (e.g., Bleomycin, Elspar, Cis-Platin, and Etoposide).
- ▲ When adverse drug reaction is suspected, stop infusion; administer emergency drugs as prescribed; notify physician; take and record vital signs; maintain KVO IV with normal saline (NS) solution; reassure patient.
- See also Anaphylactic shock, p. 156.

High Risk for Injury

RISK FACTORS

Extravasation
Infiltration or leakage of chemotherapeutic drug from vein

EXPECTED OUTCOMES

Patient is free of complications of drug extravasation, as evidenced by absence of pain/ discomfort at infusion site, adequate blood return from peripheral or central venous catheter, prompt reporting of early signs/symptoms.

ONGOING ASSESSMENT

- Assess at frequent intervals per established hospital policy/procedure: blood return, patency of vein/catheter, signs of infiltration (*defective or malpositioned indwelling central venous catheter/access device into local subcutaneous tissue surrounding administration site*).
- Observe injection/infusion site closely during chemotherapy administration.

THERAPEUTIC INTERVENTIONS

- Select veins most suitable for administration of chemotherapeutic agents. *These are cephalic, median brachial, and basilic vein in midforearm area.*
- Avoid veins in anticubital fossa, near wrist, or dorsal surface of hand. *Damage to underlying tendons/nerves may occur in event of drug extravasation.*
- Instruct patient to report tenderness, stinging, burning, or other unusual sensation at IV site immediately.
- Evaluate patient complaints of "painful infusion"; rule out source extravasation versus other causes of pain (may include chemical composition of drug, venous spasm, phlebitis, and/or psychogenic factors).

Continued.

Hematolymphatic and Oncologic Care Plans

NURSING DIAGNOSES	EXPECTED OUTCOMES AND NURSING INTERVENTIONS / *RATIONALE* (■ = INDEPENDENT; ▲ = COLLABORATIVE)
	THERAPEUTIC INTERVENTIONS— cont'd
	▪ Know local toxicity of chemotherapeutic agent(s) administered and hospital policy/procedure of intervention in event of extravasation.
	▲ Keep extravasation kit accessible. *Contents vary according to hospital policy.*
	▲ When drug extravasation is suspected: stop infusion; initiate extravasation management appropriate for chemotherapeutic drug infiltrated; notify physician; reassure patient; document incident per institutional policy/procedure. *Management of site after extravasation remains a controversial issue in chemotherapy administration. However, most hospitals/agencies have developed care standards in management of extravasation of drugs classified as "vesicants." These agents potentially cause cellular damage, ulceration, and tissue necrosis. Plastic surgeon may be consulted for consideration of débridement/skin grafting.*

See also:
Anxiety/Fear, p. 5, 23.
Impaired Oral Mucous Membranes, p. 46.
Diarrhea, p. 19.
Fluid Volume Deficit, p. 25.
Fluid Volume Excess, p. 26.
Tumor Lysis Syndrome, p. 429.
Central Venous Access, p. 408.

By: Christa M. Schroeder, RN, MSN

Central venous access devices

Indwelling silicone rubber catheter placed in the right atrium, or an infusion port consisting of a metal or plastic chamber with a self-sealing silicone rubber septum (attached to a silicone catheter) implanted beneath the skin. Common catheters include the Broviac, Hickman and Groshong catheters and implantation of an infusion port (Port-a-cath).

NURSING DIAGNOSES	EXPECTED OUTCOMES AND NURSING INTERVENTIONS / *RATIONALE* (■ = INDEPENDENT; ▲ = COLLABORATIVE)
High Risk for Injury: Impaired Catheter Function	**EXPECTED OUTCOMES** Patient's catheter function is maintained, as evidenced by patency with acceptable two-way function (in and outflow).
RISK FACTORS Mechanical impairment (e.g., clotting of catheter) Catheter break/malposition	**ONGOING ASSESSMENT** ▪ Inspect for catheter integrity: check for patency; observe for kinks; note leakage or resistance when flushing line; observe gravitational flow (e.g., in transfusion of blood products); check clamp; check patency of Huber needle.
	THERAPEUTIC INTERVENTIONS ▪ Avoid use of scissors; use noncrushing clamps/hemostats when needed *to prevent catheter damage.* ▲ Flush catheter per established institutional policy/procedure *to prevent catheter clotting:* at the end of every blood drawing procedure, at completion of each IV solution and blood product, before capping catheter. ▪ Avoid coadministration of incompatible solutions *as this may cause precipitation within the catheter and eventual obstruction.*

NURSING DIAGNOSES	EXPECTED OUTCOMES AND NURSING INTERVENTIONS / *RATIONALE* (■ = INDEPENDENT; ▲ = COLLABORATIVE)

THERAPEUTIC INTERVENTIONS— cont'd

- Use mechanical IV pumps *to prevent "dry" IVs and backing up of blood into catheter.*
- Troubleshoot catheter/port for common problems (i.e., sluggish inflow and inability to draw blood).

 Alternate irrigation and aspiration of catheter using 15 ml of normal saline solution in a 30-cc syringe with patient in a lying, arm-raised, sitting, or side-lying position.

 Obtain prescription for use of Abbokinase-Open Cath for clearance of occuded catheter/port if other measures to restore catheter function are unsuccessful.

- ▲ Repair external damage per manufacturing company recommendations or established procedures.
- ▲ Notify physician of suspected internal catheter damage.

Pain

RELATED FACTORS

Difficult/traumatic insertion
Needle displacement from port
Tunnel phlebitis
Deep vein thrombosis

DEFINING CHARACTERISTICS

Report of discomfort
Edema of neck and extremity
Limited movement of extremity

EXPECTED OUTCOMES

Patient verbalizes relief of pain.
Patient appears comfortable.

ONGOING ASSESSMENT

- Check insertion site q4hr or prn for signs of inflammation or discomfort.
- Check site for swelling. If swelling is present, assess for catheter displacement, needle displacement from port, infection, deep vein thrombosis. *Check hand, arm, and neck on affected side for edema; compare to unaffected side.*

THERAPEUTIC INTERVENTIONS

- Maintain optimal position of extremity. Elevate distal portion of extremity.
- Avoid tight bandaging of affected extremity. Use occlusive but nonconstricting dressing *to allow adequate circulation.*
- *Promote circulation to affected extremity* by performing active/passive ROM, noting limitation of catheter.
- If pain, phlebitis, or inflammation occurs, facilitate removal of catheter; apply warm compresses.
- ▲ Administer analgesic before pain becomes severe.

High Risk for Infection

RISK FACTORS

Indwelling catheter
Manipulation of catheter connecting tubing
Prolonged use of catheter

EXPECTED OUTCOMES

Patient is free of infection, as evidenced by normal temperature, no signs of redness, warmth, or drainage.

ONGOING ASSESSMENT

- Check catheter site for signs of infection. *Redness, warmth, tenderness, "streaking" over subcutaneous tunnel and exudate from exit/portal pocket/or needle insertion site are signs of infection.*
- Assess vital signs q4hr as needed.

THERAPEUTIC INTERVENTIONS

- ▲ Follow institutional policy/procedure *to reduce possibility of contamination when performing the following:* changing IV solution, tubing, adapters or caps; changing site care and dressings; drawing blood; accessing/deaccessing port; flushing/heparinizing catheter.
- ▲ If infection is suspected, notify physician for culturing, treatment, and possible catheter removal *to prevent spread of infection.*

High Risk for Injury

RISK FACTORS

Blood vessel (vein/artery) injury at time of insertion
Irritation of ventricular endocardium by catheter during insertion/repositioning
Lodging of catheter tip in tricuspid valve
Use of subclavian insertion site
Less than optimal positioning during insertion

EXPECTED OUTCOMES

Patient is free of complications, as evidenced by normal cardiac rhythm, clear breath sounds, no shortness of breath, normal chest movement, absence of bleeding.

ONGOING ASSESSMENT

- Assess for signs of subclavian or carotid artery injury. *These may manifest as complaints of shortness of breath, hemoptysis, hypertension, swelling on affected side.*
- Observe patient for dysrhythmias after catheter insertion.
- ▲ Verify catheter position on chest radiograph and whenever dysrhythmias occur.
- If dysrhythmias occur:

 Assess patient for complaints of dizziness, palpitations, lightheadedness, shortness of breath.

 Observe contributing factors that may have potentiated dysrhythmias (e.g., patient/catheter position; other medical problems) *to correct/intervene as early as possible.*

Continued.

NURSING DIAGNOSES	EXPECTED OUTCOMES AND NURSING INTERVENTIONS / *RATIONALE* (▪ = INDEPENDENT; ▲ = COLLABORATIVE)
	ONGOING ASSESSMENT—cont'd ▪ Assess for signs of pneumothorax. *These may be manifested as shortness of breath, decreased breath sounds on affected side, unequal thoracic wall movement, or shift of trachea toward unaffected side.* ▲ When checking for catheter placement on radiograph, note lung expansion. **THERAPEUTIC INTERVENTIONS** ▪ Keep patient still during procedure, especially for subclavian site. Provide sedative, local anesthesia, and reassurances as needed. ▪ Provide optimal positioning at time of insertion (towel roll in back/shoulder/subclavian region) *to minimize risk of accidental puncture of pleura.* ▲ If pneumothorax symptoms noted, refer to physician and anticipate chest tube insertion. ▲ Provide oxygen as needed. ▲ Administer antidysrhythmia medications (usually lidocaine) as prescribed.

See also:
Anxiety/Fear, p. 5, 23.
Knowledge Deficit, p. 41.

By: Christa M. Schroeder, RN, MSN

Disseminated intravascular coagulation (DIC)

(COAGULOPATHY; DEFIBRINATION SYNDROME)

Inappropriate, accelerated consumption of coagulation factors resulting in hemorrhage. Disseminated intravascular coagulation always occurs secondary to some other abnormality and is associated with infection, neoplastic disorders, obstetric complications, tissue trauma, and burns.

NURSING DIAGNOSES	EXPECTED OUTCOMES AND NURSING INTERVENTIONS / *RATIONALE* (▪ = INDEPENDENT; ▲ = COLLABORATIVE)
High Risk for Injury: Bleeding/Fluid Deficit **RISK FACTORS** Depleted coagulation factors Adverse effects of heparin: excess heparin, insufficient heparin	**EXPECTED OUTCOMES** Patient's side effects of heparin therapy are reduced through ongoing assessment and early intervention. Patient experiences reduced episodes of bleeding/hematomas. Patient maintains optimal fluid balance, as evidenced by normotensive blood pressure, urine output >30 ml/hr. **ONGOING ASSESSMENT** ▲ Monitor coagulation profile: *prothrombin time (PT) >15 sec, partial thromboplastin time (PTT) >60-90 sec, hypofibrinogenemia, thrombocytopenia, elevated fibrin split products, prolonged bleeding time. All put patient at risk for increased bleeding.* ▲ Monitor Hct and Hb. ▪ Examine skin surface for signs of bleeding. Note petechiae, purpura, hematomas, oozing of blood from IV sites, drains, and wounds, and bleeding from mucous membranes. ▪ Observe for signs of bleeding from GI/GU tracts. ▪ Note any hemoptysis or blood obtained during suctioning. ▪ Observe for changes in mental status; institute neurologic checklist. *Mental status changes may occur with the decreased fluid volume or with decreasing Hb.* ▪ Monitor vital signs. Assess correlation of arterial line blood pressure to cuff blood pressure. ▪ Observe for signs of orthostatic hypotension (drop of greater than 15 mm when changing from supine to sitting position). *This indicates reduced circulating fluids.*

Ongoing Assessment—cont'd

- Note any adverse effects of heparin therapy *(Note that heparin aborts clotting process by blocking thrombin production)*:

    Any increase in bleeding from IV sites, GI/GU tracts, respiratory tract, wounds

    Development of new purpura, petechiae, or hematomas

- If bleeding is increased, notify physician of possible need to decrease drip.
- ▲ Monitor PTT. *The goal is to maintain PTT at twice the control level.*

Therapeutic Interventions

- Institute precautionary measures:

    Use only compressible vessels for IV sites.

    Avoid IM injections: *any needle stick is a potential bleeding site.*

    Draw all laboratory specimens through an existing line: arterial line or venous hep-lock line.

    Apply pressure to any oozing site.

    Prevent stable clots from dislodging through careful handling of patient; if clot dislodges, apply pressure and cold compress.

    Prevent trauma to catheters/tubes by proper taping; minimize pulling.

    Minimize number of cuff blood pressures; maintain arterial line.

    Use gentle suctioning *to prevent trauma to respiratory mucosa.*

    Provide gentle oral care.

    If patient is confused/agitated, pad side rails *to prevent bruising.*

- ▲ Administer heparin therapy as prescribed *to interrupt abnormal accelerated coagulation. Heparin interferes with production of thrombin, which is necessary for clot formation.*

    Infuse continuous heparin drip on infusion device (usually 1000-1500 U/hr).

    Maintain PTT at 2 times normal.

    Consider dosage alteration in patients with hepatic or renal failure.

    Titrate dose to lab values and clinical situation. *As clinical situation improves, heparin need decreases. Challenge lies in differentiating the blood loss as an untoward effect of heparin therapy from a worsening of DIC.*

- ▲ Administer parenteral fluids as prescribed. Anticipate the need for an IV fluid challenge with immediate infusion of fluids, for patients with abnormal vital signs.
- ▲ Administer blood products as prescribed; monitor patient response. Observe for transfusion reaction.

Impaired Gas Exchange

Related Factors

Inappropriate coagulation resulting in blood loss with decreased available hemoglobin

Generalized systemic microvascular clot formation

Defining Characteristics

Confusion

Somnolence

Restlessness

Irritability

Hypercapnia

Hypoxia

Expected Outcomes

Patient maintains optimal gas exchange as evidenced by normal ABGs, alert responsive mentation/or no further reduction in mental status.

Ongoing Assessment

- Assess respiratory rate, rhythm, and depth. *Rapid shallow respirations may result from hypoxia or from the acidosis with the shock state. Development of hypoventilation indicates that immediate ventilator support is needed.*
- Assess for any increase in work of breathing: shortness of breath, use of accessory muscles.
- Assess breath sounds.
- Assess for changes in orientation and behavior. *Early signs of cerebral hypoxia are restlessness and anxiety, which lead on to agitation and confusion.*
- ▲ Monitor ABGs and note changes.

Therapeutic Interventions

- Position patient with proper body alignment *for optimal lung expansion.*
- Change position q2hr *to facilitate movement and drainage of secretions.*
- Suction as needed *to clear secretions.*
- Provide reassurance and allay anxiety by staying with patient during acute episodes of respiratory distress. *Air hunger can produce an extremely anxious state.*
- ▲ Maintain O$_2$ delivery system *so that the appropriate amount of oxygen is applied continuously and the patient does not become desaturated.*
- ▲ Anticipate the need for intubation and mechanical ventilation. See also Mechanical ventilation, p. 202; ARDS, p. 183, as needed.

Continued.

Disseminated intravascular coagulation (DIC)—cont'd

NURSING DIAGNOSES	EXPECTED OUTCOMES AND NURSING INTERVENTIONS / *RATIONALE* (▪ = INDEPENDENT; ▲ = COLLABORATIVE)
High Risk for Altered Peripheral Perfusion **RISK FACTORS** DIC with peripheral thromboembolus formation in capillaries and arterioles resulting in possible interruption of arterial flow Hypovolemia	**EXPECTED OUTCOMES** Patient's peripheral circulation is optimized through ongoing assessment and early intervention. **ONGOING ASSESSMENT** ▪ Assess color, warmth, movement, and sensation of extremities. *Acute occlusion results in a numb cold limb, with pain aggravated by movement of the limb.* ▪ Assess peripheral pulses and mark with skin marker if diminished. Use Doppler ultrasound as needed to assess for presence of pulses. Notify physician immediately of signs of decreasing perfusion to an extremity. ▪ Assess blood pressure. **THERAPEUTIC INTERVENTIONS** ▪ Elevate extremities *to promote venous return and prevent edema formation. Edema formation could further add to a decrease in peripheral perfusion.* ▲ Maintain fluids and medications as needed to prevent hypotension. *Hypotension will lead to a further decrease in perfusion to extremities.*
Knowledge Deficit **RELATED FACTORS** Lack of familiarity with procedures Unfamiliar environment **DEFINING CHARACTERISTICS** Increased questioning Lack of questions **See also:** Anxiety, p. 5. Pain/comfort, p. 49. Decreased Cardiac Output, p. 12. Knowledge Deficit, p. 41.	**EXPECTED OUTCOMES** Patient/significant others verbalize basic understanding of DIC and its management. **ONGOING ASSESSMENT** ▪ Assess present knowledge of DIC. **THERAPEUTIC INTERVENTIONS** ▪ Instruct patient to notify nurse of bleeding from wounds, IV sites, etc. *This can aid in achieving early intervention to bleeding sites.* ▪ Instruct patient to try to avoid trauma *(may precipitate further bleeding).* ▪ Explain purpose of drug/transfusion therapy. ▪ Explain rationale for therapy to significant others; encourage them and other visitors to remain calm while visiting.

By: Audrey Klopp, RN, PhD, ET
Susan Galanes, RN, MS, CCRN

Granulocytopenia: risk for infection

(DISORDER OF NEUTROPHILS)

There are three types of granulocytes: basophils, eosinophils, and neutrophils. Granulocytopenia and its complications actually center around the neutrophilic granulocyte. A substantial decrease in the number of circulating neutrophils may result in overwhelming, potentially life-threatening infection. Neutrophils constitute 60% to 70% of all white blood cells. Their primary function is phagocytosis, the digestion and subsequent destruction of microorganisms, and as such, they form one of the body's most powerful defenses against infection.

NURSING DIAGNOSES	EXPECTED OUTCOMES AND NURSING INTERVENTIONS / *RATIONALE* (■ = INDEPENDENT; ▲ = COLLABORATIVE)

High Risk for Infection

RISK FACTORS

Granulocytopenia, secondary to:
  Radiation therapy
  Chemotherapy
  Hypersplenism
  Bone marrow depression/
    failure
  Autoimmune responses

EXPECTED OUTCOMES

Patient is at reduced risk of local/systemic infection as evidenced by normal temperature/ vital signs, chest radiograph result within normal limits, negative results of blood/ surveillance cultures, prompt reporting of early signs of infection.

ONGOING ASSESSMENT

▲ Monitor WBC (especially neutrophils/bands). *To determine relative risk of bacterial infections associated with absolute neutrophil count (ANC): 1000/mm^3 = minimal risk, 500/ mm^3 = moderate risk, <500/mm^3 = severe risk. The chance of developing a serious infection is related not only to the absolute level of circulating granulocytes but also to the length of time the patient is neutropenic. Prolonged duration (greater than 1 wk) predisposes patients to a higher risk of infection. Granulocytopenia not only predisposes one to infection, but when an infection occurs causes it to be more severe. The ANC can be calculated by using the following formula:*

$$ANC = total\ WBC \times \frac{(\%\,segs\,+\,\%\,bands)}{100}$$

- Identify source(s) of low WBC if unknown. Review drug profile for medications that can potentially cause granulocytopenia (i.e., tegradol, propylthiouracil, methimazole, bactrim, indocin, gold injections for rheumatoid arthritis).
- Inspect body sites with high potential for infection (e.g., orifices, catheter sites, skin folds).
- Note abnormalities in color/character of sputum, urine/stool that might indicate presence of infection.
- Monitor for increased temperature, heart rate, respirations; decreased blood pressure.
- Observe closely for fever/chills *(may be initial presentation of infection since in absence of granulocytes, locus of infection may develop without characteristic inflammation/pus formation at site).*
- Assess for local/systemic infection signs/symptoms (e.g., fever, chills, diaphoresis, local redness, warmth, pain, tenderness, excessive malaise, sore throat, dysphagia, retrosternal burning, or cellulitis). *Inflammation and exudate may be absent because of decrease or lack of neutrophils.*
- Identify medication patient may have taken that would mask infection signs/symptoms (e.g., steroids, antipyretics).
▲ Send cultures as prescribed for temperature >38.5° C *to determine organism causing the infection and antibiotic sensitivity.*

THERAPEUTIC INTERVENTIONS

- Wash hands thoroughly with antimicrobial cleanser before physical contact with patient *(removes transient and resident bacteria from hands and prevents transmission to patient). Because microorganisms can also be transmitted from one site of infection to other portals of entry, thorough handwashing is also important between patient care activities (central line dressing change, mouth care, perineal care, etc.).*
- Use sterile technique with dressing changes and catheter care.
▲ Observe isolation protocol *to protect patient from exposure to environmental contagions.*
- Limit visitors. Discourage anyone with current or recent infection from visiting.
- Encourage daily shower. Explain need for perineal care (with soap and water) after urination and defecation. *(Perineal area is source of many pathogens, frequent portal of entry for microorganisms).*
- Apply lotion to body after bath and as needed *to preserve skin integrity. The skin and mucous membranes are the first line of defense for the body; when this barrier is weakened or interrupted (e.g., dryness, cracking, abrasions), the site becomes a potential portal of entry for microorganisms and a source of infection.*

Continued.

Granulocytopenia: risk for infection—cont'd

NURSING DIAGNOSES	EXPECTED OUTCOMES AND NURSING INTERVENTIONS / *RATIONALE* (▪ = INDEPENDENT; ▲ = COLLABORATIVE)
	THERAPEUTIC INTERVENTIONS— cont'd

▪ Encourage meticulous oral hygiene before and after each meal and at bedtime (*important in prevention of periodontal disease as locus of infection*).

▪ Encourage oral fluids *to assist in meeting hydration requirement (particularly during fever episodes)*.

▲ Initiate low-bacterial diet (e.g., no fresh fruits/vegetables, only well-cooked foods) *to reduce the microbial level in foods, which could colonize and infect the GI tract.*

▲ Assist patient in selection of high-protein, high-vitamin, high-calorie diet (refer to dietitian as needed). *For maintenance of optimal health status, which promotes improvement of host resistance and provides nutrients necessary to meet energy demands for bone marrow recovery and tissue repair.*

▪ Avoid unnecessary invasive procedures *to minimize risk of infection.*

▲ Initiate measures for fever control (e.g., cool sponge bath, blanket, light covers, antipyretics).

▲ Initiate IV broad-spectrum antibiotic therapy as per hospital protocol *to prevent early dissemination of suspected infection. Once infection causing organism is determined, antimicrobial therapy may be adjusted to type of organism and infection and clinical response.*

▲ Administer stool softeners/high-fiber foods *to prevent constipation, which could traumatize the intestinal mucosa and increase the risk of perirectal abscess/fistula formation.*

Knowledge Deficit

RELATED FACTORS

Unfamiliarity with nature, treatment of condition

DEFINING CHARACTERISTICS

Multiple questions
Lack of questions
Misconceptions
Request for information

EXPECTED OUTCOMES

Patient/significant others verbalize understanding of medical diagnosis, treatment plan, safety measures, and follow-up care.

ONGOING ASSESSMENT

▪ Assess knowledge of infection (recognition of, plan of care for, evaluation of care).

THERAPEUTIC INTERVENTIONS

▪ Explain factors that contribute to low neutrophil count (e.g., chemotherapy, drug sensitivity).

▪ Explain that low neurophil counts produce high susceptibility to infection.

▪ Explain plan of care (e.g., need for private room, isolation) *to decrease fear/anxiety about therapeutic regimen.*

▪ Explain signs/symptoms of infection; instruct patient to contact appropriate health team member immediately if any occurs or is suspected.

▪ Instruct about:

Use of prescribed medications after discharge (indications, dosages, side effects), which may include G-CSF (Filgrastim), which stimulates the bone marrow to produce granulocytes; Acyclovir to prevent/treat viral infection; Diflucan to prevent/treat fungal infection.

Need for frequent blood draws to monitor neutrophil/WBC status.

Avoidance of activities that may result in trauma to mucosa. Suggest alternatives where appropriate (e.g., oral/axillary temperatures instead of rectal, electric razor instead of razor blades, sanitary napkins instead of tampons, tooth sponge instead of toothbrush).

Avoidance of crowds and persons with current or recent infection.

Avoidance of shared drinking and eating utensils; need to wash food well.

Avoidance of contact with cat litter boxes, fish tanks, human/animal excreta.

Importance of good handwashing.

Importance of meticulous body/oral hygiene.

▪ Instruct patient to make routine dental visits *to decrease the opportunity for infection to begin in oral cavity.*

By: Christa M. Schroeder, RN, MSN

Hemophilia

(BLEEDERS)

An inherited disorder of the clotting mechanism caused by diminished or absent factors necessary to the formation of prothrombin activator (the catalyst to clot formation). Classic hemophilia (type A) is caused by the lack of factor VIII; it is the most common and usually most severe type of hemophilia. Type B (Christmas disease) and type C hemophilia are caused by the lack of factors IX and XI respectively. Symptom severity is directly proportional to the plasma levels of available clotting factors; depending on these levels, the disease is classified as mild, moderate, or severe. Patients with close to normal factor levels may only experience frequent bruising and slightly prolonged bleeding times. This care plan addresses the more severe symptoms of hemophilia.

NURSING DIAGNOSES	EXPECTED OUTCOMES AND NURSING INTERVENTIONS / *RATIONALE* (■ = INDEPENDENT; ▲ = COLLABORATIVE)

High Risk for Injury: Hemorrhage

RISK FACTORS

Decreased concentration of clotting factors circulating in the blood; identified as factor VIII, factor IX, or factor XI

EXPECTED OUTCOMES

Risk of injury caused by hemorrhage is reduced through early assessment and intervention.

ONGOING ASSESSMENT

- Perform physical assessment to determine sites of bruising and bleeding.
- Assess extent of bleeding by measuring bruises, and counting or weighing blood-soaked dressings. *Bleeding can be life-threatening to these patients.*
- Assess for pain and swelling over the entire body. *Abdominal pain may signal internal hemorrhage. Headache, in the presence of a trauma history, may be indicative of intracranial hemorrhage. Bleeding into a joint is often reported as a peculiar tingling sensation felt well before pain or swelling is detected.*
- ▲ Monitor vital signs, Hb, and Hct.
- Assess history of previous reactions to blood components.
- ▲ Assess for inhibitor antibody to factor VIII. *Patients who require frequent transfusions may develop inhibitor antibody and require a subsequent change in coagulation therapy to factor VIIa.*
- Monitor for blood component transfusion reaction (see also Blood component therapy, p. 384).

THERAPEUTIC INTERVENTIONS

- Apply sterile dressings to wounds and apply pressure if active bleeding is present.
- ▲ Anticipate need for blood replacement. *Volume expanders and O-negative blood should be immediately available in event of life-threatening hemorrhage.*
- If bleeding is in a joint (hemarthrosis), elevate and immobilize the affected limb. Use ice packs *to control bleeding.*
- Establish IV access.
- ▲ Control hemorrhage by administering factor VIII or Autoplex either by IV push or in a continuous infusion.
- ▲ Administer plasma-derived factor VIIa (PFVIIa) for patients with antibodies against factor VIII.
- Document blood product transfusion per hospital policy.
- Maintain universal precautions. *Hemophiliacs who received blood products before 1986 are at risk for becoming human immunodeficiency virus–(HIV)-positive.*

Pain

RELATED FACTORS

Bleeding into joint (hemarthrosis)
Traumatic injury to muscles

EXPECTED OUTCOMES

Patient verbalizes relief of pain.
Patient appears relaxed and comfortable.

ONGOING ASSESSMENT

- Assess location and character of pain.
- Have patient note pain intensity on a scale of 1 to 10.
- Assess for ability to move affected limb.
- Assess for parasthesias.
- Assess for soft tissue hemorrhage. *This results in compartment syndrome, a condition in which increased pressure within a confined space results in circulatory compromise.*

Continued.

Hematolymphatic and Oncologic Care Plans

NURSING DIAGNOSES	EXPECTED OUTCOMES AND NURSING INTERVENTIONS / *RATIONALE* (■ = INDEPENDENT; ▲ = COLLABORATIVE)
	THERAPEUTIC INTERVENTIONS ▲ Administer prescribed pain medications. ▲ Administer factor VIII or other prescribed factor component immediately. *This treatment controls the bleeding that is causing the pain.* ▪ Apply cold treatment. ▲ Anticipate possible surgical procedure (faciotomy) if compartment syndrome evolves despite blood factor therapy.
High Risk for Injury **RISK FACTORS** Complications secondary to clotting factor concentrates.	**EXPECTED OUTCOMES** Patient does not develop inhibitors or blood borne viruses. **ONGOING ASSESSMENT** ▲ Assess for evidence of factor VIII inhibitors. ▪ Assess for transmission of blood-borne viruses. *This population is at high risk for hepatitis and HIV infection.* **THERAPEUTIC INTERVENTIONS** ▲ Administer recombinant factor VIIa in prescribed doses *to achieve hemostatic effect.* ▲ Administer hepatitis B vaccine to any person not showing Hbs antibodies. ▪ Explain need for HIV testing. *If a hemophiliac patient has a positive result, a CD4 count should be made and an asymptomatic patient followed at 6-mo intervals.*
High Risk for Impaired Physical Mobility **RISK FACTORS** Hemarthrosis Joint degeneration	**EXPECTED OUTCOMES** Patient maintains optimal physical mobility as evidenced by normal ROM, ADLs within ability. **ONGOING ASSESSMENT** ▪ Assess current limitations. *Patients who have active bleeding should have restricted mobility.* ▪ When bleeding is controlled, assess for limited ROM, contractures, and bony changes in joints. *Repeated joint bleeds cause bone destruction, permanent deformities, and crippling.* **THERAPEUTIC INTERVENTIONS** ▪ Provide gentle, passive ROM exercise when patient's condition is stable. ▪ Encourage progression to active exercise as tolerated. ▪ Provide assistive devices when needed. ▲ Refer for physical therapy/occupational therapy and orthopedic consultations as required. ▪ Instruct on preventive measures, including administration of factor products and application of protective gear. *Prevention of injury and hemarthrosis is best method of maintaining joint/limb mobility and use.*
High Risk for Ineffective Airway Clearance **RISK FACTORS** Bleeding in or around airway, nose, pharynx, esophagus (blood may or may not be seen, depending on site). Obstruction caused by tissue swelling.	**EXPECTED OUTCOMES** Patient maintains patent airway, as evidenced by no nosebleeds, clear breath sounds, normal respiratory rate. **ONGOING ASSESSMENT** ▪ Assess time, pattern, and character of nosebleed. ▪ Assess for history of head and neck trauma. ▪ Observe for bleeding that could obstruct airway. ▪ Monitor vital signs, respiratory rate, breath sounds, and any reported difficulty in breathing. **THERAPEUTIC INTERVENTIONS** ▲ Administer prescribed IV clotting factors. *Again, control of bleeding is the priority.* ▲ Anticipate need for nasal packing if bleeding does not stop with conservative pressure measures. ▪ If neck or pharyngeal injury is suspected, keep an oral airway and suction apparatus nearby; keep tracheostomy apparatus available; prepare for intubation.

NURSING DIAGNOSES	EXPECTED OUTCOMES AND NURSING INTERVENTIONS / *RATIONALE* (■ = INDEPENDENT; ▲ = COLLABORATIVE)

Knowledge Deficit Regarding Disease Management, Changes in Therapy, and Prevention of Complications

RELATED FACTORS

Lack of resources
Unfamiliarity with aspects of disease management

DEFINING CHARACTERISTICS

Many questions.
Lack of questions.
Misconceptions

EXPECTED OUTCOMES

Patient verbalizes understanding of hemophilia and its treatment and home care.

ONGOING ASSESSMENT

- Assess patient's knowledge of his or her individual disease course.
- Assess history of bleeding episodes and treatment protocols.
- Assess patient's reported behaviors to prevent trauma or injury.

THERAPEUTIC INTERVENTIONS

- Provide information about disease severity, treatment plans, and measures to prevent injury.
- Explain genetic transference. Refer for genetic counseling if needed. *Hemophilia is a recessive sex-linked disease, transmitted by females and seen almost exclusively in males.*
- When condition is stable, discuss construction of a safe environment with possible use of protective devices.
- Emphasize need to avoid aspirin products.
- Discuss need for *prophylactic* treatment with coagulation factors if need for surgery or dental manipulation occurs.
- Instruct to avoid contact sports, use caution when working with tools/devices that can readily cut or injure (saws, cutting shears), wear protective gloves, avoid walking barefooted.
- Encourage wearing of Medic Alert bracelet. Provide phone numbers for emergency help.

Fear

RELATED FACTORS

Potential trauma
Threat of acquired immunodeficiency syndrome (AIDS)
Threat of death

DEFINING CHARACTERISTICS

Verbalized concern or fear
Irritability
Difficulty concentrating
Palpitations
Loss of appetite

EXPECTED OUTCOMES

Patient verbalizes ability to cope with threat of complications from disease.

ONGOING ASSESSMENT

- Assess degree of fear.
- Identify risk factors for AIDS.
- Assess available supportive relationships.

THERAPEUTIC INTERVENTIONS

- Allow expression of fears, anger, and other feelings.
- Discuss actual fears, likelihood of occurrence, preventive measures if available.
- ▲ Provide psychiatric referral if necessary. *Hemophiliacs may need help in controlling fears and anxiety. Fear of AIDS is especially destructive; assistance may be needed to prevent fear from controlling life.*
- If patient's HIV status is negative, reinforce need for safe sexual behaviors and avoidance of IV drug use.
- If patient has positive HIV status, provide more detailed information about disease progression and self-care measures.
- Refer to support group such as a chapter of the National Hemophilia Society. *Groups that come together for mutual support and information exchange can aid in coping with this chronic disease.*

By: Mary T. McCarthy, RN, MSN, CS

Lead poisoning

(PLUMBISM)

Symptoms of lead poisoning are a result of chronic ingestion or inhalation of lead-bearing products. Lead poisoning is most commonly seen in children exhibiting pica behaviors but also occurs in adults who have chronically inhaled fumes from motor fuels, batteries, and paints. Accidental ingestion can result from serving acidic liquids from lead-glazed pottery, antique pewter, and lead crystal. Lead salts are absorbed by the blood, interfere with hemoglobin production, and destroy kidney and brain tissue. Symptoms of lead poisoning in adults mimic anemia and/or leukemia. About 30% of children treated for lead poisoning suffer irreversible damage to the nervous system, including mental retardation, hyperactivity, cerebral palsy, seizures, and optic atrophy.

NURSING DIAGNOSES	EXPECTED OUTCOMES AND NURSING INTERVENTIONS / *RATIONALE* (■ = INDEPENDENT; ▲ = COLLABORATIVE)

High Risk for Injury: Poisoning

RISK FACTORS

Internal
Verbalized lack of safeguards in occupational setting.
Lack of safety, education, or proper precaution.

External
Dangerous products stored within reach of children or confused persons
Chemical contamination of food, water.
Unprotected contact with heavy metal.
Inhalation of paint, lacquer fumes.

EXPECTED OUTCOMES

Patient maintains serum lead level below 50 μg/dl, preferably less than 15 μg/dl.

ONGOING ASSESSMENT

- Check vital signs.
- Observe skin for pallor/anemia.
- ▲ Monitor daily lead levels. *Increased lead level is level greater than 15-50 mg/100 ml.*
- ▲ Monitor daily Hb and Hct.
- Assess for history of pica.
- Monitor for side effects/complications of chelating agents.
- ▲ Obtain repeat lead level after 5 days of chelation therapy. *Should be below 50 μg/dl. Lead levels over 50 μg/dl indicate a need for further chelation. Lead level may rebound as a result of absorption of lead into circulating blood from soft tissue deposits.*

THERAPEUTIC INTERVENTIONS

- ▲ Administer chelating agents as prescribed: *These agents form highly soluble compound that causes free lead to be readily excreted in urine.*
  IM injections: dimercaprol (BAL in oil), edetate calcium disodium (CaEDTA)
  Oral chelator: succimer (chemet). *This will decrease circulating lead and diminish amount absorbed by soft tissues.*
- ▲ Assist with exchange transfusion if needed.
- ▲ Provide oxygen therapy for patients with significant decreases in Hct/Hb.

High Risk for Injury: Neurologic complications

RISK FACTORS

Poisoning, chronic lead ingestion
Tissue hypoxia
Altered mobility

EXPECTED OUTCOMES

Patient maintains optimal neurologic functioning, as evidenced by clear mentation, alertness, good coordination and balance, absence of seizures.
Patient does not incur injury.

ONGOING ASSESSMENT

- Assess level of consciousness (LOC) q4hr, more frequently if deterioration, increased toxicity, or encephalopathy noted.
- Assess for neurologic changes: drowsiness, irritability, clumsiness, falling, peripheral nerve palsy, headache, vomiting, seizures.
- Compare present neurologic assessment to previous level from history.
- Document serial assessments. *Patterns of deterioration/improvement are more easily recognized using serial assessments. Treatment can be adjusted to patient response.*
- Assess vital signs, especially respiratory status.

THERAPEUTIC INTERVENTIONS

- Use seizure precautions and safety measures (i.e., side rails up and padded). *Seizure activity, loss of coordination, drowsiness may occur.*
- ▲ If actual LOC alteration is noted: obtain emergency equipment; place Ambu bag at bedside; report to physician; consult neurologic clinical specialist.

| NURSING DIAGNOSES | EXPECTED OUTCOMES AND NURSING INTERVENTIONS / *RATIONALE*
(■ = INDEPENDENT; ▲ = COLLABORATIVE) |

High Risk for Fluid Volume Excess

RISK FACTORS
Compromised regulatory mechanisms
Toxic BAL/CaEDTA levels

EXPECTED OUTCOMES
Patient maintains urine output of at least 30 ml/hr or greater, based on fluid intake.

ONGOING ASSESSMENT
- Monitor vital signs (especially for increased heart rate and change in blood pressure).
- Monitor I & O for decreased urine output. *Chelating agents are nephrotoxic.*
- Check specific gravity and dipstick for protein/blood every void.
▲ Monitor lab results (urinalysis, electrolytes, blood urea nitrogen [BUN], and creatinine); *chelating agents are toxic to kidneys.*
- Assess for edema, shortness of breath.

THERAPEUTIC INTERVENTIONS
- Review potential renal side effects of all drugs used before administration.
- Do not administer CaEDTA to dehydrated patients. *Decreased kidney function severely limits chelation therapy effectiveness.*
- Ensure adequate PO/IV intake. *Fluids assure lead excretion via urine.*

Pain

RELATED FACTORS
Multiple injections
Viscosity of medication

DEFINING CHARACTERISTICS
Irritability
Swelling, inflammation, and redness at injection sites
Verbalized complaint

EXPECTED OUTCOMES
Patient verbalizes relief of or reduction in pain

ONGOING ASSESSMENT
- Observe injection areas for swelling, redness, inflammation, abscess formation. *Viscosity of med and large amount to be injected increase irritation to injection site.*
- Inspect skin of patient receiving chemet. *May cause rash.*

THERAPEUTIC INTERVENTIONS
- Palpate muscle area before preparing site *to locate/avoid fibrous tissue from previous injections.*
- Rotate all injection sites; use large muscle groups.
▲ Obtain order for use of local anesthetic with injection (draw up last in syringe; do not mix); *helps lessen pain during administration.*
▲ Administer BAL and CaEDTA by deep IM injection *for adequate absorption.*
- Apply warm soaks to injection sites as necessary *to relieve discomfort.*
- Consider IV route for CaEDTA *to avoid painful IM injections.*
- Notify physician of any complications.

Knowledge Deficit

RELATED FACTORS
Unfamiliarity with diagnosis, source of exposure

DEFINING CHARACTERISTICS
Verbalized lack of understanding of diagnosis, cause
Multiple questions/comments
Repeated episodes of ingestion

EXPECTED OUTCOMES
Patient verbalizes/demonstrates understanding of lead poisoning, environmental hazards, long-term complications, medications, and follow-up care.

ONGOING ASSESSMENT
- Assess knowledge of lead poisoning, source of ingestion.
- Assess for pica behavior and general nutrition.
- Elicit information for possible lead sources.
- Screen family members for increased lead levels if exposure is in the home.

THERAPEUTIC INTERVENTIONS
- Explain cause of lead poisoning (i.e., pica, improperly glazed pottery, toxic fumes [paint], lead pipes).
- Explain environmental factors that contribute to lead poisoning. *Environment must be controlled or effective safety precautions performed to decrease risk of poisoning.*
    Poorly maintained older swellings
    Water pipes made of lead
    Fumes from toxic waste
    Job-related exposure (e.g., paint fumes)
- Review, emphasize hazards of lead, signs of lead intoxication, and long-term complications.
- Inform of importance of proper home medication administration. *Poor compliance will result in ineffective therapy and continued lead poisoning.*
▲ Initiate referrals with social worker, public health nurse, board of health, and other agencies that can assist in overall management.
- Emphasize need for continuing follow-up observation, lead level monitoring.
- Provide telephone number for local emergency room, poison control.

By: Michele Puzas, RN, MHPD

Leukemia

Leukemia is a malignant disorder of the blood-forming system. The proliferation of immature white blood cells (WBCs) interferes with the production/function of the red blood cells (RBCs) and platelets. Leukemia can be characterized by identification of the type of leukocyte involved: granulocyte or lymphocyte. In acute lymphocytic leukemia (ALL) there is a proliferation of lymphoblasts; in acute myelocytic leukemia (AML) there is a proliferation of myeloblasts. In chronic lymphocytic leukemia there are increased lymphocytes; in chronic myelocytic leukemia there are increased granulocytes. Depending on the type of leukemia, therapeutic management may consist of combined chemotherapeutic agents, radiation therapy and/or bone marrow transplantation. The goals of nursing care are to prevent complications and provide educational and emotional support.

NURSING DIAGNOSES	EXPECTED OUTCOMES AND NURSING INTERVENTIONS / *RATIONALE* (■ = INDEPENDENT; ▲ = COLLABORATIVE)

Knowledge Deficit

RELATED FACTORS
New disease
Lack of information resources

DEFINING CHARACTERISTICS
Many questions
Lack of questions
Misconceptions

EXPECTED OUTCOMES
Patient verbalizes understanding of diagnosis, treatment strategies, and prognosis.

ONGOING ASSESSMENT
- Assess knowledge of disease, diagnosis, treatment strategies, and prognosis.

THERAPEUTIC INTERVENTIONS
- Describe the etiology of leukemia:
  Not well understood; probably multifactorial
  May be related to genetic factors, viruses, exposure to radiation or chemical agents, immunologic deficiencies, antineoplastic drugs
- Explain the blood-forming changes that occur with leukemia:
  Bone marrow failure; leukemic infiltrates
  Anemia from reduced RBC production
  Granulocytopenia from reduced number of WBCs
  Thrombocytopenia from decreased platelet production
- Clarify the difference between acute and chronic leukemia:
  Acute leukemia is abnormal proliferation of immature leukocytes or blasts with rapid onset of symptoms.
  Chronic leukemia is characterized by disease of mature WBCs with a progressive, gradual onset of symptoms.
- Describe the patient's specific type of leukemia. *Four major kinds of leukemia are known, as described in the Definition.*
- Explain the diagnostic process: bone marrow aspiration/examination, peripheral blood evaluation.
- Describe common approaches to treatment. *Treatment is guided by current research findings and definitive protocols.*
  Combination chemotherapy. *Has reduced side effects and improved response.*
  Radiation therapy
  Bone marrow transplantation
- Explain common complications:
  Bleeding. *From decreased platelet production*
  Infection. *From immature WBC production*
- Discuss prognosis:
  The prognosis is hopeful, with the treatment goal being a curative attempt, though at times the treatment may only result in prolonged remission.
  Patients may be in remission for a long time

NURSING DIAGNOSES	EXPECTED OUTCOMES AND NURSING INTERVENTIONS / *RATIONALE* (■ = INDEPENDENT; ▲ = COLLABORATIVE)

High Risk for Ineffective Coping

RISK FACTORS

Situational crisis
Inadequate support system
Inadequate coping methods

EXPECTED OUTCOMES

Patient demonstrates positive coping strategies, as evidenced by expression of feelings/fears/hopes; realistic goal setting for long-term future, life-style, and roles; use of available resources and support systems.

ONGOING ASSESSMENT

- Assess patient's concept and knowledge of disease. *Because leukemia is cancer, patients may expect to die.*
- Assess for:
  Events/illnesses preceding hospitalization
  Awareness and comprehension of illness, importance of procedures, importance of hospitalization
  Coping mechanisms used in previous illnesses and hospitalization experiences
  Dynamics of relationship with significant others

THERAPEUTIC INTERVENTIONS

- Establish open lines of communication; define your role as patient informant and advocate.
- Understand grieving process, respect patient's feelings as they ensue.
- Assist patient/significant others in redefining hopes, components of individuality (e.g., roles, values, and attitudes).
- Introduce new information about disease treatment. *At this time there is no cure for leukemia. However, remission is possible and long-term survival is feasible.*
- Describe community resources available to meet unique demands of leukemia, its treatment, and survival (i.e., Leukemia Society of America, American Cancer Society, National Coalition for Cancer Survivorship).
- Explain need for compliance with treatment regimen *to optimize chances for remission.*

High Risk for Infection

RISK FACTORS

Altered immunologic responses related to disease process
Immunosuppression secondary to chemotherapy

EXPECTED OUTCOMES

Patient has reduced risk of local/systemic infection, as evidenced by afebrile state, compliance with preventive measures, prompt reporting of early signs of infection.

ONGOING ASSESSMENT

- Auscultate lung fields for rales, rhonchi, decreased breath sounds. *Pulmonary infections are common.*
- Observe patient for coughing spells, sputum character.
- Observe for changes in color, character, frequency of urine and stool.
- Inspect body sites with high infection potential (mouth, throat, axilla, perineum, rectum).
- Inspect IV/central catheter sites for redness/tenderness. *In absence of granulocytes, site of infection may develop without characteristic pus formation.*
- Monitor vital signs as needed.
- ▲ Obtain cultures as prescribed *to determine antibiotic sensitivity and presence of fungi.*

THERAPEUTIC INTERVENTIONS

- Explain definition, cause, and effects of leukopenia: normal range of blood count, function of leukocytes and neutrophils.
- ▲ Place patient in protective isolation if lab results indicate neutropenia (WBC < 1000mm^3).
  Screen visitors to minimize room traffic.
  Implement thorough handwashing of staff/visitors before physical contact with patient *to remove transient and resident bacteria from hands, thus minimizing/preventing transmission to patient.*
- Administer antibiotic/antifungal/antiviral drugs on time *to maintain therapeutic drug level(s).*
- Observe strict aseptic technique when changing dressings: avoid wetting central catheter dressings *to prevent bacterial growth.*
- Instruct patient to maintain personal hygiene:
  To bathe with chlorhexidine (Hibiclens) before initially entering room and every day thereafter *to remove skin surface bacteria that may play a role in secondary infection*
  To wash hands well before eating and after using bathroom
  To wipe perineal area from front to back.
- Instruct patient to brush teeth with soft toothbrush qid and as necessary, to remove dentures at night, to rinse mouth after each emesis or when expectorating phlegm.

Continued.

■ **Leukemia—cont'd**

NURSING DIAGNOSES	EXPECTED OUTCOMES AND NURSING INTERVENTIONS / *RATIONALE* (■ = INDEPENDENT; ▲ = COLLABORATIVE)

THERAPEUTIC INTERVENTIONS— cont'd

- Teach patient to inspect oropharyngeal area daily for white patches in mouth, coated/encrusted oral ulcerations, swollen and erythematous tongue with white/brown coating, infected throat and pain on swallowing, debris on teeth, ill-fitting dentures, amount and viscosity of saliva, changes in vocal tone.
- Teach patient to avoid mouthwashes that contain alcohol *(drying effect on mucous membranes),* avoid irritating foods/acidic drinks.
- Teach patient to use prescribed topical medications (e.g., nystatin [Nilstat] and lidocaine [Xylocaine]).
- Instruct patient to observe for fever spikes, flulike symptoms (malaise, weakness, and myalgia); notify nurse/physician if they occur; avoid crowds or contact with contagious persons; take oral and axillary temperature.
- Explain importance of regular medical and dental checkups.
- ▲ Refer patient to dietitian for instructions on maintenance of well-balanced diet.

High Risk for Injury: Bleeding

RISK FACTORS

Bone marrow depression secondary to chemotherapy
Proliferation of leukemic cells

EXPECTED OUTCOMES

Patient's risk for bleeding is reduced as evidenced by platelet count within acceptable limits, compliance with preventive measures, prompt reporting of early signs/symptoms.

ONGOING ASSESSMENT

- ▲ Monitor platelet count daily *to determine risk for bleeding. Mild thrombocytopenia: platelets 50,000-100,000/mm³; moderately severe: platelets 20,000-50,000/mm³; severe: platelets 20,000/mm³ or less.*
- Assess for signs/symptoms of bleeding. *May include petechiae and bruising; hemoptysis; hematemesis; hematochezia; melena; vaginal bleeding; dizziness; orthostatic changes; decreased blood pressure; headaches; changes in mental and visual acuity; increased pulse rate.*
- Note bleeding from puncture sites (e.g., venipuncture, bone marrow aspiration sites).

THERAPEUTIC INTERVENTIONS

- ▲ Institute bleeding precautions for platelet count <50,000/mm³:
- Explain to patient/significant others definition, etiology, and symptoms of thrombocytopenia and functions of platelets:
   Normal range of platelet count
   Effects of thrombocytopenia
   Rationale of bleeding precautions
- Avoid IM/SC injections. If necessary, use small-bore needles for injections; apply ice to site for 5 min. Observe for oozing from site.
- Place sign over patient's bed as reminder to apply pressure after venipunctures.
- Avoid fingerstick if possible. Coordinate lab work so all tests are done at one time.
- Apply pressure/dressing/sandbag to bone marrow aspiration site. *To prevent excessive pressure when compressing soft tissues and deeper structures of the arm as this may lead to bruising/hematomas.*
- Inflate blood pressure cuff as little as possible to get accurate reading.
- ▲ Apply ice or topical thrombin promptly as prescribed for bleeding mucous membranes *to promote clot formation.*
- Maintain safe environment for patient, especially during episodes of chills, fever, confusion, and weakness. Assist patient during ambulation and shower/tub bath to prevent falls/injury.
- Encourage rest to decrease pulse rate, *thus assisting clot formation.*
- ▲ Ensure availability and readiness of platelets for transfusion *to prevent spontaneous or excessive bleeding (generally for count <20,000/mm³ or per institutional protocol).*
- ▲ Administer antacids as prescribed for patients taking steroids.
- Instruct patient to:
   Use soft toothbrush and nonabrasive toothpaste.
   Inspect gums for oozing.
   Avoid use of toothpicks and dental floss *to prevent gum trauma.*

THERAPEUTIC INTERVENTIONS— cont'd

Avoid rectal suppositories, thermometers, enemas, vaginal douches, and tampons *to reduce mucosal trauma.*

Avoid aspirin or aspirin-containing products, nonsteroidal antiinflammatory drugs (NSAIDs) and anticoagulants. *These interfere with platelet function.*

Avoid straining with bowel movements, forceful nose blowing, coughing, sneezing *to prevent risk of bleeding.*

Count used sanitary pads during menstruation. Report menstrual cycle changes.

Use electric razor for shaving (not razor blades) *to prevent accidental break in skin.*

Avoid sharp objects such as scissors/knives. *To prevent cuts, which would not only bleed but become portals of entry for microorganisms, leading to infection in the presence of neutropenia.*

Use emery boards.

Avoid wearing tight/constrictive clothing. *to prevent pressure to body areas.*

Lubricate nostrils with saline solution drops as necessary *to prevent drying/cracking;* avoid picking nose.

Lubricate lips with petroleum jelly as needed.

Practice gentle sex; use water-based lubricant before sexual intercourse *to prevent mucosal trauma.*

Protect self from injury/trauma (e.g., falls, bumps, strenuous exercise, contact sports).

- At time of discharge give patient/family at least two phone numbers to call in case of bleeding.

High Risk for Social Isolation

RISK FACTORS

Protective isolation
Impaired mobility secondary to disease entity

EXPECTED OUTCOMES

Patient maintains optimal socialization, as evidenced by attention to personal appearance, involvement in hobbies or pleasurable activities, interaction with staff.

ONGOING ASSESSMENT

- Recognize early verbal/nonverbal communication cues reflecting need to socialize.
- ▲ Monitor blood counts to determine duration of isolation. *Usually maintained for WBC <1000/mm³.*
- Observe patient closely for behavioral changes. *Withdrawal, outbursts, reduced social interaction, lack of interest in mobility/ability to ambulate may be such signs.*

THERAPEUTIC INTERVENTIONS

- Visit and talk with patient frequently *to minimize social isolation.* Avoid using intercom when responding to patient's call.
- Provide normal aids for interaction (e.g., eyeglasses, hearing aids, writing materials).
- Encourage participation of significant others through visits and telephone calls.
- ▲ Provide diversional therapy/activities (e.g., radio, television, magazines, audio/videotapes, cards, puzzles, knitting) and occupational therapy *to decrease feelings of boredom or apathy.*
- Provide a clock and calendar *for concrete reminders of time.*
- Ask significant others to bring in familiar objects (e.g., pictures and pillows).
- Leave patient's door open if allowed by isolation precautions.
- Encourage patient to ambulate during course of protective isolation as permitted by physician and physical limitations.
- Assist patient in grooming when entertaining visitors. *Wearing makeup, wig, may increase self-esteem and foster more interest in interaction.*
- Acknowledge patient's efforts in maintaining sense of well-being.

See also:
Altered Nutrition: Less than Body Requirements, p. 11.
Fluid Volume deficit, p. 25.
Activity Intolerance, p. 2.
Grief over Long-term Illness/ Disability, p. 30.
Anxiety/Fear, p. 5, 23.
Cancer Chemotherapy, p. 403.
Bone Marrow Transplantation, p. 386.

By: Christa M. Schroeder, RN, MSN

Multiple myeloma

(PLASMACYTOMA; MYELOMATOSIS; PLASMA CELL MYELOMA)

Seen mostly in the elderly, this terminal disease is characterized by infiltration of bone and marrow by malignant plasma cells. This infiltration causes demineralization, fractures, and pain. Late stages of the disease involve kidney, liver, spleen, and lymph node infiltration. Occasionally this disease converts to acute leukemia. Cause is unknown.

NURSING DIAGNOSES	EXPECTED OUTCOMES AND NURSING INTERVENTIONS / *RATIONALE* (■ = INDEPENDENT; ▲ = COLLABORATIVE)

Pain

RELATED FACTORS

Invasion of marrow and bone by plasma cells
Pathologic fractures

DEFINING CHARACTERISTICS

Constant, severe bone pain on movement
Low back pain
Abdominal pain
Swelling, tenderness
Guarding behavior
Decreased physical activity
Moaning, crying
Pacing, restlessness, irritability, altered sleep pattern

EXPECTED OUTCOMES

Patient reports reduction in or relief of pain.
Patient appears comfortable.

ONGOING ASSESSMENT

- Assess pain characteristics. *Back pain, especially in lower back, occurs most commonly.*
- Assess effectiveness of relief measures and adjust dosage, drug, or route as needed.

THERAPEUTIC INTERVENTIONS

▲ Anticipate need for pain medication. Administer analgesics early *to prevent severe pain.*
▲ Provide analgesics in dosage, route, and frequency best suited to individual patient. Consider around-the-clock schedule, continuous infusion, or patient-controlled analgesia (PCA) *to control pain.*
▲ Consider combination analgesics *to arrest pain cycle at varied levels.*
- Schedule pain-inducing procedures/activities during peak analgesic effect.
▲ Notify physician if pain medications are ineffective *so other methods may be implemented; braces and splints may be used for support and/or radiation therapy may be required to decrease size of lesions causing pain.*
- Implement nonpharmacologic measures for comfort: decreased noise and activity, relaxation techniques/distraction techniques, good body alignment, additional rest and sleep periods, ambulation unless contraindicated (e.g., by spinal lesions).

Impaired Physical Mobility

RELATED FACTORS

Bone weakness
Generalized weakness caused by chemotherapy
Pain

DEFINING CHARACTERISTICS

Inability to move purposefully within physical environment
Decrease in ADLs
Reluctance to attempt movement
Limited ROM
Decreased muscle strength or control
Restricted movement and impaired coordination

EXPECTED OUTCOMES

Patient maintains optimal state of mobility as evidenced by participation in ADLs within ability, necessary life-style adaptations.

ONGOING ASSESSMENT

- Assess ability to carry out ADL. *Progressive weakness and malaise are common symptoms of this disease.*
- Assess ROM and muscle strength.

THERAPEUTIC INTERVENTIONS

- Assist patient with ADLs.
- Change position in bed q1-2hr.
- Perform ROM *to prevent contractures of upper and lower extremities.*
- Maintain uncluttered environment *to prevent bumping into objects or falls. Bone weakening can readily result in fractures.*
- Encourage ambulation *to prevent further bony demineralization.*
- Provide assistive devices (e.g., walker, cane, back brace) as needed.
- Allow rest periods after ambulation.

High Risk for Injury: Anemia/Thrombocytopenia

Risk Factors

Bone marrow depression or failure

Replacement or invasion of bone marrow by neoplastic plasma cells

Abnormal hepatic or renal function

Bleeding

Expected Outcomes

Patient maintains Hb/Hct/platelets within normal limits.

Patient complies with measures to prevent bleeding.

Ongoing Assessment

▲ Identify factors that lower platelet/RBC count or predispose patient to bleeding such as impaired bone marrow function caused by infiltration by plasma cells that disrupt normal platelet/RBC production.

▲ Monitor lab values: Hb, Hct, platelet count.

- Check current chemotherapy regimens for potential myelosuppression.
- Identify drugs interfering with platelet function.
- Observe and report signs/symptoms of spontaneous or excessive bleeding.

Therapeutic Interventions

- Avoid unnecessary trauma:

  Draw all blood for lab work with one daily venipuncture.

  Avoid IM injection; if necessary, use smallest needle possible.

  Apply direct pressure for 3-5 min after IM injection, venipuncture, and bone marrow aspiration.

  Avoid rectal temperatures and enemas. *Axillary route may be least harmful.*

  Prevent constipation by increased oral fluid/fiber intake/stool softeners as prescribed. *Straining causes breakage of small blood vessels around anus.*

  Use soft toothbrushes.

  Use electric razor, not blades.

- Avoid aspirin, aspirin-containing compounds. *These drugs interfere with hemostatic platelet function.*
- Place sign near patient informing other health team members of bleeding precautions.

▲ Transfuse platelet/packed red cells as prescribed for platelet count <20,000/mm^3, Hb <10, Hct < 30%.

▲ Administer hormones (steroids/androgens) and colony-stimulating factor (EPO) *to stimulate red cell production.*

High Risk for Infection

Risk Factors

Decrease in synthesis of immunoglobulin by plasma cells secondary to:

  Bone marrow depression/failure

  Decrease in normal circulating antibodies

  Decreased autoimmune response

  Chemotherapy

Expected Outcomes

Patient's risk of infection is reduced or prevented, as evidenced by normal temperature, absence of skin, urine, pulmonary infection.

Ongoing Assessment

- Check body for: open wounds, skin breakdown, swelling, redness.
- Monitor temperature.

▲ Obtain urine, sputum, and blood for culture and sensitivity testing if temperature >37.7° C.

- Monitor for signs of urine infection.
- Observe for coughing (productive and nonproductive), and changes in color and odor of sputum. *Bronchopneumonia is a common complication.*
- Review medications. *Patient taking steroids may not have overt infection symptoms.*

Therapeutic Interventions

- Use good handwashing technique before and after each patient contact. Use universal precautions.
- Use sterile technique for dressing change and catheter care.

▲ Maintain reverse isolation per unit policy.

- Discourage visitors with current or recent infection (e.g., family member who has upper respiratory infection but must visit wears mask and limits stay to 10 min).
- Avoid unnecessary invasive procedures.
- Maintain normal or near-normal body temperature with medications as prescribed, tepid bath, cooling blanket.
- See also Cancer chemotherapy, p. 403.

Continued.

NURSING DIAGNOSES	EXPECTED OUTCOMES AND NURSING INTERVENTIONS / *RATIONALE* (■ = INDEPENDENT; ▲ = COLLABORATIVE)

High Risk for Altered Urinary Elimination

RISK FACTORS

Immunoglobulin precipitates
Hypercalcemia/hypercalcuria
Hyperuricemia
Pyelonephritis
Myeloma kidney
Renal vein thrombosis
Spinal cord compression

EXPECTED OUTCOMES

Patient maintains optimal renal function as evidenced by serum/urine lab values within normal limits, balanced intake and output, normal blood pressure.

ONGOING ASSESSMENT

▲ Monitor serum laboratory values. *Increased BUN, creatinine, Ca, K^+, and uric acid levels are signs of renal dysfunction.*
· Monitor I & O for signs of decreased urine output.
· Assess for bladder distention *(may indicate spinal cord compression).*
· Monitor urine for specific gravity, color, odor, and blood.
· Observe for dyspnea, tachycardia, pulmonary edema, distended neck veins, peripheral edema; monitor weight daily *to evaluate for fluid retention.*
· Assess blood pressure for hypertensive changes.

THERAPEUTIC INTERVENTIONS

▲ Provide renal diet if prescribed; restrict sodium and protein.
▲ Provide IV fluids if necessary *to prevent dehydration, which may precede acute renal failure.*
▲ If hypercalcemia is present, push fluids 2500-3000 ml/day as prescribed.
▲ Administer medications *Didronel, Aredia, Mithracin, Calcimar/calcitonin, Ganite, aggressive IV hydration with 0.9% normal saline (NS) solution and Lasix, or oral phosphates may be used for hypercalcemia; allopurinol for hyperuricemia.*
▲ Place indwelling catheter *to determine I & O and decrease bladder distention.*
▲ Prepare for dialysis if renal failure impending.

See also:
Renal failure, acute, p. 436
Hypercalcemia, p. 436.

Knowledge Deficit

RELATED FACTORS

New diagnosis
Unfamiliarity with disease process, treatment, and discharge/follow-up care

DEFINING CHARACTERISTICS

Questions
Lack of questions
Confusion over disease and outcome

EXPECTED OUTCOMES

Patient/significant others describe diagnosis and treatment plan, side effects of medications, follow-up care.

ONGOING ASSESSMENT

· Assess knowledge of pain and medications; possible infection; bleeding disorders; mobility, including restrictions if indicated; dietary and fluid restriction.

THERAPEUTIC INTERVENTIONS

· Provide information on the following: nature of disease and its effect on target organs (i.e., renal damage, bone marrow impairment, skeletal manifestations); pain control; infection signs and prevention; diet and fluid therapy; bleeding tendencies; need for continued mobility; tests and procedures; treatment plan and possible side effects of medications and radiation therapy; discharge planning/follow-up care.
· Involve family/significant other so they can effectively provide support on discharge.
· Refer patient to U.S. Department of Health and Human Services (for information on multiple myeloma) and American Cancer Society.

See also:
Impaired Individual Coping, p. 18.
Anticipatory Grieving, p. 28.
Altered Nutrition: Less than Body Requirements, p. 44.
Anxiety, p. 5.
Fear, p. 23.

By: Christa M. Schroeder, RN, MSN
    Michele Knoll Puzas, RN,C, MHPE

Sickle cell pain crisis

(VASOOCCLUSIVE CRISIS: SICKLE CELL ANEMIA)

Sickle cell anemia is a severe genetic hemolytic anemia caused by a defective hemoglobin molecule. This disease is found in Africans, black Americans, and people from Mediterranean countries. Sickle cell pain crisis is defined as pain of sufficient severity to require medical attention and hospitalization. The severe pain, usually in the extremities, is caused by the occlusion of small blood vessels by sickle-shaped red blood cells. This chronic disease can cause impaired renal, pulmonary, nervous system, and spleen function; increased susceptibility to infection; and ultimately decreased life span. Persons with low socioeconomic status appear to have more frequent episodes of painful crisis.

NURSING DIAGNOSES	EXPECTED OUTCOMES AND NURSING INTERVENTIONS / *RATIONALE* (■ = INDEPENDENT; ▲ = COLLABORATIVE)

Pain

RELATED FACTORS

Vasooclusive crisis hypoxia, which causes cells to become rigid and elongated, thus forming crescent shape
Stasis of RBCs

DEFINING CHARACTERISTICS

Complaint of generalized or localized pain
Tenderness on palpation
Inability to move affected joint
Swelling to area
Deformity to joint
Warmth, redness

EXPECTED OUTCOMES

Patient verbalizes relief from pain.
Patient appears relaxed and comfortable.

ONGOING ASSESSMENT

- Assess for pain characteristics:
  Severity (use 1-10 scale). *The lack of objective criteria by which sickle cell disease and even occurrence of crises can be judged makes evaluation difficult. However, patient's report of pain should be believed and treated appropriately.*
  Location. *Usually described as bone or joint pain, less often as muscle pain. May include abdominal or back pain.*
  Type. *May be reported as tenderness or inability to move. Physical manifestations may include swelling, warmth, or redness, or fever.*
- Assess the pattern of previous hospitalizations for pain management. *Patterns of addiction or deviant psychological behavior may emerge, necessitating management by the psychiatric team.*
- ▲ Check laboratory values (e.g., Hb electrophoresis for amount of sickling and RBC count). *A severe decrease in functioning RBCs may indicate the need for replacement transfusion of packed RBCs.*

THERAPEUTIC INTERVENTIONS

- ▲ Administer pain medications as prescribed. *Initial pain crisis requires parenteral (IM or IV) administration on an around-the-clock schedule.*
  Meperidine (Demerol) or morphine sulfate by IM injection or via patient-controlled analgesia (PCA) pump. *These are more often prescribed.*
  Nonsteroidal inflammatory drugs (NSAIDs) with narcotics. *New parenteral agents such as ketorolac (Torodol) are used to decrease inflammation and, ideally, lessen patient's narcotic requirement.*
- ▲ As pain control is achieved, begin titration of medication as prescribed. *Both oral narcotics and NSAIDs may be prescribed for home care.*
- ▲ Administer prescribed IV fluids (3-5 L/day). *Fluids promote hemodilution, which reverses agglutination of sickled cells within the microcirculation. Hydration and reversal of viscous blood flow in small blood vessels work to reestablish blood flow so that tissue necrosis does not occur.*
- Use additional comfort measures such as positioning devices and splints for joint discomfort. Use foam overlay mattresses.
- Use distractional devices such as TVs and VCRs as well as relaxation techniques. *These can facilitate pain control.*
- Provide rest periods. *Facilitate comfort, sleep, and relaxation, which make it easier to cope with discomfort.*

Continued.

Sickle cell pain crisis—cont'd

NURSING DIAGNOSES	EXPECTED OUTCOMES AND NURSING INTERVENTIONS / *RATIONALE* (■ = INDEPENDENT; ▲ = COLLABORATIVE)

High Risk for Ineffective Management of Therapeutic Regimen

RISK FACTORS

Economic difficulties
Social support deficits
Family patterns of health care
Excessive demands on individual or family
Knowledge deficit
Decisional conflicts
Perceived seriousness
Perceived powerlessness

EXPECTED OUTCOMES

Patient verbalizes understanding of sickle cell disease, prevention of crisis, and appropriate treatment.
Patient identifies appropriate resources.
Patient describes intention to follow prescribed regimen.

ONGOING ASSESSMENT

- Assess pattern of compliance with treatment plan.
- Assess for related factors that may negatively affect success in following regimen. *Knowledge of causative factors provides direction for subsequent intervention.*
- Assess individual's perception of health problem. *Patient may not understand the chronicity of this disease nor his or her ability to control some of the precipitating factors.*
- Assess ability to learn desired regimen.

THERAPEUTIC INTERVENTIONS

- Explain causes of sickle cell disease and the pain of crisis.
- Inform of benefits of adherence to prescribed life-style. *May involve significantly less hospitalization and pain.*
- Instruct on preventable/treatable situations that can precipitate crisis:
   decreased fluid intake, infection, strenuous physical exertion, emotional stress, extreme fatigue, cold exposure, hypoxia, trauma.
- Instruct on the necessity of contacting a physician at the first sign of infection.
- Instruct on importance of drinking at least 4-6 L of fluid daily. *Reduces blood viscosity.*
   Dressing appropriately in severe cold weather.
   Taking prescribed medications such as folic acid. *Replaces depleted folic acid stores in the bone marrow.*
   Keeping physician/clinic appointments.
- Inform of support groups. *Groups that meet for mutual information can be beneficial.*
- Inform of the need for genetic counseling in family planning. *Pregnancy has increased risks for women with sickle cell disease.*
- Inform of new medications under investigation such as hydroxyurea. *Raises Hb F levels, which reduce sickling and crisis episodes.*

High Risk for Ineffective Coping

RISK FACTORS

Chronicity of disease
Inadequate psychologic resources (e.g., self-esteem)
Personal vulnerability
Situational crises
Unsatisfactory support system
Inadequate coping method

EXPECTED OUTCOMES

Patient identifies own maladaptive coping behaviors.
Patient identifies available resources/support systems.
Patient initiates alternative coping strategies.

ONGOING ASSESSMENT

- Assess patient's ability to openly express feelings about disease.
- Assess family's and significant other's support for disease management.
- Assess number of emergency room visits for crisis management. *Provides information on the patient's ability to follow prevention/treatment plan.*
- Assess use of controlling behaviors by patients with frequent hospital admissions. *Patients frequently need to escalate their "controlling" behaviors to gain attention by health care providers, who may see the patient as "only seeking medication."*

THERAPEUTIC INTERVENTIONS

- Set aside time to talk with patient when the pain is controlled. *During crisis the patient is distracted by the pain and may not be receptive to counseling.*
- Assist patient in understanding the chronicity of this disease and the need to follow suggested treatment plan.
- Provide information on coping strategies.
- Establish a working relationship with patient through continuity of care. *An ongoing relationship facilitates trust.*
- Involve social services, psychiatric liaison, pastoral care for additional and ongoing support resources.
- Avoid placing patient with crisis in same hospital room with another crisis patient. *Contact with patients with similar maladaptive behaviours may only intensify behavior.*
- Inform patient of existing community resources such as the National Association of Sickle Cell Anemia.

See also:
High Risk for Infection, p. 40.
Ineffective Individual Coping, p. 18.

By: Mary T. McCarthy, RN, MSN, CS

Tumor lysis syndrome

Rapid necrosis of malignant tumor cells induced by chemotherapy/radiation therapy resulting in hyperkalemia, hyperphosphatemia with hypocalcemia, azotemia, and hyperuricemia. Seen in patients receiving therapy for tumors with very high growth rates and rapid cell turnover (e.g., leukemias and malignant lymphomas).

NURSING DIAGNOSES	EXPECTED OUTCOMES AND NURSING INTERVENTIONS / *RATIONALE* (■ = INDEPENDENT; ▲ = COLLABORATIVE)

Altered Body Fluid Composition

RELATED FACTORS

Renal impairment
Chemotherapy
Radiation therapy

DEFINING CHARACTERISTICS

Potassium level >5.1 mEq/L
Calcium level <8.6 mg/dl
Cardiac dysrhythmias: bradycardia, ventricular dysrhythmias
Changes in ECG: prolonged PR and QT intervals; depressed ST segments; tall, peaked T waves; widened QRS complex

EXPECTED OUTCOMES

Patient maintains normal body fluid composition as evidenced by K^+ 4-5 mEq/L, calcium between 8.5-11, absence of cardiac dysrhythmias, normal ECG complexes.

ONGOING ASSESSMENT

- Assess cardiac status, noting rate and regularity of heart beat.
- If ECG monitoring is available, observe for common dysrhythmias and for ECG changes (see Defining Characteristics). *Of total body K^+ 98% is normally intracellular. In tumor cell lysis, intracellular K^+ is released into the blood, potentially causing elevation of K^+. Excess K^+ exerts a depressant effect on the cardiac conduction system, resulting in potentially life-threatening cardiac manifestations.*
- ▲ Assess serum potassium, sodium, and calcium levels daily. *The effects of hyperkalemia on the heart are more severe in the presence of hypocalcemia/hyponatremia.*

THERAPEUTIC INTERVENTIONS

- ▲ Restrict K^+-containing foods *to decrease K^+ intake* (e.g., restrict bananas, grapes, dried fruits, chocolate, meats).
- ▲ Encourage Na intake *(promotes K^+ loss if not restricted)*.
- ▲ Administer diuretics as prescribed; monitor intake/output q8hr.
- ▲ Administer cation-exchange resins (Kayexelate) *(exchanges Na^+ ions for K^+ ions through GI mucosa, then excretes K^+)*.
- ▲ Administer calcium gluconate IV as prescribed.
- ▲ Administer $NaHCO_3$/IV glucose with insulin. *Causes temporary shift of K^+ back into cell.*
- ▲ Prepare patient for dialysis if other measures are unsuccessful.

High Risk for Injury: Neuromuscular System

RISK FACTORS

Hyperphosphatemia
Chemotherapy
Radiation therapy
Hypocalcemia

EXPECTED OUTCOMES

Patient remains injury-free, as evidenced by neurologic status within normal limits, serum calcium and phosphate levels within normal limits.

ONGOING ASSESSMENT

- Assess patient for neuromuscular changes. *Hypocalcemia is associated with nervous system changes.* Observe for overt tetany (i.e., carpopedal spasms); latent tetany: Chvostek's sign *(tapping face over facial nerve in front of temple causes face to twitch);* Trousseau's sign *(inflating blood pressure cuff above systolic pressure for 3 min causes contraction of hand).*
- Assess for changes in mental status (confusion).
- Monitor for seizure activity.
- ▲ Monitor serum calcium and phosphate levels daily. *Serum phosphate and calcium are reciprocally related. Increase in phosphate causes decrease in calcium because of calcium-phosphate salt formation.*

THERAPEUTIC INTERVENTIONS

- Teach patient signs/symptoms of hypocalcemia (muscle cramps, paresthesias). Instruct patient to notify staff if they occur.
- Teach patient to avoid putting direct pressure on motor nerves (e.g., by crossing legs), *which exacerbates tetany.*
- Teach patient the importance of relaxation. *Tetany can be potentiated by stress.*
- If confusion present, reorient as needed; assist with ADLs; maintain safety precautions *to prevent injury.*
- Maintain seizure precautions: airway at bedside, padded side rails.
- ▲ Administer aluminum hydroxide, *which binds dietary phosphate from small bowel.* Monitor for constipation.
- ▲ Provide stool softeners.
- ▲ Administer calcium gluconate IV *to treat acute calcium deficit.*

Continued.

Tumor lysis syndrome—cont'd

NURSING DIAGNOSES	EXPECTED OUTCOMES AND NURSING INTERVENTIONS / *RATIONALE* (■ = INDEPENDENT; ▲ = COLLABORATIVE)
High Risk for Injury: Renal Damage **RISK FACTORS** Uric acid nephropathy resulting from increased uric acid precipitation in renal tubules; release of nucleic acids from tumor cell lysis	**EXPECTED OUTCOMES** Patient maintains normal renal function, as evidenced by balanced I & O, urine pH > 7.0, serum BUN, creatinine, uric acid within normal limits. **ONGOING ASSESSMENT** · Monitor intake and output, observing for decreasing output. · Monitor urine pH. *Urine should remain alkalized with pH greater than 7.* ▲ Monitor serum lab values: uric acid, BUN, creatinine. · If allopurinol is administered, observe for side effects: rash, fever, GI upset, abnormal liver function test findings, diarrhea, and acute renal failure. **THERAPEUTIC INTERVENTIONS** ▲ Administer fluids as prescribed. IV hydration should begin 1-2 days before chemotherapy, continue 2-3 days after chemotherapy is completed *to prevent uric acid precipitation in urine.* ▲ If urine is acidic, administer allopurinol *to reduce uric acid production and reduce chance of nephropathy.* · See also Renal failure, acute, p. 436, as needed.
High Risk for Fluid Volume Overload **RISK FACTORS** IV hydration Chemotherapy	**EXPECTED OUTCOMES** Patient maintains normal fluid volume, as evidenced by stable weight, balanced I & O, clear breath sounds, no JVD, no signs of edema. **ONGOING ASSESSMENT** · Monitor vital signs for tachycardia, increased or decreased blood pressure, increased RR · Monitor daily weight after breakfast; weigh patient on same scale every day. *Monitoring weight helps assess changes in fluid shifts and effectiveness of therapy.* · Observe for edema: pedal, sacral, generalized. · Monitor I & O. Notify physician if intake exceeds output by 1 L/24 hr. · Observe for jugular vein distention. *Present with right-sided fluid overload.* · Assess lungs for signs of fluid overload: tachypnea, rales, shortness of breath at rest/with exertion. **THERAPEUTIC INTERVENTIONS** · Apply elastic stockings (TED hose) *to prevent venous pooling.* ▲ Restrict fluids as necessary: set up 24-hr schedule for fluid intake. Restrict Na⁺ intake. · Place patient in semi- to high Fowler's position; encourage ambulation (*improves lung expansion).* · Encourage frequent rest periods *to conserve energy.* ▲ Administer diuretics as prescribed *to decrease fluid retention.*

Knowledge Deficit
 	
RELATED FACTORS
 	
Change in body function
Unfamiliarity with disease process
Misinterpretation of disease process
 	
DEFINING CHARACTERISTICS
 	
Multiple questions
Noncompliance with medications and diet
	EXPECTED OUTCOMES
	Patient/family verbalize understanding of condition, procedures, and treatment.
	
	ONGOING ASSESSMENT
	· Assess understanding of condition, procedures, and treatments.
	
	THERAPEUTIC INTERVENTIONS
	· Inform patient of severity of condition and necessary treatments.
	· Prepare patient and family members for possible dialysis, if necessary:
	    Teach about venous access: peripheral/vascular.
	    Teach about rationale for dialysis:
	        To decrease K⁺, Ca⁺, phosphate, and uric acid levels.
	        To reverse acute renal failure caused by hyperphosphatemia.
	    Teach about signs, symptoms, and complications of TLS.
	    Discuss nursing/medical treatment
	    Discuss early signs/symptoms to report to health care team.

By: Christa M. Schroeder, RN, MSN
    Sharon Flucus, RN, BSN
    Carol Nawrocki, RN, BSN

Vulvectomy

A vulvectomy is surgical removal of the vulva, which is done to remove cancer. Rarely, it is performed as a result of Paget's disease, leukoplakia, or intractable pruritis. A simple vulvectomy involves removal of the labia majora and minora, and sometimes the clitoris. A radical vulvectomy involves removal of tissue from just above the anus to just above the symphysis pubis, in addition to labia majora and minora, and clitoris; groin lymph node dissection may also be performed

NURSING DIAGNOSES	EXPECTED OUTCOMES AND NURSING INTERVENTIONS / *RATIONALE* (■ = INDEPENDENT; ▲ = COLLABORATIVE)

Knowledge Deficit, Preoperative

RELATED FACTORS

Unfamiliarity with proposed surgical procedure
Lack of previous surgical experience

DEFINING CHARACTERISTICS

Anxiety
Questioning
Lack of questions
Misconceptions

EXPECTED OUTCOMES

Patient is able to verbalize purpose and nature of vulvectomy, and describe aspects of postoperative nursing care.

ONGOING ASSESSMENT

- Assess patient's knowledge of proposed procedure. *The type and amount of information the patient knows or is able to verbalize are related to several factors, including: the type and amount of information given, appropriateness of teaching to patient's cognitive ability, and the patient's readiness to "hear" certain information that is disturbing or frightening.*
- Assess knowledge of preoperative preparation.
- Assess postoperative expectations regarding condition.
- Assess appropriateness of/patient's desire for having a significant other present during teaching. *Since this surgery has implications for altered sexuality, having the spouse/ significant other present may be useful to postoperative coping and adaptation.*

THERAPEUTIC INTERVENTIONS

- Using pictures, charts, videos, etc., and language that is appropriate to patient's level of understanding and readiness for learning, describe/reinforce surgeon's description of the proposed surgical procedure: explain/show in pictures the tissue to be removed (a simple vulvectomy *involves removal of the labia majora and labia minora, and possibly the* clitoris; a radical vulvectomy *involves removal of labia minora and majora, the clitoris, plus tissue from just above the anus to just above the symphysis pubis, and possibly lymph tissue from the groin area*).
- Explain that the wound will be covered with dressings but most likely left open (*unsutured, not covered by skin*) to heal. *Since the wound is in the perineum, the risk of infection is high; this method of wound healing is often chosen for such wounds.*
- Explain that postoperatively, drains (Jackson-Pratt, Hemovac) from the surgical site will be in place, especially for radical procedures involving lymph dissection. *When lymph drainage is interrupted, drains are placed to reduce edema and collection of fluid that could become infected.*
- Explain the need for IV feeding. *Until bowel sounds return and oral fluids are tolerated (usually 3-4 days postoperatively), IV fluid will provide hydration and access for the administration of parenteral antibiotics.*
- Explain the need for a Foley catheter. *A Foley catheter will allow for drainage of urine even though edema around the urethra can be severe; additionally, drainage of urine away from the surgical site reduces the risk of infection.*
- Explain the need for early postoperative ambulation and use of TED hose and/or sequential compression devices on the legs, *to reduce the risk of deep vein thrombosis and pulmonary emboli. Patients with pelvic malignancies are often hypercoagulable.*

High Risk for Infection

RISK FACTORS

Open surgical wound
Proximity of wound to rectal area
Reduced lymphatic flow
Cancer
Postoperative immobility
Indwelling catheter
IV catheter

EXPECTED OUTCOMES

Patient remains free of infection as evidenced by clean, healing wound; clear yellow urine; clear lungs on auscultation; normal temperature; normal WBC.

ONGOING ASSESSMENT

- Assess appearance of wound, noting any redness, swelling, purulent/foul-smelling drainage, or increased complaint of pain. *A healthy wound will be pink and moist and produce a small amount of clear serous fluid.*
- Check temperature q4hr. *Temperature elevation to 38.2° C is a normal postoperative stress response; temperatures above 38.2° C usually indicate infection (typically, pulmonary atelectasis is the site, but an open surgical wound must be highly suspect.)*

Continued.

NURSING DIAGNOSES	EXPECTED OUTCOMES AND NURSING INTERVENTIONS / *RATIONALE* (■ = INDEPENDENT; ▲ = COLLABORATIVE)

ONGOING ASSESSMENT—cont'd

- Observe color, clarity, and odor of urine. *Cloudy urine with a strong foul odor indicates urinary tract infection.*
- ▲ Monitor WBC. *Elevated WBC may indicate infection.*
- Assess peripheral and/or central IV sites for redness, swelling, or purulent drainage.
- Auscultate lungs to detect crackles, *which may indicate postoperative atelectasis and increased risk of pulmonary infection.*

THERAPEUTIC INTERVENTIONS

- Wash hands before each contact with the patient. *Handwashing remains the single most effective method of reducing nosocomial infection.*
- Maintain asepsis in wound care. *Sterile saline or prescribed antibiotic solutions may be used in wound care; irrigation of the wound using a bag of IV fluid with tubing attached may be helpful. Any irrigation device (e.g., Water Pik) is useful in thoroughly cleaning the wound.*
- ▲ Administer antibiotics as prescribed.
- Maintain patency of Foley catheter *to prevent leakage of urine from around catheter into surgical site.*
- Provide low-fiber, high-fluid intake *to reduce straining at stool and fecal contamination of surgical site.*
- Provide meticulous perineal care after each bowel movement *to minimize amount of bacteria in the perineum.*
- Maintain suction to drains as ordered *to reduce risk of stasis of drainage.* Empty drainage collectors as needed using aseptic technique.
- See also Infection, high risk for, p. 40.

High Risk for Sexual Dysfunction

RISK FACTORS

Surgery involving genital/ gynecologic structures
Altered body image
Altered self-esteem related to surgery
Removal of clitoris

EXPECTED OUTCOMES

Patient discusses issues related to sexuality and begins to incorporate changes into self-concept.

ONGOING ASSESSMENT

- Explore patient's knowledge of human sexuality. *Understanding normal sexual functioning and the role of structure and function of anatomic structures is fundamental to correcting misconceptions/providing realistic information.*
- Assess patient's understanding of how self-esteem and expectations for role performance affect sexuality; involve spouse/significant other as appropriate/as desired by patient. *The degree of importance assigned to the ability to perform sexually will affect the patient's sense of altered sexuality.*
- Assess degree to which patient fears/expects to experience unsatisfying, unrewarding, or inadequate sexual functioning postoperatively. *Any genital/gynecologic surgery has potential for creating fears/feelings that sexuality will be altered. Since vulvectomy often involves removal of the clitoris, the patient's orgasmic ability may be altered (although some women report reaching orgasm without clitoral stimulation).*
- Assess value systems/beliefs that may have impact on patient's ability to discuss/learn/ try alternate methods of achieving sexual satisfaction.

THERAPEUTIC INTERVENTIONS

- Encourage patient to discuss concerns/fears about potential changes in sexuality related to vulvectomy.
- Acknowledge patient's difficulty in discussing issues related to sexuality.
- Clarify language (patient's and nurse's) *so that there is common understanding throughout discussion; a great deal of slang exists in the language of sexuality and can complicate/render ineffective a helpful discussion unless common language is established.*
- Give realistic information; avoid creating false hope or notion that "everything will be OK" but avoid destroying hope. *A straightforward discussion of sexuality, including discussion of structures, function, role of self-esteem, and impact of existing relationships, will be most helpful. This can only be undertaken successfully if there is rapport between the patient and the nurse, and is tempered by nurse's own comfort level and knowledge of sexuality.*

NURSING DIAGNOSES	EXPECTED OUTCOMES AND NURSING INTERVENTIONS / *RATIONALE* (■ = INDEPENDENT; ▲ = COLLABORATIVE)

THERAPEUTIC INTERVENTIONS—cont'd

▲ Refer patient/significant other for sex counseling/other psychological therapy if needed/desired.

■ Arrange visit from a successfully recovered sexually functioning patient, if patient desires. *Interaction with a nonprofessional person who has "survived" similar surgery is often very reassuring and provides a positive role model for patient; often, long-term supportive relationships develop through these meetings that serve the patient and the visitor well for long periods. Consider timing of such visit, and ask patient's preference. Some patients benefit more from visit after surgery; both preoperative and postoperative visits may be desired. Telephone contact is useful for patients who verbalize discomfort at suggestion of face-to-face visit.*

■ See also Altered sexuality, p. 58; Self-Esteem Disturbance, p. 55.

High Risk for Pain

RISK FACTORS

Open perineal wound
Indwelling catheters (Foley, IV)

EXPECTED OUTCOMES

Patient verbalizes relief of or reduction in pain.
Patient appears comfortable.

ONGOING ASSESSMENT

■ Assess postoperative pain, including verbal and nonverbal cues indicating pain.
■ Assess effectiveness of pain relief measures.
■ Assess impact of pain on ability to carry out necessary postoperative treatment, such as turning, coughing, deep-breathing, early ambulation, being able to begin coping with altered body part and function.

THERAPEUTIC INTERVENTIONS

▲ Provide pain relief measures. *Early and aggressive use of techniques such as positioning, massage, use of heat/cold modalities, sitz baths as ordered, and distraction/guided imagery techniques will reduce the amount of pain medication required and enhance patient's ability to participate effectively in postoperative care.*

▲ Administer pain medication/reinforce use of patient-controlled analgesia (PCA) as needed. *Assure the patient that the dosage of pain medication used postoperatively is not addictive, and that the benefits of being comfortable enough to participate effectively in postoperative care far outweigh adverse effects of analgesia. It is also most effective to manage pain before it becomes severe.*

■ Assure patient that pain medication will be given before dressing changes or ambulation. *This will reduce the fear/anxiety that accompanies the prospect of unpleasant procedures and increase the patient's sense of control; this in turn may positively impact the patient's perception of pain during procedures.*

■ Provide a bed cradle *to prevent linen from coming into contact with perineal area.*

■ Tape urinary catheter and any surgical drains securely *to prevent painful movement or inadvertent dislodgment.*

▲ Administer stool softeners *to prevent straining at stool.*

Knowledge Deficit: Postoperative

RELATED FACTORS

Need for care after discharge
Partially healed perineal wound

DEFINING CHARACTERISTICS

Anxiety about discharge
Questions about home care/activity
Lack of questions about home care/activity
Verbalized misconceptions about home care/activity

EXPECTED OUTCOMES

Patient verbalizes and demonstrates home care before discharge from the hospital.

ONGOING ASSESSMENT

■ Assess patient's understanding of the wound healing process. *Wounds that are left open to heal by secondary intention granulate from the bottom up and from the sides toward the middle. Progress in healing demands a moist healing environment, lack of infection, adequate nutrition, and care to prevent mechanical disruption of the wound (pulling the wound apart, overaggressive local wound care [dressing changes] that disturb delicate new tissue).*

■ Assess understanding of signs/symptoms of infection.

■ Assess knowledge of the relationship between body position and development of edema.

Continued.

Hematolymphatic and Oncologic Care Plan

NURSING DIAGNOSES	EXPECTED OUTCOMES AND NURSING INTERVENTIONS / *RATIONALE* (■ = INDEPENDENT; ▲ = COLLABORATIVE)

	THERAPEUTIC INTERVENTIONS
	• Teach patient/significant other to care for perineal wound:
	  Dressings using clean technique (handwashing before and after, clean gloves for handling of soiled dressing, use of a cleaned surface for new dressings).
	  Cleansing of the perineal wound using a Water Pik or hand-held shower head
	  Shower rather than bath *to prevent soaking in dirty water*
	  Wiping from front to back and using perineal cleansing wipe or solution (e.g., Peri-Wash) after bowel movement and/or urination
	• Teach patient/significant other the signs of perineal wound infection: *increased drainage, yellow or greenish drainage with a foul odor, increased pain in perineal wound, fever, malaise, loss of appetite, which should be reported to physician/nurse immediately.*
	• Teach patient/significant other about medications to be taken after discharge *(typically analgesics and antibiotics).*
	• Teach patient/significant other the importance of continuing a high-fluid, low-residue diet *to prevent constipation and straining, which could be painful and which could mechanically damage the healing wound.*
	• Teach patient/significant other about the ongoing need for high-calorie, high-protein dietary intake *while the wound continues to heal.*
	• Teach the patient about body position and edema formation. Instruct patient to avoid long periods of sitting (driving, desk work), avoid strenuous walking, continue to wear support stockings. *Pelvic surgery, particularly if lymph node dissection was done, puts the patient at high risk for formation of pelvic and lower extremity edema.*
	• Teach patient/significant other that sexual activity can be gradually resumed. *Resumption of sexual activity will depend on patient's general well-being, comfort level of partner, condition of perineal wound, and patient/significant other's willingness to try alternate methods of sexual expression. Positions that reduce pressure and friction on the perineal area (such as side and woman on top) are preferable, with the use of water-soluble lubricant; vaginal intercourse may be avoided altogether and alternate methods used.*

See also:
Anticipatory Grieving, p. 28.

By: Audrey Klopp, RN, PhD, ET

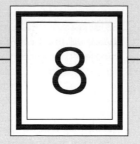

Renal Care Plans

Acute renal failure

(ACUTE TUBULAR NECROSIS [ATN]; RENAL INSUFFICIENCY)

In acute renal failure the kidneys are incapable of clearing the blood of the waste products of metabolism. This may occur as a single acute event with return of normal renal function or result in chronic renal insufficiency or chronic renal failure. During the period of loss of renal function hemodialysis or peritoneal dialysis is used to clear the accumulated toxins from the blood. Renal failure can be divided into three major types: prerenal failure (resulting from a decrease in renal blood flow), postrenal failure (caused by an obstruction), and intrarenal failure (caused by a problem within the vascular system, the glomeruli, the interstitium, or the tubules). Hospital-acquired renal failure is most likely acute tubular necrosis (ATN), which results from nephrotoxins or an ischemic episode.

NURSING DIAGNOSES	EXPECTED OUTCOMES AND NURSING INTERVENTIONS / *RATIONALE* (■ = INDEPENDENT; ▲ = COLLABORATIVE)

Altered Patterns of Urinary Elimination

RELATED FACTORS

Severe renal ischemia secondary to sepsis, shock, or severe hypovolemia with hypotension (usually after surgery or trauma)
Nephrotoxic drugs or antibiotics such as amphotericin and gentamicin
Renal vascular occlusion
Hemolytic blood transfusion reaction

DEFINING CHARACTERISTICS

Increased blood urea nitrogen (BUN) and creatinine
Urine specific gravity fixed at or near 1.010
Hematuria, proteinuria
Urine output <400 ml/24 hr (in absence of inadequate fluid intake or fluid losses by other route)

EXPECTED OUTCOMES

Patient achieves optimal urinary elimination, as evidenced by:
Urine output ≥30 ml/hr
Electrolytes/BUN within/near normal levels
Normal specific gravity

ONGOING ASSESSMENT

- Assess for alteration in urinary elimination.
- Monitor and record I & O; include all fluid losses (e.g., stool, emesis, and wound drainage). Report output < 30 ml/hr.
- Monitor urine specific gravity. *Specific gravity measures the ability of the kidneys to concentrate urine. The ability to concentrate urine is lost in intrarenal failure.*
- ▲ Check for protein and blood in urine. *The presence of protein or blood indicates an abnormal state.*
- Palpate bladder for distention to assess for urinary retention.
- ▲ Monitor blood and urine lab tests as prescribed, electrolytes (Na, K, Cl, Ca, P, Mg); urinalysis, urine electrolytes; BUN, creatinine. *(Both BUN and creatinine are elevated in renal failure. However, creatinine is more specific because it is not affected by diet, blood in the gut, or metabolism.)*
- Obtain daily weights.

THERAPEUTIC INTERVENTIONS

- ▲ Administer fluids and diuretics as prescribed.
- ▲ Maintain patency of Foley catheter. If urine output decreases, irrigate catheter with sterile saline solution *to ensure patency. Maintaining catheter patency excludes low urinary tract obstruction as a cause of decreased urine output.*
- ▲ When administering medications (e.g., antibiotics) metabolized by kidneys, remember that excretion of these drugs may be altered. Dosages, frequency, or both may require adjustment.

Fluid Volume Excess

RELATED FACTORS

Inability to excrete fluid and electrolytes properly
Excessive administration of oral/IV fluids during periods of decreased renal function

DEFINING CHARACTERISTICS

Increased central venous pressure
Increased blood pressure
Acute weight gain, edema
Signs/symptoms of congestive heart failure (jugular vein distention, crackles [rales])
Shortness of breath, dyspnea

EXPECTED OUTCOMES

Patient's optimal fluid balance is maintained as evidenced by stable weight, vital signs within normal range, clear breath sounds.

ONGOING ASSESSMENT

- Assess for signs of circulatory overload *(increased central venous pressure [CVP], increased blood pressure (BP), weight gain, edema)*, congestive heart failure *(jugular vein distention, crackles)*, and pulmonary congestion *(shortness of breath, dyspnea, crackles).*
- Monitor heart rate, BP, CVP, and respiratory rate. *Edematous patients may actually be intravascularly depleted; similarly, when fluids begin to shift, overload can occur quickly, requiring management adjustments.*
- Monitor and record I & O. Include all stools, emesis, and drainage. *Close monitoring of all losses/output is necessary to determine adequate replacement needs.*
- Weigh patient daily (before and after dialysis); record. *Patient weights are the best monitor of fluid status.*
- Auscultate breath sounds and heart sounds for signs of fluid overload.

THERAPEUTIC INTERVENTIONS

▲ Administer oral and IV fluids as prescribed *to replace sensible and insensible losses. Note: Not all patients enter the oliguria phase of renal failure. If urine output remains high, volume replacement can be considerable.*

▲ Administer medications (e.g., diuretics) as prescribed.

▲ Administer IV medications in least amount of fluid possible *to minimize fluid intake during periods of decreased renal function with fluid overload.*

■ If peripheral edema is present, handle extremities/move patient gently *to prevent shearing.*

▲ Prepare patient for hemodialysis, ultrafiltration, or peritoneal dialysis if indicated *to clear body of excess fluid and waste products. Even when patient reaches diuretic phase of renal failure, dialysis is needed to clear solutes.*

■ See also Vascular access for hemodialysis, p. 456; Peritoneal dialysis, p. 449.

High Risk for Decreased Cardiac Output

RISK FACTORS

Dysrhythmias caused by electrolyte imbalance from acute renal failure:

Primary hyperkalemia: Decreased renal elimination of electrolytes: K, P, Mg, Na

Metabolic acidosis (present with acute renal failure) exacerbates hyperkalemia by causing cellular shift of H^+ and K^+. Excess H ions traded intracellularly with K ions, causing increased extracellular K^+

Hyponatremia results from excessive extracellular fluid (dilutional effect), edema, and restricted IV or dietary intake

Hypocalcemia can also occur; exact cause unknown

Volume overload leading to congestive failure.

EXPECTED OUTCOMES

Patient maintains adequate cardiac output as evidenced by: BP within normal limits for patient, strong regular pulses, absence of JVD.

ONGOING ASSESSMENT

■ Assess for signs of decreased cardiac output: change in BP, heart rate, CVP, peripheral pulses; jugular venous distension (JVD); decreased urine output; abnormal heart sounds; dysrhythmias; anxiety/restlessness.

■ Monitor vital signs.

▲ Monitor serum electrolytes as prescribed, assessing for electrolyte disturbances:

Hyperkalemia (K > 5.5 mEq/L):
ECG changes:
Widened QRS segment, increased T waves
Prolonged PR interval
Bradycardiac dysrhythmias, cardiac arrest

Hyponatremia (Na <115 mEq/L):
Nausea/vomiting
Lethargy, weakness
Seizures (with severe deficit)

Hypocalcemia (Ca <6.0 mg/dl):
Perioral paresthesia
Twitching, tetany, seizures
Cardiac dysrhythmias

■ Monitor cardiac rhythm. Determine patient's hemodynamic response to dysrhythmias.

■ Auscultate heart sounds for presence of third heart sound *(indicating heart failure)* or pericardial friction rub *(indicating uremic pericarditis). If either is present, the patient may require prompt dialysis.*

THERAPEUTIC INTERVENTIONS

▲ Administer oral and IV fluids as prescribed *to maintain optimal fluid balance;* note effects.

▲ Administer medications as prescribed *to equilibrate electrolyte disturbances temporarily* (e.g., sodium bicarbonate [$NaHCO_3$] *to correct acidosis or hyperkalemia;* calcium salts *to treat hypocalcemia;* glucose/insulin drip *to drive K^+ into the cell;* K^+ exchange resins *to exchange K^+ for Na^+ in the GI tract, thereby decreasing serum K^+ levels).* Note patient's response.

▲ Administer inotropic agent (e.g., digoxin) as prescribed *to increase myocardial contractility.*

▲ Administer O_2 as needed.

■ Provide calm environment with minimal stressors.

■ Restrict activity *to conserve O_2.*

▲ Prepare patient for dialysis or ultrafiltration when indicated.

Continued.

Acute renal failure—cont'd

NURSING DIAGNOSES	EXPECTED OUTCOMES AND NURSING INTERVENTIONS / *RATIONALE* (■ = INDEPENDENT; ▲ = COLLABORATIVE)

Altered Nutrition: Less than Body Requirements

RELATED FACTORS

Stomatitis
Anorexia, decreased appetite
Nausea, vomiting
Diarrhea
Constipation
Melena, hematemesis

DEFINING CHARACTERISTICS

Loss of weight
Documented inadequate caloric intake
Caloric intake inadequate to keep pace with abnormal disease/metabolic state

EXPECTED OUTCOMES

Patient's nutritional state is maximized as evidenced by maintenance of weight and adequate caloric intake.

ONGOING ASSESSMENT

- Assess for possible cause of decreased appetite or GI discomfort.
- Assess actual oral intake; obtain calorie counts as necessary.
- ▲ Monitor serum laboratory values (e.g., electrolytes, albumin level).
- Record emesis and stool output. Observe all stools/emesis for gross blood; test for occult blood.
- Assess weight gain pattern.

THERAPEUTIC INTERVENTIONS

- Administer small, frequent feedings as tolerated.
- ▲ Consult dietitian *to assist in providing a low-potassium, high-carbohydrate diet as indicated.*
- ▲ Limit dietary protein intake *to prevent additional elevations of blood urea nitrogen.*
- ▲ Administer enteral/parental feedings as prescribed.
- Provide frequent oral hygiene *to freshen mouth.*
- Offer ice chips/hard candy if not contraindicated.
- ▲ Offer antiemetics as prescribed.
- Make meals look appetizing; try to eliminate other procedures at mealtime if possible and focus on eating.

High Risk for Injury: Anemia

RISK FACTORS

Bone marrow suppression secondary to insufficient renal production of erythropoietic factor
Increased hemolysis leading to decreased life span of red blood cells secondary to abnormal chemical environment in plasma
Bleeding tendencies: decreased platelets and defective platelet cohesion, inhibition of certain clotting factors

EXPECTED OUTCOMES

Patient's risk of injury from anemia is reduced through ongoing assessment and early intervention.

ONGOING ASSESSMENT

- Observe, document signs of fatigue, pallor, bleeding from puncture sites and incisions and bruising tendencies.
- ▲ Monitor results of studies (Hb, Hct, platelets, coagulation studies).
- Check for guaiac in all stools and emesis.
- Observe for signs of fluid overload and adverse reactions during transfusion.

THERAPEUTIC INTERVENTIONS

- ▲ Administer O_2 as prescribed *to maintain oxygenation.*
- ▲ Administer blood transfusions as prescribed.
- ▲ If fluid overload is a problem after transfusion, administer diuretics as prescribed.
- ▲ Administer erythropoietin (recombinant human erythropoietin) as prescribed *to decrease the effects of the anemia. This helps to reduce the need for frequent blood transfusions by maintaining Hb/Hct.*
- Institute precautionary measures for patients with a tendency to bleed:
  Use only compressible vessels for IV sites.
  Avoid IM injections: *any needle stick is a potential bleeding site*
  Draw all laboratory specimens through an existing line: arterial line or venous access line.
  Provide gentle oral care.

High Risk for Systemic or Local Infection

RISK FACTORS

Uremia resulting in decreased immune response
Debilitated state with poor nutrition
Use of indwelling catheters, subclavian lines, Foley catheters, endotracheal (ET) tubes, etc.

EXPECTED OUTCOMES

Patient's risk of systemic/local infection is reduced through ongoing assessment and early intervention.

ONGOING ASSESSMENT

- Assess for potential sites of infection: urinary, pulmonary, wound, or IV line.
- Monitor temperature. *Note: Caused by the decreased immune response, an elevated temperature may not be present with infection.*
- ▲ Monitor WBC count.
- Note signs of localized or systemic infection; report promptly. *Infection is the leading cause of death in acute renal failure.*
- ▲ If infection is suspected, obtain specimens of blood, urine, sputum, etc., for culture and sensitivity as prescribed.

THERAPEUTIC INTERVENTIONS

- Provide scrupulous perineal and catheter care.
- Provide meticulous skin care *to prevent skin breakdown over pressure areas.*
- Use aseptic technique during dressing changes, wound irrigations, catheter care, and suctioning.
- Avoid use of indwelling catheters or IV lines whenever possible.
- ▲ If indwelling catheters or IV lines are mandatory, change them per unit/hospital policy.
- Protect patient from exposure to other infected patients.
- ▲ If infection is present, administer antibiotics as prescribed.

Knowledge Deficit

RELATED FACTORS

New condition
New procedures

DEFINING CHARACTERISTICS

Verbalized confusion about treatment
Lack of questions
Request for information

EXPECTED OUTCOMES

Patient/significant others verbalize understanding of acute renal failure and associated treatments.

ONGOING ASSESSMENT

- Assess knowledge and understanding of acute renal failure.

THERAPEUTIC INTERVENTIONS

- Encourage expression of feelings and questioning.
- Discuss need for monitoring equipment and frequent assessment.
- Explain all tests and procedures *before* they occur. Use terms the patient can understand; be clear and direct.
- Explain purpose of fluid and dietary restrictions.
- Explain need for dialysis as appropriate and what to expect during procedure.
- Instruct the patient to perform deep-breathing and coughing exercises *to promote lung expansion and clearing.*
- Involve the patient's family in care as much as possible (when appropriate). Discuss the need for follow-up visits. *Return of renal function may occur over a 12-month period, necessitating changes in medications, diet, and fluid restriction.*
- ▲ Encourage family conferences with members of patient's health care team (e.g., physician, nurses, rehabilitation personnel, social workers) as necessary. *This will facilitate family involvement in multidisciplinary planning.*
- ▲ Consult appropriate resource persons (e.g., rehabilitation personnel, physicians, social workers, psychologists, clergy, occupational therapists, and clinical specialists) as needed.

See also:
Ineffective Breathing Pattern, p. 10.
Decreased Level of Consciousness, p. 252.

By: Deborah Lazzara, RN, MSN, CCRN
Susan Galanes, RN, MS, CCRN

End-stage renal disease (ESRD)

(CHRONIC RENAL FAILURE)

End-stage renal disease (ESRD) is defined as irreversible kidney disease causing chronic abnormalities in the body's homeostasis and necessitating treatment with dialysis or renal transplantation for survival. Uremia or the uremic syndrome consists of the signs, symptoms, and physiologic changes that occur in renal failure. These changes are related to fluid and electrolyte abnormalities, accumulation of uremic toxins that cause physiologic changes and alter function of various organs, and regulatory function disorders (hypertension, renal osteodystrophy, anemia, and metastatic calcifications).

NURSING DIAGNOSES	EXPECTED OUTCOMES AND NURSING INTERVENTIONS / *RATIONALE* (■ = INDEPENDENT; ▲ = COLLABORATIVE)

Fluid Volume Excess

RELATED FACTORS

Excess fluid intake
Excess sodium intake
Compromised regulatory mechanisms

DEFINING CHARACTERISTICS

Edema
BP elevated (above patient's normal BP) before dialysis
Weight gain
Distended neck veins
Orthopnea
Tachycardia
Restlessness

EXPECTED OUTCOMES

Patient experiences normal fluid balance as evidenced by normotensive BP, weight gain ≤ 1 kg between visits, eupnea.

ONGOING ASSESSMENT

- Assess vital signs.
- Assess respiratory pattern and work of breathing.
- Check for distended neck veins.
- Auscultate for crackles, *which would signify the presence of fluid in the small airways.*
- Assess amount of edema by palpating area over tibia, at ankles, sacrum, back, and assessing appearance of face.
- Assess patient's compliance with dietary and fluid restrictions at home.

THERAPEUTIC INTERVENTIONS

- Weigh at every visit before and after dialysis (weight gain not to exceed 1 kg between visits).
▲ Restrict fluid intake as required by patient's condition.
▲ Restrict dietary sodium. *Sodium intake produces feeling of thirst. By restricting sodium intake, the amount of fluid a patient drinks can be reduced.*
- Advise patient to elevate feet when sitting down *to prevent fluid accumulation in lower extremities.*
- Instruct about necessity to follow prescribed fluid/dietary restriction.
▲ Give antihypertensive medications if prescribed.
- Maintain optimal positioning for air exchange. Have patient sit up if he/she complains of shortness of breath.

High Risk for Decreased Cardiac Output

RISK FACTORS

Fluid volume overload
Electrolyte imbalances
Hypoxia
Accumulated toxins

EXPECTED OUTCOMES

Patient achieves adequate cardiac output as evidenced by strong peripheral pulses, normal vital signs, warm dry skin, alert responsive mentation or no further reduction in mental status.

ONGOING ASSESSMENT

- Monitor vital signs with frequent monitoring of BP.
- Assess skin warmth and peripheral pulses. *Peripheral vasoconstriction causes cool, pale, diaphoretic skin.*
- Assess level of consciousness. *Early signs of cerebral hypoxia are restlessness and anxiety, leading on to agitation and confusion.*
- Monitor for dysrhythmias. *Cardiac dysrhythmias may result from the low perfusion state, acidosis, or hypoxia.*
- Assess for presence of fluid volume overload: *edema, elevated BP, weight gain, distended neck veins, orthopnea.*
▲ Monitor laboratory study findings for serum K^+, BUN, creatinine, etc., *to assess for presence of electrolyte imbalances and accumulated toxins.*
- Auscultate heart sounds for presence of third heart sound (*indicating heart failure*) or pericardial friction rub (*indicating uremic pericarditis*). *If either is present, the patient may require prompt dialysis.*
- Assess for jugular venous distention, distant or muffled heart sounds, and hypotension. *Chronic renal failure patients on dialysis are at high risk for development of pericarditis, increasing the risk for pericardial effusion and pericardial tamponade. See also Cardiac tamponade, p. 169, as appropriate.*

NURSING DIAGNOSES	EXPECTED OUTCOMES AND NURSING INTERVENTIONS / *RATIONALE* (■ = INDEPENDENT; ▲ = COLLABORATIVE)

THERAPEUTIC INTERVENTIONS

▲ Administer oral and IV fluids as prescribed *to maintain optimal fluid balance.* Use fluid restriction as appropriate.

▲ Administer medications as prescribed *to equilibrate electrolyte disturbances temporarily* (e.g., sodium bicarbonate [NaHCO] *to correct acidosis* or hyperkalemia; calcium salts *to treat hypocalcemia;* glucose/insulin drip *to drive K^+ into the cell;* K^+ exchange resins *to exchange K^+ for Na^+ in the GI tract, thereby decreasing serum K^+ levels).* Note patient's response.

▲ Administer inotropic agents (e.g., dobutamine HCl [Dobutrex], dopamine, digoxin, or amrinone [Inocor]) as prescribed *to increase myocardial contractility.*

▲ Administer oxygen as needed.

■ Provide a calm environment with minimal stressors and restrict activity *to conserve O_2.*

▲ Prepare patient for dialysis or ultrafiltration when indicated.

High Risk for Injury: Hypocalcemia

RISK FACTORS

Increased phosphorus level
Renal failure

EXPECTED OUTCOMES

Patient's risk of injury is diminished through ongoing assessment and early intervention. Patient follows appropriate ambulation and safety measures.

ONGOING ASSESSMENT

■ Assess for signs/symptoms of hypocalcemia: tingling sensations at ends of fingers, muscle cramps and carpopedal spasms, tetany, convulsion.

■ Observe for signs/symptoms of calcium-phosphorus imbalance: pruritus, blurred vision, cardiac dysrhythmias.

▲ Monitor calcium and phosphorus levels every week/month *to determine whether patient is at risk of metastatic calcification from high-calcium and high-phosphate product.*

■ Assess for signs/symptoms of extremity pain and joint swelling.

■ Observe patient's gait, ambulation, and movement of extremities.

■ Assess history for tendency to fracture easily. *The decreased blood calcium level causes a demineralization of the bones that makes them brittle, porous, and thinner.*

THERAPEUTIC INTERVENTIONS

▲ Administer phosphate-binding medications as prescribed *so ingested phosphorus will not be absorbed but can bind with medication and be excreted via feces.*

■ Apply lotion for itchiness; recommend use of scratcher rather than fingernails.

■ Provide safety measures: side rails, uncluttered room, orientation to surroundings, proper lighting. *Bones becomes so fragile that they break easily even from mild trauma.*

▲ Refer to rehabilitation medicine department as indicated for use of crutches, transport from wheelchair to chair or vice versa.

High Risk for Injury: Anemia

RISK FACTORS

Bone marrow suppression secondary to insufficient renal production of erythropoietic factor
Increased hemolysis leading to decreased life span of red blood cells secondary to abnormal chemical environment in plasma
Bleeding tendencies: decreased platelets and defective platelet cohesion, inhibition of certain clotting factors.

EXPECTED OUTCOMES

Patient's risk for injury is reduced through ongoing assessment and early intervention.

ONGOING ASSESSMENT

■ Observe, document signs of fatigue, pallor, bleeding from puncture sites and incisions, and bruising tendencies.

▲ Monitor results of studies (Hb, Hct, platelets, coagulation studies) as prescribed.

■ Check for guaiac in all stools and emesis.

■ Observe for signs of fluid overload and adverse reactions during transfusion.

THERAPEUTIC INTERVENTIONS

▲ Administer oxygen as prescribed *to maintain oxygenation.*

▲ Administer blood transfusions as prescribed.

▲ If fluid overload is a problem after transfusion, administer diuretics as prescribed.

▲ Administer erythropoietin (recombinant human erythropoietin) as prescribed *to decrease the effects of the anemia. This helps to reduce the need for frequent blood transfusions by maintaining Hb/Hct.*

■ Institute precautionary measures for patients with a tendency to bleed: use only compressible vessels for IV sites; avoid IM injections; *any needle stick is a potential bleeding site;* draw all laboratory specimens through an existing arterial or venous access line; provide gentle oral care.

Continued.

End-stage renal disease (ESRD)—cont'd

NURSING DIAGNOSES	EXPECTED OUTCOMES AND NURSING INTERVENTIONS / *RATIONALE* (■ = INDEPENDENT; ▲ = COLLABORATIVE)

High Risk for Impaired Skin Integrity

RISK FACTORS

Edema related to end-stage renal disease

Peripheral neuropathy from end-stage renal disease

EXPECTED OUTCOMES

Patient's optimal skin integrity is maintained as evidenced by the absence of breakdown.

ONGOING ASSESSMENT

- Assess skin integrity for pitting of extremities on manipulation, demarcation of clothing and shoes on patient's body.
- Assess for presence of peripheral neuropathy, *which results in changes in sensation.*

THERAPEUTIC INTERVENTIONS

- Instruct the patient to wear loose-fitting clothing when edema is present. *Restrictive clothing can increase risk of skin breakdown.*
- Teach factors important to skin integrity: nutrition, mobility, hygiene, early recognition of skin breakdown.
- Use caution when heating or cooling devices are applied to the patient and also instruct the patient. *The peripheral neuropathy can impair sensation, especially in the lower extremities.*

High Risk for Self-esteem Disturbance

RISK FACTORS

Prolonged outpatient dialysis
Loss of body function
Financial cost of chronic dialysis
Change in perceptions as autonomous and productive individual

EXPECTED OUTCOMES

Patient manifests more positive self-esteem, as evidenced by verbalization of positive feelings about self.

ONGOING ASSESSMENT

- Assess for signs of reduced self-esteem: self-negating verbalizations, depression, expressed anger, withdrawal; expressions of shame/guilt; evaluation of self as unable to deal with events.

THERAPEUTIC INTERVENTIONS

- Talk with patient, significant others, and friends, if possible, about chronic outpatient dialysis.
- Discuss problems and possible solutions with patient. Explore strengths and resources with patient.
- Allow patient time to voice concerns and express anger related to condition.
- ▲ Have social workers see patient regularly as a preventive measure. *Social worker can give psychological support and assist in financial arrangements.*
- ▲ Refer to psychiatric consultant as necessary. *Most dialysis patients experience some degree of emotional imbalance. With professional psychiatric consultant, most can gradually accept changed self-esteem.*
- Provide/encourage discussions with other patients with renal failure *to share their responses to illness.* Encourage use of support groups.
- Assist patient in identifying major areas of concern related to altered self-esteem. Use problem-solving technique with patient to explore ways of minimizing these concerns. *The nurse-patient relationship can provide strong basis for implementing other strategies to assist patient/family with adaptation.*
- Assist patient in incorporating changes into ADLs, social life, interpersonal relationships, and occupational activities.

Sexual Dysfunction

RELATED FACTORS

Effects of uremia on the endocrine system: amenorrhea, failure to ovulate, and decreased libido in females; azoospermia, atrophy of testicles, impotence, decreased libido, and gynecomastia in males

Psychosocial effects of renal failure and its treatment

EXPECTED OUTCOMES

Patient's sexual functioning is enhanced as evidenced by ability to discuss concerns and verbalization of improved sexual outlook.

ONGOING ASSESSMENT

- Assess patient's perception of change/lack of sexual development.
- Assess patient's behavior in terms of actual or perceived change/lack of development.
- Assess impact of changes in sexual function on patient.
- Explore meaning of sexuality with patient.

NURSING DIAGNOSES	EXPECTED OUTCOMES AND NURSING INTERVENTIONS / *RATIONALE* (■ = INDEPENDENT; ▲ = COLLABORATIVE)

DEFINING CHARACTERISTICS

Verbalization of concern about sexual functions

Expressed decrease in sexual satisfaction

Reported change in relationship with partner

THERAPEUTIC INTERVENTIONS

- Encourage patient to verbalize feelings about change/lack of sexual development.
- Discuss alternate methods of sexual expression with patient/significant others. *Emphasize that intercourse is not the only method for satisfying sexual relationship.*
- Emphasize importance of giving and receiving love and affection, as opposed to "performing."
- ▲ Confer with physician about medical treatments and procedures that may alleviate some sexual dysfunction: discuss possibility of penile implant/prosthesis; if patient has low zinc levels, discuss possible replacement therapy for male patients.

High Risk for Noncompliance

RISK FACTORS

Knowledge deficit

Lack of resources

Side effects of treatment, diet, and medications

Poor relationship with health care team

Denial

EXPECTED OUTCOMES

Patient demonstrates adherence to therapy, evidenced by: attendance at appointments, lab values within normal range, verbalization of compliance.

ONGOING ASSESSMENT

- Assess for signs of noncompliance: missed appointments, unused medications, abnormal laboratory values, acknowledgment of noncompliance.
- Elicit patient's understanding of treatment regimen.
- Explore with patient his/her feelings about illness and treatment.

THERAPEUTIC INTERVENTIONS

- Maintain consistency of care givers (*helps develop therapeutic relationship*).
- Promote decision making and ADL management; use social support systems. *Social support has been closely linked to compliance with dialysis; it is necessary to manage the role demands of daily living and especially important in coping with stressful life events and transitions.*
- ▲ Explore alternatives with health care team to reduce side effects.
- Contract with patient for behavioral changes.
- ▲ Consult social work department as appropriate.

Knowledge Deficit

RELATED FACTORS

Lack of interest in learning

Unfamiliarity with disease process

Information misinterpretation

EXPECTED OUTCOMES

The patient verbalizes a general understanding of chronic renal failure, prevention of complications, medications, and necessary dietary restrictions.

ONGOING ASSESSMENT

- Assess understanding of end-stage renal disease.
- Observe for dietary deviations and noncompliance when patient is on unit.

THERAPEUTIC INTERVENTIONS

- Discuss end-stage renal failure with patient, including the need for dialysis for survival.
- Instruct patient in methods to relieve dry mouth and maintain fluid restriction:

   Allow ice chips as needed. *One cup of ice equals only ½ cup of water. Sucking cup of ice takes much longer than drinking cup of water; patient can attain more satisfaction.*

   Suggest keeping hard candy on hand to alleviate dry mouth (*stimulates secretion of saliva and alleviates some mouth dryness*).

   Suggest frequent mouth rinses with ½ cup mouthwash mixed with ½ cup of ice water. *Rinses can produce freshness in mouth and alleviate thirst temporarily.*
- Instruct patient in dietary restrictions. *Diet needs to be individualized according to the impairment of renal function.*
- Involve significant others in instruction sessions on special diets and fluid restrictions. *They may prepare patient's food.*
- Instruct patient in recognition of signs of fluid volume excess. *Patients can adjust sodium and water intake independently if they know how to assess for signs of fluid overload.*
- Teach to observe for signs/symptoms of hypocalcemia. Provide list of symptoms on discharge.
- Discuss importance of taking prescribed medications.
- Discuss thoroughly, before discharge, patient's medications, dosages, and side effects.

Continued.

End-stage renal disease (ESRD)—cont'd

NURSING DIAGNOSES	EXPECTED OUTCOMES AND NURSING INTERVENTIONS / *RATIONALE* (■ = INDEPENDENT; ▲ = COLLABORATIVE)

See also:
Powerlessness, p. 52.
Altered Family Processes, p. 23.
Activity Intolerance, p. 2.
Impaired Gas Exchange, p. 27.
Grieving, p. 30.
Body Image Disturbance, p. 7.

By: Susan Galanes RN, MS, CCRN

Glomerulonephritis

POSTSTREPTOCOCCAL GLOMERULONEPHRITIS (ACUTE GLOMERULONEPHRITIS [AGN]; RAPIDLY PROGRESSIVE GLOMERULONEPHRITIS [RPGN])

Glomerulonephritis (GN) is caused by an immune response to bacterial or viral infection, drugs, immunizations, or systemic disease (i.e., lupus erythematosus, scleroderma). An antigen-antibody reaction causes immune complexes that become trapped with antibodies and antigens in the glomerular basement membrane. An inflammatory response occurs, resulting in decreased plasma filtration and increased membrane permeability to large protein molecules. Although rapidly progressive glomerulonephritis (RPGN) has a 50% rate of development of renal failure and chronic glomerulonephritis (which is often undetected and can result in renal failure after many years), prognosis is very good for complete recovery from common forms of the disorder (i.e., poststreptococcal GN).

NURSING DIAGNOSES	EXPECTED OUTCOMES AND NURSING INTERVENTIONS / *RATIONALE* (■ = INDEPENDENT; ▲ = COLLABORATIVE)

Fluid Volume Excess

RELATED FACTORS

Diminished glomerular filtration
Increased Na^+ retention

DEFINING CHARACTERISTICS

Periorbital edema
Facial puffiness
Generalized edema
Dark urine, dysuria
Decreased output, oliguria
Hematuria
Proteinuria
Specific gravity ≥1.020
Serum electrolytes within normal limits
Anorexia
Mild/moderate hypertension

EXPECTED OUTCOMES

Patient maintains fluid volume within normal limits, as evidenced by absence of edema, increased urinary output, urinalysis results within normal limits.

ONGOING ASSESSMENT

- Assess for facial/periorbital edema in A.M. *Generalized edema appears later in disease course and late during day.*
- Measure I&O. *Patient may become oliguric; persistent anuria/oliguria may indicate acute renal failure. A slight increase in output usually indicates increasing kidney function with diuresis following in 3 to 4 days.*
- Evaluate pulse, respiration, and blood pressure (BP).
- Weigh daily.
- ▲ Evaluate lab results: urinalysis, serum electrolytes, blood urea nitrogen (BUN), creatinine, erythrocyte sedimentation rate (ESR), and ASO titer. *ESR reflects acute inflammation and can be used to follow disease course. ASO titer (antistreptolysin O) can be used to detect streptococcal antibodies 4 to 6 wk after infection. Urinalysis may reveal 3+ to 4+ hematuria and proteinuria with increasing specific gravity.*
- ▲ Review test results: renal biopsy, magnetic resonance imaging (MRI), ultrasound.
- ▲ Assess for hyperlipidemia, hypoalbuminemia, massive proteinuria, and fatty casts in urine. *Presence indicates development of nephrotic syndrome, seen in approximately 20% of adult cases of glomerulonephritis.*

NURSING DIAGNOSES	EXPECTED OUTCOMES AND NURSING INTERVENTIONS / *RATIONALE* (■ = INDEPENDENT; ▲ = COLLABORATIVE)

THERAPEUTIC INTERVENTIONS

▲ Restrict fluid intake to equal urinary and insensible loss when signs of hypertension, renal, or cardiac failure are present.

▲ Provide a no-added-salt diet. Restrict K^+ only if oliguric.

▲ Restrict protein if azotemia, elevated BUN, oliguria is present. *Because of anorexia, dietary restrictions are seldom needed.*

▲ Administer antihypertensives and in severe cases furosemide (Lasix) as prescribed, *to control blood pressure and fluid volume. Other diuretics have not been useful.*

■ Keep patient on bedrest *(enhances diuresis).*

Infection

RELATED FACTORS

Group A β-hemolytic strepto-
 coccus
Pharyngitis
Impetigo
Upper respiratory infection
Scarlet fever
Recent immunizations
Known systemic disorder

DEFINING CHARACTERISTICS

Pain
Redness
Skin rash
Fever
Lethargy
Positive culture result

EXPECTED OUTCOMES

Patient remains free of infection, as evidenced by negative culture results and afebrile status.

ONGOING ASSESSMENT

■ Assess for physical evidence of infection. *Infections must be treated to stop the immune response.*

▲ Review results of specimen cultures.

■ Obtain recent history for signs and symptoms of infection or exposure to infected individuals. *Symptoms of AGN appear 10-14 days after initial streptococcal illness.*

THERAPEUTIC INTERVENTIONS

■ Provide comfort measures as needed.

▲ Administer antibiotics *(usually not prescribed unless culture findings are positive).*

High Risk for Decreased Cardiac Output

RISK FACTORS

Hypervolemia
Cardiac decompensation

EXPECTED OUTCOMES

Patient maintains adequate cardiac output, as evidenced by clear mentation, normal vital signs, clear breath sounds, warm dry skin.

ONGOING ASSESSMENT

■ Monitor for signs of compromised cardiac output: rales, tachypnea, dyspnea; frothy sputum; weight gain, edema, oliguria; anxiety, restlessness; weakness, fatigue; abnormal heart sounds; decreased peripheral pulses; cold, clammy skin; decreased mentation.

▲ Evaluate chest radiographs for pulmonary edema.

▲ Monitor ABGs, electrolytes.

THERAPEUTIC INTERVENTIONS

■ Place on cardiopulmonary monitor.

■ Position for comfort and ease of respiration.

▲ Restrict fluids as prescribed.

▲ Administer humidified oxygen and restrict activity *to decrease cardiac demands.*

▲ Administer corticosteroids if prescribed. *Although not usually used in the treatment of AGN, it may have a positive antiinflammatory effect in RPGN.*

▲ Prepare patient for possible dialysis. *Patients at risk for significant complications and renal failure can benefit from early initiation of dialysis.*

High Risk for Injury: Seizures

RISK FACTOR

Hypertensive encephalopathy

EXPECTED OUTCOMES

Risk of injury is reduced, as evidenced by reduced/normal BP, clear mentation, absence of signs of encephalopathy.

ONGOING ASSESSMENT

■ Assess for central nervous system changes such as headache, dizziness, vomiting, vision changes, disorientation, hemiparesis. *Signs of encephalopathy must be detected and treated early to prevent seizure/stroke. This can be a medical emergency.*

■ Assess for history of seizure activity.

Continued.

Glomerulonephritis—cont'd

NURSING DIAGNOSES	EXPECTED OUTCOMES AND NURSING INTERVENTIONS / *RATIONALE* (■ = INDEPENDENT; ▲ = COLLABORATIVE)
	THERAPEUTIC INTERVENTIONS ▲ Administer anticonvulsants as prescribed. ▲ Administer antihypertensives *to control blood pressure and decrease risk of encephalo-pathic changes.*
Pain **RELATED FACTORS** Inflammatory response Infection **DEFINING CHARACTERISTICS** Verbal complaint Tenderness on examination	**EXPECTED OUTCOMES** Patient verbalizes relief or reduction in pain. Patient appears comfortable. **ONGOING ASSESSMENT** • Assess for complaints of flank pain. • Assess for tenderness at the costovertebral angle. **THERAPEUTIC INTERVENTIONS** • Explain cause of pain. • Encourage bedrest; assist with repositioning. • Provide warm or cool packs as desired. ▲ Do not administer pain medications unnecessarily. *As the inflammation diminishes, so will the pain. Medications can be nephrotoxic and pose an unnecessary risk.*
Knowledge Deficit **RELATED FACTORS** New diagnosis Hospitalization **DEFINING CHARACTERISTICS** Stated lack of understanding Many questions Appearance of confusion **See also:** Acute Renal Failure, p. 436. Seizures, p. 281. Nephrotic Syndrome, p. 447.	**EXPECTED OUTCOMES** Patient verbalizes understanding of disease process and follow-up care required. **ONGOING ASSESSMENT** • Assess for knowledge of disease process and current status **THERAPEUTIC INTERVENTIONS** • Provide information about course of disease and all treatments, procedures. • Explain home care measures: I&O, BP measurement. • Explain need for follow-up care. *Although most patients recover completely (70%) there may be persistent hematuria and above-average BUN for some weeks. A small percentage may progress to chronic GN or acute renal failure.*

Michele Knoll Puzas, RNC, MHPE

Nephrotic syndrome

NEPHROSIS, RENAL INSUFFICIENCY

Nephrotic syndrome refers to a group of symptoms (edema, severe proteinuria, hypoalbuminemia, and hyperlipidemia) that occur in response to profound glomerular permeability caused by any condition that seriously damages the glomerular capillary membrane. Severe plasma protein loss stimulates hepatic lipoprotein synthesis, fluid shift to extracellular spaces, hypovolemia, sodium retention, and severe edema. Symptoms may or may not become chronic, depending on the underlying disease/cause. As nephrotic syndrome worsens, treatment becomes similar to that for renal failure. A complication of nephrotic syndrome is hypercoagulability, leading to renal vein thrombosis and pulmonary embolism.

NURSING DIAGNOSES	EXPECTED OUTCOMES AND NURSING INTERVENTIONS / *RATIONALE* (■ = INDEPENDENT; ▲ = COLLABORATIVE)

Fluid Volume Excess

RELATED FACTORS

Decreased renal filtering capacity
Fluid loss into interstitial spaces
Activation of renin-angiotensin system

DEFINING CHARACTERISTICS

Total body edema
Low BP
Puffy eyelids
Severe proteinuria
Hypoalbuminemia
Hyperlipidemia
Elevated BUN and creatinine levels
Abnormal electrolytes

EXPECTED OUTCOMES

Patient maintains adequate fluid volume as evidenced by vital signs within normal limits, absence of orthostatic BP changes, absence of edema.
Patient maintains normal electrolyte levels.

ONGOING ASSESSMENT

- Obtain historical data that may help in identifying cause (i.e., medications, drug use, recent illness, hereditary illness).
- Monitor pulse, respirations, and postural BP.
- Assess for edema.
- Monitor I&O.
- Obtain weight; compare with estimated dry weight.
- Measure abdominal girth every day.
- Check urine specific gravity and dipstick for protein, blood, pH.
- ▲ Monitor lab results: serum albumin, triglycerides, electrolytes, urinary protein, WBCs, RBCs, BUN, creatinine.

THERAPEUTIC INTERVENTIONS

- ▲ Prepare for needle biopsy of kidney. *This is necessary for definitive diagnosis of glomerulonephritis.*
- ▲ Limit IV and oral fluid intake as prescribed.
  Use IV infusion device *for accuracy.*
  Limit free water oral intake *to allow increased intake of nutritious fluids with or between meals.*
  Provide medication with fluids other than water.
- ▲ Administer steroids. *Used to treat antigen-antibody and inflammatory reactions and decrease edema and protein loss.*
- ▲ Administer electrolytes as prescribed.
- ▲ Administer salt-poor albumin and diuretics as prescribed. *Albumin causes shift of fluids into vascular system, enhancing the diuretic effects. Used to treat severe edema, orthostatic hypotension, and hypovolemia.*
- ▲ Provide a low-sodium, high-protein diet. *Protein loss causes hypovolemia and activation of the renin-angiotensin system. Hepatic lipoproteins cannot compensate for the severe loss. The renin-angiotensin system causes sodium retention and further contributes to the edema.*
- ▲ Administer cyclophosphamide (Cytoxin) as prescribed. *Cyclophosphamide is nephrotoxic and scleroses the glomeruli, resulting in decreased dumping of proteins into the urine.*

Altered Nutrition: Less Than Body Requirements

RELATED FACTORS

Impaired renal function and protein loss
Poor appetite

EXPECTED OUTCOMES

Nutrition is adequate, as evidenced by good skin, hair condition; good muscle development; weight gain or no further weight loss.

ONGOING ASSESSMENT

- Monitor food intake.
- ▲ Monitor proteinuria.
- Perform calorie count if needed.

Continued.

Nephrotic syndrome—cont'd

NURSING DIAGNOSES	EXPECTED OUTCOMES AND NURSING INTERVENTIONS / *RATIONALE* (■ = INDEPENDENT; ▲ = COLLABORATIVE)

DEFINING CHARACTERISTICS
Hypoalbuminemia
Proteinuria
Muscle wasting
Weight loss

THERAPEUTIC INTERVENTIONS
- ▲ Obtain dietary consultation.
- ▲ Administer vitamin supplements.
- ■ Offer small, frequent meals of preferred foods; allow favored foods from home if within diet regimen.
- ▲ Provide diet:
  High in protein, calories (CHO), and potassium
  Low in sodium, fat. *Protein is required for tissue growth, carbohydrates to spare protein and for energy. Potassium is needed because of high loss with interstitial fluid shift and diuresis.*
- ▲ Consider tube feeding supplements and/or total parenteral nutrition (TPN) if condition warrants.

High Risk for Infection

RISK FACTORS
Immunosuppression of steroid therapy
Anemia

EXPECTED OUTCOMES
Patient is free of infection, as evidenced by normal WBC count, afebrile status.

ONGOING ASSESSMENT
- ■ Assess for signs of infection.
- ■ Assess vital signs, especially temperature. *Fever may not be present because of reduced immune response.*
- ▲ Monitor WBC.
- ■ Observe visitors for any obvious symptoms of infection.
- ■ Assess for signs of anemia: stools for blood, pallor. *Blood is lost in urine and the GI tract, and red cell production is decreased as a result of poor erythropoetin production.*

THERAPEUTIC INTERVENTIONS
- ■ Screen roommates or consider private room.
- ■ Limit visitors and staff contact.
- ■ Report signs of infection immediately *to ensure prompt treatment and prevent exacerbation of renal symptoms.*

High Risk for Impaired Skin Integrity

RISK FACTORS
Tissue edema

EXPECTED OUTCOMES
Patient's optimal skin integrity is maintained as evidenced by the absence of breakdown.

ONGOING ASSESSMENT
- ■ Assess dependent areas for skin breakdown.
- ■ Assess for pitting edema. *Pitting edema is manifested by a depression that remains after one's finger is pressed over an edematous area and then removed.*
- ■ Observe open wounds for proper healing.

THERAPEUTIC INTERVENTIONS
- ■ Change position frequently if immobile.
- ■ Use pillows for support when positioning *to relieve pressure areas and prevent tissue breakdown.*
- ■ Keep skin clean and dry.
- ■ Avoid tight clothing *to reduce venous pooling.*
- ■ Elevate edematous extremities, *to increase venous return and in turn lessen edema.*
- ■ Provide pressure-relieving devices *as prophylactic measures.*

NURSING DIAGNOSES	EXPECTED OUTCOMES AND NURSING INTERVENTIONS / *RATIONALE* (■ = INDEPENDENT; ▲ = COLLABORATIVE)

Knowledge Deficit

RELATED FACTORS

New diagnosis
Chronicity of disease
Long-term medical management

DEFINING CHARACTERISTICS

Lack of questions
Excessive anxiety
Inability to talk about present status

See also:
Acute Renal Failure, p. 436.
Glomerulonephritis, p. 444.

EXPECTED OUTCOMES

Patient verbalizes disease process and follow-up care.

ONGOING ASSESSMENT

- Assess knowledge base and readiness for learning.
- Assess support system and ability to provide home/self-care.

THERAPEUTIC INTERVENTIONS

- Explain nephrotic syndrome, all tests, and procedures.
- Instruct to observe for increased edema by daily weights, periorbital edema, abdominal distention, ankle edema.
- Provide instruction on use of dipsticks for protein check, signs of infection, dietary needs/restrictions, medication therapy.
- Provide follow-up appointments and encourage compliance.

By: Michele Knoll Puzas, RNC, MHPE

Peritoneal dialysis

(INTERMITTENT PERITONEAL DIALYSIS [IPD]; CONTINUOUS CYCLIC PERITONEAL DIALYSIS [CCPD]; CONTINUOUS AMBULATORY PERITONEAL DIALYSIS [CAPD])

Hemodialysis, peritoneal dialysis, or transplantation are necessary to maintain life in patients with absence of kidney function. Peritoneal dialysis is indicated for patients in renal failure who have vascular access problems and/or cannot tolerate the hemodynamic alterations of hemodialysis. A peritoneal catheter is placed through the anterior abdominal wall to achieve access. During peritoneal dialysis the peritoneum functions as the membrane by which molecules flow from the side of high concentration to the side of lower concentration. This procedure removes excess fluid and waste products from the body during renal failure. Peritoneal dialysis may be performed as intermittent perioneal dialysis (IPD), continuous ambulatory peritoneal dialysis (CAPD), or continuous cyclic peritoneal dialysis (CCPD).

NURSING DIAGNOSES	EXPECTED OUTCOMES AND NURSING INTERVENTIONS / *RATIONALE* (■ = INDEPENDENT; ▲ = COLLABORATIVE)

Fluid Volume Excess

RELATED FACTORS

Renal insufficiency
Increased peritoneal permeability to glucose, H_2O, protein

DEFINING CHARACTERISTICS

Acute weight gain
Elevated BP
Peripheral edema
Shortness of breath
Orthopnea
Crackles
Elevated serum glucose

EXPECTED OUTCOMES

Patient's fluid volume excess is reduced as evidenced by vital signs within normal limits, clear breath sounds.

ONGOING ASSESSMENT

- Monitor BP, pulse, respirations, and patient response during dialysis.
- Obtain history of estimated dry weight, BP, and dialysate solution used. *Elevated BP and weight gain can be caused by dialysate reabsorption.*
- Obtain baseline weight when peritoneal cavity is empty, then every day.
- Measure inflow/outflow of dialysate with each exchange and maintain record of cummulative fluid balance.
- Assess work of breathing and for presence of orthopnea.
- Auscultate breath sounds. *Increased fluid absorption can lead to pulmonary congestion.*
- Check for sacral and peripheral edema.
- Monitor I/Os.
- ▲ Monitor serum glucose *(glucose absorption may occur with dialysate)* and use of hypertonic dialysate *(may lead to fluid volume deficit if not closely monitored).*

Continued.

NURSING DIAGNOSES	EXPECTED OUTCOMES AND NURSING INTERVENTIONS / *RATIONALE* (■ = INDEPENDENT; ▲ = COLLABORATIVE)
	THERAPEUTIC INTERVENTIONS ▲ Institute fluid restrictions as appropriate. ▲ Collaborate with the pharmacist to concentrate IVs and medications maximally *in order to decrease unnecessary fluids.* ▲ Administer IVs via an infusion pump, if possible, *to assure accurate delivery.* ■ Elevate edematous extremities *to increase venous return and in turn lessen edema.* ■ Reduce constriction of vessels (use appropriate garments; avoid crossing of legs or ankles) *to prevent venous pooling.*
High Risk for Injury **RISK FACTORS** Complications of peritoneal dialysis: decreased outflow leading to increased abdominal pressure, electrolyte imbalance	**EXPECTED OUTCOMES** Patient remains free of injury as evidenced by eupnea, electrolytes within normal limits. **ONGOING ASSESSMENT** ■ Obtain baseline vital signs and dry weight. ■ Monitor patient's BP periodically during dialysis. ■ Record fluid I & O. ■ Measure abdominal girth daily at end of drain time. ■ Auscultate breath sounds. ■ Monitor patient for tachypnea, retractions, nasal flaring. *If dialysate fluid is retained in the abdomen, it may cause pressure on the diaphragm, resulting in a decrease in lung expansion and possible respiratory distress.* ▲ Monitor patient's electrolyte levels, especially K^+. ■ Observe for nausea, vomiting, edema, or disorientation. ■ Monitor each exchange, checking that outflow is equal to or greater than inflow. ■ Check catheter for kinks, fibrin, or clots, *which could obstruct outflow of fluid from the catheter, resulting in retained fluid in the abdomen.* **THERAPEUTIC INTERVENTIONS** ■ Change position frequently *to maximize drainage.* Elevate HOB at 45 degrees and turn patient from side to side. *Position changes will also help to prevent pulmonary complications by preventing an upward displacement of the diaphragm, which can result from inadequate drainage.* ■ Discontinue dialysis if signs of hypokalemia are present and notify physician. ▲ Notify physician and change dialysate concentration when patient reaches dry weight *so as not to dehydrate patient by removing too much fluid.* ■ Stop dialysis if drainage is inadequate. *Overinfusion causes pain, dyspnea, nausea, and electrolyte imbalance.* ■ Assure proper functioning if using automatic cycler.

High Risk for Infection
 	
 RISK FACTOR
 	
 Possible contamination of peritoneal catheter entry site
	EXPECTED OUTCOMES
	 Patient's risk for infection is reduced through ongoing assessment and early intervention.
	
	 ONGOING ASSESSMENT
	 ■ Assess patient for signs/symptoms of infection: fever; generalized malaise; complaints of abdominal pain, tenderness, warm feeling, chills; rigid abdominal wall, peritoneal catheter site reddened with discharge; cloudy returned dialysate; positive culture and sensitivity results; nausea; vomiting; diarrhea.
	 ■ Assess peritoneal drainage with each exchange (normal is clear); cloudiness: *indicates increased WBC, chyle;* volume: *decreased volume noted with increased peritoneal permeability;* fibrin: *increased production noted with peritonitis.*
	 ▲ Collect effluent as appropriate for:
	     WBC with differential: *cell count >100 cells/mm³ with >50% polys indicates peritonitis.*
	     Culture/sensitivity with Gram's stain: *indicates need of appropriate antibiotic. Gram's stain may reveal fungus, which takes 5-7 days to grow.*
	 ■ Assess area around catheter site; should be clean with no signs of inflammation.
	 ■ Assess patient for complaint of abdominal tenderness.
	 ■ Palpate abdomen for rebound tenderness and pain along catheter tunnel tract. *Rebound tenderness or pain along tunnel tract indicates inflammation.*

ONGOING ASSESSMENT—cont'd

- Auscultate abdomen for bowel sounds. *Absent bowel sounds may indicate ileus from bacterial toxins.*
- Assess vital signs, including temperature.
- Ask patient to describe how he/she feels during exchanges. *Early detection and treatment of infection minimize complications of infection.*
▲ Notify nephrologist and/or dialysis staff for any signs of infection. *Treatment can be instituted quickly and more serious complications can be prevented.*

THERAPEUTIC INTERVENTIONS

- Use strict aseptic technique when setting up dialysis and hooking up patient. *Poor hygiene and improper technique during hook-up can lead to catheter site infection, the most common complication of peritoneal dialysis.*
- Maintain drainage receptacle below level of peritoneum *to prevent backflow of dialysate.*
- Ensure aseptic handling of peritoneal catheter and connections.
- Anchor connections and tubing securely *to prevent inadvertent disconnection.*
▲ Send any purulent drainage from exit site for culture and sensitivity.
▲ If peritonitis is suspected:
  Assist with peritoneal lavage as prescribed *to remove products of inflammation and relieve pain.*
  Administer antibiotics intraperitoneally as prescribed, using shortened dwell periods for first 24 hr *(puts medications at source of infection). Shortened dwell periods are used so dialysate reabsorption is decreased.*
▲ If aminoglycosides are administered, obtain blood levels after 48 hr as prescribed. *Ototoxicity can occur with prolonged use.*
▲ Add heparin to dialysate, as prescribed, *to decrease fibrin production.*
▲ Perform exit site care per unit protocol.

High Risk for Pain

RISK FACTORS

Length of procedure
Actual infusion of dialysate
Distended abdomen

EXPECTED OUTCOMES

Patient verbalizes relief of/absence of pain.
Patient appears comfortable.

ONGOING ASSESSMENT

- Assess continually for signs of discomfort.
- Assess need for pain medications and evaluate their effect.
- Assess for pain in the scapula region. *Referred pain to the scapula occurs when air is inadvertently infused into the peritoneal cavity.*

THERAPEUTIC INTERVENTIONS

- Remain at bedside during initiation of dialysis. Do not allow air inflow; always use warm fluids. *Cool fluids can cause cramping.*
- Allow/encourage family involvement during dialysis *to provide comfort.*
- Change patient's position *to relieve discomfort during inflow.*
▲ Allow ambulation if permitted.
- Lessen or eliminate source of discomfort if possible. *May need to reduce flow.*
- Explain reasons for inflow pain: *pH of fluid lower than body causes discomfort until equilibration; air in cavity causes discomfort; pressure on organs and diaphragm causes discomfort until patient becomes accustomed to procedure; cold or hot solution.*
- If patient experiences scapula pain, allow adequate drain time and position patient on side with knees to chest *to assist in removal of any air from the peritoneal cavity.*
- Provide diversional activities *to direct focus away from pain/procedure.*

Knowledge Deficit

RELATED FACTORS

Unfamiliarity with peritoneal dialysis and its complications

EXPECTED OUTCOMES

Patient becomes proficient at performing peritoneal dialysis and is able to verbalize signs/symptoms of infection.

ONGOING ASSESSMENT

- Identify existing misconceptions about peritoneal dialysis.
- Assess ability to perform tasks related to peritoneal dialysis.

Continued.

Peritoneal dialysis—cont'd

NURSING DIAGNOSES	EXPECTED OUTCOMES AND NURSING INTERVENTIONS / *RATIONALE* (■ = INDEPENDENT; ▲ = COLLABORATIVE)

DEFINING CHARACTERISTICS
Verbalizes inaccurate information
Requests information
Acknowledges noncompliance
Expresses frustration/ confusion when performing task
Performs task incorrectly
	THERAPEUTIC INTERVENTIONS
	■ Review patient diagnosis and need for peritoneal dialysis.
	▲ Discuss dietary/fluid requirements and restrictions: low sodium, low potassium, adequate protein, high calories, free fluids. Arrange dietary consultation if necessary.
	■ Discuss medications and use.
	■ Demonstrate and request return demonstration of peritoneal catheter care.
	■ Demonstrate and have patient perform repeat demonstration:
	    Appropriate handwashing techniques
	    Steps to peritoneal dialysis:
	      Assuring a clean work area
	      Using appropriate supplies
	      Checking dialysate for expiration date, dextrose concentration, correct volume, pinhole leaks, and foreign particles
	      Wearing mask during the procedure
	      Clamping tubing; using sterile technique when spiking or unspiking from dialysate
	■ When instructing in continuous ambulatory peritoneal dialysis (CAPD), review the use of commercially available devices that help maintain the sterility of the system during tubing connections. *It is of critical importance to maintain sterile technique to prevent infection.*
	■ Instruct the patient, as appropriate, that an orthopedic binder and the use of a regular low back exercise program can be helpful for low back pain aggravated by the increase in intraabdominal pressure.
	■ Work collaboratively with the patient to fine-tune the length of dialysis, diet regulations, pain and diversion needs *to achieve optimum benefit of the treatment.*
	■ Describe signs/symptoms of infection/peritonitis, including basis of occurrence and when to call physician.
	■ Discuss return appointments, follow-up care, emergency numbers.
	▲ Arrange social service consultation if necessary.

See also:
Noncompliance, p. 42.

By: Adrian Cooney, RN, BSN
    Susan Galanes, RN, MS, CCRN

Renal transplantation, postoperative

(KIDNEY TRANSPLANTATION)

Renal transplantation is the surgical implantation of a renal allograft from either a cadaver or a live donor into a patient with end-stage renal failure. Most frequently transplant candidates are on chronic hemodialysis or peritoneal dialysis, exhibiting symptoms of azotemia, anemia, fluid overload, and oliguria. After a successful operative course, the renal transplantation recipient recovers in the intensive care unit or stepdown unit, where fluid shifts and vital signs are monitored.

NURSING DIAGNOSES	EXPECTED OUTCOMES AND NURSING INTERVENTIONS / *RATIONALE* (■ = INDEPENDENT; ▲ = COLLABORATIVE)

High Risk for Fluid Volume Deficit/Excess

RISK FACTORS

Variable time for initial renal function:

Immediately after renal transplantation patient may vacillate between fluid depletion and fluid overload

Prolonged transport time causing acute tubular necrosis (ATN): Patients may experience diuresis several days postoperatively

EXPECTED OUTCOMES

Patient's risk for development of fluid volume deficit/excess is reduced through ongoing assessment and early intervention.

ONGOING ASSESSMENT

- Weigh daily. Use same scale *to prevent discrepancies in measuring device.*
- Monitor I & O hourly in the ICU and q4hr on general unit.
- Note and document presence of peripheral or sacral edema.
- Auscultate lungs to assess for rales (crackles).
- Assess skin turgor and hydration of mucous membranes. *During assessment of the patient, keep in mind the signs of fluid volume deficit (polyuria, weight loss, dry mucous membranes, weakness, and thirst) and the signs of fluid volume excess (edema, weight gain, shortness of breath, orthopnea, intake greater than output, abnormal breath sounds such as crackles).*

THERAPEUTIC INTERVENTIONS

- ▲ Replace fluids ml per ml plus 30 ml/hr *to account for insensible loss or according to unit protocol (may vary among institutions). ATN patients may have diuresis several days after surgery, exceeding 200-400 ml/hr. Living-related transplantation recipients have greater urine volumes in early postoperative period (may exceed 400-600 ml/hr). Fluid replacement must match output so patient does not become dehydrated.*
- ■ Notify physician if urine output <30 ml/hr.
- ▲ Administer diuretics and restrict fluids as indicated.
- ▲ Begin progressive ambulation *to facilitate adequate tissue perfusion to edematous body areas.*
- ▲ Prepare for hemodialysis, as necessary, until the transplanted kidney is functioning.

High Risk for Urinary Retention

RISK FACTOR

Obstructed Foley catheter

EXPECTED OUTCOMES

Patient's risk of urinary retention is decreased as evidenced by patency of Foley catheter or patient request to void q1-2hr.

ONGOING ASSESSMENT

- Obtain preoperative history of patient's pattern of urinating. *If patient was oliguric, urinary bladder may be atrophied and/or reduced in size.*
- Assess urine for color, amount, sediment, and presence of clots. *Depending on volume of urine, bladder capacity, muscle tone, and degree of hematuria, indwelling catheter will remain in place 2-7 days.*
- Assess for abdominal/bladder distention resulting from clotted Foley catheter or anastomosis leak.
- Record accurate I & O (q1h in ICU or q4hr on general unit).
- After discontinuing Foley catheter, assess color, clarity, sediment, and blood in voided urine.

THERAPEUTIC INTERVENTIONS

- ■ Maintain Foley catheter drainage, preventing kinks, *which would obstruct flow.*
- ▲ If gross hematuria is evident, strain urine for clots. Irrigate Foley catheter with physician approval. *Bleeding from anastomosis can cause clotted Foley catheter.*
- ■ After discontinuing Foley catheter, ask patient to void q1-2hr *to prevent urinary retention and urinary bladder overdistention. If bladder capacity is significantly compromised, patient will need to empty bladder more often. Full bladder causes additional strain on ureteral anastomosis.*
- ■ Instruct patient to record daily urine output and notify transplantation physician if output decreases or color, clarity, or consistency changes.

Continued.

Renal transplantation, postoperative—cont'd

NURSING DIAGNOSES	EXPECTED OUTCOMES AND NURSING INTERVENTIONS / *RATIONALE* (■ = INDEPENDENT; ▲ = COLLABORATIVE)

High Risk for Local/Systemic Infection

RISK FACTORS

Immunosuppression with antirejection medications (*decrease circulating lymphocytes and ability to fight infectious organism*)

EXPECTED OUTCOMES

Patient's risk of infection is reduced through ongoing assessment and early intervention.

ONGOING ASSESSMENT

- Monitor temperature 1-3 times/day. *A fever may be a sign of infection or rejection.*
- Inspect wound twice daily for local erythema, purulent drainage, or dehiscence; notify transplant physician if they occur.
- ▲ Culture wound for aerobic organisms if drainage purulent, green, or foul-smelling.
- ▲ Culture urine if patient is febrile or dysuric or if urine turns cloudy.
- ▲ Monitor all culture reports.
- Assess respiratory rate and rhythm and check for signs of increased work of breathing.
- Assess breath sounds.

THERAPEUTIC INTERVENTIONS

- Wash hands before and after touching patient. *Bacteria, viruses, fungi, and protozoa indigenous in nontransplantation populations may be infectious in immunosuppressed transplantation patient.*
- ▲ Obtain private room for patient. *Patients do not require isolation, but a private room is recommended.* Restrict visitors and flowers at transplantation team's discretion.
- Encourage deep breathing, coughing, and turning *to prevent associated respiratory complications.*
- Encourage postoperative use of incentive spirometry. *A respiratory infection can result in postop mortality when maximum doses of immunosuppressive are being given.*
- ▲ Administer antibiotics as prescribed.
- Teach patient/significant other about avoidance of infectious crowds, importance of good hygiene, signs/symptoms of infection. *Patient must understand increased infection risk and importance of calling transplantation physician for signs of infection.*

Pain

RELATED FACTORS

Incisional pain
Ineffective analgesia
Pain exacerbated by straining and early ambulation

DEFINING CHARACTERISTICS

Facial mask of pain
Crying/moaning
Complaints of pain
Guarding behavior
BP and pulse rate change

EXPECTED OUTCOMES

Patient verbalizes relief/reduction in pain
Patient appears relaxed and comfortable.

ONGOING ASSESSMENT

- Assess for verbal and nonverbal pain symptoms.
- Observe and record vital sign changes indicating increased pain.
- Assess prescribed analgesia's effectiveness.

THERAPEUTIC INTERVENTIONS

- Reinforce relaxation techniques and position changes *to alleviate incisional or muscular pain, thereby reducing need for narcotic analgesia.*
- Encourage patient to splint abdominal incision *to reduce pain.*
- ▲ Titrate prescribed analgesia as needed.
- ▲ Premedicate patient 20 min before ambulating, performing ADLs, or having large dressing changes *to minimize movement-induced pain.*
- Assist with ambulation and ADLs until patient can resume self-care.

High Risk for Anxiety/Fear

RISK FACTORS

Change in health status:
  End of dialysis
  Postoperative need for dialysis
  Threat of rejection or infection
Change in role functioning

EXPECTED OUTCOMES

Patient's anxiety/fear is reduced as evidenced by cooperative behavior and calm appearance.

ONGOING ASSESSMENT

- Assess for signs of anxiety/fear: apprehension, feelings of inadequacy, facial tension, restlessness, worry. *Occasionally the patient must be dialyzed postoperatively until the transplanted kidney begins functioning. This can be very anxiety-provoking for the patient.*
- Assess patient's/family's dependent/independent behaviors.
- Assess available support systems and functional coping mechanisms.
- Assess patient's ability to accept self-care responsibility.

NURSING DIAGNOSES	EXPECTED OUTCOMES AND NURSING INTERVENTIONS / *RATIONALE* (■ = INDEPENDENT; ▲ = COLLABORATIVE)

THERAPEUTIC INTERVENTIONS

- Allow patient time to ventilate fears and anxiety. *After surgery, the transplantation patient must maintain health and cannot rely on the dialysis staff. This independence is often frightening, especially with the potential for rejection or infection.*
- Assist with identifying available support systems.
- ▲ Offer emotional support. *If the patient is anxious about the need for postoperative dialysis, reassure the patient that this is not uncommon (especially with cadaver-donated kidneys). Consult social service staff as indicated.*
- Set limits for regressive and aggressive behavior.

Knowledge Deficit:

RELATED FACTOR

New condition

DEFINING CHARACTERISTICS

Verbalized confusion about treatment
Lack of questions
Request for information

EXPECTED OUTCOMES

The patient/significant other states an understanding of renal transplantation, including postoperative self-care.

ONGOING ASSESSMENT

- Assess patient's/family's readiness to discuss transplantation surgery, postoperative course, and potential life-style changes. *Teaching begins before surgery. Patients often do not understand impact of transplantation until several months after surgery. Thus teaching begins during dialysis; staff proceeds gradually, taking into account patient's learning style, educational level, and readiness to learn.*
- Assess previous knowledge of transplantation; clarify misconceptions.

THERAPEUTIC INTERVENTIONS

- Prepare and use visual aids and logs for record keeping (e.g., medication charts, I & O sheets, vital sign log).
- Provide information on:
  Signs/symptoms of graft rejection
  Signs/symptoms of local and systemic infection. *Transplant recipients are at increased risk for developing infection because of immunosuppressive therapy.*
  Medication teaching:
     Instruct patient to take medication *every day* for life. *Immunosuppressive medications must be taken daily as long as patient has kidney transplant, to prevent rejection.*
     Instruct patient to wear medical alert bracelet *stating that he/she uses antirejection medications and is a transplantation patient.*
     Instruct and supervise medication self-administration at bedside, *to prepare for self-administration at home.*
     Instruct reasons for *all* medications, side effects, schedule, complications associated with medications, when to be concerned, and when to report to transplantation/nephrology team (i.e., fine tremors associated with cyclosporine A; however, sudden increase may signal toxicity).
  Diet restrictions, if any
  Physical self-examination: 24 hr I & O; BP, pulse, temperature (twice/day); daily weight; daily self-assessment for graft tenderness
- Instruct patient on appropriate course of action for suspected rejection or infection.

See also:
Ineffective Breathing Pattern, p. 10.
Powerlessness, p. 52.

By: Gina Marie Petruzzelli, RN, BSN

Vascular access for hemodialysis

(INTERNAL ARTERIOVENOUS FISTULA OR
EXTERNAL CATHETER [SUBCLAVIAN,
INTRAJUGULAR, FEMORAL, QUINTON PERMCATH])

Dialysis is the diffusion of solute molecules and fluids across a semipermeable membrane. Dialysis is often necessary to sustain life in people with no, or very little, kidney function. The purpose of dialysis is to remove excess fluids, toxins, and metabolic wastes from the blood during renal failure. Hemodialysis requires a vascular access. This can be accomplished by surgically creating an arteriovenous (A-V) fistula or graft (synthetic material used to connect an artery and a vein) or by insertion of an external catheter into the subclavian, internal jugular, or femoral vein. The internal A-V fistula is made surgically by creating an anastomosis between an artery and a vein, thus allowing arterial blood to flow through the vein, causing engorgement and enlargement. Placement may be in either forearm, using the radial artery and cephalic vein or branchial artery and cephalic vein. The internal A-V fistula must mature before it may be used for access in hemodialysis. The external catheter may be either single- or double-lumen. A single-lumen catheter serves as the arterial source, and the venous return is made via a peripheral vein or by the use of an alternating flow device. A double-lumen catheter is used for both the arterial source and the venous return. Femoral catheters are used only with inpatients on a short-term basis, because of their location and low durability. The subclavian or intrajugular catheters can be used for weeks or even months on an outpatient basis. External A-V shunts are currently considered obsolete and are rarely used today.

NURSING DIAGNOSES	EXPECTED OUTCOMES AND NURSING INTERVENTIONS / *RATIONALE* (■ = INDEPENDENT; ▲ = COLLABORATIVE)

High Risk for Infection

RISK FACTORS

Hemodialysis catheter
A-V access cannulation

EXPECTED OUTCOMES

Patient's risk for infection is reduced through ongoing assessment and early intervention.

ONGOING ASSESSMENT

- Assess for signs and symptoms of infection: pain around the catheter site/over access site; fever; red, swollen, warm area around catheter exit site/access site; drainage from catheter exit site/access site.
- ▲ Obtain blood and catheter exit site culture if evidence of infection.
- Visually inspect and palpate the areas around and over intact dressing each shift for phlebitis, tenderness, inflammation, and infiltration.
- Assess perfusion of affected limb. Check for proper blanching and absence of cyanosis.
- Notify physician of any signs of decreased perfusion to affected limb.

THERAPEUTIC INTERVENTIONS

Subclavian and intrajugular catheters

- ▲ Maintain asepsis with the subclavian/intrajugular catheters during dialysis:
  Clean area with antiseptic. *Povidone-iodine (Betadine) solution is recommended.*
  Change sterile dressing over catheter exit site before each dialysis treatment.
  Use sterile technique when initiating or discontinuing dialysis.
  Instill heparin into catheter and secure placement of catheter and caps after dialysis.
  Do not use catheter for any purpose but hemodialysis.
- Explain importance of maintaining asepsis with catheter. *Because of its location and long-term use, infection is almost inevitable. Infection may be localized at exit site, but septicemia can occur.*
- Instruct to keep the dressing clean and dry at all times. *Meticulous care of catheter site and maintenance of dry intact dressing lessen infection risk.*
  Protect catheter dressing during bathing.
  Advise against swimming.
  If dressing loosens, reinforce with tape.
  If dressing comes off or becomes *wet,* go to dialysis unit as soon as possible for sterile catheter site care if incapable of performing at home.

NURSING DIAGNOSES	EXPECTED OUTCOMES AND NURSING INTERVENTIONS / *RATIONALE* (■ = INDEPENDENT; ▲ = COLLABORATIVE)

THERAPEUTIC INTERVENTIONS—cont'd

Femoral catheters

▲ Maintain asepsis with femoral catheter during dialysis:
Use sterile technique when initiating or discontinuing dialysis.
Instill heparin into catheter, secure placement of catheter end caps after dialysis.
If intravenous line cannot be started in peripheral vessel, femoral catheter may be used with extreme caution.

▲ Maintain femoral catheter:
Change *all* dressings q48hr or more often if soiled.
Notify physician if infection is suspected.
Anticipate need to change femoral catheter q48-72hr *to lessen infection risk.*
Maintain strict bed rest if patient has femoral catheter, with cannulated leg flat *to prevent kinking of intravenous catheter.*

A-V fistula

▲ Maintain asepsis with A-V access during dialysis:
3-minute surgical scrub of access area (povidone-iodine scrub or Hibiclens). Wipe area with antiseptics. *Povidone-iodine is recommended agent.*
Apply povidone-iodine ointment to cannulation sites.
Cover cannulation sites with sterile bandages.
Allow only dialysis staff to cannulate A-V access. *This is the patient's lifeline* and is not for general use.
Stress good hygiene.
Remove bandages 4-6 hr after dialysis.

High Risk for Altered Peripheral Tissue Perfusion

RISK FACTOR

Interruption in arteriovenous (A-V) access blood flow

EXPECTED OUTCOMES

Patient's A-V access remains patent as evidenced by palpable pulse/thrill, bruit on auscultation, adequate color/temperature to extremity.

ONGOING ASSESSMENT

■ Assess A-V access for presence of adequate blood flow:
Palpate for pulse and thrill *(absence of pulse above venous site, or absence of thrill over anastomosis is a sign of inadequate blood flow).*
Auscultate for bruit; "swishing" sound should be audible. *When artery is connected to vein, blood is shunted from artery into vein, causing turbulence. This may be palpated above venous side of access for "thrill" or buzzing.*
Check for blanching of nailbeds of affected limb.
Check for mottling of skin and temperature of affected limb.
Assess for pain over access area.

THERAPEUTIC INTERVENTIONS

■ Promote the following preventive measures to ensure adequate blood flow: do not take BP in access limb; do not draw blood specimens from access limb.

■ Instruct patient to *avoid* devices and activities that endanger access patency, including:
Sleeping on access limb
Wearing tight clothing over limb with access
Carrying bags, purses, or packages over access arm
Participating in activities or sports that involve active use of and/or trauma to access limb. *Thrombosis is a common complication of vascular access. Causes include thrombi (caused by venipuncture), extrinsic pressure (BP cuff, tourniquet, sleeping on limb or tight clothes), or trauma to access limb (related to activities or sports that involve active use of limb).*

■ Maintain proper positioning of access limb. Consider elevating limb postoperatively *to reduce dependent edema.* Consider arm sling for support when patient is ambulatory. Encourage normal use of access limb *as this also promotes healing and reduced edema.*

Continued.

Renal Care Plans

NURSING DIAGNOSES	EXPECTED OUTCOMES AND NURSING INTERVENTIONS / *RATIONALE* (■ = INDEPENDENT; ▲ = COLLABORATIVE)

Knowledge Deficit

RELATED FACTORS

New procedure
New diagnosis
Home management

DEFINING CHARACTERISTICS

Questions
Confusion about treatment
Inability to comply with treat-
ment
Lack of questions

EXPECTED OUTCOMES

Patient/significant others are able to verbalize home care of intravenous catheter access or A-V fistula, recognize signs and symptoms of infection, and know how to notify the physician/dialysis staff if infection is suspected.

ONGOING ASSESSMENT

- Assess current knowledge level of dialysis access catheter and home maintenance.

THERAPEUTIC INTERVENTIONS

- Review diagnosis.
- Review dialysis and rationale.
▲ Discuss dietary/fluid requirements and restrictions: low sodium, low potassium, ade-
  quate protein, high calories, free fluids. Arrange dietary consultation if necessary.
- Discuss medications and use.
- Demonstrate and request return demonstration of access care before discharge.
- Discuss return appointments, follow-up care, emergency numbers.
▲ Arrange social service consultation if necessary.
- Teach how to check for adequate blood flow through fistula:
    Demonstrate how to feel for pulses and thrill.
    Designate specific areas to feel for pulses and thrill.
      *Absence of pulses and thrill may indicate clotting of access with the need to inform
      nephrologist or dialysis staff immediately.*
      *Waiting to declot access may result in inability to "save access" and require surgery
      to establish new vascular access.*
    Allow adequate time for return demonstration.
- Instruct patient to inform nephrologist or dialysis staff immediately of any signs and
  symptoms of infection: pain over access site; fever; red, swollen, and warm access site;
  drainage from access; red streaks along access area.
- Explain importance of maintaining asepsis with external catheter. *Infection is almost an
  inevitable complication of external vascular device. Infection may be localized cellulitis,
  but septicemia can occur. Meticulous daily care and avoidance of trauma to area prevent
  risk of infection.*
- Instruct to keep dressing clean and dry at all times:
    Protect catheter dressing while bathing (tub and sponge baths only); no swimming; no
    showers.
    Keep entire catheter under occlusive dressing; reinforce as necessary.
- Teach how to manage accidental separation or dislodgment of external access connections. *Information given to the patient/significant other of the medical condition and
  proper care of external access will increase awareness of his/her condition and decrease
  anxiety concerning ADL with renal failure.*
- Instruct patient/significant other in care of dressings if applicable.
- Recommend Medic-Alert bracelet.
▲ Inform patient that A-V fistula maturation may be hastened by exercising:
    Resistance exercise may begin 10-14 days after surgery.
    Apply light tourniquet to upper arm to impede venous flow and distend forearm ves-
    sels; use care not to occlude blood flow with tourniquet; apply tightly enough to dis-
    tend vessels.
    Instruct patient to open and close fist to pump arterial blood against venous resis-
    tance caused by tourniquet. Patient's squeezing rubber ball, tennis ball, hand grips,
    or rolled up pair of socks will help exert pressure.
    Repeat exercises for 5-10 min, 4-5 times/day. Patient may do exercises while watch-
    ing TV. *Resistance exercises cause vessels to stretch and engorge with blood.*

See also:
Anxiety/fear, p. 5, 23.

By: Susan Pische RN, BSN, MBA
    Susan Galanes RN, MS, CCRN

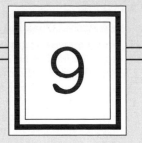

Genitourinary/Gynecologic Care Plans

Benign prostatic hypertrophy/prostate cancer/prostatectomy

([BPH]; TRANSURETHRAL RESECTION [TUR])

Disorders of the prostate gland are common in men over age 40. Benign prostatic hypertrophy (BPH) occurs in 75% of men over age 70. BPH is an overgrowth of muscle and connective tissue which causes obstructive urinary symptoms; it is treated by one of four surgical approaches to remove the excess tissue. Cancer of the prostate is one of the most common cancers in men; it is typically asymptomatic until advanced to metasasis. Prostate cancer depends on the presence of androgens (male hormones); in addition to orchiectomy and surgeries that are similar to those performed for BPH, prostatic cancer is also treated hormonally and with radiation therapy.

NURSING DIAGNOSES	EXPECTED OUTCOMES AND NURSING INTERVENTIONS / *RATIONALE* (■ = INDEPENDENT; ▲ = COLLABORATIVE)

Altered Patterns of Urinary Elimination

Related Factors
Hypertrophied prostatic tissue
Malignant tissue

Defining Characteristics
Diminished urinary stream
Incomplete bladder emptying
Dribbling at the end of a void
Hesitancy in starting stream
Recurrent urinary tract infections caused by obstruction
Nocturia
Hematuria
Hydronephrosis
Hydroureters

Expected Outcomes
Patient has unobstructed flow of urine, either by catheterization or after surgical removal of hypertrophied or cancerous prostatic tissue.

Ongoing Assessment
- Assess patterns of elimination; inquire about/observe urination: symptoms include difficulty starting a stream, dribbling at the end of a void, nocturia. *The male urethra is surrounded by the prostate gland; when the prostate gland is enlarged, as a result of either prostatic hypertrophy or cancer, the urethra is compressed.*
- Assess history of urinary tract infections. *Because the flow of urine is chronically obstructed, stasis of urine occurs and infections are common.*
- Assess for hematuria, *which can result from distention of the bladder with resultant rupture of small blood vessels.*
▲ Review radiograph findings: *hydroureters (distended ureters) and hydronephrosis (enlarged, overdistended kidneys) may result from long-standing obstruction caused by prostatic disease.*

Therapeutic Interventions
▲ Encourage oral fluids/administer IV fluids *for adequate hydration,* but do not push fluids/overhydrate *because rapid filling of the bladder can precipitate complete urinary retention.*
▲ Restore flow of urine by inserting an indwelling catheter. *Indwelling catheterization is used to allow free drainage of the bladder. Chronic urinary obstruction can result in severe damage to the kidneys and ultimate renal failure.*
   Note: When prostatic hypertrophy or cancer makes catheterization difficult or dangerous, the urologist or surgeon may opt to perform the catheterization. Special catheters with curved or firm tips may be requested and should be on hand.
▲ Administer antibiotics as prescribed *to treat/prevent urinary tract infection resulting from obstruction and stasis.*
- Prepare the patient for surgery.
   Transurethral resection (prostatectomy) (TURP): *This procedure is done through an instrument passed through the urethra; no incision is made. Excess prostate tissue or cancerous tissue is removed through the instrument.*
   Suprapubic resection: *An abdominal incision that extends through the bladder is used to remove the prostate gland completely.*
   Retropubic resection: *A low abdominal incision is made, but the bladder is not opened. The prostate gland is completely removed; this approach also allows for removal of lymph nodes, if necessary.*
   Perineal resection: *An incision is made in the perineum; the prostate gland is removed through the perineal incision. This type of surgical approach is common for cancer of the prostate.*
   Orchiectomy: *The testes are surgically removed to eliminate the production of androgens, on which prostate cancer is dependent for growth.*

NURSING DIAGNOSES	EXPECTED OUTCOMES AND NURSING INTERVENTIONS / *RATIONALE* (■ = INDEPENDENT; ▲ = COLLABORATIVE)

High Risk for Fluid Volume Deficit

RISK FACTORS

Postoperative hemorrhage

EXPECTED OUTCOMES

Patient maintains normal fluid volume as evidenced by stable BP, heart rate; absence of gross hematuria.

ONGOING ASSESSMENT

- Monitor blood pressure (BP) and heart rate.
- Monitor amount and severity of hematuria and clots in the urine. *Bright red blood in the urine is expected over the first 24 hr but should irrigate to clear pink, without clots, during that period. Continuous irrigation of the bladder with normal saline solution is usually carried out for 24-72 hr postoperatively, to remove clots and wash away debris that has been resected.*
- Monitor I & O. *Intake and output should include careful record of any irrigation fluid instilled.*
▲ Monitor Hb and Hct. *Decreases indicate significant blood loss.*

THERAPEUTIC INTERVENTIONS

▲ Perform irrigation of the bladder (continuous or intermittent) as prescribed.
▲ Ensure that catheter is patent and free of clots; readjust flow of continuous bladder irrigation, if necessary, *to maintain urine pink to clear.*
- Position tubing and collection system in gravity-dependent fashion *to ensure drainage away from patient and to prevent clotting.*
▲ Irrigate the catheter manually with small amount of normal saline solution as prescribed; do not irrigate against resistance.
▲ Administer IV fluids as prescribed *to restore fluid balance.*
▲ Push oral fluids as prescribed/tolerated by the patient.

Pain

RELATED FACTORS

Bladder spasm
Surgical incision
Surgical drains

DEFINING CHARACTERISTICS

Verbal reports of pain/spasm
Escape of urine from around catheter
Facial grimacing
Pulling/tugging at catheter

EXPECTED OUTCOMES

Patient verbalizes absence of pain/spasms or ability to tolerate discomfort.

ONGOING ASSESSMENT

- Assess severity, location, and quality of pain. *The most severe pain after prostate surgery is caused by spasm of the bladder. The patient is usually able to differentiate this pain from incisional pain.*
- Assess concurrence of spasms/pain with irrigation or catheter care. *Manipulation of catheter or activity by the patient can stimulate painful bladder spasms.*

THERAPEUTIC INTERVENTIONS

▲ Anticipate need for analgesics and antispasmodics *to prevent peak pain periods.*
- Maintain traction on catheter *to prevent movement (can stimulate spasm).*
- Teach and encourage use of splinting incision *to minimize incisional pain during movement and coughing.*
- Stabilize other tubes/drains securely to minimize inadvertent movement.

High Risk for Infection

RISK FACTORS

Surgical resection
Instrumentation
Open incision (except for transurethral procedure)
Indwelling catheter
Bladder irrigation
Space drains
Underlying malignancy

EXPECTED OUTCOMES

Patient remains free of infection as evidenced by normal temperature, clear urine, clean, dry incisions.

ONGOING ASSESSMENT

- Assess incisions for redness, swelling, pain, and purulent drainage. *These are signs of local wound infection.*
- Monitor color and odor of urine. *Cloudy, foul-smelling urine may be infected.*
▲ Obtain culture of cloudy, foul-smelling urine *to determine pathogens present.*
▲ Monitor urinalysis for presence of WBCs, *which indicate urinary tract infection.*
- Monitor temperature. *A temperature of up to 38.5° C for 48 to 72 hr postoperation is expected. Fever beyond that point may indicate an infection.*

THERAPEUTIC INTERVENTIONS

- Maintain sterile, closed urinary drainage/irrigation system *to prevent bacterial invasion of compromised urinary tract.*
- Change dressings by aseptic technique.
- Provide and encourage intake of high-protein, high-calorie diet *to promote healing.*
- Provide meatal care every shift *to reduce pathogens at site of catheter entrance.*
▲ Administer antibiotics and antipyretics as prescribed.

Continued.

Genitourinary/Gynecologic Care Plans

NURSING DIAGNOSES	EXPECTED OUTCOMES AND NURSING INTERVENTIONS / *RATIONALE* (▪ = INDEPENDENT; ▲ = COLLABORATIVE)

High Risk for Sexual Dysfunction

RISK FACTORS

Injury to perineal nerves during surgery
Incontinence after removal of catheter

EXPECTED OUTCOMES

Patient/significant other express comfort discussing concerns about sexual functioning.

ONGOING ASSESSMENT

- Assess patient's and significant other's expectations for sexual function. *Although many men undergoing prostatectomy are older, do not assume that sexual functioning is unimportant.*
- Assess patient's and significant other's understanding of potential impact that surgery may have had on sexual functioning. *A discussion of the possible negative impact of prostatectomy on sexual functioning should occur preoperatively, but frequently the patient is too anxious or preoccupied with other information (i.e., fear about surgery, prognosis with cancer diagnosis) to comprehend fully and may benefit from postoperative discussion. Not all patients who have had prostatectomy have sexual dysfunction. Orchiectomy renders the patient sterile but not necessarily impotent.*
- Assess whether patient and significant other need/want information during the postoperative period or prefer to wait a few weeks.
- Assess for urinary incontinence after removal of catheter. *Dribbling may occur for as long as a few months after prostatectomy and catheter removal. The psychological impact of urinary incontinence can negatively impact patient's perceived ability to perform sexually.*

THERAPEUTIC INTERVENTIONS

- Teach patient about nerves necessary for erection and ejaculation; distinguish between sterility and impotence. Clarify all language; use diagrams, models as needed, depending on patient's learning style.
- Offer suggestions for alternatives to usual sexual practices to patient and significant other.
- Inform patient that retrograde ejaculation often occurs after prostatectomy. *Retrograde ejaculation means that ejaculate goes into the bladder, rather than into the urethra; this is harmless and results in a cloudy discoloration of the urine. This is of no consequence in terms of sexual performance or satisfaction.*
- Discuss urinary incontinence as a consequence of prostatectomy; teach Kegel exercises to strengthen related muscles to achieve continence. Explain that dribbling may occur up to months and then resolve. *Occasionally incontinence after prostatectomy is permanent.*
- Refer for sexual counseling as indicated.

Knowledge Deficit

RELATED FACTORS

Need for home management
Lack of previous experience with prostate surgery

DEFINING CHARACTERISTICS

Questions
Lack of questions
Verbalized misconceptions

EXPECTED OUTCOMES

Patient verbalizes understanding of need for follow-up care, wound care, and management of incontinence and/or sexual dysfunction.

ONGOING ASSESSMENT

- Assess understanding of need for follow-up care:
    Patients who have had incomplete prostatecomy: *remain at risk for developing prostate cancer because management of benign prostatic hypertrophy does not alter the possibility of later development of cancer of the prostate.*
    Patients who have had surgery to remove prostatic cancer or orchiectomy to remove the glands that produce hormones on which prostatic cancers are dependent *may require further treatment (i.e., chemotherapy, radiation therapy) as part of the overall management of their cancer to eliminate cancer cells that were not removed at surgery.*
- Assess ability to care for surgical wounds.
- Assess understanding of potential dribbling and methods for improving and dealing with incontinence.
- Assess knowledge of resources for sexual dysfunction.

| NURSING DIAGNOSES | EXPECTED OUTCOMES AND NURSING INTERVENTIONS / *RATIONALE* (■ = INDEPENDENT; ▲ = COLLABORATIVE) |

THERAPEUTIC INTERVENTIONS

- Teach wound care:

  Suprapubic and retropubic wounds: *Stitches/staples are usually removed by the time of discharge. Daily cleaning of the wounds with soap and water is sufficient.*

  Perineal wounds: *Stitches/staples are usually removed by the time of discharge; these wounds, however, remain tender longer than abdominal wounds because of their location. They are also at higher risk for infection because of proximity to the anus. Warm Sitz baths/tub baths once or twice daily are recommended until the wound has healed completely and soreness is gone.*

- Teach patient the following about incontinence:

  Remind patient that urinary incontinence may resolve up to 1 yr postoperation.

  Encourage use of Kegel exercises *to improve perineal musculature and control over urinary stream.*

  Refer patient to self-help incontinence group if incontinence is a problem.

- Teach patient to report any of the following:

  Signs of infection: fever; unusual drainage from incisions; unusual drainage from urethra, especially in patients having TURP

  Signs of urinary tract infection (cloudy, foul-smelling urine; frequency)

  Hematuria

  Unresolved incontinence

  Bone pain *(may indicate metastatic cancer in patients with prostatic cancer)*

- Encourage patient to seek help for sexual dysfunction as appropriate.

See also:
Urinary Incontinence, p. 71.

By: Nancy Ruppman, RN, BSN, CURN
Encaracion Mendoza, RN, BSN
Audrey Klopp, RN, Ph.D, ET

Hysterectomy (salpingectomy, oophorectomy)

A surgical procedure that involves the complete excision of the uterus. It may also include removal of the ovaries (oophorectomy) and the fallopian tubes (salpingectomy). Surgery can be performed via the abdominal or vaginal approach. Indications for hysterectomy include endometreosis, uterine fibroids, cancer, elective sterilization, uterine dysfunction/bleeding, and ectopic pregnancy.

| NURSING DIAGNOSES | EXPECTED OUTCOMES AND NURSING INTERVENTIONS / *RATIONALE* (■ = INDEPENDENT; ▲ = COLLABORATIVE) |

Knowledge Deficit

RELATED FACTORS

Unfamiliarity with surgical treatment and recovery process

Lack of experience

DEFINING CHARACTERISTICS

Verbalized lack of knowledge

Increased questions

EXPECTED OUTCOMES

Patient verbalizes understanding of reason for hysterectomy, surgical procedures anticipated, postoperative recovery, discharge instructions, and follow-up care.

Patient verbalizes knowledge of advantages and disadvantages of hormone replacement therapy.

ONGOING ASSESSMENT

- Assess understanding of indications for patient's surgery.
- Assess knowledge of loss of reproductive ability with hysterectomy.
- Assess knowledge of surgical menopause and possible hormone replacement therapy.

THERAPEUTIC INTERVENTIONS

- Provide preoperative instruction: rationale for planned surgical approach, explanation of procedures, activity restrictions.
- Provide discharge instruction on incision care, avoidance of vaginal invasion until operative site is healed in 4-6 wk, need to inform physician of signs of infection.

Continued.

NURSING DIAGNOSES	EXPECTED OUTCOMES AND NURSING INTERVENTIONS / *RATIONALE* (■ = INDEPENDENT; ▲ = COLLABORATIVE)

THERAPEUTIC INTERVENTIONS— cont'd

- Provide instruction on resumption of home activities. *Women usually feel very fatigued during early recovery when trying to maintain usual household activities. They need to pace activities and consider temporary help as indicated.*
- Provide information on surgical menopause and indications for and side effects related to hormone replacement therapy. *The risks for osteoporosis and heart disease increase with menopause. Women need to discuss the advantages versus disadvantages with their health care provider in order to make the best decision regarding replacement therapy.*
- Provide information on possible changes in sexual response. *Some women are relieved that intercourse can no longer result in pregnancy and may find sex more enjoyable. Others may have difficulty reaching orgasm post procedure.*
- Instruct of the need to continue with frequent gynecologic examinations. *Women often assume that removal of the uterus is the end to female health problems. However, periodic examination of the breasts and ovaries and Papanicolaou tests are still recommended.*

Pain

RELATED FACTORS

Incision
Reduced mobility
Ineffective pain control

DEFINING CHARACTERISTICS

Verbal complaints of pain
Tachycardia
Facial grimacing
Guarding of abdomen
Withdrawal

EXPECTED OUTCOMES

Patient verbalizes relief or reduction in pain.
Patient appears comfortable.

ONGOING ASSESSMENT

- Assess patient's pain.
- Assess response to pain medication.
- Assess effectiveness of other pain-relief measures: position change, back-rub, heat application, relaxation and breathing modifications.

THERAPEUTIC INTERVENTIONS

- Teach ways to prevent tension on suture line during leg exercises, position changes, and ambulation.
- ▲ Administer pain medications as needed. Consider epidural morphine or patient-controlled analgesia (PCA). *Individual patients react to pain differently; therefore, selection of pain relief is individual. Epidural morphine delays incisional pain for about 18-24 hr, thereby facilitating early ambulation and preventing many postsurgical complications. PCA provides a continuous basal dose of analgesia while allowing the patient to self-medicate up to a preprogrammed maximum dose.*
- Initiate measures to reduce likelihood of pain (e.g., ice packs, abdominal binder).

Body Image Disturbance

RELATED FACTORS

Perceived body image
  changes
Loss of childbearing capability
Fears of loss of sexuality and
  femininity

DEFINING CHARACTERISTICS

Self-deprecating remarks
Poor eye contact
Weeping
Decreased attention to grooming
Verbalized negative feelings
  about body

EXPECTED OUTCOMES

Patient verbalizes positive statements about body/self.
Patient identifies available resources to aid in coping.

ONGOING ASSESSMENT

- Assess patient's feelings about self and body. *Loss of reproductive capability may cause disappointment and coping difficulties. The age of the woman, the reason for the hysterectomy, and religious/cultural childbearing expectations will impact on the extent of body image changes.*
- Assess usual coping mechanisms and their previous effectiveness.
- Assess patient's/spouse's understanding of effect of hysterectomy on sexual activity. *Physical recovery from hysterectomy requires abstinence from sex during healing period (4-6 wks). Psychosocial impact of hysterectomy may affect subsequent sexual relations. Exploring these common concerns may promote normal adaptation.*

THERAPEUTIC INTERVENTIONS

- Provide accurate information about physiology, treatment, and recovery process. *Clarifying misconceptions may help women resume normal life.*
- Encourage patient/significant other to express feelings. Explore misconceptions.
- Discuss physiologic and emotional influences on sexual functioning.
- Stress the importance of spouse/significant other support. *Expressed acceptance can help the body image and self-image of the woman.*
- ▲ Refer for sexual counseling as indicated.

NURSING DIAGNOSES	EXPECTED OUTCOMES AND NURSING INTERVENTIONS / *RATIONALE* (■ = INDEPENDENT; ▲ = COLLABORATIVE)

High Risk for Fluid Volume Deficit

RISK FACTORS

Excessive blood loss during surgery

Dysfunctional uterine bleeding that preceeded surgery

EXPECTED OUTCOMES

Patient maintains normal fluid volume as evidenced by urine output greater than 30 ml/hr, normal blood pressure and heart rate.

Patient maintains normal hemoglobin and hematocrit levels.

ONGOING ASSESSMENT

- Assess for bleeding from abdominal or vaginal incision. If extensive, initiate pad count. *Some serosanguinous drainage is expected with these procedures.*
- Monitor blood loss by weighing perineal or abdominal dressings.
- Monitor intake and output.
- Monitor for signs of hypovolemia: restlessness, rapid pulse, drop in blood pressure, reduced urine output.
- ▲ Monitor Hb and Hct for evidence of bleeding.

THERAPEUTIC INTERVENTIONS

- Reinforce dressings as needed.
- Maintain bedrest if blood pressure falls or patient becomes orthostatic.
- Anticipate need for vitamin and iron supplements/iron-rich diet. Provide patient instruction.
- ▲ Administer parenteral fluids, blood, and blood components as indicated.

High Risk for Constipation

RISK FACTORS

Bowel manipulation during surgery

Immobility

Abdominal pain

Paralytic ileus

EXPECTED OUTCOMES

Patient has normal bowel movement.

Patient passes gas without difficulty.

ONGOING ASSESSMENT

- Assess for presence or absence of bowel sounds, belching, or passing flatus *to determine onset/delay of peristalsis.*
- Assess dietary fluid intake and tolerance as patient progresses from NPO to regular diet.

THERAPEUTIC INTERVENTIONS

- Encourage sitting up and progressive ambulation *to relieve abdominal distention and promote return of peristalsis.*
- Restrict food and fluids until peristalsis resumes.
- Encourage fruit juice, high-roughage foods when tolerated.
- ▲ Administer laxatives as prescribed.
- Use rectal tube *to relieve flatus.*

See also:

High Risk for Infection, p. 40.

Sexual Dysfunction, p. 58.

Urine Retention, p. 74.

Ineffective Coping, p. 18.

Ineffective Breathing Pattern—Postoperative, p. 10.

By: Rosaline L. Roxas, RN
    Deidre Gradishar, RNC, BS

Ovarian cancer

Cancer of the ovary generally occurs between the ages of 40 and 65; it is linked to familial history and endometriosis. Early ovarian cancer is typically asymptomatic; this accounts for its high mortality rate. Later signs include increased abdominal girth, caused by either tumor bulk or ascites; pain; urinary urgency and frequency; and constipation. Treatment depends on the stage; early stages are treated with surgical removal of the uterus, ovaries, and fallopian tubes, along with the tumor; later stages are treated with radiation therapy and chemotherapy. Prognosis is poor. This care plan does not address surgical management; see also Hysterectomy, p. 463.

NURSING DIAGNOSES	EXPECTED OUTCOMES AND NURSING INTERVENTIONS / *RATIONALE* (■ = INDEPENDENT; ▲ = COLLABORATIVE)

Pain

RELATED FACTORS

Increased abdominal pressure caused by tumor or metastasis to abdominal structures

DEFINING CHARACTERISTICS

Verbal expression of pain
Inability to rest
Facial grimacing

EXPECTED OUTCOMES

Patient reports absence of pain or tolerable pain.

ONGOING ASSESSMENT

- Assess severity, quality, and location of pain. *Typically pain is abdominal, but it may radiate to the back. Pain is due to pressure on abdominal structures as the tumor enlarges.*
- Assess factors patient perceives as precipitating or relieving pain.
- Assess effect of pain on patient's ability to carry out ADLs and activities patient deems meaningful.
- Assess degree to which psychological factors contribute to pain. *Pain is accentuated when the patient feels loss of control, and when self-concept or role is threatened. Women with ovarian cancer often have a poor prognosis and may be grieving in anticipation of death.*

THERAPEUTIC INTERVENTIONS

- ▲ Administer analgesics as prescribed; establish a schedule for use of pain medications *to alleviate peak pain periods.*
- Position patient for comfort. *Positioning is helpful in many instances because pain is related to pressure; positions that alleviate pressure (e.g., side lying with knees bent, Fowler's position) may reduce pain.*
- Eliminate additional stressors or sources of discomfort whenever possible.
- Instruct patient in the use of one or a combination of the following techniques:
    Imagery: *Mental picture or imagined event that involves use of the five senses to distract oneself from painful stimuli*
    Distraction: *Heightening of concentration on nonpainful stimuli to decrease one's awareness and experience of pain*
    Relaxation: *Techniques used to bring about a state of physical and mental awareness and tranquility to reduce tension and pain*
- Massage back and shoulders if patient perceives that it lessens pain.

High Risk for Ineffective Breathing Pattern

RISK FACTORS

Presence of ascites

EXPECTED OUTCOMES

Patient maintains an effective breathing pattern, as evidenced by absence of dyspnea, normal ABGs.

ONGOING ASSESSMENT

- Assess for signs of ineffective breathing pattern: altered chest excursion, shallow breathing, verbal complaints of dyspnea. *Women with ovarian cancer frequently develop ascites, which can become severe to the point that breathing is impaired.*
- Assess for presence of ascites (*the collection of protein-rich fluid in the peritoneal cavity*):
    Measure abdominal girth daily, taking care to measure at the same point consistently.
    Percuss abdomen daily; *percussion over the abdomen sounds dull when fluid is present.*
    Check for ballottement (*fluid wave*) *caused by shifting of ascitic fluid.*
- Assess position patient assumes for easiest breathing. *Patients are typically able to breathe best in an upright position, because the ascitic fluid assumes a gravity-dependent position and pressure on the thoracic cavity is relieved.*
- ▲ Monitor ABGs for deterioration as ascites progresses.
- Monitor effect of ineffective breathing pattern on patient's ability to perform ADLs.

NURSING DIAGNOSES	EXPECTED OUTCOMES AND NURSING INTERVENTIONS / *RATIONALE* (■ = INDEPENDENT; ▲ = COLLABORATIVE)

THERAPEUTIC INTERVENTIONS

- Place patient in Fowler's position *to relieve pressure from ascitic abdomen on thoracic cavity.*
- ▲ Assist with paracentesis as needed *to drain ascitic fluid from the peritoneal cavity.*
- ▲ If patient has peritoneovenous shunt (LeVeen shunt, Denver shunt), facilitate shunt function. *Although paracentesis (removal of peritoneal fluid by needle) effectively removes ascitic fluid, fluid reaccumulates rapidly. Peritoneovenous shunting returns ascitic fluid to the vascular space and functions continuously to relieve ascites.*
    Apply abdominal binder.
    Encourage use of blow bottle or incentive spirometer. *Inspiring against pressure and using an abdominal binder increase intraperitoneal pressure, causing valve in the shunt to open, allowing ascitic fluid to shunt into vascular space.*
- ▲ Administer diuretics as prescribed to the patient with a peritoneovenous shunt *to facilitate excretion of excess fluid.*
- ■ Pace activities and nursing care *to prevent dyspnea resulting from fatigue.*
- ▲ Administer O$_2$ as prescribed *to improve oxygenation.*

High Risk for Altered Nutrition: Less than Body Requirements

RISK FACTORS

Cancer
Poor appetite secondary to disease, side effects of therapies, pressure from ascites
Depression
Fear

EXPECTED OUTCOMES

Patient maintains an adequate nutritional intake, as evidenced by stable weight, calorie intake of at least 1800 cal/day.

ONGOING ASSESSMENT

- Obtain weight history and current weight.
- Determine weight distribution; check limbs for wasting. *Weight loss may seem insignificant until the weight of the ascitic abdomen is considered.*
- Assess appetite and factors patient believes improve or hinder appetite. *Appetite is a complex phenomenon involving physiologic well-being as well as psychologic, psychosocial, and environmental factors. A woman with ovarian cancer may lose her appetite as a result of the disease, treatments in progress, complications of the disease, and/or the emotional turmoil of coping with a disease that may be terminal.*
- Document I & O and complete calorie counts *to quantify amount of nourishment taken.*

THERAPEUTIC INTERVENTIONS

- ■ Involve patient in selection of menu
- ▲ Consult dietician *to assist in providing high-calorie, high-protein, high-fiber diet that is palatable to patient. Calories and protein are necessary for strength and healing; fiber combats constipation, which may result from inactivity and increased intraabdominal pressure.*
- ■ Encourage family/friends to bring foods patient likes. *This may serve to enhance the social aspect of eating, as well as providing food the patient enjoys eating.*
- ■ Encourage activity/exercise, as tolerated. *Activity enhances appetite by stimulating peristalsis.*
- ■ Provide company and a pleasant atmosphere during mealtimes.
- ▲ Give antiemetics as prescribed *to combat nausea and vomiting.*
- ■ Provide oral hygiene *to maintain clean, moist mouth.*

High Risk for Impaired Home Maintenance Management

RISK FACTORS

Potentially terminal disease
Lack of resources
Inadequate support system

EXPECTED OUTCOMES

Patient participates in discharge planning and verbalizes understanding of need for follow-up care.

ONGOING ASSESSMENT

- Assess patient's perception of ability to care for self and household at time of discharge. *A major stressor for a woman with terminal disease can be her integral role in managing a household and caring for a family; these concerns often supersede her recognition of needing help caring for herself.*
- Assess need for special equipment in the household *to accommodate patient's needs* (e.g., a hospital bed, bedside commode).
- Assess need for professional caregiver or homemaker *to provide care in the home.*
- Assess resources patient may be able to use (family, friends).

Continued.

NURSING DIAGNOSES	EXPECTED OUTCOMES AND NURSING INTERVENTIONS / *RATIONALE* (■ = INDEPENDENT; ▲ = COLLABORATIVE)

THERAPEUTIC INTERVENTIONS

- Help patient to identify those areas in which she may require help.
- Involve patient in arranging/mobilizing support systems and resources before discharge from the hospital.
- Respect patient's wishes/preferences in arranging for home assistance. *Loss of ability to carry out usual roles is very distressing; allowing the patient to make and carry out decisions supports an intact self-concept and aids the patient in coping with disease, treatment, and outcomes.*
- ▲ Involve social worker early in hospitalization *to provide psychosocial support and to arrange discharge planning services well in advance of planned discharge.*
- Teach patient the importance of follow-up care. *Patients with stage I ovarian cancer need follow-up with gynecologist-oncologist q3-6mo to monitor progress/recurrence of disease. Patients with advanced stages require chemotherapy and/or radiation therapy to control disease and complications of disease.*

See also:
Grieving, Anticipatory, p. 28.
Constipation, p. 16.

By: Audrey Klopp, RN, Ph.D, ET

Pelvic inflammatory disease (PID)

(ACUTE SALPINGITIS)

A sexually transmitted process involving the endocervix, endometrium, and endosalpinx, with subsequent spill of tubal exudate into the peritoneal cavity, causing pain, inflammation, and tissue destruction. If untreated or frequently recurrent, can become a chronic condition; tissue destruction can lead to infertility.

NURSING DIAGNOSES	EXPECTED OUTCOMES AND NURSING INTERVENTIONS / *RATIONALE* (■ = INDEPENDENT; ▲ = COLLABORATIVE)

Pain

RELATED FACTORS
Pelvic cavity inflammation
Excoriated perineal area

DEFINING CHARACTERISTICS
Lower abdominal pain and tenderness on rebound
Abdominal distention
Back pain

EXPECTED OUTCOMES
Patient verbalizes relief of or reduction in pain.
Patient appears comfortable.

ONGOING ASSESSMENT

- Assess patient for lower abdominal and back pain. *Characteristically pain associated with PID may be experienced as crampy, bilateral lower abdominal pain that is continuous. Pain is usually increased when the uterus is moved, as during vaginal examination.*
- Measure abdominal girth every shift. *Expanding girth may indicate progression of PID to peritonitis.*
- Assess bowel sounds. *Cessation may indicate progression to peritonitis.*
- Assess for medication effects/side effects.

THERAPEUTIC INTERVENTIONS

- ▲ Administer oral and topical analgesics for pain as prescribed. *Some patients experience extreme discomfort and may require narcotic analgesia. Effective antibiotic management will eventually treat the causative factors, thereby relieving pain.*
- Provide external comfort measures: heating pad at low temperature, positioning with extra pillows, sitz baths, perineal care.

NURSING DIAGNOSES	EXPECTED OUTCOMES AND NURSING INTERVENTIONS / *RATIONALE* (■ = INDEPENDENT; ▲ = COLLABORATIVE)

Actual Infection

RELATED FACTORS

Gram-positive cocci:
  Chlamydia trachomatis
  Neisseria gonorrhoeae
  Mycoplasma hominis
Gram-negative cocci:
  Escherichia coli
  Hemophilus influenzae

DEFINING CHARACTERISTICS

Edematous vaginal mucosa
Copious/malodorous greenish/
  yellow vaginal discharge
Fever
Positive culture results
Abnormal vaginal bleeding

EXPECTED OUTCOMES

Patient manifests signs of treated infection, as evidenced by absence of fever, absence of pain, absence of vaginal discharge, negative culture results.

ONGOING ASSESSMENT

- Monitor vital signs. Note spiking temperatures.
- Assess for malodorous vaginal discharge (may be present, copious).
- Assess inflammation of the vulva.
▲ Monitor cultures.
- Assess history of last menstrual period, abnormal menses, sexual contacts, and pregnancy status.
- Assess for past sexually transmitted diseases. *More than one STD may be present at the same time.*

THERAPEUTIC INTERVENTIONS

- Institute universal precautions:
    Discard soiled perineal pads per policy.
    Maintain strict handwashing for all persons in contact with patient.
    Cleanse all equipment (i.e., bedpan, tub, and toilet seat) with disinfectant.
    Use utensil/gloves when handling soiled materials.
- Administer perineal care after each pad change and after bedpan is used *to prevent skin excoriation.* Change perineal pads often *to reduce risk of reinfection from exudate on the pad.*
▲ Administer antibiotics as prescribed. *Aggressive antibiotic therapy may prevent tubal damage that will predispose patient to ectopic pregnancy/infertility.*
- Ensure that patient does not use tampons *(can be medium for further bacterial growth; inhibit drainage).*
- Position patient in sitting position as often as possible *to promote drainage and comfort.*

Knowledge Deficit

RELATED FACTORS

Unfamiliarity with cause of
  disease, medical management, prevention
Embarrassment about topic

DEFINING CHARACTERISTICS

Questioning
Lack of questions
Anxiety

EXPECTED OUTCOMES

Patient verbalizes understanding of PID process, complications, medical treatment, and prevention of recurrence.

ONGOING ASSESSMENT

- Assess knowledge of PID.
- Assess past experiences with sexually transmitted diseases (STDs).
- Obtain a sexual history. *Multiple sex partners or contact with infected partner increases risk of PID.*

THERAPEUTIC INTERVENTIONS

- Explain how PID is transmitted. *Acute or chronic PID may be transmitted during sexual intercourse or during pelvic surgery, including abortion or childbirth. Infections may occur secondary to use of an intrauterine device.*
- Abolish misconceptions about STD. *Some people believe only "bad people" have STDs.*
- Be supportive and nonjudgmental about patient's behavior. *Patient must not be penalized for seeking medical attention.*
- Explain that sexual contact(s) may have to be notified to obtain treatment *to prevent transmission and reinfection.*
- Instruct on importance of proper administration of medication *to prevent ineffective treatment and recurrence of symptoms:*
- Encourage patient to complete course of treatment even if symptoms disappear.
    Explain all tests and procedures to patient before performed *to alleviate apprehension and promote cooperation:* blood and urine test, pregnancy test, gynecologic examination, radiographic studies.
- Inform patient of importance of refraining from sexual intercourse until after follow-up visit *to prevent transmission to partners.* Stress importance of test of cure *to confirm adequate treatment.*
- Discuss contraceptive use. *Condoms can reduce the transmission of certain sexually transmitted diseases.*

Continued.

Pelvic inflammatory disease (PID)—cont'd

NURSING DIAGNOSES	EXPECTED OUTCOMES AND NURSING INTERVENTIONS / *RATIONALE* (■ = INDEPENDENT; ▲ = COLLABORATIVE)
	THERAPEUTIC INTERVENTIONS— cont'd ▪ Instruct patient to notify physician of reappearance of symptoms, lack of menstruation, nonmenstrual bleeding, severe abdominal cramps, presence of purulent, malodorous vaginal discharge. ▲ Refer to STD clinic, social worker as appropriate.

See also:
Ineffective Coping, p. 18.
Body Image Disturbance,
  p. 7.
Altered Sexual Patterns,
  p. 58.

By: Denise Talley-Lacey, RN, BSN

Penile prosthesis

The implantation of silicone into penile tissue to replace erectile tissue in the impotent man. These may be rigid, semirigid, or inflatable

NURSING DIAGNOSES	EXPECTED OUTCOMES AND NURSING INTERVENTIONS / *RATIONALE* (■ = INDEPENDENT; ▲ = COLLABORATIVE)

Pain

RELATED FACTORS

Penile incision
Postoperative edema
Indwelling catheter
Initial movement/inflation of
  prosthesis

DEFINING CHARACTERISTICS

Verbalized pain
Guarded movement
Grimacing
Sleep disturbance

EXPECTED OUTCOMES

Patient is pain-free or verbalizes ability to tolerate pain.

ONGOING ASSESSMENT

▪ Assess pain.
▪ Monitor edema of penis and scrotal area.

THERAPEUTIC INTERVENTIONS

▲ Anticipate need for pain medications or patient-controlled analgesia (PCA).
▪ Use bed cradle *to keep linens off operative area.*
▪ Use nonadherent (Telfa) dressing *to prevent trauma to suture line.*
▪ Postpone initial movement/inflation until edema subsides, usually 3-5 days after operation.
▪ Tape indwelling catheter to abdomen *to keep penis perpendicular to body;* do not tape penis or prosthesis to bed cradles or other objects.
▪ See also Pain, p. 49.

High Risk for Infection

RISK FACTOR

Implanted prosthesis

EXPECTED OUTCOMES

Patient is free of infection as evidenced by normal temperature, normal WBC, absence of pain, swelling, redness at operative site.

ONGOING ASSESSMENT

▪ Assess condition of infrapubic, perineal, penile, or suprapubic incision; note redness, excessive swelling, or suspicious drainage.
▲ Obtain culture of suspicious drainage.
▪ Monitor temperature.
▲ Monitor WBC; *elevated WBC indicates infection*

THERAPEUTIC INTERVENTIONS

▪ Wash hands before contact with patient.
▪ Use aseptic technique for dressing changes.
▪ Provide meticulous perineal care after bowel movements *to prevent fecal contamination of operative area.*
▪ Provide daily or more frequent meatal care if indwelling catheter in place *to reduce pathogens.*
▲ Administer antibiotics and antipyretics as ordered.

NURSING DIAGNOSES	EXPECTED OUTCOMES AND NURSING INTERVENTIONS / *RATIONALE* (■ = INDEPENDENT; ▲ = COLLABORATIVE)

High Risk for Body Image Disturbance

RISK FACTORS

Penile prosthesis
Need for manipulation of genitalia

EXPECTED OUTCOMES

Patient begins to resolve body image issues as evidenced by ability to discuss surgery, participation in own care.

ONGOING ASSESSMENT

- Assess feelings about altered body part and function. Note verbalization about prosthesis, focusing on genitalia, refusal to discuss/participate in care, embarrassment.
- Assess degree to which patient's preoperative expectations are met/unmet by surgical result. *Patients are often distressed by swelling.*
- Assess perceived impact of implant on significant relationships.

THERAPEUTIC INTERVENTIONS

- Encourage patient to discuss feelings; convey normality of both positive and negative feelings about implant. *Body image issues may take months to resolve.*
- Include significant other in discussion when appropriate *so patient and partner accept changed body structure and function.*
- See also Body image disturbance, p. 7.

Altered Sexuality Patterns

RELATED FACTORS

Impotence
Placement of prosthesis
Expectations of self/partner after surgery

DEFINING CHARACTERISTICS

Verbalized concern about sexual functioning
Reported change in relationship with partner(s)
Expressed increased or decreased satisfaction with sexual performance
Inappropriate behavior or conversation related to sexual functioning

EXPECTED OUTCOMES

Patient verbalizes readiness to resume sexual functioning.

ONGOING ASSESSMENT

- Assess preoperative impotence and impact on relationships and perceived sexuality. *Unsatisfactory sexual functioning caused by psychogenic factors may not be improved by prosthetic surgery.*
- Inquire about other methods of impotence therapy.
- Ask patient/partner about expectations of implant. *Correcting misconceptions will decrease unrealistic expectations.*

THERAPEUTIC INTERVENTIONS

- Provide undisturbed private place/time to discuss altered sexuality with patient/partner.
- Encourage patient/partner to verbalize concerns and feelings.
- Help patient/partner differentiate concepts of erection, ejaculation, fertility, and orgasm. *Prosthetic implant restores erectile capability but has no impact on ejaculation, fertility, or orgasm.*
- Arrange for patient/significant other to talk with another patient/couple who has had penile prosthesis.
- See also Sexuality patterns, altered, p. 58.

Knowledge Deficit

RELATED FACTORS

Postoperative care/ management of penile prosthesis

DEFINING CHARACTERISTICS

Multiple questions
Lack of questions
Demonstrated inability to care for/manipulate prosthetic device

EXPECTED OUTCOMES

Patient/significant other verbalize knowledge of and demonstrate appropriate care/use of penile prosthesis.

ONGOING ASSESSMENT

- Assess knowledge about care and use of penile prosthesis.

THERAPEUTIC INTERVENTIONS

- Teach patient type and name of prosthesis implanted. *Possible future need for genitourinary and/or prostatic procedures is more difficult because of penile implants; patients need accurate, complete information.*
- Inform patient that pain and edema are expected for 5-14 days.
- Teach perineal care to prevent infection.
- Inform patient/partner about use of prosthesis:
    Sexual activity may resume 6-8 wk after surgery unless pain is present.
    Lubricant should be used liberally *to prevent penile trauma, soft tissue perforation.*
    Teach inflation/deflation of inflatable devices.
- Offer to arrange talk with someone successfully functioning with implant.
▲ Refer patient to sexual counseling if appropriate.

By: Dorothy Rhodes, RN
    Nancy Ruppman, RN, BSN, CURN

Renal calculi

(KIDNEY STONES, UROLITHIASIS,
NEPHROLITHIASIS, STAGHORN CALCULI)

Renal stones are a common problem, affecting men more frequently than women, whites more frequently than blacks. People in hotter climates are more commonly affected. Stones may form anywhere in the urinary tract but most commonly form in the kidney; they frequently move to other parts of the urinary tract, causing pain, infection, and obstruction. Approximately 90% of stones pass spontaneously. Stones may be treated medically, mechanically (by nephroscopic technique or by lithotripsy [use of shock waves to crush the stones]), or surgically (by pyelolithotomy or nephrolithotomy). Renal stones may be made up of calcium phosphate, calcium oxalate, uric acid, cystine, magnesium ammonium phosphate (so-called struvite stones), or combinations of these substances. Staghorn calculi are large stones that fill and obstruct the renal pelvis. Recurrence of stones is a problem; patients face lifelong need for preventative management. This care plan addresses management of the patient hospitalized with kidney stones; it also addresses postoperative and postlithotripsy care.

NURSING DIAGNOSES	EXPECTED OUTCOMES AND NURSING INTERVENTIONS / *RATIONALE* (■ = INDEPENDENT; ▲ = COLLABORATIVE)

Knowledge Deficit

RELATED FACTORS

Factors related to urolithiasis
Potential courses of management

DEFINING CHARACTERISTICS

Multiple questions
Lack of questions
Anxiety about management
Recurrence of urolithiasis

EXPECTED OUTCOMES

Patient verbalizes understanding of factors contributing to the development of renal calculi, and discusses possible courses of treatment.

ONGOING ASSESSMENT

- Assess understanding of factors that predispose to formation of renal stones:
    Family history of kidney stones
    Dietary factors, including low fluid intake, intake of foods high in purine, calcium, and *oxalate*
    Medical conditions, including hyperparathyroidism, Paget's disease; breast, lung, and prostate cancer, and Cushing's disease.
    Prolonged immobility, *resulting in stasis of urine*
- Assess understanding of the possible courses of therapy to treat kidney stones.
- Assess history of renal stone formation. *Recurrence may indicate knowledge deficit regarding prevention.*

THERAPEUTIC INTERVENTIONS

- Teach patient the following about possible courses of treatment:
    Medical management: *90% of stones pass spontaneously; there may be considerable pain, nausea, and vomiting. If it is felt that the stone is moving and will pass, management will consist of fluid therapy, pain management, and antibiotics to prevent/treat infection caused by stasis of urine and/or obstruction caused by the stone.*
    Mechanical intervention: *Percutaneous catheters may be used to instill chemicals to dissolve the stone. Nephroscopic procedures using a basket to catch and crush the stone may be used. Use of shock waves, either passed through percutaneous catheters or transmitted through a fluid medium from outside the body (extracorporeal shock wave lithotripsy), may be used to pulverize stones so that the fragments can pass.*
    Surgical intervention: *Surgical procedures include ureterolithotomy (an incision into a ureter to remove a stone), pyelolithotomy (incision into the renal pelvis to remove a stone), and nephrolithotomy (incision into the calyx of the kidney to remove a stone). Partial or complete nephrectomy may be done if damage or infection from the stone is severe.*

NURSING DIAGNOSES	EXPECTED OUTCOMES AND NURSING INTERVENTIONS / *RATIONALE* (■ = INDEPENDENT; ▲ = COLLABORATIVE)

Pain

RELATED FACTORS

Irritation by presence of, obstruction by, or movement of the stone
Obstruction of flow of urine caused by stone

DEFINING CHARACTERISTICS

Verbal reports of pain
Restlessness
Grimacing
Sleeplessness

EXPECTED OUTCOMES

Patient verbalizes relief of pain or ability to tolerate pain.

ONGOING ASSESSMENT

- Assess severity, location, and duration of pain. *Pain associated with kidney stones is typically located in the flank region and may radiate to the pelvic/abdominal area. Pain subsides when/if the stone passes into the bladder.*
- Assess symptoms related to severe pain. *Pain related to kidney stone obstruction/movement is commonly severe and may be associated with profuse diaphoresis, nausea, and vomiting.*
- Assess patency of drains or catheters. *Obstructed flow of urine will result in increased renal pressure and cause/intensify pain.*

THERAPEUTIC INTERVENTIONS

- ▲ Anticipate need for analgesics *to prevent peak periods of pain;* evaluate effectiveness.
- Explore and use nonpharmacologic pain management methods successful for patient in past.
- Minimize gross motor movement.
- See also Pain, p. 49.

High Risk for Infection

RISK FACTORS

Obstructed flow of urine
Stasis
Instrumentation of urinary tract
Percutaneous punctures communicating with renal pelvis
Long-term use of collection devices
Incisions
Presence of gravel

EXPECTED OUTCOMES

Patient remains free of infection as evidenced by normal temperature, normal WBC, clear urine.

ONGOING ASSESSMENT

- Monitor I & O. *Desired urine output is 2000 to 3000 ml/24 hr. The more dilute and the higher the flow of urine, the less stasis there is; this lessens the possibility of further stone formation and increases the possibility that the stone will pass spontaneously.*
- Observe urine for hematuria. *Hematuria results from trauma to the urinary tract as the stone moves.*
- Observe for changes in elimination pattern: dysuria: *painful elimination;* frequency: *need to void frequently, passing small amounts each time;* hesitancy: *difficulty or delay in starting the stream of urine;* retention: *inability to start urinary stream.*
- Monitor temperature. *Urinary tract infection can result in very high fever.*
- ▲ Monitor WBC. *Elevated WBC is a sign of infection.*
- Observe percutaneous sites and/or incisions for redness, swelling, pain, *which may indicate infection.*
- ▲ Obtain culture of urine and drainage from around catheters (meatal or percutaneous) *to determine presence of pathogens.*
- Check pH of urine. *Urine with a pH > 6.0 (i.e., alkaline urine) is more prone to infection than acidic urine.*

THERAPEUTIC INTERVENTIONS

- Strain all urine *to detect passage of stone, stone fragments, or gravel. If the type of stone (e.g., composition) is unknown, the stone may be sent to laboratory for analysis. This assists in planning therapy to prevent the recurrence of stones.*
- Encourage fluid intake of 3000 to 4000 cc of fluid daily *to keep urine dilute and flow of urine high.*
- Clean and/or replace leg bags, gravity collection bags, and any other collection system daily *to prevent accumulation of pathogens.*
- Provide meatal care every shift for patients with indwelling catheters.
- ▲ Change dressings over percutaneous nephrostomy tubes and incisions as prescribed, using good handwashing and aseptic technique.
- Encourage measures to acidify urine, *since acidic urine inhibits the growth of pathogenic bacteria:* vitamin C (ascorbic acid) 500-1000 mg/day, cranberry juice, 4-6 8 oz glasses per day. *Cranberry juice yields hippicuric acid as it metabolizes and is excreted.*
- ▲ Administer antibiotics and antipyretics as prescribed.
- If a catheter is removed, encourage patient to continue pushing fluids; notify physician if patient has not voided 6 hr after catheter removal.
- Instruct patient to report changes in pain, fever, chills.

Continued.

NURSING DIAGNOSES	EXPECTED OUTCOMES AND NURSING INTERVENTIONS / *RATIONALE* (■ = INDEPENDENT; ▲ = COLLABORATIVE)

High Risk for Fluid Volume Deficit

RISK FACTORS

Nausea, vomiting
Blood loss (hematuria, post-operative hemorrhage)

EXPECTED OUTCOMES

Patient maintains normal fluid balance, as evidenced by stable BP, heart rate; diminishing hematuria.

ONGOING ASSESSMENT

- Monitor BP, heart rate.
- Measure and record the amount of any emesis.
- Monitor amount and severity of hematuria. *Blood loss can be significant as the stone passes through the urinary tract. After urinary tract instrumentation to crush or remove a stone or after urinary tract surgery, postoperative hemorrhage can occur.*
- Monitor I & O. *Intake and output should include careful record of any irrigation fluid instilled or used for irrigation.*

THERAPEUTIC INTERVENTIONS

▲ Administer IV fluids as prescribed *to replace losses and maintain hydration.*
▲ Push oral fluids as tolerated. *Fluid intake, oral and IV combined, should be 3000 to 4000 cc/day to keep urine dilute and flow high.*

Knowledge Deficit

RELATED FACTORS

Home management
Need for prevention of recurrence of renal calculi

DEFINING CHARACTERISTICS

Questions
Lack of questions
History of recurrence

EXPECTED OUTCOMES

Patient verbalizes understanding of factors related to development/recurrence of renal calculi.

ONGOING ASSESSMENT

- Assess understanding of relationship of diet to development/recurrence of renal stones.
- Assess knowledge of the relationship between development of renal stones and the climate/fluid intake. *Persons in the southeastern and southwestern United States are more likely to develop calculi; this is believed to be due to warmer weather, higher chance for dehydration, more concentrated urine.*
- Assess understanding of activity and development of renal stones. *Persons who have a sedentary life-style or limited mobility are at higher risk for development of calculi, because of calcium loss from bones combined with urinary stasis.*

THERAPEUTIC INTERVENTIONS

- Teach patient the following regarding diet:
  For patients with stones related to hypercalcuria:
    Calcium intake should be limited; *this includes dairy products, beans, nuts, and chocolate.*
    Vitamin D intake should be limited *because vitamin D intake enhances calcium uptake from the GI tract.*
  For patients with stones related to oxalate:
    Foods containing oxalate (*green leafy vegetables, coffee, tea, and chocolate, colas, peanuts, peanut butter*) should be restricted.
  For patients with stones related to uric acid:
    An alkaline-ash diet should be followed. *Foods encouraged on an alkaline-ash diet include dairy products; fruits, except cranberries, plums, and prunes; vegetables, especially beans; and meats.*
  For patients with struvite stones:
    An acid-ash diet is recommended. *Foods encouraged on an acid-ash diet include meat, eggs, poultry, fish, cereals, and most fruits and vegetables.*
- Teach patient the importance of maintaining a fluid intake of 3000-4000 cc/day *to maintain high-flow, low-solute (dilute) urine and to prevent stasis.*
- Teach patient about medications used to prevent the recurrence of renal calculi:
  Sodium cellulose phosphate (*SCP*): *binds calcium so that GI absorption of calcium is decreased*
  Diuretic agents (*thiazide*): *increase tubular reabsorption of calcium, making less available for calculi formation in the urinary tract*
  Cholestyramine: *binds oxalate and enhances GI excretion.*
  Allopurinol: *reduces uric acid production.*
  Antibiotics: *used long-term to prevent chronic urinary tract infections that can be precursors to renal calculus formation.*

NURSING DIAGNOSES	EXPECTED OUTCOMES AND NURSING INTERVENTIONS / *RATIONALE* (■ = INDEPENDENT; ▲ = COLLABORATIVE)

THERAPEUTIC INTERVENTIONS— cont'd

- Teach patients to increase mobility *to prevent stasis of urine.*
- Teach postoperative patients about care of incisions:

  Incisions should be cleaned using clean technique and dressed with sterile gauze or vapor-permeable membrane dressings. *Vapor-permeable membrane dressings (e.g., Op-Site, Tegaderm) allow showering and bathing without risk of infection.*
- Teach patient to report any of the following: pain not relieved by medication; fever accompanied by nausea, vomiting, chills; changes in appearance or odor of urine.
- Instruct patients that stone fragments may continue to pass for weeks after stone crushing or lithotripsy.

By: Audrey Klopp, RN, Ph.D, ET

Urinary diversion

Urinary diversion, diversion of urinary flow from its usual path through the urinary tract, may be performed for a variety of reasons, including cancer, obstruction, destruction of structures by trauma, and neurogenic bladder caused by disease or injury. Some procedures result in incontinence and necessitate the wearing of a collection system or pouch; other procedures reroute the urinary flow to another structure (e.g., surgically created internal reservoir, colon) from which the urine is eventually excreted (so-called continent procedures). This care plan addresses those procedures that result in urinary incontinence.

NURSING DIAGNOSES	EXPECTED OUTCOMES AND NURSING INTERVENTIONS / *RATIONALE* (■ = INDEPENDENT; ▲ = COLLABORATIVE)

Knowledge Deficit: Preoperative

RELATED FACTOR

Lack of previous surgical experience

DEFINING CHARACTERISTICS

Questions
Lack of questions
Verbalized misconceptions

EXPECTED OUTCOMES

Patient verbalizes understanding of proposed surgical procedure, including loss of urinary continence and postoperative need for a collection system.

ONGOING ASSESSMENT

- Assess what information about the proposed surgical procedure has been given to the patient. *Options depend on nature of disease/disorder that makes the urinary diversion necessary:*

  Ileal conduit (or ileal loop): *The most common type of urinary diversion performed, using a piece ("loop") of small intestine as a conduit to which the ureters are attached; one end of the conduit is brought to the anterior abdominal surface as a stoma, over which a pouch must always be worn. Usually done with cystectomy (removal of the bladder) for bladder cancer.*

  Nephrostomy: *Percutaneous catheterization of one or both kidneys, usually done when the urinary path is obstructed distally; often a palliative measure for urinary diversion. Necessitates wearing one or two leg bags for collection of urine.*

  Ureterostomy (unilateral or bilateral): *Implantation of one or both ureters to the anterior abdominal wall as small stomas; usually done when reestablishment of normal urinary flow is anticipated.*

  Vesicostomy: *Usually a temporary urinary diversion performed when the lower urinary tract must be bypassed (e.g., urethral trauma); an opening is made into the bladder wall, which is attached to the lower anterior abdomen. A pouch must be worn over the vesicostomy stoma to collect the urine.*
- Assess patient's understanding of the proposed surgical procedure and its relationship to urinary continence. *It is very important that the patient understand that the proposed surgical procedure will make him/her incontinent of urine and necessitate the wearing and maintenance of an external collection device, because postoperative adaptation will require management of the collection system and incorporation of the altered function and the collection system into the body image/self-concept of the person.*

Continued.

Genitourinary/Gynecologic Care Plans

NURSING DIAGNOSES	EXPECTED OUTCOMES AND NURSING INTERVENTIONS / *RATIONALE* (■ = INDEPENDENT; ▲ = COLLABORATIVE)

ONGOING ASSESSMENT—cont'd

- Assess patient's knowledge about whether the urinary diversion proposed is temporary or permanent. *The patient's ability to cope with changes in ADLs necessitated by wearing an external collection device is facilitated when the patient understands that the diversion is permanent; patients having temporary diversion may decline involvement in self-care and defer care to a family member or outside caregiver.*
- Ask whether patient has had contact with another person who has a urinary diversion. *Previous contact, either positive or negative, influences the patient's perception of what his/her experience will be like.*

THERAPEUTIC INTERVENTIONS

- Reinforce and reexplain proposed procedure. *Preoperative anxiety frequently makes it necessary to repeat instructions/explanations several times in order for patient to comprehend.*
- Use diagrams, pictures, and models to explain anatomy and physiology of the GU tract, pathophysiology necessitating urinary diversion, proposed location of stoma:
  Ileal conduit: *usually located in the lower right quadrant of the abdomen.*
  Nephrostomy: *tubes exit on one or both flanks, just below the costal margin(s).*
  Ureterostomy: *anywhere on the anterior abdominal surface, preferably below the waistline.*
  Vesicostomy: *on the anterior abdomen, suprapubic area.*
- Show patient the pouch or collection system that will be used postoperatively. *Allowing the patient to wear the pouch or collection device is also helpful and may identify need for relocation of proposed stoma.*
- Offer the patient a visit with a rehabilitated ostomate. *Often contact with another individual who has "been there" is more beneficial than factual information given by a health professional.*

High Risk for Self-Care Deficit: Toileting

RISK FACTORS

Presence of poorly placed stoma
Presence of pouch
Poor hand-eye coordination

EXPECTED OUTCOMES

Patient performs self-care (emptying/changing pouch) independently as a result of preoperative stoma site selection.

ONGOING ASSESSMENT

- Assess for the following: presence of old abdominal scars, presence of bony prominences on anterior abdomen, presence of creases/skin folds on abdomen, extreme obesity, scaphoid abdomen, pendulous breasts, ability to see and handle equipment. *Stoma placement is facilitated by a flat abdomen that has no scars, bony prominences, or extremes of weight. Stoma site selection may need to be altered when these factors are present in order to locate the stoma where the patient can see and reach it and where a relatively flat surface for pouching exists.*

THERAPEUTIC INTERVENTIONS

- ▲ Consult ET nurse or surgeon to mark proposed stoma site indelibly in an area that patient can easily see and reach where scars, bony prominences, skinfolds are avoided; where hip flexion does not change contour. *Stoma location is a key factor in self-care. A poorly located stoma can delay/preclude self-care abilities.*
- Note usual sites for placement: *ileal conduit:* right lower quadrant; *nephrostomy:* flank(s); *ureterostomy:* anterior abdomen, preferably below waist; *vesicostomy:* suprapubic.
- If possible, have patient wear a collection device over proposed site; evaluate effectiveness in terms of patient's ability to see, handle equipment, and wear normal clothing.

NURSING DIAGNOSES	EXPECTED OUTCOMES AND NURSING INTERVENTIONS / *RATIONALE* (■ = INDEPENDENT; ▲ = COLLABORATIVE)

High Risk for Body Image Disturbance

RISK FACTORS

Presence of stoma
Loss or urinary continence
Presence of pouch/collection system
Primary disease (often cancer)
Fear of offensive odor
Fear of appearing different

EXPECTED OUTCOMES

Patient begins to verbalize about stoma and body image.

ONGOING ASSESSMENT

- Assess perception of change in body structure and function.
- Assess perceived impact of change. *The patient's response to real or perceived changes in body structure and/or function are related to the importance the patient places on the structure or function (i.e., a very fastidious person may experience the presence of a urine-filled pouch on the anterior abdomen as intolerable, or a person who works out, swims, etc., may find the presence of visible tubes protruding from flanks as intolerable). On the other hand, some patients will express that such changes are "a small price to pay" for absence of disease.*
- Note verbal/nonverbal references to stoma. *Patients frequently "name" stomas as an attempt to separate the stoma from self. Others may look away or totally deny the presence of the stoma until able to cope.*
- Note patient's ability/readiness to look at, touch, care for stoma and ostomy equipment.

THERAPEUTIC INTERVENTIONS

- Acknowledge appropriateness of emotional response to perceived change in body structure and function. *Because control of elimination is skill/task of early childhood and a socially private function, loss of control precipitates a body image change and possible self-concept change.*
- Assist patient in looking at, touching, and caring for stoma when ready. *Patients look for reactions, both positive and negative, from caregivers. Share positive reactions, such as "The stoma looks pink and healthy" or "The urine is clear and yellow, as it should be."*
- Assist patient in identifying specific actions that could be helpful in managing perceived loss/problem related to stoma. *Leakage of contents from the pouch with resultant embarrassment about odor, loss of control is a major concern. Assuring the patient that skill will develop and that accidents are preventable will go a long way in helping him or her adapt to the altered structure/function.*

High Risk for Altered Stoma Tissue Perfusion

RISK FACTORS

Surgical manipulation of small intestine (ileal conduit), bladder (vesicostomy), ureters (ureterostomy)

EXPECTED OUTCOMES

Patient's stoma remains pink and moist.

ONGOING ASSESSMENT

- Assess the stoma for adequate arterial perfusion at least q4hr:
  Color of ileal conduit stoma: *Ileal conduit stoma is a piece of rerouted small intestine with attached mesentery (blood supply); it should appear pink and moist if perfusion is adequate.*
  Appearance of ureterostomy stoma: *Because the ureters have a small diameter, manipulation at surgery or edema of surrounding tissue can compress the ureters at the skin line and compromise perfusion; ureteral stomas should appear pink and moist if perfusion is adequate.*
  Vesicostomy stoma: *This stoma is constructed of inverted bladder that has been surgically sewn to abdominal skin; normal appearance is pink and moist. This stoma is least susceptible to altered tissue perfusion.*
- Assess stoma for edema at least q4hr. *Some postoperative edema is expected and will subside over a period of 2 to 6 wk. When edema becomes severe, venous congestion, evidenced by a purplish discoloration of the stoma, may occur.*

THERAPEUTIC INTERVENTIONS

- Ensure that faceplate of pouch is correctly fitted. *A faceplate that is tightly fitted to the stoma can reduce blood flow to the stoma and impede venous drainage, resulting in further edema and increasing the risk of ischemia.*
- Remove the faceplate and notify the surgeon immediately if stoma appears dusky, black, or dry. *A stoma that is dusky blue, black, or dry is receiving inadequate blood supply; usually the patient returns to surgery for stoma revision.*

Continued.

NURSING DIAGNOSES	EXPECTED OUTCOMES AND NURSING INTERVENTIONS / *RATIONALE* (■ = INDEPENDENT; ▲ = COLLABORATIVE)

High Risk for Infection

RISK FACTORS

Surgical incision

Small bowel anastomosis (ileal conduit)

Anastomoses of ureters to small bowel (ileal conduit), abdominal wall (ureterostomy)

Percutaneous access to renal pelvis (nephrostomy)

Direct opening into bladder (vesicostomy)

EXPECTED OUTCOMES

Patient remains free of infection, as evidenced by normal temperature, normal WBC, absence of signs of local wound infection, absence of purulent drainage from around nephrostomy tubes.

ONGOING ASSESSMENT

- Assess surgical incisions and areas around percutaneous nephrostomies for redness, swelling, suspicious drainage, *which indicate wound infection.*
- Monitor temperature. *Temperature above 38.5° C after the third postoperative day is an indication of infection. In addition to usual causes of postoperative infections (i.e., lungs, invasive lines), possible sites of infections in patients who have had urinary diversion surgeries include the following:*
  Incision
  Anastomosis of ureters to small bowel. *As the ileal conduit is fashioned, ureters are anastomosed into the segment of small bowel designated for the conduit; breakdown of these anastomoses results in peritonitis because urine spills into the peritoneal cavity instead of traveling to the conduit and out through the stoma.*
  Areas where ureters are attached to abdomen
  Percutaneous puncture sites *where nephrostomy tubes have been placed*
  Bladder *because in patients with a vesicostomy, the bladder communicates with the outside*
- Monitor urine output. *Diminishing amounts of urine output in patients with an ileal conduit may indicate spillage of urine into the peritoneal cavity.*
- ▲ Send any suspicious drainage from surgically placed drains to the laboratory for analysis *to determine internal urine leak.*
- ▲ Monitor WBC. *Elevated WBC is a sign of infection.*
- ▲ Obtain culture of urine.
- Check pH of urine. *Urine with a pH above 6.0 (i.e., alkaline urine) is more prone to infection than acidic urine.*

THERAPEUTIC INTERVENTIONS

- ▲ Provide wound care to incisions and areas around percutaneous sites, vesicostomy outlet, and ureterostomies as prescribed, using aseptic technique.
- Wash hands before handling any tubes, drains *to reduce pathogens.*
- Maintain closed drainage systems and change leg bags, gravity collection bags, and any other collection systems daily *to prevent accumulation of pathogens.*
- Encourage measures to acidify urine *since acid urine inhibits the growth of pathogenic bacteria:* vitamin C (ascorbic acid) 500-1000 mg/day, cranberry juice, 4-6 8 oz glasses per day. *Cranberry juice yields hippicuric acid as it metabolizes and is excreted.*
- ▲ Encourage fluid intake of 3000 to 4000 cc of fluid daily *to keep urine dilute and to flush out bacteria.*
- ▲ Administer antibiotics and antipyretics as prescribed.
- Instruct patient to report pain, fever, chills.

NURSING DIAGNOSES	EXPECTED OUTCOMES AND NURSING INTERVENTIONS / *RATIONALE* (■ = INDEPENDENT; ▲ = COLLABORATIVE)

High Risk for Impaired Home Maintenance Management

RISK FACTORS

Presence of new stoma
Presence of ureterostomy
Presence of percutaneous nephrostomy
Presence of vesicostomy

EXPECTED OUTCOMES

Patient demonstrates ability to provide care for ostomy, nephrostomy tubes, and/or skin.

ONGOING ASSESSMENT

- Assess patient's perception of ability to care for self at time of discharge.
- Assess resources (family member, friend) who may be available and willing to assist patient with care after discharge.
- Assess ability to empty and change pouch (ileal conduit, vesicostomy). *Most patients will be independent in emptying pouch by time of discharge; many will still need assistance and may require outpatient follow-up or in-home care.*
- Assess ability to care for peristomal skin.
- Assess ability to identify peristomal skin problems:
  Excoriation: *Appears as sore, reddened area, most typically the result of a poorly fitted faceplate that allows urine to contact the skin, too frequent changing of pouch, or frequent accidents in which urine comes into contact with the skin.*
  Crystal formation: *Appears as collection of white crystals around stoma or on skin around stoma or tubes; forms when urine is highly alkaline. Acts as an abrasive, resulting in excoriation.*
  Yeast infection: *Appears as a beefy-red, itchy area around stoma or tubes. Tends to spread by "satellite," small round extensions at the perimeter of the main area of redness.*
  Contact dermatitis: *Usually the result of allergy to some product in use around stoma or tubes. Appears as a continuous reddened area; may itch, may feel painful. Contact dermatitis can develop even after years of successful use of products. Is characterized by its size and shape, which approximate the area of contact with the offending product.*
- Assess knowledge about:
  Diet: *Patients with urinary diversion are instructed to drink 3000 to 4000 cc of fluid per day to prevent stasis and infection.*
  Activity: *Patients may bathe or shower with pouch on or off; patients with nephrostomy tubes should cover dressings with waterproof dressing (e.g., Op-Site, Tegaderm) or with waterproof tape. Other activities are governed by patient's desire and energy level. Patients may be afraid to engage in usual activities, such as sports, sex. The lack of confidence in abilities diminishes as the patient gains control over management of the urinary diversion and fear of an "accident" diminishes.*

THERAPEUTIC INTERVENTIONS

- Provide teaching during first and subsequent pouch changes, or opportunities to care for nephrostomy tubes. *Even before patients are able to participate actively, they can observe and discuss ostomy care.*
- Include one (or more) significant other as appropriate/desired by patient. *It is beneficial to teach others alongside the patient, so long as all realize that the goal is for the patient to become independent in self-ostomy care. Patients with nephrostomy tubes cannot reach the flank and will need to rely on another person to provide care.*
- Gradually transfer responsibility for care to patient/family.
- Allow at least one opportunity for supervised return demonstration of pouch change before discharge from the hospital. *Self-ostomy care requires both cognitive and psychomotor skills; postoperatively, learning ability may be decreased, requiring repetition and opportunity for return demonstration.*
- Teach patient how to care for peristomal skin or skin around nephrostomy tube:
  Wash and dry skin around stoma, tubes using soap and water.
  Apply a liquid barrier film (Bard Protective Barrier Film, Skin Prep) *to protect skin from moisture and any adhesives used in the area.*
  Change pouch no more frequently than q3-6days. *Frequent changing strips away epithelial cells and can lead to excoriation.*
- Discuss odor control and acknowledge that odor (or fear of odor) can impair social functioning. *Odor control is best achieved by attention to pouch hygiene; urinary equipment can be rinsed with a half-and-half solution of water and vinegar to reduce urinary odor. Certain foods (e.g., asparagus, coffee) cause a disagreeable urinary odor and can be eliminated to control odor.*
- Discuss availability of ostomy support groups *for ongoing peer support.*
- Instruct patient to maintain contact with an ET nurse *for follow-up care and problem solving.*

By: Audrey Klopp, RN, PhD, ET

Urinary tract infection/pyelonephritis

(UTI, CYSTITIS, URETHRITIS, NEPHRITIS)

Urinary tract infection (UTI) is an invasion of all or part of the urinary tract (kidneys, bladder, urethra) by pathogens that cause infection. Pyelonephritis is inflammation of the kidney; it may be acute or chronic and typically follows chronic UTIs.

NURSING DIAGNOSES	EXPECTED OUTCOMES AND NURSING INTERVENTIONS / *RATIONALE* (▪ = INDEPENDENT; ▲ = COLLABORATIVE)

Infection

RELATED FACTORS

Instrumentation
Indwelling catheter
Improper toileting
Pregnancy
Chronically alkaline urine
Stasis

DEFINING CHARACTERISTICS

Burning on urination
Frequency of urination
Fever
Cloudy urine
Elevated WBCs
Low back pain
Suprapubic tenderness
Hematuria
Bacteria in urine
Flank pain
Fever
Chills

EXPECTED OUTCOMES

Patient is free of urinary tract infection as evidenced by clear urine, pain-free urination, normal WBC, absence of fever, chills, flank pain.

ONGOING ASSESSMENT

▪ Assess for signs/symptoms of UTI: frequency and burning/pain on urination, cloudy or bloody urine. *Patients with UTI may be asymptomatic, especially those with recurrent infection.*
▲ Assess for signs/symptoms of pyelonephritis: frequent and/or painful urination, flank pain, fever, chills.
▪ Assess laboratory data:
    Urinalysis: hematuria, pyuria
    Urine culture: Causative organism
    WBC: Polymorphonuclear leukocytosis >mm^3.
▪ Assess for prior UTI history. *Patients with chronic history of UTIs are at risk for development of pyelonephritis.*

THERAPEUTIC INTERVENTIONS

▪ Encourage patient to drink extra fluid *to promote renal blood flow and flush bacteria from urinary tract.*
▪ Instruct patient to void frequently (q2-3hr during day) and empty bladder completely *to enhance bacterial clearance, reduce urine stasis, and prevent reinfection.*
▪ Suggest cranberry or prune juice *to acidify urine.*
▲ Give prescribed antibiotic; note effectiveness. *Patients with pyelonephritis typically require a 3 or 4 day course of parenteral antibiotics.*

Pain

RELATED FACTOR

Infection

DEFINING CHARACTERISTICS

Pain, cramps, or spasm in lower back and bladder area; dysuria; body malaise
Facial mask of pain
Guarding behavior
Protective decreased physical activity

EXPECTED OUTCOMES

Patient verbalizes relief of pain or ability to tolerate pain.

ONGOING ASSESSMENT

▪ Solicit patient's description of pain.
▪ Assess pain characteristics.

THERAPEUTIC INTERVENTIONS

▪ Apply heating pad to lower back for back pain.
▪ Instruct patient in use of sitz bath for perineal pain.
▲ Administer analgesics and antispasmodics as prescribed; note effectiveness.
▪ Use distractions and relaxation techniques whenever appropriate.
▪ See also Pain, p. 49.

Knowledge Deficit

RELATED FACTORS

Unfamiliarity with nature and treatment of UTI/pyelonephritis

DEFINING CHARACTERISTICS

Lack of questions
Apparent confusion about events
Expressed need for more information
Noncompliance with medical treatment

EXPECTED OUTCOMES

Patient verbalizes knowledge of causes and treatment of UTI/pyelonephritis.

ONGOING ASSESSMENT

- Assess knowledge of nature of UTI.
- Assess preventive measures patient may currently use to minimize UTI.

THERAPEUTIC INTERVENTIONS

- Provide health teaching and discharge planning *to prevent recurrence of infection.* Instruct patient in:

    Having follow-up urine studies *to determine whether asymptomatic infection is present (thus marked tendency to recomence)*

    Following hygienic measures *to decrease introital concentration of pathogens by washing in shower or while standing in tub and washing perineum with soap and water from front to back after each bowel movement*

    Voiding immediately after sexual intercourse *to clear urethra of pathogens*

    Voiding at first urge *to prevent urinary distention*

    Changing underpants daily and wearing well-ventilated clothes (e.g., cotton underpants, cotton-crotched pantyhose)

    Taking medication for long-term antimicrobial therapy before bedtime *to ensure overnight concentration of drug*

By: Caroline Sarmiento, RN, BSN

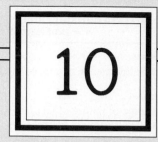

Endocrine and Metabolic Care Plans

Addison's disease

(ADRENOCORTICAL INSUFFICIENCY; ADDISONIAN CRISIS)

An abnormality of the adrenal glands with the destruction of the adrenal cortex and impairment of glucocorticoid and mineralocorticoid production. Patients using steroids may also manifest adrenocortical insufficiency. Addisonian crisis is the most dangerous component of Addison's disease. It is a life-threatening emergency with severe hypotension that may occur during stress, sudden withdrawal of replacement therapy, adrenal surgery, or sudden pituitary gland destruction.

NURSING DIAGNOSES	EXPECTED OUTCOMES AND NURSING INTERVENTIONS / *RATIONALE* (■ = INDEPENDENT; ▲ = COLLABORATIVE)

Fluid Volume Deficit

RELATED FACTORS

Addison's disease results in reduced aldosterone secretion, causing an increase in sodium and water excretion with potassium retention
Gastrointestinal disturbances, e.g., nausea, vomiting, diarrhea which can be manifestations of Addison's disease

DEFINING CHARACTERISTICS

Decreased urinary output
Concentrated urine
Output greater than intake
Sudden weight loss
Decreased venous filling
Hypotension
Hyponatremia
Hyperkalemia
Hypoglycemia

EXPECTED OUTCOMES

Patient experiences adequate fluid volume and electrolyte balance as evidenced by urine output > 30 ml/hr, normotensive BP, heart rate < 100/min, consistent weight, normal skin turgor.

ONGOING ASSESSMENT

- Assess skin turgor and mucous membranes for signs of dehydration.
- Assess vital signs, especially noting BP and pulse rate for orthostatic changes *(a BP drop of greater than 15 mm Hg when changing from supine to sitting position, with concurrent elevation in HR). This indicates reduced circulating fluids.*
- Assess color and amount of urine. Report urine output < 30 ml/hr for 2 consecutive hours.
- Weigh patient daily.
- Assess for fatigue, sensory deficits, muscle weakness, and paralysis, *which are signs of hyperkalemia.*
- Assess ECG rhythm, as available, for signs of hyperkalemia *(sharp peaked T wave and widened QRS complex).*
- Document baseline mental status and record during each nursing shift. *Dehydration can alter mental status.*
- ▲ Assess serum glucose levels. *Hypoglycemia results from the decrease in cortisol secretion.*
- Assess for bowel sounds and for presence of nausea, vomiting, or diarrhea, which would add to the fluid losses and electrolyte disturbances.

THERAPEUTIC INTERVENTIONS

- Encourage oral fluids as patient tolerates.
- Instruct patient in ingesting salt additives in conditions of excess heat or humidity.
- ▲ Obtain and maintain a large-bore IV.
- ▲ Administer parenteral fluids as prescribed. Anticipate the need for an IV fluid challenge with immediate infusion of fluids, for patients with abnormal vital signs. IV saline solution should be given *to replace Na$^+$ deficit,* and glucose may be added *to correct hypoglycemia.*
- ▲ Institute measures to control excessive electrolyte loss (e.g., resting the GI tract, administering antipyretics as prescribed).
- ▲ Administer replacement medications as prescribed/indicated: oral cortisone (Cortone), hydrocortisone (Cortef), or prednisone *(to replace cortisol deficits, which will promote sodium resorption);* fludrocotison (Florinef) *(a mineralocorticoid for patients who require aldosterone replacement to promote sodium and water replacement).*

High Risk for Decreased Cardiac Output

RISK FACTORS

Any situations requiring increased corticosteroids (e.g., stress, infection, GI upsets) may lead to shock or vascular collapse

EXPECTED OUTCOMES

Patient achieves adequate cardiac output as evidenced by strong peripheral pulses, normal vital signs, urine output > 30 ml/hr, warm dry skin, alert responsive mentation.

ONGOING ASSESSMENT

- Assess skin warmth and peripheral pulses. *Peripheral vasoconstriction causes cool, pale, diaphoretic skin.*
- Assess level of consciousness. *Early signs of cerebral hypoxia are restlessness and anxiety, leading on to agitation and confusion.*
- Monitor vital signs with frequent monitoring of BP. Include assessment for orthostatic hypotension. *Sudden development of profound hypotension may indicate Addisonian crisis. Direct intraarterial monitoring of pressure should be anticipated for a continuing shock state. Auscultory BP may be unreliable secondary to vasoconstriction.*

Continued.

Endocrine and Metabolic Care Plans

NURSING DIAGNOSES	EXPECTED OUTCOMES AND NURSING INTERVENTIONS / *RATIONALE* (■ = INDEPENDENT; ▲ = COLLABORATIVE)

ONGOING ASSESSMENT—cont'd

- Monitor for dysrhythmias. *Cardiac dysrhythmias may result from the low perfusion state, acidosis, hypoxia, or electrolyte imbalance. Hyperkalemia is present in Addison's disease.*
- ▲ If hemodynamic monitoring is in place, assess CVP, PAP, PCWP, and CO. *CVP provides information on filling pressures of right side of the heart; PAP and PCWP reflect left-sided fluid volumes.*
- Monitor urine output. *Oliguria is a classic sign of inadequate renal perfusion.*
- ▲ Monitor arterial blood gas (ABG) results.
- Monitor temperature. *Hyperpyrexia can result from the hormonal and fluid imbalance and may be an early sign of crisis if accompanied by a sudden drop in BP.*

THERAPEUTIC INTERVENTIONS

- Minimize stressful situations and promote a quiet environment. *Patient's normal response to stress is not functioning since he or she cannot produce corticosteroids. Stress can result in a life-threatening situation with addisonian crisis.*
- Provide rest periods *to prevent overexertion.*
- Assist patient with activities as needed. *The patient in crisis should be helped with all activities (e.g., turning, feeding, cleansing) to prevent overexertion.*
- ▲ If hypotension develops with signs of decreased cardiac output, administer IV fluids rapidly *to restore patient's circulating blood volume;* administer glucocorticoid (e.g., hydrocortisone [Solu-Cortef] IV) *to stabilize the hypotension. Circulatory collapse does not respond to usual treatment (inotropes and vasopressors), and ultimately these patients require glucocorticoids to correct the shock state.*
- ▲ Administer antipyretics as needed for fever.

High Risk for Altered Nutrition: Less than Body Requirements

RISK FACTORS

Decreased GI enzymes, causing loss of appetite and decreased oral intake tolerance
Decreased gastric acid production
Nausea, vomiting, diarrhea

EXPECTED OUTCOMES

Patient's nutritional status is maintained as evidenced by maintenance of weight, adequate dietary intake

ONGOING ASSESSMENT

- Assess GI function and appetite. *Cortisol deficit can impair GI function, causing anorexia, nausea, and vomiting.*
- Monitor and record weight daily.
- Assess foods patient can tolerate.

THERAPEUTIC INTERVENTIONS

- Provide foods patient can tolerate. Prevent fasting.
- Offer frequent small meals. *Inadequate caloric intake in meals may precipitate hypoglycemia. Promotion of oral intake maintains adequate blood glucose levels and nutrition.*
- Create environment conducive to eating.
- Encourage rest periods.
- ▲ Encourage high-protein, low-carbohydrate, high-sodium diet.
- Explain need for diet supplements. *Patient tires because of inadequate production of the hepatic glucagon. Recommended diet prevents fatigue, hypoglycemia, and hyponatremia.*

High Risk for Ineffective Management of Therapeutic Regimen

RISK FACTORS

Lack of experience with adrenocortical insufficiency
Complexity of regimen
Knowledge deficits

EXPECTED OUTCOMES

Patient verbalizes understanding of Addison's disease and guidelines for replacement therapy.

ONGOING ASSESSMENT

- Assess knowledge of Addison's disease, including the need for lifelong medication.
- Assess available support systems and the ability to comply with treatment.
- Assess ability to identify/verbalize signs/symptoms that require physician consultation: fever, nausea/vomiting, weight gain, diaphoresis, progressive weakness, dizziness.

| NURSING DIAGNOSES | EXPECTED OUTCOMES AND NURSING INTERVENTIONS / *RATIONALE*
(■ = INDEPENDENT; ▲ = COLLABORATIVE) |

THERAPEUTIC INTERVENTIONS

- Instruct patient in self-administration of steroids, including expected effects and dosage. *Steroidal replacement may be oral or IM. Knowledge of disease process and drug regimen will promote compliance.*
- Offer information about need to adjust dosage when under stress.
- Emphasize need for morning or evening dose. *Patient must identify personal stressors and learn to adjust steroidal drugs to compensate for stress response. Twice-daily dosing is encouraged to prevent crisis.*
- Stress importance of regular physician visits. *Drug levels may be adjusted to patient's requirements during visits.*
- Discuss signs/symptoms requiring physician consultation.
- Explain how to obtain medical identification tag and importance of wearing it.
- Inform patient of availability of injectable cortisol with sterile syringe. *Patients should carry a readily injectable syringe of cortisol at all times.*

See also:
Noncompliance, p. 42.
Self-esteem Disturbance, p. 53.
Altered Thought Processes, p. 65.

By: Susan Galanes RN, MS, CCRN

Cushing's syndrome

(EXCESS CORTICOSTEROIDS)

Cushing's syndrome reflects an excess of corticosteroids, especially glucocorticoids. Depending on the cause of the syndrome, mineralocorticoids and androgens may also be secreted. The syndrome may be primary (an intrinsic adrenocortical disorder, e.g., neoplasm), secondary (from pituitary or hypothalmic dysfunction with increased ACTH secretion resulting in glucocorticoid excess), or iatrogenic (from prolonged or excessive administration of corticosteroids). The syndrome results in fluid and electrolyte disturbances, suppressed immune response, altered fat distribution, and disturbances in protein metabolism.

| NURSING DIAGNOSES | EXPECTED OUTCOMES AND NURSING INTERVENTIONS / *RATIONALE*
(■ = INDEPENDENT; ▲ = COLLABORATIVE) |

High Risk for Fluid Volume Excess

RISK FACTORS

Retention of sodium and water caused by glucocorticoid excess

Marked sodium and water retention if mineral corticoids are also in excess

EXPECTED OUTCOMES

Patient experiences a normal fluid balance as evidenced by normotensive BP, weight gain ≤ 1 kg, eupnea, clear lungs.

ONGOING ASSESSMENT

- Monitor and record heart rate, BP, CVP, and respiratory rate. *Cushing's syndrome may result in hypertension caused by the expanded fluid volume with Na and H_2O retention.*
- Assess patient for signs of circulatory overload: (elevated CVP, hypertension, weight gain, edema), congestive heart failure (CHF) (jugular vein distention, crackles), pulmonary congestion (shortness of breath, dyspnea, crackles).
- Assess ECG for changes in rhythm and regularity. *Unexplained hypokalemia is associated with excessive glucocorticoids, which can result in cardiac dysrhythmias.*
- Monitor and record I & O.
- Weigh patient daily and record. *Excessive glucocorticoid and mineralocorticoid secretion predisposes patient to fluid and sodium retention.*
- ▲ Monitor lab results (especially potassium and sodium). *Excessive glucocorticoids cause Na and H_2O retention, edema, and hypokalemia. Mineralocorticoids regulate Na and K secretion, and excess levels cause marked Na and H_2O retention as well as marked hypokalemia.*

Continued.

Cushing's syndrome—cont'd

NURSING DIAGNOSES	EXPECTED OUTCOMES AND NURSING INTERVENTIONS / *RATIONALE* (■ = INDEPENDENT; ▲ = COLLABORATIVE)

THERAPEUTIC INTERVENTIONS

▲ Encourage diet low in calories, carbohydrates, and sodium with ample protein and potassium *to help control development of hyperglycemia, edema, and hypokalemia. An increase in blood sugar with glucose intolerance occurs in the presence of excessive glucocorticoids.* See also Diabetes, p. 490, as needed.

▪ Instruct patient to reduce fluid intake as required by condition.

▪ Advise patient to elevate feet when sitting down *to prevent fluid accumulation in the lower extremities.*

▲ Administer antihypertensive medications as prescribed.

Body Image Disturbance

RELATED FACTORS

Increased production of androgens [giving rise to virilism in women; hirsutism (abnormal growth of hair)]

Disturbed protein metabolism resulting in muscle wasting, capillary fragility, and wasting of bone matrix: ecchymosis, osteoporosis, slender limbs, striae (usually purple)

Abnormal fat distribution along with edema resulting in moon face, cervicodorsal fat (buffalo hump), trunk obesity

DEFINING CHARACTERISTICS

Verbal identification of feeling about altered body structure

Verbal preoccupation with changed body

Refusal to discuss or acknowledge change

Change in social behavior (withdrawal, isolation, flamboyancy)

Compensatory use of concealing clothing, other devices

EXPECTED OUTCOMES

Patient's body image is enhanced as evidenced by patient verbalization, use of appropriate coping mechanisms.

ONGOING ASSESSMENT

▪ Assess for changes in personal appearance caused by the glucocorticoid excess. *These may include obesity, thin extremities with muscle atrophy, moon face, red cheeks, buffalo hump, increased body and facial hair.*

▪ Assess for presence of pronounced acne, *which may result from adrenal androgen excess.*

▪ Assess patient's feelings about changed appearance and coping mechanisms.

THERAPEUTIC INTERVENTIONS

▪ Promote coping methods to deal with patient's change in appearance, (e.g., adequate grooming, flattering clothes).

▪ Reassure the patient that the physical changes are a result of the elevated hormone levels and will resolve when those levels return to normal.

▪ Anticipate the need to discuss/reinforce the probable treatment in correcting the hypersecretion of hormone:

If an intrinsic adrenocortical disorder: probable surgery for removal of the adenoma, tumor, or adrenal glands

If a disorder secondary to pituitary hypersecretion: transphenoidal pituitary tumor resection or irradiation.

If iatrogenic: gradual discontinuation of excessive administration of corticostroids as the patient's condition permits.

High Risk for Infection

RISK FACTORS

Increased cortisol secretion keeping body in chronic stress state

Increased cortisol suppressing leukocyte adherence to endothelial surface

Increased cortisol decreasing leukocyte accumulation at injury site

Increased cortisol impairing WBC migration, antibody formation, and lymphocyte proliferation

Increased cortisol increasing protein breakdown

EXPECTED OUTCOMES

Patient is free of infection as evidenced by normal temperature, WBC count within normal limits, absence of purulent drainage.

ONGOING ASSESSMENT

▪ Assess potential infection sites: urinary, pulmonary, wound, or IV line.

▪ Monitor and record temperature.

▲ Monitor WBC count.

▪ Note signs of localized or systemic infection; report promptly. *Increase in glucocorticoids inhibits the immune response with a suppression of allergic response, as well as inhibition of inflammation. Note: An elevated temperature may not be present with infection because of the decreased immune response. Assess for purulent drainage. Other signs of infection may be minimized by inhibition of the immune response as well as inhibition of inflammation.*

▪ Assess for areas of skin breakdown and assess wound healing. *Wound healing is prolonged in Cushing's syndrome.*

▲ Obtain specimens of blood, urine, serum, and so on, for culture and sensitivity if infection is suspected.

THERAPEUTIC INTERVENTIONS

- Use strict aseptic technique when performing dressing changes, wound irrigations, catheter care, or suctioning.
- ▲ Avoid use of indwelling catheters or IV lines whenever possible. *Limited immune response predisposes patients to infection. Avoidance of catheters, IV lines decreases risk of potential infection.*
- ▲ Administer antibiotics as prescribed.
- Protect patient from bumping and bruising. *Bruising occurs readily in Cushing's syndrome.* Change patient's position. *Protection from injury decreases susceptibility to infection.*
- Pad bony prominences. *Protection/position changes promote peripheral tissue perfusion.*
- Provide a private room if possible, *to decrease the patient's exposure to possible pathogens.*
- Cleanse any open skin areas and maintain them clean and dry *to allow for healing.*

High Risk for Injury: Fracture

RISK FACTORS

As protein catabolism increases, protein synthesis decreases, leading to osteoporosis from bone matrix wasting. In children this can lead to retarded linear growth.

EXPECTED OUTCOMES

Patient's risk for fractures is reduced through ongoing assessment and early intervention.

ONGOING ASSESSMENT

- Assess patient's ability to ambulate; observe gait.
- Observe for loss of muscle mass and osteoporosis after minor trauma. *Muscle wasting, fatigue, weakness, and osteoporosis are associated with excess glucocorticoids.*
- Assess patient for signs of kyphosis or height loss.
- Assess fat distribution. *Chronic cortisol hypersecretion redistributes body fat with fat from arms and legs deposited on back, shoulder, trunk, and abdomen.*
- Measure actual height at time or admission; compare with past medical records. *Identifies possibility of minor fractures, disk or hip injury.*

THERAPEUTIC INTERVENTIONS

- Orient patient to surroundings.
- Keep floor in patient's room clean, dry, and uncluttered *to decrease risk of injury by providing a safe environment.*
- Encourage use of cane or walker if patient's gait is unsteady. Provide necessary aids *to promote independence with mobility.*

Knowledge Deficit

RELATED FACTORS

Lack of experience with Cushing's syndrome

DEFINING CHARACTERISTICS

Questioning, especially if repetitive
Silence
Anxiety
Repeated hospital admissions for complications
Verbalized misconceptions

EXPECTED OUTCOMES

Patient verbalizes an understanding of Cushing's syndrome and guidelines for therapy.

ONGOING ASSESSMENT

- Assess level of knowledge of Cushing's syndrome.
- Assess patient's resources, strengths and weaknesses.

THERAPEUTIC INTERVENTIONS

- Explain all tests to patient. *Patient/family must understand disease process and receive specific instructions related to treatment, methods to control symptoms, signs of infections, complications, and indicators of when to notify physician.*
- Answer all questions honestly.
- Explain methods, rationale, and expected effects of appropriate treatment: surgery, radiation therapy *(may be used to combat nonoperable tumors)*, drug therapy *(replacement may be temporary or permanent)*, diet restrictions.
- Review signs and symptoms of infection and instruct patient to report promptly. Inform patient that Cushing's syndrome may mask infection from the suppressed inflammatory response.
- Instruct in behavior modification techniques to assist in diet alterations: low-calorie, high-nutrition diet.
- Arrange for follow-up care as appropriate.
- Explain how to obtain a medical identification tag and the importance of wearing it.

See also:
Impaired Skin Integrity, p. 59.
Activity Intolerance, p. 2.
Self-esteem Disturbance, p. 55.

By: Susan Galanes, RN, MS, CCRN

Diabetes insipidus

(DI; NEUROGENIC DIABETES)

Diabetes insipidus (DI) is a disturbance of water metabolism caused by a failure of vasopressin (antidiuretic hormone [ADH]) synthesis or release resulting in the excretion of a large amount of dilute urine. Diabetes insipidus may also have a nephrogenic or psychogenic cause.

NURSING DIAGNOSES	EXPECTED OUTCOMES AND NURSING INTERVENTIONS / *RATIONALE* (■ = INDEPENDENT; ▲ = COLLABORATIVE)

Fluid Volume Deficit

RELATED FACTORS

Compromised endocrine regulatory mechanism
Neurohypophyseal dysfunction
Hypopituitarism
Hypophysectomy

DEFINING CHARACTERISTICS

Polyuria
Polydypsia (increased thirst)
Sudden weight loss
Urine specific gravity <1.005
Hypernatremia (Na$^+$ >145 mEq/L)
Change in mental status
Urine osmolality: <300 mOsm/L
Requests for cold/ice water
Output exceeds intake

EXPECTED OUTCOMES

Patient experiences normal fluid volume as evidenced by absence of thirst, normal serum Na$^+$ level, stable weight.

ONGOING ASSESSMENT

- Monitor I & O. Report urine volume > 200 ml for each of 2 consecutive hr or 500 ml in 2-hr period.
- Monitor for increased thirst (polydypsia). *If the patient is conscious and the thirst center is intact, thirst can be a reliable indicator of fluid balance. Polyuria and polydypsia strongly suggest DI.*
- Weigh daily to detect excessive fluid loss, especially in incontinent patients with inaccurate I & O.
- Monitor urine specific gravity every shift *(may be 1.005 or less).*
- ▲ Monitor serum and urine osmolality. *Urine osmolality is less than 300 mOsm/L in DI, whereas serum osmolality is normal or only moderately elevated if the patient is allowed to ingest large amounts of water to compensate for the urinary loss.*
- ▲ Monitor for serum Na$^+$ levels > 145 mEq/L. *Dehydration is a hyperosmolar state in which serum Na$^+$ level rises.*
- ▲ Monitor serum K$^+$. *Hypokalemia may result from the increase in urinary output.*
- Monitor for signs of hypovolemic shock (e.g., tachycardia, tachypnea, hypotension). *Frequent assessment can detect changes early for rapid intervention.*
- Assess bowel pattern. *Constipation may stem from the fluid losses with DI.*

THERAPEUTIC INTERVENTIONS

- Allow patient to drink at will. *Patients with intact thirst mechanisms may maintain fluid balance by drinking huge quantities of water to compensate for the amount they urinate. Patients prefer cold or iced water.*
- Provide easily accessible fluid source, keeping adequate fluids at bedside.
- ▲ If patient has decreased LOC or impaired thirst mechanism, obtain parenteral fluid prescription.
- ▲ Administer medication as prescribed. *Aqueous vasopressin is usually used for DI of short duration (e.g., postoperative neurosurgery or head trauma). Pitressin Tannate in Oil (the longer-acting vasopressin) is used for longer-term DI. Patients with milder forms of DI may use chlorpropamide (Diabinese), clofibrate (Atromid), or carbamezepine (Tegretol) to stimulate release of ADH from the posterior pituitary and enhance its action on the renal tubules. Hydrochlorthiazide (Hydrodiuril) may also be used for nephrogenic DI.*
- ▲ If vasopressin is given, monitor for water intoxication/rebound hyponatremia. *Overmedication can result in volume excess.*

High Risk for Altered Skin Integrity

RISK FACTORS

Urinary frequency with high volume output and the potential for incontinence

EXPECTED OUTCOMES

Patient's skin remains intact.

ONGOING ASSESSMENT

- Inspect skin every shift; document condition and changes in status. *Early detection and intervention may prevent progression of impaired skin integrity.*
- Assess for continence/incontinence. Evaluate the need for an indwelling urinary catheter. *Urinary output can be excessive in DI.*
- Assess other risks of patient's skin integrity (e.g., immobility, nutritional status).

THERAPEUTIC INTERVENTIONS

- Provide easy access to bathroom/urinal/bedpan.
- Use skin barriers as needed *to prevent redness/excoriation from urinary frequency.*

| NURSING DIAGNOSES | EXPECTED OUTCOMES AND NURSING INTERVENTIONS / *RATIONALE*
(■ = INDEPENDENT; ▲ = COLLABORATIVE) |

Knowledge Deficit

RELATED FACTORS

Disease process
Medications and treatments

DEFINING CHARACTERISTICS

Questions
Requests for more information
Verbalized misconceptions/
  misinterpretation

EXPECTED OUTCOMES

Patient verbalizes correct understanding of DI, medications, and treatments.

ONGOING ASSESSMENT

- Assess level of knowledge of DI.
- Assess level of understanding of medications and treatments.

THERAPEUTIC INTERVENTIONS

- Explain DI and treatment(s) in simple, brief terms to patient/family/significant others.
- Teach patient the necessity of closely monitoring fluid balance, including daily weights (same time of day with same amount of clothing), fluid I & O, measurement of urine specific gravity.
- For patient going home with long-term ADH replacement, instruct in medication self-management:
    How to administer:
        Desmopressin acetate (DDAVP) *usually taken bid intranasally*
        Lypressin nasal spray *usually 3-4 times/day*
        Pittressin tannate in oil, given IM; The patient or significant other will need instruction/return demonstration in giving own injections
    Signs of overdosage
    Signs of underdosage
    Signs of fluid volume excess
- Discuss when to seek further medical attention.
- Instruct patient to wear a Medic-Alert, listing DI and the treatment patient is using.

See also:
Constipation, p. 16.
Altered Skin Integrity, p. 59.
Fear, p. 23.
Sleep Pattern Disturbance,
  p. 61.

By: Susan Galanes RN, MS, CCRN

Diabetes mellitus

(TYPE I, TYPE II, ADULT ONSET, JUVENILE
DIABETES, INSULIN-DEPENDENT [IDDM],
NON-INSULIN-DEPENDENT [NIDDM])

A pancreatic disorder in which the β cells of the islets of Langerhans do not secrete enough insulin, if any. Insulin, a hormone usually secreted after meals, facilitates glycogen storage in the liver and transport of glucose into muscle and fat cells and maintains blood glucose at normal levels. Inadequate insulin causes hyperglycemia and glycosuria, which lead to fluid and electrolyte imbalance. Gluconeogenesis (use of protein and fat stores) causes ketoacidosis, muscle wasting, and weight loss.

NURSING DIAGNOSES	EXPECTED OUTCOMES AND NURSING INTERVENTIONS / *RATIONALE* (■ = INDEPENDENT; ▲ = COLLABORATIVE)

Altered Nutrition: Less than Body Requirements

RELATED FACTORS

Decreased number or function of pancreatic islet cells
Increased blood glucose level by poor cell uptake
Glycosuria caused by exceeding renal tubular capacity limits

DEFINING CHARACTERISTICS

Polydipsia
Polyphagia
Polyuria
Weight loss

EXPECTED OUTCOMES

Patient experiences resolution of polydipsia, polyuria, and polyphagia as glucose levels approach normal.

ONGOING ASSESSMENT

- Assess for signs of hyperglycemia. *Hyperglycemia results when inadequate insulin is present to use glucose; excess glucose in the bloodstream creates an osmotic effect, which results in the following: polydipsia (thirst), polyphagia (excessive hunger), polyuria (frequent urination).*
- ▲ Monitor blood glucose levels at least every shift; compare to laboratory results at least daily. *The availability of on-unit blood glucose monitoring allows timely assessment of blood glucose by clinicians; care must be taken, however, to assure validity of findings. Capillary samples may test higher than venous samples. Normal blood glucose levels: 70-110 mg/dl.*
- ▲ Monitor the following laboratory results:
  Na: normal: 136-147 mEq/L
  Cl: normal: 95-110 mEq/L
  CO_2: normal: 21-32 mEq/L
  Electrolyte imbalances occur in diabetes because of the osmotic diuresis caused by hyperglycemia. Ketone formation, secondary to breakdown of fats and proteins, can cause acidosis.
- ▲ Monitor glycosylated hemoglobin, if available. *This relatively new blood test is an adjunct in determining glucose control over the preceeding 120 days. Note: Glycosylated hemoglobin may not be useful for patients with wide ranges in blood glucose levels.*
- Monitor BP and heart rate. *Unchecked diuresis with loss of fluid and electrolytes can cause fluid volume deficit.*
- Check color and temperature of skin. *Cool, clammy skin is symptomatic of fluid volume deficit secondary to hyperglycemia.*
- Obtain a weight history. *Patients typically demonstrate weight loss. This is due to chronic breakdown of fats and protein for use as energy because glucose cannot be used.*

THERAPEUTIC INTERVENTIONS

- ▲ Administer insulin as prescribed. *Insulin, a hormone, facilitates use of glucose by allowing transport across cell membranes. Typically the need for insulin is a lifelong one. A variety of insulin administration schemes may be chosen, depending on the patient's clinical picture/need:*
  Insulin drip: delivers a continuous, easily titratable dose; switched to sub-Q when control is achieved
  Regular insulin: usually given subcutaneously before meals
  Regular/NHP A.M. and P.M. split mixed dose: maximizes the benefits of short- and long-acting insulins.
- Rotate injection sites. *The purpose of rotating sites is to enhance absorption of insulin. Some practitioners advocate rotating sites with every administration; others feel that rotating site once each month is acceptable.*
- ▲ Administer oral hypoglycemic agents as prescribed. *Oral hypoglycemic agents act by increasing the release of insulin from the pancreas and can be an effective part of therapy for patients with non-insulin-dependent diabetes mellitus.*
- ▲ Provide appropriate diet: obtain dietary consultation; reinforce need to consume all foods on tray, not save for later; check each meal tray for proper identification.
- Give all meals and snacks on time.

High Risk for Ineffective Individual Coping

RISK FACTORS

Diagnosis and treatment course
New problem
Chronic disease

EXPECTED OUTCOMES

Patient demonstrates effective coping strategies in approach to new disease/complications, as evidenced by identification of specific stressors, identification of available support systems and resources.

ONGOING ASSESSMENT

- Assess for the following signs that coping is/may be ineffective:
  Patient verbalizes inability to cope or to make decisions.
  Patient behaves in ways known to be harmful (overeating, dependence on alcohol or other chemical substances, excessive smoking).
  Patient is depressed.
  Patient is unable to sleep.
  Patient is generally irritable.
  A new diagnosis of diabetes or an admission for complications related to diabetes can precipitate/may indicate ineffective coping, as the patient attempts to incorporate chronic disease management and significant restriction into his/her life.
- Assess for anger, noncompliance, regressive behaviors. *These behaviors may be protective and should be anticipated and allowed when the diagnosis is new.*
- Assess past coping mechanisms. *Patient may be able to identify techniques that were helpful in another/similar situation.*
- Assess support systems *that may be helpful as patient begins to cope with a new diagnosis or new or altered management.*
- Ask patient to identify specific stressors. *The patient is best served when the health care professional understands clearly what the patient finds stressful. This technique also can guide the plan of care.*

THERAPEUTIC INTERVENTIONS

- Encourage patient to verbalize feelings about disease, treatment, chronicity, whatever the patient perceives as stressful.
- Allow and reinforce that feelings are a normal part of coping.
- Involve support person/significant other in efforts aimed at improving patient's coping skills. *This should be done with the patient's permission, since some individuals feel very private about coping with own problems.*
- Assist patient in determining what assistance is needed in order for coping to occur. *Some patients may feel better simply verbalizing feelings; others may benefit from detailed teaching to gain mastery over disease. Still others will benefit from contact with another patient who has successfully coped with a similar illness.*
- Encourage patient to set realistic goals *to prevent disappointment/feelings of failure.*
- Point out/praise positive progress of changes. *This can be accomplished by breaking large tasks (e.g., self insulin administration) into smaller tasks (e.g., selecting a site, preparing injection, giving injection) so that there are multiple opportunities for success and praise.*
- Encourage patient to engage in activities that have been satisfying and successful in the past (e.g., hobbies).

Continued.

NURSING DIAGNOSES	EXPECTED OUTCOMES AND NURSING INTERVENTIONS / *RATIONALE* (■ = INDEPENDENT; ▲ = COLLABORATIVE)

High Risk for Ineffective Management of Therapeutic Regimen

RISK FACTORS

Initial diagnosis of chronic disease

Multifaceted treatment involved in controlling diabetes and potential complications

Lack of familiarity with resources

Need for information about hyperglycemia/hypoglycemia

Complexity of health care system

Perceived powerlessness

Perceived inability to take/ meet responsibility for health needs

EXPECTED OUTCOMES

Patient demonstrates knowledge of and compliance with treatment regimen.

ONGOING ASSESSMENT

- Assess knowledge of diabetes.
- Assess for ability to learn. *Mental status changes/other impairments to learning may require an adapted teaching approach and/or the involvement of a significant other.*
- Assess physical abilities, including sight, hand-eye coordination. *Insulin administration requires a combination of cognitive and psychomotor skills. Management of blood glucose monitoring and diet requires cognitive abilities and judgment.*
- Assess willingness to learn about diabetes, medications (oral agents, insulin), dietary management, blood glucose level monitoring, management of complications.
- Assess knowledge of signs and symptoms of hypoglycemia and hyperglycemia. *Even in well-controlled diabetes, hyperglycemia (high blood glucose level) and hypoglycemia (low blood glucose level) can occur; it is essential that patients recognize symptoms.*
- Assess need for individual or family counseling. *Patients who are unable to accept the permanence/need for long-term management will have difficulty learning management.*

THERAPEUTIC INTERVENTIONS

▲ Contact diabetes teaching service.
- Explain definition of diabetes, including signs and symptoms.
  Reinforce fact that diabetes is chronic incurable condition that can be controlled by diet, insulin, and exercise.
  Explain need for diet-controlled exchange system and importance of strict adherence.
  Explain that daily exercise is important to lower blood sugar level and also allows for normal socialization. *Exercise increases body's sensitivity to insulin and decreases serum cholesterol and triglyceride levels, decreasing risk factors for developing cardiovascular complications of diabetes.*
- Reinforce and encourage progress toward independence at blood glucose level monitoring and insulin administration techniques:
  Define insulin; discuss different types, action, duration, especially split-mixed insulin regimen.
  Demonstrate accurate method of drawing up and administering insulin; explain rationale for rotating injection sites.
  Explain that blood glucose level monitoring is necessary for diabetic control; *normal glucose level is 70-110 mg/dl.*
  Demonstrate accurate method of obtaining and interpreting blood glucose Chemstrips or Accu-Chek system (or other electronic device).
- Instruct in recognition of signs/symptoms of altered glucose metabolism:
  Hypoglycemia:
    Hunger, sweating, pallor, tremor, feelings of nervousness or anxiety, lethargy, irritability, tingling or numbness in lips or tongue (early), blurred or double vision, mental dullness, change in behavior, fatigue, confusion, dizziness, slurred speech, slow or uncoordinated movement (gradual).
  Hyperglycemia:
    Polydipsia, polyphagia, polyuria, nocturia, nausea, vomiting, dim or blurred vision, headache (early), abdominal pain, GI cramps, constipation, drowsiness, headache, weakness, flushed/dry skin, rapid labored or deep breathing, weak rapid pulse, elevated temperature, acetone breath odor, hypotension, coma (gradual). *Overall goal of patient care is to regulate glucose levels (to decrease risk of complications). Secondary goal is to disrupt patient's life as little as possible with management regimens.*
- Instruct patient/family about treatment regimen for altered glucose levels.
  Hypoglycemia:
    Administration of 10-15 g carbohydrate *to raise blood glucose levels to target range of 70-110 mg/dl.* Source: 4 oz fruit juice, 2 tsp honey, 5 life savers, or 1 glass soft drink or milk, or 1-2 glucose tablets.
    If no response to treatment, oral carbohydrate may be repeated.
    IV glucose source may be required.

THERAPEUTIC INTERVENTIONS— cont'd

Hyperglycemia:

If patient is conscious, sugar-free fluids should be taken; (10-12 oz/hr); *water decreases hyperosmolar state.*

Blood specimens obtained q2hr *to monitor glucose levels.*

Parenteral fluids/insulin may be required *to decrease glucose levels and replace fluids. When diabetes successfully regulated, patient prevents complications of hyperglycemia/hypoglycemia.*

▲ Reinforce information provided by diabetic teaching service/physician/other nursing staff.

▲ Provide patient variety of resources in diabetes education as appropriate *to ensure health maintenance, diabetes control, and support network.*

■ Discuss/define diabetic ketoacidosis and need for immediate medical attention. *Family must learn basic survival skills of diabetes mellitus (DM) management to prevent complications (see also Diabetic ketoacidosis, p. 494).*

■ Discuss need for careful blood sugar level monitoring during illness (may require insulin adjustment).

■ Reinforce need for regular follow-up care (e.g., of eyes, feet, and teeth) *to prevent microvascular complications of diabetes (e.g., reduced vision, blindness, foot problems, and renal failure).*

See also:
Altered Health Maintenance,
p. 31.
Health Seeking Behaviors,
p. 33.
High Risk for Noncompliance,
p. 42.
High Risk for Infection, p. 40.
High Risk for Altered Sexuality Patterns, p. 58.

By: Linda Rosen-Walsh, RN, BSN
Charlotte Niznik, RN, BSN, CDE
Margaret A. Cunningham, RN, MS
Eileen Raebig, RN,C
Lynne Wentz, RN, BSN, MHS, CDE

Diabetic ketoacidosis (DKA)

(HYPERGLYCEMIA; DIABETES MELLITUS; DIABETIC COMA)

Diabetic ketoacidosis (DKA) is an acute, potentially life-threatening complication of diabetes mellitus. Normally the body metabolizes glucose for energy needs. In the diabetic, glucose metabolism does not occur because of absent or ineffective insulin that is necessary for migration of glucose into cells. Diabetic ketoacidosis (DKA) results from cellular metabolism of fat to produce energy. By-products of this metabolic process are ketone bodies (organic acids) that cause metabolic acidosis.

NURSING DIAGNOSES	EXPECTED OUTCOMES AND NURSING INTERVENTIONS / *RATIONALE* (■ = INDEPENDENT; ▲ = COLLABORATIVE)

High Risk for Injury: Ketoacidosis

RISK FACTORS

Omission/reduction of insulin
Inability of cells to recognize/ use available insulin
Initial onset of diabetes
Infection/intercurrent illness
Acute pancreatitis
Stress

EXPECTED OUTCOMES

Patient experiences resolution of electrolyte imbalance and restoration of normal acid-base balance.

ONGOING ASSESSMENT

▲ Monitor laboratory tests for signs of ketoacidosis:
    Serum glucose level >300 mg/dl and <900 mg/dl
    Serum ketones
    Decreased serum pH, phosphate, bicarbonate
■ Monitor and record urine glucose and ketone levels. *Presence of ketone denotes ketoacidotic state.*
■ Assess for clinical signs of ketoacidosis: polydipsia, polyuria; weakness, anorexia, polyphagia; abdominal pain; lethargy; acetone breath; blurred vision; nausea, vomiting
■ Monitor and record respiratory rate, depth, and presence of Kussmaul respirations: *Deep, rapid respirations indicate increased acidic state. Carbon dioxide and acetone are blown off with each breath in an attempt to compensate acidosis.*
■ Auscultate for bowel sounds. Assess for abdominal pain; check intensity and location of pain. *Abdominal pain, nausea, vomiting result from ketoacidosis.*
▲ Monitor potassium level when therapy begins. *With metabolic and fluid correction, K^+ returns intracellularly and serum hypokalemia may result from K^+ loss with diuresis.*
▲ Monitor ABGs as ordered.
▲ Monitor for signs of hypoglycemia: confusion, tremors, pallor, weakness, diaphoresis, serum glucose level <60 mg/dl. *Hypoglycemia can occur as ketoacidosis is aggressively treated.*

THERAPEUTIC INTERVENTIONS

▲ Administer and record IV fluids and additives as prescribed.
    Use normal saline solution to correct volume depletion. *Restriction of glucose solutions is desired until blood glucose level drops to 250 mg/dl.*
    Initiate K^+ therapy if indicated.
▲ Administer sodium bicarbonate only in cases of severe, life-threatening acidosis. *Early or overzealous use of $NaHCO_3$ often causes rebound metabolic alkalosis when rehydration has occurred.*
▲ Administer and record insulin injection/drip as prescribed. Follow hospital/unit procedure for preparing insulin drip. *Short-acting insulin (IV infusion) allows glucose transport to cells and promotes fat/protein storage.*
■ If signs of hypoglycemia are present, administer glucose gel or milk sugar under tongue if NPO; or orange juice if patient tolerates oral fluids. *With decrease of blood glucose level and IV infusion, patient is at risk for hypoglycemia and cerebral edema.*
■ If vomiting occurs, elevate head of bed (HOB) 30 degrees; prepare for possible nasogastric tube placement.
▲ Administer antiemetics as prescribed.

Fluid Volume Deficit

RELATED FACTORS

Osmotic diuresis from hyperglycemia
Vomiting
Kussmaul respirations

EXPECTED OUTCOMES

Patient achieves normal fluid volume, as evidenced by normal BP, normal heart rate, urine output 30 ml/hr.

NURSING DIAGNOSES	EXPECTED OUTCOMES AND NURSING INTERVENTIONS / *RATIONALE* (■ = INDEPENDENT; ▲ = COLLABORATIVE)

DEFINING CHARACTERISTICS

Abdominal pain
Hypotension, tachycardia
Dilute urine
Output greater than intake
Increased Hb, Hct, glucose, BUN levels
Increased sodium, creatinine levels
Oliguria or anuria possible in severe dehydration and shock

ONGOING ASSESSMENT

- Monitor vital signs. *Severe hypotension and tachycardia precede hypovolemic shock.*
- Assess skin turgor, *an indication of hydration.*
- Monitor and record I & O. Report if urine output <30 ml for 2 consecutive hr. *Urinary output should be at least 30 ml/hr. Lower output indicates decreased renal perfusion.*
- Monitor and record urine specific gravity (*early indicator of dehydration and/or electrolyte imbalance*).
- Weigh patient daily; record.
- ▲ Monitor serum Hct, Hb, osmolality, BUN, glucose, and urine laboratory values (*increased because of hemoconcentration*).

THERAPEUTIC INTERVENTIONS

- ▲ Administer isotonic IV fluid (saline solution) followed by glucose IV fluid when glucose levels drop. *Isotonic saline solution is administered to increase volume quickly and maintain sodium balance. Restrict glucose only until serum glucose level begins to drop to prevent hypoglycemia.*
- Reassure patient during episodes of abdominal pain and vomiting. *These symptoms are thought to be related to severe dehydration and electrolyte imbalance; should subside when fluid volume corrected.*

Altered Levels of Consciousness

RELATED TO

Acid-base imbalance
Ineffective breathing pattern
Dehydration

DEFINING CHARACTERISTICS

Change in alertness, orientation, ability to respond verbally, decreased motor response, decreased pupillary reaction
Kussmaul respirations
Agitation
Impaired judgment
Lethargy/Drowsiness
Coma

EXPECTED OUTCOMES

Patient returns to baseline level of consciousness.

ONGOING ASSESSMENT

- Assess level of consciousness (LOC) by using coma scale on neurologic flow sheet. *Flow sheet documentation quickly identifies immediate changes in trends in patient's neurologic status.*
- ▲ Assess serum electrolytes, glucose, pH levels.
- Monitor respiratory rate, tidal volume, quality. *Change in quality of respirations may lead to decreased sensorium, ultimate respiratory arrest.*

THERAPEUTIC INTERVENTIONS

- ▲ Correct serum electrolytes, fluid, glucose levels, and pH imbalance.
- Ensure safety as necessary: side rails, restraints.

High Risk for Decreased Cardiac Output

RISK FACTORS

Cardiac dysrhythmias secondary to hyperkalemia/hypokalemia

EXPECTED OUTCOMES

Patient maintains normal cardiac output as evidenced by normal BP; alert, responsive state; warm skin.
Patient maintains normal cardiac rhythm.

ONGOING ASSESSMENT

- Monitor ECG for early signs of potassium imbalance. *Electrolyte abnormalities exhibit specific ECG effects. Recognition of hyperkalemia/hypokalemia can alert nurse to life-threatening situation.*

  Progressive signs of hyperkalemia: high-peaked T waves; flat P waves; prolonged PR interval; atrial arrest; prolonged QRS, slow ventricular rate; ventricular fibrillation; asystole.

  Signs of hypokalemia: prolonged low-amplitude T waves, prominent U waves, ectopic beats.

- Monitor for changes in cardiac output; check BP regularly. *BP and pulses reflect cardiac output.*

THERAPEUTIC INTERVENTIONS

- ▲ Provide accurate administration of fluids and electrolytes *to correct fluid, acid-base imbalance. Acidosis is associated with hyperkalemia, which causes slowed conduction. In contrast, aggressive treatment can cause hypokalemia, which causes ectopic cardiac rhythms.*
- Place patient on cardiac monitor if indicated. *Patient in mild DKA may not require monitoring if clinically stable.*

Continued.

Diabetic ketoacidosis (DKA)—cont'd

NURSING DIAGNOSES	EXPECTED OUTCOMES AND NURSING INTERVENTIONS / *RATIONALE* (■ = INDEPENDENT; ▲ = COLLABORATIVE)

Altered Nutrition: Less than Body Requirements

RELATED FACTORS

Lack of glucose metabolism caused by absence of effective insulin
Use of fat/protein for energy needs *(Protein metabolism may occur but only when fat stores are depleted)*
Protein loss caused by diuresis

DEFINING CHARACTERISTICS

Weight loss
Ketoacidosis
Hyperglycemia
Abdominal discomfort
Flushed skin
Nausea/vomiting
Diuresis

EXPECTED OUTCOMES

Patient maintains normal nutritional balance, as evidenced by normal glucose level, maintenance of weight.

ONGOING ASSESSMENT

- Obtain weight; compare with usual weight if possible.
- Assess for muscle wasting, weakness. *This indicates chronic nutritional derangement.*
- Assess dietary habits, especially for new onset diabetes.
- Monitor I & O, including calorie and carbohydrate intake.
- Monitor urine for sugar, protein, and ketone levels.
▲ Monitor blood sugar level routinely once DKA is resolved.

THERAPEUTIC INTERVENTIONS

▲ Administer insulin (short-acting) *to allow glucose transport to cells. Glucose metabolism for energy requirements spares fat and protein for cell growth and maintenance and allows fat/protein storage.*
▲ Notify physician when serum glucose level has dropped to 250 to 300 mg/dl. *At this time glucose IV should be administered and insulin therapy halted to prevent hypoglycemia and cerebral edema.*
- Provide oral intake when nausea and vomiting abate and LOC has stabilized.
▲ Obtain dietary consultation *to prevent recurrence of DKA.*
- Provide instruction on American Dietetic Association meal planning when oral nutrition is tolerated and IV is discontinued.
▲ Continue to administer subcutaneous insulin on routine, daily basis *to prevent recurrence of DKA.*
- Allow patient to test own blood sugar, self-administer insulin, and make menu selections when able.
- See also Diabetes p. 490.

High Risk for Ineffective Management of Therapeutic Regimen

RISK FACTORS

Unfamiliarity with disease process and treatment
Noncompliance with medications, testing of urine and blood, and follow-up care
Complexity of therapeutic regimen
Social support deficits

EXPECTED OUTCOMES

Patient/significant others demonstrate knowledge of disease process and importance of medications, urine and blood testing.
Patient follows prescribed treatment plan, as evidenced by glucose levels within patient's recommended range, no further episodes of ketoacidosis.

ONGOING ASSESSMENT

- Assess understanding of causes and consequences of diabetic ketoacidosis.
- Assess feelings about health status.
- Assess for contributing factors to DKA.

THERAPEUTIC INTERVENTIONS

- Explain to patient/significant others:
    Symptoms of early acute diabetic ketoacidosis (drowsiness, nausea, vomiting, flushed skin, thirst, excessive urination, glycosuria, ketonuria). *Patient and family must identify signs/symptoms of impending hyperglycemia/ketoacisosis to prevent complications and future hospitalizations.*
    Factors that predispose patient to diabetic ketoacidosis (illness, stress, infection, insufficient insulin, decreased activity and exercise).
    Importance of balanced diet, routine exercise, weight control, accurate medication administration, regular urine ketone and blood testing, and follow-up care.
    Management of diabetes during other illness: importance of taking insulin even if feeling ill and not eating, appropriate diet and insulin dosage modifications, need to inform physician of status, frequent testing for ketonuria and hypoglycemia/hyperglycemia.
▲ Refer for psychological counseling, if needed, *to improve acceptance of chronic disease.*
▲ Refer to diabetic teaching service.
- See also Diabetes p. 490.

See also:
Noncompliance, p. 42
Ineffective Coping, p. 18
Altered Health Maintenance, p. 31

By: Charlotte Niznik, RN, BSN, CDE
   Lynne Wentz, RN, BSN, MHS, CDE

Hyperglycemic hyperosmotic nonketotic syndrome (HNKS)

(DIABETIC COMA; NONKETOTIC HYPEROSMOLAR COMA)

Hyperglycemic hyperosmotic nonketotic syndrome (HNKS) can be a complication of diabetes but may also result from hyperalimentation, dialysis, IV fluids, steroid therapy, diuretic administration, pancreatitis, diabetes insipidus, and severe burns. The severe hyperglycemia persists because of ineffective or inadequate insulin levels and results in osmotic diuresis and severe dehydration.

NURSING DIAGNOSES	EXPECTED OUTCOMES AND NURSING INTERVENTIONS / *RATIONALE* (■ = INDEPENDENT; ▲ = COLLABORATIVE)

Fluid Volume Deficit

RELATED FACTORS

Hyperglycemia
Osmotic diuresis

DEFINING CHARACTERISTICS

Increased urine output
Sudden weight loss
Hemoconcentration
Increased BUN/creatinine ratio
Hypotension
Thirst/dry skin and mucous membranes
Poor skin turgor
Decreased cardiac output
Hypokalemia
Hypernatremia
Change in LOC
Ventricular dysrhythmias

EXPECTED OUTCOMES

Patient's fluid volume is normal, as evidenced by normal vital signs, electrolyte balance.

ONGOING ASSESSMENT

▲ Monitor status of fluid volume: increased urine output *(caused by osmotic load from hyperglycemia),* sudden weight loss, hemoconcentration *(increase in Hb and Hct values as circulating volume decreases),* increased BUN/creatinine ratio, thirst/dry skin and mucous membranes, poor skin turgor, decreased cardiac output, hypokalemia *(K⁺ is lost with diuresis),* hypernatremia, change in LOC.

▪ Monitor BP and heart rate. *Hypotension and compensatory heart rate increase occur as fluid volume deficit progresses.*

▲ Monitor serum osmolarity, *a relative indicator of fluid to solute ratio. As dehydration worsens, osmolarity increases.*

▪ Auscultate lungs for rhonchi, rales (crackles) *(may result from circulatory overload caused by aggressive fluid therapy).*

▪ Monitor cardiac function. *Ventricular dysrhythmias may occur as hypokalemia worsens.*

THERAPEUTIC INTERVENTIONS

▲ Administer isotonic IV fluids *to increase cardiac output and tissue perfusion along with correcting fluid imbalance.*

▲ Administer insulin according to blood glucose levels. *Insulin therapy is essential to decrease serum glucose level and osmolarity. This will allow extracellular fluid to shift to intracellular fluid, alleviating intracellular dehydration.*

Altered Nutrition: Less than Body Requirements

RELATED FACTORS

Insulin deficiency
Ineffective metabolism of available glucose

DEFINING CHARACTERISTICS

Weight loss
Muscle weakness
Hyperglycemia
Abdominal pain

EXPECTED OUTCOMES

Patient maintains ability to metabolize glucose, as evidenced by normal blood glucose level, weight maintenance.

ONGOING ASSESSMENT

▲ Monitor blood glucose levels q2-4hr until stable. *Aggressive fluid therapy and insulin management can cause precipitous changes that must be monitored closely.*

▪ Observe for abdominal pain. *Nausea and vomiting may result from fluid/electrolyte imbalance as well as ketonemia. Ketonemia is not necessarily present until later in disease course.*

THERAPEUTIC INTERVENTIONS

▲ Administer continuous low-dose insulin infusion. *Rapid infusion of insulin may result in hypoglycemia.*

▪ Promote nutrition. *When electrolyte and glucose imbalances are corrected, appetite is restored.*

▲ Provide fluids and progress diet as tolerated.

▲ Obtain dietary consultation if needed.

Continued.

Hyperglycemic hyperosmotic nonketotic syndrome (HNKS)—cont'd

NURSING DIAGNOSES	EXPECTED OUTCOMES AND NURSING INTERVENTIONS / *RATIONALE* (■ = INDEPENDENT; ▲ = COLLABORATIVE)

Altered Level of Consciousness

RELATED FACTORS

Dehydration
Electrolyte imbalance

DEFINING CHARACTERISTICS

Change in orientation, verbal response, motor response, pupillary action
Agitation
Impaired judgment
Seizure activity
Positive Babinski's sign

EXPECTED OUTCOMES

Patient maintains a normal level of consciousness, as evidenced by alert, responsive state; normal motor responses; absence of seizures.

ONGOING ASSESSMENT

- Monitor LOC. Maintain neurologic flow sheet.
▲ Monitor vital signs, fluid volume, and electrolyte balance.
- Assess for potential for injury secondary to seizure activity.
- See also Consciousness, altered level of, p. 252.

THERAPEUTIC INTERVENTIONS

- Protect from injury caused by impaired neurologic function:
  Keep side rails up and bed in low position at all times.
  Maintain oral airway.
  Reorient patient to surroundings as needed (*patient may be unaware of past events and limitations*).
▲ Restore fluid volume. *As dehydration and hyperglycemia resolve, LOC improves.*

Altered Health Maintenance

RELATED FACTORS

Cognitive limitations
Lack of interest
Ineffective coping
Lack of/impaired motor skills

DEFINING CHARACTERISTICS

Demonstrated lack of knowledge
Reported inability to take responsibility
Lack of health-seeking behaviors

EXPECTED OUTCOMES

Patient verbalizes understanding of cause of HNKS and measures to prevent recurrence.

ONGOING ASSESSMENT

- Assess for predisposing factors and most current cause of HNKS.
- If patient is diabetic, assess level of knowledge and home care practices *to identify factors interfering with health maintenance.*

THERAPEUTIC INTERVENTIONS

- Describe HNKS, its cause and treatment.
- If the patient is diabetic, review effective self-care practices and introduce new information/skills as necessary. *Note:* For more information on diabetes teaching, see also Diabetes, p. 490.
- Inform patient of available resources.
- Assist patient in establishing appropriate contacts.

See also:
Ineffective Coping, p. 18.

By: Charlotte Niznik, RN, BSN, CDE
    Michele Knoll Puzas, RN,C, MHPE

Syndrome of inappropriate antidiuretic hormone (SIADH)

(DILUTIONAL HYPONATREMIA)

A syndrome characterized by the continued synthesis and release of antidiuretic hormone (ADH) unrelated to plasma osmolarity; water retention and dilutional hyponatremia occur. Potential causes include head trauma, brain tumor, subarachnoid hemorrhage, and systemic cancer.

NURSING DIAGNOSES	EXPECTED OUTCOMES AND NURSING INTERVENTIONS / *RATIONALE* (■ = INDEPENDENT; ▲ = COLLABORATIVE)

Fluid Volume Excess

RELATED FACTORS

Compromised endocrine regulatory mechanisms
Neurohypophysial dysfunction
Inappropriate ADH syndrome
Excessive fluid intake
Renal failure
Steroid therapy

DEFINING CHARACTERISTICS

Intake greatly exceeding output
Sudden weight gain
Cellular edema
Absence of peripheral edema
High specific gravity
Serum hyponatremia
Serum hypoosmolality
Urine hypernatremia
Urine hyperosmolality

EXPECTED OUTCOMES

Patient's fluid volume, serum sodium level, and osmolarity are within normal limits.

ONGOING ASSESSMENT

- Carefully monitor intake and output and urine specific gravity.
- Weigh daily. *A sudden weight gain of 2.2 lb can indicate retention of 1 L water. SIADH patients can retain 3-5 L.*
- Assess patient for signs of hyponatremia: apprehension, confusion, muscle twitches/cramps, convulsions, nausea/vomiting, anorexia, abdominal cramps.
- Assess for signs of cerebral edema: headache, decreased mental status, seizures, vomiting. *Gradual onset results in mild signs and symptoms. Rapid onset of SIADH may result in severe effects leading to seizures, coma, and death.*
- Check for fingerprint edema over sternum, reflecting cellular edema. *Water diffuses from hypoosmotic intravascular space to intracellular space.*
- Monitor for symptoms of increased ICP (e.g., slow bounding pulse, increased pulse pressure, irritability, lethargy, increased BP, vomiting).
- Monitor for symptoms of water intoxication (e.g., change in mentation, confusion, incoordination). *Brain cells are particularly sensitive to increased intracellular H_2O.*
- ▲ Monitor serum Na^+ level and serum osmolality, urine Na^+, and urine osmolality, specific gravity. *Serum Na level < 130 mEq/L and serum osmolality < 275 mOsm/L suggest SIADH. In addition, urine osmolality is usually above 900 mOsm/L with urine sodium inappropriately high compared to the low serum Na^+ level.*
- ▲ Assess serum K^+, Ca^+, BUN, and creatinine levels. *Hypokalemia and hypocalcemia are present with SIADH from dilutional effects. BUN and creatinine levels are usually normal.*
- ▲ Assess patient's medications for potential drugs that have been known to increase the risk of developing SIADH: *chloropropamide, clofibrate, carbamazepine, cyclophosphamide, isoproterenol, morphine, oxytocin, phenothiazines, thiazide diuretics, tricyclic antidepressants, vasopressin, vincristine.*

THERAPEUTIC INTERVENTIONS

- ▲ Restrict fluid intake to 1-1.5 L/day.
- Provide ice chips and frequent mouth care *to alleviate thirst.*
- ▲ Administer diuretic agents as prescribed (e.g., Lasix, *a potent loop diuretic that may help to diurese the excess water*).
- ▲ Administer hypertonic saline solution (3% NaCl) *as a sodium replacement.*
- Position patient with HOB flat, as patient tolerates, *to increase LA pressure through enhancing venous return to the heart and in turn decrease ADH release.*
- ▲ Administer medications (e.g., demeclocycline hydrochloride [Declomycin]), as prescribed, *to suppress the activity of ADH. Lithium carbonate (Lithonate) may also be used, but serious side effects are possible.*

High Risk for Impaired Thought Processes

RISK FACTOR

Severe hyponatremia

EXPECTED OUTCOMES

Patient's LOC and orientation remain normal or without further impairment, and injury is prevented.

ONGOING ASSESSMENT

- Monitor LOC and orientation.
- ▲ Assess serum Na^+ levels (normal: 135-145 mg/L). *Neurologic signs in patients with head injury may be caused by hyponatremia. When serum Na^+ level drops below 118, seizure activity may occur.*
- Monitor for disorientation, hostility, decreased deep tendon reflexes, drowsiness, lethargy, headache.

Continued.

Syndrome of inappropriate antidiuretic hormone (SIADH)—cont'd

NURSING DIAGNOSES	EXPECTED OUTCOMES AND NURSING INTERVENTIONS / *RATIONALE* (■ = INDEPENDENT; ▲ = COLLABORATIVE)
	THERAPEUTIC INTERVENTIONS ▲ Administer hypertonic saline solution as prescribed, *to replace Na$^+$*. ■ Reduce stimuli to maintain calm environment. ■ Explain reasons for altered thought processes to family/significant others. ■ Maintain bed in low position, side rails up. ▲ Maintain Posey vest/soft restraints as indicated *to prevent injury to patient during confused episodes.* ■ Provide assistance/supervision with ambulation.
High Risk for Diarrhea **RISK FACTORS** Fluid volume excess Hyponatremia	**EXPECTED OUTCOMES** Patient's normal bowel elimination is maintained. **ONGOING ASSESSMENT** ■ Assess usual bowel habits and patterns, including any deviations from normal. ■ Assess characteristics of stool (i.e., color, consistency, amount). *Diarrhea may signal water intoxication.* ■ Assess bowel sounds. *Hyperactive bowel sounds may occur with diarrhea.* ■ Observe and report skin condition. *Frequent diarrhea stools may lead to irritation and excoriation.* **THERAPEUTIC INTERVENTIONS** ■ Instruct patient to report episodes of diarrhea. ▲ Administer medications as prescribed; observe and report effectiveness.
Knowledge Deficit **RELATED FACTORS** New disease process Unfamiliarity with medications and treatments **DEFINING CHARACTERISTICS** Request for information Verbalized misconceptions	**EXPECTED OUTCOMES** Patient verbalizes understanding of SIADH and rationale for medications and treatments. **ONGOING ASSESSMENT** ■ Assess level of knowledge of SIADH, including understanding of medications and treatments. **THERAPEUTIC INTERVENTIONS** ■ Explain SIADH/treatments in simple, brief terms to patient/family/significant others. ■ Ask patient/family/significant others to verbalize explanations of SIADH/treatments (*will indicate misconceptions or misinterpretations*). ■ If SIADH is a chronic condition, teach patient the necessity of closely monitoring fluid balance and maintaining fluid balance at home: daily weights (same time of day with same amount of clothing), strict fluid intake restrictions, including instructions about fluid contained in foods. ■ Instruct patient on medications (e.g., democlocycline or lithium chloride) in treatment of chronic SIADH and the importance of close follow-up care because of potential side effects. ■ Instruct patient to wear a Medic-Alert listing SIADH and the treatment patient is using.

See also:
Fear/Anxiety, p. 5, 23.
Pain, p. 49.
Nutrition, p. 44.
Skin Integrity, p. 59.

By: Susan Galanes RN, MS, CCRN

Thyroidectomy

Surgical removal of the thyroid gland performed for benign or malignant tumor, hyperthyroidism, thyrotoxicosis, or thyroiditis, in patients with very large goiters, or for patients unable to be treated with radioiodine or thionamides.

NURSING DIAGNOSES	EXPECTED OUTCOMES AND NURSING INTERVENTIONS / *RATIONALE* (■ = INDEPENDENT; ▲ = COLLABORATIVE)

High Risk for Ineffective Breathing Pattern

RISK FACTORS

Hematoma
Laryngeal edema
Vocal cord paralysis
Tracheal collapse

EXPECTED OUTCOMES

Patient's breathing pattern is maintained as evidenced by eupnea, regular respiratory rate/pattern.

ONGOING ASSESSMENT

- Observe respiratory rate, rhythm.
- Note voice quality. *Edema may result in changes in voice quality such as hoarseness, for 3 to 4 days after surgery. However, paralysis of the vocal cord may result from recurrent laryngeal nerve damage. Be alert for this possibility, which could result in closure of the glottis and the need for emergency tracheostomy.*
- Observe neck for swelling or tightness, *which may be indicative of edema and/or internal bleeding/hematoma formation. Patient may complain of fullness at the incision site.*
- Examine wound for evidence of hematoma, oozing. Assess dressing both anterior and posterior and assess behind the neck for pooling. *Gravity tends to pull the drainage posterior.*
- Observe for presence of stridor.
- Assess for work of breathing, presence of dyspnea, or presence of intercostal rib retractions.

THERAPEUTIC INTERVENTIONS

- ▲ Keep tracheostomy tray at bedside. *If airway becomes totally occluded, an emergency tracheostomy is necessary.*
- Keep HOB elevated to 45 degrees *to limit the formation of edema at the surgical site.*
- ▲ Use ice collar as appropriate *to decrease edema formation.*
- Encourage deep breathing q1hr.
- Instruct patient to cough only as needed to clear secretions. *Coughing can irritate the incisional area, so is used only to clear secretions and not as a routine.*
- Suction as needed to clear secretions if patient unable to clear airway.
- Instruct the patient to minimize speaking *in order to rest the vocal cords and throat.*
- ▲ Administer humidified oxygen as needed.

High Risk for Injury: Hypocalcemia

RISK FACTORS

Inadvertent surgical removal of parathyroid glands or trauma to parathyroid glands (hypoparathyroidism)
Blood supply to parathyroids is damaged (usually temporary but may be permanent)

EXPECTED OUTCOMES

Patient's risk for injury is decreased as evidenced by serum calcium level in normal range, absence of signs of hypocalcemia.

ONGOING ASSESSMENT

- ▲ Monitor serum calcium level. *Hypocalcemia may occur postoperatively as a result of inadvertent surgical removal or trauma to the parathyroid glands.*
- Assess for presence of circumoral and peripheral (fingers and toes) paresthesia. Instruct patient to report development of these signs immediately.
- Observe for tremors in extremities and any seizure activity.
- Assess for lethargy, headache, and confusion, *which are additional signs of hypocalcemia.*
- Check for presence of Chvostek's sign *(tapping the cheek over the facial nerve; a positive sign results in a twitch of the lip or facial muscles that is indicative of tetany)* and for Trousseau's sign *(carpal spasm induced by inflation of the BP cuff 20 mm Hg above the patient's systolic BP for 3 mins; also indicative of tetany).*
- Assess for laryngeal stridor, *which may result from tetany.*
- ▲ Monitor serum K$^+$ and Mg$^+$ levels. *Hyperkalemia and hypomagnesemia potentiate cardiac and neuromuscular irritability in the presence of hypocalcemia.*

Continued.

NURSING DIAGNOSES	EXPECTED OUTCOMES AND NURSING INTERVENTIONS / *RATIONALE* (■ = INDEPENDENT; ▲ = COLLABORATIVE)

THERAPEUTIC INTERVENTIONS

▲ Maintain IV access and keep calcium gluconate at bedside *to treat dangerously low serum calcium levels. Normal level is 8.8-10.8 mg/100 ml.* Notify physician if Ca$^+$ < 8.0 mg/100 ml.

▲ Administer/monitor infusions of calcium gluconate; also administer oral calcium, vitamin D, as prescribed. Use caution in patients receiving digitalis preparations. *Ca$^+$ enhances the toxic effects of digitalis.*

· Institute seizure precautions as appropriate.

High Risk for Injury: Thyroid Storm, Hyperthyroidism

RISK FACTORS

Inadequate preoperative preparation (euthyroid state not achieved)

Increased release of thyroid hormone

EXPECTED OUTCOMES

Patient is free of thyroid storm as evidenced by vital signs within normal limits, no decrease in mentation.

ONGOING ASSESSMENT

· Assess vital signs for presence of increased pulse (up to 200 beats/min), dysrhythmias, elevated temperature, and increased BP. *Any rise in temperature and heart rate without a specific known cause should be considered thyroid storm. Thyroid storm can occur postoperatively as the result of increased hormone release from manipulation of the gland intraoperatively.*

· Assess for presence of heat intolerance.

· Assess for GI distress. *Elevated thyroid hormone level increases GI tract motility, possibly resulting in diarrhea.*

· Assess for restlessness and changes in LOC. *As thyroid storm progresses, LOC decreases and the patient may enter into a coma.*

THERAPEUTIC INTERVENTIONS

· Provide quiet environment (control noise level).

▲ Maintain IV infusion *for hydration, nutrition, electrolyte balance.*

▲ Maintain adequate nutritional intake, especially of protein, carbohydrates, vitamins; avoid caffeine. *Hypermetabolic states increase basal metabolic demand.*

▲ Promote rest; administer sedatives as prescribed; assist with ADLs.

▲ Protect patient from adverse effects of excess thyroid hormone:
  Lower temperature by keeping covers off; use hypothermia blanket; administer nonsalicylate antipyretic agents; give sponge bath.
  Administer antithyroid drug (iodine) *to inhibit thyroid hormone release,* β-receptor blocking agent (propranolol) *to decrease the cardiovascular and neuromuscular effects,* adrenal corticosteroid *to block thyroid hormone secretion.*

High Risk for Pain

RISK FACTORS

Postoperative surgical pain
Hematoma formation
Improper positioning, movement resulting in excessive strain on suture line
Wound infection

EXPECTED OUTCOMES

Patient's pain is relieved/prevented as evidenced by patient verbalization, relaxed appearance.

ONGOING ASSESSMENT

· Assess for presence/description of pain. *Pain may be routine postoperative surgical discomfort or may result from pressure of an expanding hematoma.*

· Assess patient's position. *Improper positioning can result in pain caused by tension to the surgical site.*

· Assess neck incision for approximated edges, redness, swelling, drainage, presence of staples/sutures.

THERAPEUTIC INTERVENTIONS

▲ Administer analgesics, throat sprays/lozenges as needed.

· Use relaxation techniques as appropriate. Administer cool liquids and soft foods when patient begins eating *to lessen the difficulty in swallowing.*

· Protect neck incision by instructing patient to:
  Avoid neck flexion/hyperextension. *Neck flexion (bending forward) would compress the trachea. Hyperextension would cause pulling/tension on the incision line.*
  Avoid rapid head movements.
  Support head with hands when rising *to prevent suture-line tension.*

NURSING DIAGNOSES	EXPECTED OUTCOMES AND NURSING INTERVENTIONS / *RATIONALE* (■ = INDEPENDENT; ▲ = COLLABORATIVE)

Knowledge Deficit

RELATED FACTOR

Lack of previous experience

DEFINING CHARACTERISTICS

Multiple questions
Lack of questions
Expressed need for further
  information

EXPECTED OUTCOMES

Patient/significant other verbalize understanding of postoperative care for thyroidectomy.

ONGOING ASSESSMENT

- Assess knowledge of thyroidectomy and postoperative care.

THERAPEUTIC INTERVENTIONS

- Instruct patient to inform physician if the following develop:
  Circumoral, peripheral paresthesia; tremors *that may result from low serum calcium level.*
  Signs of infection: excessive or continual drainage from incisional line, incision open and/or red
  Signs of hematoma/increase in edema formation: difficulty in breathing, alteration in voice, sensation of pressure, tightness, fullness in neck
  Signs/symptoms of thyroid storm
- Instruct patient to avoid abrupt head, neck movements.
- Instruct patient in dosage, schedule, desired effects, and side effects of medication(s) sent home. *If a total thyroidectomy was completed, the patient must develop a basic understanding of the long-term need for thyroid replacement therapy and the consequences of failure to take the medication.*
- ▲ Instruct in wound care:
  Incisional care: cleansing; dressings as needed for drainage; keeping wound dry, patient may shower when approved by physician.
  Scar appearance and resolution over time: use of scarves, high collars, etc., to camouflage the scar until normal healing occurs.
- Instruct patient in ROM exercises *for the neck to strengthen, return full ROM, and aid in the healing process.*
- Encourage regular exercise *to help stimulate the remaining thyroid gland to function.*
- Instruct the partial thyroidectomy patient in dietary measures.
  During hypothyroid period patient should reduce caloric intake *to prevent weight gain.*
  Avoid foods that contain thyroid-inhibiting substances (goitrogens): turnips, rutabagas, soybeans. *These foods inhibit the return of thyroid activity.*

See also:
Airway Clearance, p. 3.
Nutrition, p. 44.
Communication, p. 14.
High Risk for Infection,
  p. 40.

By: Susan Galanes, RN, MS, CCRN

11

Integumentary Care Plans

Burns

(SKIN LOSS—PARTIAL THICKNESS/FULL-THICKNESS)

Burns cause more than 10,000 deaths each year in the United States. Most commonly, burns occur in homes and result from careless smoking. Children and those over age 70 are at highest risk for death from burns. Survival rates for burned patients have improved dramatically, as a result of advances in ventilatory management, nutritional support, and use of early burn wound excision. Types of burns are flame, scald, electrical, and chemical. Full-thickness burns cannot reepithelialize and require grafting.

NURSING DIAGNOSES	EXPECTED OUTCOMES AND NURSING INTERVENTIONS / *RATIONALE* (■ = INDEPENDENT; ▲ = COLLABORATIVE)

Impaired Skin Integrity

RELATED FACTORS

Burns
Thrombocytopenia purpura
Anaphylaxis

DEFINING CHARACTERISTICS

Blanching of skin
Redness
Leathery appearance
Skin color changes: brown to black
Blistering, weeping skin
Pain/absence of pain
Skin loss

EXPECTED OUTCOMES

Patient's burns are accurately assessed; unburned skin remains intact.

ONGOING ASSESSMENT

- Assess percentage of body surface burned. Use age-appropriate body surface chart to determine total body surface area (TBSA) involved. *For adults, the "Rule of Nines" is commonly used to estimate extent of burn.*
- Identify and document location of burns.
- Assess depth of wounds: *epidermal:* painful, pink, not blistered; *partial thickness:* painful, red/pink, often blistered; *full-thickness:* anesthetic (*not painful because of destruction of nerves*), charred, gray, white.
- Note areas where skin is intact. *These areas must be cared for and preserved, as they may serve as graft donor sites later.*
- Assess degree of pain.
- Assess for adherent debris/hair.
- Take photos for later comparison.

THERAPEUTIC INTERVENTIONS

- Use burn pack or nonadherent sheeting *to prevent sticking.*
- ▲ Use hydrotherapy tub as prescribed *to aid in cleansing and loosening slough, exudate, eschar.*
- Prevent trauma to area (*can increase tissue destruction*).
- ▲ Apply topical bacteriostatic substances as prescribed. Use extreme care when removing topical ointments during dressing change *to prevent removal of granulating skin.*
- Elevate extremities, if possible, *to reduce swelling.*
- Dress wounds to prevent burn-to-burn contact; keep body, limbs in correct anatomical position *to decrease improper healing and contractures.*
- Do not bandage facial burns. Apply topical ointments and leave wound open to air.

High Risk for Infection

RISK FACTORS

Impaired skin integrity
Damage to respiratory mucosa
Presence of dead skin
Poor nutrition

EXPECTED OUTCOMES

Patient remains free of infection, as evidenced by normal temperature, normal WBC, healing wounds.

ONGOING ASSESSMENT

- Monitor temperature.
- Observe potential sites of infection: burn wounds; IV sites; indwelling catheter drainage (obtain culture of urine weekly); upper respiratory tract (obtain culture of sputum that looks abnormal).
- Assess odor and wound appearance at each dressing change; obtain culture of any suspicious drainage.
- Assess for eschar (*devitalized skin and tissue*), which should be excised as soon as possible; *eschar is an excellent medium for bacterial growth.*
- ▲ Obtain and monitor wound cultures.
- ▲ Monitor WBC for sudden changes. *Initial WBC may be low because of cell destruction and inflammatory response and should increase gradually. Sudden increase may indicate infection.*
- ▲ Monitor topical agent's effectiveness via wound cultures as prescribed.
- Observe for disorientation, fever, and ileus; *may indicate impending septic shock.*

Continued.

NURSING DIAGNOSES	EXPECTED OUTCOMES AND NURSING INTERVENTIONS / *RATIONALE* (■ = INDEPENDENT; ▲ = COLLABORATIVE)

THERAPEUTIC INTERVENTIONS

- Maintain aseptic technique; wear mask and sterile gloves for physical contact *to prevent iatrogenic contamination.*
- Keep work area clean *to reduce pathogens in environment.*
- Implement isolation precautions if needed; limit visitors.
- Trim hair around wound *to decrease contamination.*
- Leave blisters intact *to form natural barrier. Blisters that affect movement or that are infected require surgical drainage.*
- ▲ Apply topical antimicrobials as prescribed *(Silvadene, Sulfamylon, Betadine, silver nitrate, gentamicin).*
- ▲ Administer IV antibiotics, *which may be prescribed prophylactically but should be specific to cultured organism when identified.*
- Provide perineal care q2hr and after each void/bowel movement *to minimize pathogens.*
- ▲ Cover wounds with graft material or dressings as prescribed *to reduce fluid loss and protect wound from invasion by bacteria. Infection is the greatest threat to survival for the burned patient; covering wounds decreases the opportunity for contamination and therefore decreases risk of infection.*
    Xenografts: skin from another species, typically porcine (pig) skin; these are temporary grafts
    Homografts: skin from the another human, typically cadaver skin
    Amnion: can be used as graft material for 48 hr per application
    Synthetic dressings: temporary dressings to cover wounds; types include Op-Site, Tegaderm, artificial skin
    Autograft: healthy skin from elsewhere on the patient's body; grafting is carried out in an operating room

---

High Risk for Fluid Volume Deficit

RISK FACTORS

Inflammatory response to burn with protein and fluid shifts
Massive fluid shifting and circulating volume loss
Hemorrhage; stress ulcer (Curling's ulcer)

EXPECTED OUTCOMES

Patient maintains normal fluid volume, as evidenced by normal BP, urine output ≥ 30 ml/hr, normal heart rate.

ONGOING ASSESSMENT

- Assess for signs/symptoms of fluid volume deficit:
  Note: Restlessness, tachycardia, hypotension, thirst *(thirst is a sensitive indicator of fluid deficit and hemoconcentration),* skin pale and cool, oliguria *(urine output < 30 ml/hr indicates inadequate renal perfusion),* hypoxia *(as interstitial spaces fill with fluid, alveolar O_2 exchange is impaired). Fluid volume deficit is directly proportional to extent and depth of burn injury.*
- ▲ Monitor lab results for: alteration in acid-base balance, catabolism (outpouring of K^+ and nitrogen), altered electrolyte levels, (especially hyperkalemia).
- Monitor urine specific gravity q4hr. *Very concentrated urine (specific gravity > 1.020) indicates fluid volume deficit.*
- Monitor for signs of bleeding: melena stools; coffee-ground emesis via nasogastric tube. *Severe physiologic stress [e.g., burns] and/or mechanical ventilation can result in gastroduodenal ulceration and life-threatening hemorrhage 48-92 hr post event.*
- ▲ Evaluate Hb and Hct, *which will be affected by hemodilution or hemoconcentration.*
- Weigh patient daily, taking care to use the same scale and bedding.

THERAPEUTIC INTERVENTIONS

- ▲ Assist with IV and central line placements. *Multiple lines or a central line may be required for rapid fluid rescue to prevent circulatory collapse.*
- ▲ Administer IV fluids, electrolytes (Na^+, K^+), plasma or plasma expanders as prescribed. *Amount and rate are calculated on the basis of TBSA and depth of wound.*
- ▲ Administer albumin and diuretic (mannitol) as prescribed *to reverse fluid shifts and decrease edema.*
- ▲ Administer antacids/H_2-receptor antagonist prophylactically *to minimize potential for gastric bleeding (cimetidine, ranitidine). Duodenal stress ulcers are seen more frequently in children than in adults but develop later in the course of treatment and recovery (approximately 4 wk).*
- See also Fluid Volume Deficit, p. 25.
- See also GI Bleeding, p. 311.

NURSING DIAGNOSES	EXPECTED OUTCOMES AND NURSING INTERVENTIONS / *RATIONALE* (■ = INDEPENDENT; ▲ = COLLABORATIVE)

High Risk for Ineffective Breathing Pattern

RISK FACTORS

Burns to head/neck
Massive edema
Inhalation of smoke/heated air

EXPECTED OUTCOMES

Patient maintains an effective breathing pattern as evidenced by normal ABGs.

ONGOING ASSESSMENT

- Assess for presence of burns to face and neck.
- Assess for history/evidence of smoke inhalation.
- Assess for edema of the head, face, neck. *As fluid shift begins to occur, oral airway and trachea become constricted, decreasing ability of patient to breathe.*
- Assess respiratory rate, rhythm, and depth; assess breath sounds.
- Assess for dyspnea, shortness of breath, use of accessory muscles, cough, and presence of cyanosis.
- ▲ Monitor ABGs. *Combined effect of edema in airway and accumulation of interstitial fluid results in decreased alveolar ventilation.*
- ▲ Assess pulse oximetry readings.
- Observe for confusion, anxiety, and/or restlessness *(signs of hypoxia).*
- ▲ Assess hemodynamic pressures if available. *Increasing pulmonary pressures may indicate pulmonary edema.*
- ▲ Review chest radiograph results.

THERAPEUTIC INTERVENTIONS

- Raise head of bed and maintain good body alignment *for optimal breathing and lung expansion.*
- ▲ Maintain humidified oxygen delivery system.
- ▲ Provide chest physical therapy if burns are not to chest *to loosen secretions caused by stasis.*
- Encourage use of incentive spirometer *to prevent alveolar collapse.*
- ▲ Be prepared for intubation and mechanical ventilation. *When edema is severe, an artificial airway may be the only means of ventilating the severely burned patient.*
- Manage fear/anxiety, *which reduces coordinated efforts to breathe.* Coach the patient to take deep, slow breaths.

High Risk for Altered Peripheral Tissue Perfusion

RISK FACTORS

Blockage of microcirculation
Blood loss
Compartment syndrome
  (edema restricting circulation)

EXPECTED OUTCOMES

Patient maintains normal tissue perfusion to extremities, as evidenced by palpable pulses in all extremities, normal sensation in extremity.

ONGOING ASSESSMENT

- Check pulses of all extremities; use Doppler if necessary. *Weak, thready pulses may not be palpable. Also, feeling pulses through extremely edematous tissue or skin covered with eschar may be difficult.*
- Monitor vital signs (BP, heart rate, and respiratory rate) for abrupt changes. *Abrupt drop in BP, heart rate can indicate decreased return blood flow secondary to severe third spacing (movement of fluid into spaces normally without fluid), which impedes venous return.*
- Assess color and temperature of extremities. *Cool discolored extremities indicate compromised tissue perfusion. This situation, if untreated, can result in limb loss.*
- Check for pain, numbness, or swelling of extremities. *Circumferential burns with eschar are most likely to cause altered tissue perfusion to extremities, because as fluid shift occurs and eschar cannot stretch, pressure is exerted on tissue, vessels, and nerves.*

THERAPEUTIC INTERVENTIONS

- Maintain good alignment of extremities *to allow adequate blood flow without compression on arteries.*
- Notify physician immediately of noted alteration in perfusion.
- Perform passive range of motion (PROM) if needed *to increase circulation.*
- ▲ Prepare for and assist with fasciotomy/escharotomy *to relieve compression of nerves/ blood vessels. Burns of chest may cause restriction/constriction that decreases chest expansion; escharotomy will be needed to alleviate constricted movement.*

Continued.

Integumentary Care Plans

NURSING DIAGNOSES	EXPECTED OUTCOMES AND NURSING INTERVENTIONS / *RATIONALE* (■ = INDEPENDENT; ▲ = COLLABORATIVE)

High Risk for Altered Nutrition

RISK FACTORS

Prolonged interference in ability to ingest or digest food
Increased basal metabolic rate
Loss of protein from dermal wounds

EXPECTED OUTCOMES

Patient maintains an adequate nutritional intake, as evidenced by stable weight.

ONGOING ASSESSMENT

- Obtain base weight; weigh daily if possible, using same scale and linens.
- Measure I & O, including oral and IV intake.
- Closely monitor caloric intake. *Patient with major burns may require 40%-100% increase in calorie intake in order to keep up with hypermetabolic state and wound protein loss.*
- ▲ Monitor skin test results for cellular immunity. *Anergic patients (those unable to muster a cellular immune response) are seriously nutritionally depleted.*
- ▲ Monitor serum albumin levels. *Serum albumin gives an indication of protein reserve. Level <2.5 g/dl indicates serious protein depletion and is linked to morbidity and mortality.*
- Check for bowel sounds. *Paralytic ileus is common in first few days after burn. If paralytic ileus fails to resolve in 48 hr, peripheral or central parenteral nutrition must be considered.*
- ▲ Monitor nitrogen balance. *If nitrogen output is greater than nitrogen intake, patient is/ will become nutritionally depleted.*
- Determine environmental/situational factors that diminish appetite.

THERAPEUTIC INTERVENTIONS

- ▲ Consult dietitian to assist in meeting nutritional needs.
- Plan dressing changes or other unpleasant situations away from mealtime.
- Involve patient in selection of menu to extent possible.
- Provide tube feeding if patient is unable to maintain oral intake *and* gut is working. *The GI tract is the most efficacious route for absorption and use of nutrients and should be used if functional.*
- ▲ Provide total parenteral nutrition as prescribed. *High-calorie, high-protein diet is required to meet metabolic needs and allow healing.*

Pain

RELATED FACTOR

Injury

DEFINING CHARACTERISTICS

Complaints of pain
Increased restlessness
Alterations in sleep pattern
Irritability
Facial grimaces
Guarding

EXPECTED OUTCOMES

Patient verbalizes relief of pain or ability to tolerate pain.

ONGOING ASSESSMENT

- Assess location, quality, and severity of pain.
- Assess factors that may contribute to an increased perception of pain (e.g., anxiety, fear).
- Assess vital signs. *Increasing pain can cause transient increases in respiratory and cardiac rates and BP.*
- Evaluate and document effectiveness of chosen pain control methods. *Changing effectiveness is expected. First- and second-degree burns are very painful; pain will decrease over time and healing. Third-degree burns do not cause pain because of nerve destruction, but as nerves regenerate, pain will increase.*

THERAPEUTIC INTERVENTIONS

- ▲ Administer sedatives and analgesics prescribed for pain.
- ▲ Consider patient-controlled analgesia use *to increase patient's sense of control over pain.*
- ▲ Apply topical anesthetics as prescribed.
- Avoid pressure on injured tissues; use bed span.
- Position patient *to promote comfort.*
- Alleviate all unnecessary stressors or discomfort sources.
- Allay fears and anxiety, *which may intensify perception of pain.*
- Turn *to help relieve pressure points;* obtain pressure-relieving mattress or beds as needed.
- ▲ Premedicate for dressing changes; allow sufficient time for medication to take effect.
- ▲ Saturate dressings with sterile normal saline solution before removal. *This will ease dressing removal by loosening adherents and decreasing pain.*
- Use distraction/relaxation techniques as indicated.

NURSING DIAGNOSES	EXPECTED OUTCOMES AND NURSING INTERVENTIONS / *RATIONALE* (■ = INDEPENDENT; ▲ = COLLABORATIVE)

High Risk for Impaired Home Maintenance Management

RISK FACTORS

Altered body image, self-concept related to deformity, disfigurement, or change in role capabilities

Need for long-term rehabilitation, follow-up care

Need for assistance with daily care

Unavailability/exhaustion of family members

EXPECTED OUTCOMES

Patient/significant other verbalize ability to care for wound, mobilize resources, get follow-up care, report signs of complication.

ONGOING ASSESSMENT

- Assess need for ongoing wound/graft site care. *Grafted skin is very delicate and at continued risk of breakdown and infection.*
- ▲ Assess need for continued rehabilitation (occupational therapy [OT], physical therapy [PT], psychosocial support). *A variety of factors (e.g., inability to cope with body image changes, guilt about injury, cause of fire/accident, need for further reconstructive surgery, use of scar prevention garments) may require care for months beyond hospital discharge.*
- Assess patient's perceived ability to care for self after discharge.
- Assess resources (environmental and human) in the home that can be tapped for assistance.

THERAPEUTIC INTERVENTIONS

- ▲ Involve social worker early in course of hospitalization *to begin early discharge planning.*
- Instruct patient/significant other in wound care of graft sites and donor sites: continue to use aseptic technique until wound is completely healed; cover open wounds with gauze; keep wounds clean and moisturized with a lanolin-based cream *to prevent drying and cracking;* avoid sun exposure of newly grafted skin.
- Instruct patient in care and use of scar-prevention garments, usually worn at all times, removed for bathing and wound care, up to 18 mo after injury. *These may need to be replaced frequently to maintain elasticity sufficient for purpose.*
- Instruct patient to report any of the following: signs/symptoms of wound infection (redness, swelling, pain, unusual drainage); limitation of movement, which can result from delayed contracture formation; inability to cope with disfigurement, role change (*depression is common after discharge, when the patient reenters society*).
- Encourage patient to maintain follow-up schedule with MD, RN, PT, OT, social services.
- Discuss fire safety/burn prevention, *taking care not to seem judgmental or to place blame/increase guilt, regardless of nature/cause of injury.*

See also:
Anxiety, p. 5.
Gas Exchange, Impaired, p. 27.
Body Image Disturbance, p. 7.

By: Linda Marie St. Julien, RN, MS

Plastic surgery for pressure ulcers

(SKIN GRAFTS, FLAP, FLAP CLOSURE, MYOCUTANEOUS FLAP)

Pressure ulcers that lack an epithelial base for healing frequently require closure by plastic surgery. Ulcers that may heal over extended periods without surgical intervention may be electively closed to hasten the rehabilitation time, or to protect the vulnerable patient from infection resulting from a long-term open wound. Skin, subcutaneous tissue, fascia, and muscle may all be relocated through a variety of procedures to achieve closure of pressure ulcers. Partial or full-thickness skin grafts may be used to close pressure ulcers, but more frequently, because of the depth of the wound and the poor circulation to the area, flap closures are performed. Flaps are categorized by either the source of blood supply or the area from which they are taken. Myocutaneous flaps are frequently performed to achieve pressure ulcer closure.

NURSING DIAGNOSES	EXPECTED OUTCOMES AND NURSING INTERVENTIONS / *RATIONALE* (■ = INDEPENDENT; ▲ = COLLABORATIVE)

High Risk for Altered Tissue Perfusion

RISK FACTORS
Skin graft
Flap closure
Anatomic location
Poor circulation
Edema

EXPECTED OUTCOMES

Patient maintains adequate tissue perfusion to graft or flap, as evidenced by normal color and warmth of graft/flap, intact suture lines.

ONGOING ASSESSMENT

- Assess skin graft or flap for the following signs of adequate circulation: color, warmth, capillary refill. *Grafts and flaps that are adequately perfused are similar in color to other skin on the patient's body. The graft or flap should feel warm to touch and should have brisk capillary refill.*
- Note anatomic area where graft or flap has been performed. *Areas where pressure occurs as patient lies in bed or sits in a chair are at risk for impaired perfusion as skin capillaries are compressed.*
- Assess for history of poor circulation, peripheral vascular disease, decreased cardiac output, or shock. *Any of these situations places the patient at risk for decreased circulation to the skin. The most dramatic complication is loss of viability of the graft/flap.*
- Assess for edema around the skin graft or flap. *Excess edema can impede venous return and compromise arterial perfusion to the area.*
- Assess patency of and output from surgically placed drains. *These drains remove serous fluid from the operative site; up to 100 cc/day for the first 72 hr is normal.*
- Assess intactness of suture lines. *Individualized prescription for wound care/dressing change is based on surgeon's preference. Care should be taken to protect suture lines from disruption.*

THERAPEUTIC INTERVENTIONS

- Position the patient off the skin graft or flap *to eliminate external pressure, which can compromise circulation to the surgical site.*
- Ensure that dressings are secure but not constrictive.
- ▲ Place the patient on an air-fluidized bed. *Air-fluidized therapy beds support the patient's weight and distribute pressure so that pressure at any point on the body is less than capillary closing pressure (usually considered to be about 32 mm Hg). The less pressure on skin grafts or flaps, the better chance the graft or flap has of remaining adequately perfused.*
- Report any signs of inadequate perfusion (discoloration, separation of suture lines, loss of warmth).

High Risk for Infection

RISK FACTORS
Surgical graft or flap
Poor nutritional status
Proximity of graft or flap to perineum
Collection of fluid beneath graft or flap
Open donor site (grafts)

EXPECTED OUTCOMES

Patient remains free of infection as evidenced by healing graft or flap free of redness, swelling, purulent drainage, normal temperature.

ONGOING ASSESSMENT

- Assess graft or flap for signs of local infection: redness, swelling, increased pain.
- Assess graft donor site and area from which flap was taken (usually sutured closed) for redness, swelling, and pain.

NURSING DIAGNOSES	EXPECTED OUTCOMES AND NURSING INTERVENTIONS / *RATIONALE* (■ = INDEPENDENT; ▲ = COLLABORATIVE)

ONGOING ASSESSMENT—cont'd

- Assess grafts or flap suture lines for drainage, color of tissue, and odor. *Small amounts of exudate that is clear to straw-colored is normal. Purulent green or yellow drainage typically indicates an infection, as does foul-smelling drainage.*
- Note any separation of suture line(s).
- ▲ Monitor wound cultures, if available.
- ▲ Monitor WBC. *Elevated WBC is a sign of infection.*
- ▲ Assess nutritional status. *Patients who are seriously nutritionally depleted (e.g., serum albumin level <2.5 mg/dl) are at risk for developing infection and are unable to heal.*
- Assess for urinary and/or fecal incontinence. *Closure of sacral wounds, because of their proximity to the perineum, are at highest risk for infection caused by urine and/or fecal contamination.*
- Monitor temperature. *Fever is an indication of infection.*

THERAPEUTIC INTERVENTIONS

- ▲ Provide local wound care as prescribed. *Xeroform, a nonadherent bismuth-saturated dressing, is often used for dressing grafts, flaps, and donor sites because it does not stick to the wound and has antimicrobial properties. It may be changed routinely or left in place to dry up and fall off.*
- Provide rigorous perineal hygiene after each episode of incontinence to *minimize pathogens in the sacral area.*
- ▲ Consult the dietician for assistance with a high-calorie, high-protein diet. *These patients, because of overall condition, frequently require enteral or parenteral nutrition in order to meet nutritional needs for healing.*
- ▲ Provide aggressive nutritional therapy.
- ▲ Administer antibiotics as prescribed.

High Risk for Impaired Home Maintenance Management

RISK FACTORS

Possible extended healing time

Lack of previous similar experience

Possible need for special equipment

EXPECTED OUTCOMES

Patient/family verbalize understanding of wound care, and pressure reduction care.
Patient is not readmitted with new pressure ulcers.

ONGOING ASSESSMENT

- Assess patient's/significant other's understanding of long-term nature of wound healing and delicacy of grafted/flapped areas. *Because grafts/flaps are frequently done in the sacral area, sitting is limited to brief intervals even after the patient is discharged; the area remains at high risk for breakdown.*
- Assess knowledge of and ability to provide local wound care. *Usually by the time of discharge, suture lines and donor sites have healed and require little more than pressure relief, cleaning, and moisturization.*
- Assess for availability of pressure reduction or pressure relief surface. *Patients may take thick, dense foam mattresses home from the hospital to place on own bed. Rental provision of low-air loss (e.g., Flexicare, Kinair) beds and air-fluidized therapy (e.g., Clinitron, Skytron, FluidAir) beds may be arranged but often pose financial difficulty because few payor sources will cover the cost of these pressure relief beds in the home. Patients who use wheelchairs must have adequate pressure reduction/relief surfaces.*
- Assess patient's understanding of and ability to shift position frequently to *relieve pressure and allow adequate circulation to grafted/flapped area(s).*
- Assess understanding of the prevention of further pressure ulcer development. *Patients who are incapable of independent movement will need frequent repositioning in order to reduce risk for breakdown in those areas that are intact.*
- Assess understanding of and ability to provide high-calorie, high-protein diet throughout the course of wound healing. *Patients may require enteral feeding (via G-tube, nasogastric feeding tubes, or the oral route), which will require knowledge of preparation, use of special equipment (e.g., feeding pumps, administration sets).*
- Assess understanding of the relationship between incontinence and further skin breakdown/complications of healing. *Managing incontinence may pose the most difficult aspect of home management and is frequently the reason decisions for nursing home placement are made.*

Continued.

NURSING DIAGNOSES	EXPECTED OUTCOMES AND NURSING INTERVENTIONS / *RATIONALE* (■ = INDEPENDENT; ▲ = COLLABORATIVE)

THERAPEUTIC INTERVENTIONS

▲ Involve social worker early in course of hospitalization *to plan for the details of discharge or to help patient/family determine whether discharge to the home is feasible or whether placement in an extended care facility is more realistic.*

▪ Teach patient/family importance of pressure reduction/relief:

Use of specialty surface: *If provision of specialty beds is a problem because of reimbursement issues, purchase of a waterbed may be a reasonable alternative.*

Use of pressure reduction/relief surface where patient sits.

Turning schedule that does not compromise other body areas.

▲ Involve dietitian to teach patient/family how to plan high-calorie, high-protein meals, or how to supplement regular meals with dietary supplements.

▪ Teach patient/family how to manage incontinence:

Use of external catheters

Intermittent self-catheterization

Use of underpads/linen protectors. *Reusable products made of cloth with a waterproof lining are better for the patient's skin and are more economical but require laundering.*

Use of moisture barrier ointments *to protect intact skin from excoriation*

Care of indwelling catheters if no other option is feasible

▲ Consider/discuss with patient/family the need for in-home nursing care, homemaker services *to provide all or part of the patient's care.*

See also:
Nutrition, Less Than Body Requirement, p. 44.
Body Image Disturbance, p. 7.
Pain, p. 49.

By: Audrey Klopp, RN, PhD, ET
Mary McCarthy, RN, MSN, C.S.

Pressure ulcers (impaired skin integrity)

(PRESSURE SORES, DECUBITUS ULCERS, BEDSORES)

Pressure ulcers are defined as any lesion caused by unrelieved pressure that results in damage to underlying tissue. Pressure ulcers usually occur over bony prominences according to the following distribution: trunk 45%, upper body 20%, and lower extremities 35%. Pressure ulcers are usually staged to classify the degree of tissue damage observed (AHCPR, 1992). Pressure ulcers stage I through III can heal with aggressive local wound treatment and proper nutritional support; stage IV pressure ulcers often require surgical intervention (e.g., flap closure, plastic surgery). Pressure ulcers affect persons, regardless of age, who are immobile, are malnourished, or have adverse environmental conditions (e.g., incontinence, decreased mental status).

NURSING DIAGNOSES	EXPECTED OUTCOMES AND NURSING INTERVENTIONS / *RATIONALE* (■ = INDEPENDENT; ▲ = COLLABORATIVE)

Impaired Skin Integrity

RELATED FACTORS

Extremes of age
Immobility
Poor nutrition
Mechanical forces (friction, shear, pressure)
Pronounced bony prominences
Poor circulation
Altered sensation
Incontinence
Environmental moisture
Radiation
Hyperthermia/hypothermia
AIDS
Chronic disease state

DEFINING CHARACTERISTICS

Stage I:
 Redness that does not resolve within 30 min of relief of pressure
 Epidermis intact
Stage II:
 Blisters (either intact or broken)
 Partial thickness skin loss (epidermis and/or dermis)
Stage III:
 Open lesion involving dermis and subcutaneous tissue
 May have adherent necrotic tissue
 Drainage usually present
 Typically presents as crater
 Undermining is common
Stage IV:
 Open lesion involving muscle, bone, joint, and/or body cavity
 Usually has adherent necrotic material (slough)
 Drainage is common
 Infection is common

EXPECTED OUTCOMES

Patient receives stage-appropriate wound care, experiences pressure reduction, and has controlled risk factors for prevention of additional ulcers.
Patient experiences healing in pressure ulcers.

ONGOING ASSESSMENT

- Determine age. *Elderly patients' skin is less elastic and has less moisture, making for higher risk of skin impairment.*
- Assess general condition of skin. *Healthy skin varies from individual to individual but should have good turgor (an indication of moisture), feel warm and dry to the touch, be free of impairment (scratches, bruises, excoriation, rashes), and have quick capillary refill (<6 sec).*
- Specifically assess skin over bony prominences (sacrum, trochanters, scapulae, elbows, heels, inner and outer maleous, inner and outer knees, back of head). *Areas where skin is stretched tautly over bony prominences are at highest risk for breakdown because the possibility of ischemia to the skin is high as a result of compression of skin capillaries between a hard surface (mattress, chair, operating room table) and the bone.*
- Assess patient's awareness of the sensation of pressure. *Normally, individuals shift their weight off pressure areas every few minutes; this occurs more or less automatically, even during sleep. Patients with decreased sensation are unaware of unpleasant stimuli (pressure) and do not shift weight.*
- Assess ability to move (shift weight while sitting, turn over in bed, move from bed to chair). *Immobility is the major risk factor in skin breakdown.*
- ▲ Assess patient's nutritional status, including weight, weight loss, and serum albumin levels. *Albumin level <2.5 g/dl is a grave sign, indicating severe protein depletion.*
- Assess for history of radiation therapy. *Irradiated skin becomes thin and friable and is at higher risk for breakdown.*
- Assess for history/presence of AIDS. *Early manifestations of HIV-related diseases may include skin lesions (e.g., Kaposi's sarcoma); additionally, because of their immunoincompetence, patients with AIDS frequently have skin breakdown.*
- Assess for fecal and/or urinary incontinence. *The urea in urine turns into ammonia within minutes and is caustic to the skin. Stool may contain enzymes that cause skin breakdown. Diapers and incontinence pads with plastic liners trap moisture and hasten breakdown.*
- Assess for environmental moisture (wound drainage, high humidity), *which may contribute to skin maceration.*
- Assess surface that patient spends majority of time on (mattress for bedridden patient, cushion for persons in wheelchairs). *Patients who spend the majority of time on one surface need a pressure reduction or pressure relief device to lessen the risk for breakdown.*
- Assess amount of shear (*pressure exerted laterally*) and friction (*rubbing*) on patient's skin. *A common cause of shear is elevating the head of the patient's bed, causing the body's weight to shift downward onto the patient's sacrum. Common causes of friction include the patient's rubbing heels/elbows against bed linen and moving the patient up in bed without the use of a lift sheet.*
- Reassess skin at least q24hr, and whenever the patient's condition or treatment plan results in an increased number of risk factors. *The incidence of skin breakdown is directly related to the number of risk factors present.*

Continued.

NURSING DIAGNOSES	EXPECTED OUTCOMES AND NURSING INTERVENTIONS / *RATIONALE* (■ = INDEPENDENT; ▲ = COLLABORATIVE)

ONGOING ASSESSMENT—cont'd

- Assess for history of preexisting chronic diseases (e.g., diabetes, malignancy, AIDS, peripheral and/or cardiovascular disease). *Patients with chronic diseases typically manifest multiple risk factors (see above) that predispose them to pressure ulceration; the number of risk factors present is directly related to the incidence of pressure ulceration.*
- Stage pressure ulcers:
    Stage I: redness that does not resolve within 30 min of relief of pressure; epidermis intact
    Stage II: blisters (either intact or broken), partial thickness skin loss (epidermis and/or dermis)
    Stage III: open lesion involving dermis and subcutaneous tissue; may have necrotic tissue adherent; drainage usually present; typically presents as crater; undermining is common
    Stage IV: open lesion involving muscle, bone, joint, and/or body cavity; usually has adherent necrotic material (slough); drainage common; infection common;
- Describe the characteristics of the ulcer(s) present:
    Location: Note exact location of pressure ulcer; examine all bony prominences.
    Diameter: Use measuring guide to determine diameter.
    Depth: Use a cotton-tipped applicator to determine depth.
    Undermining: Lateral ulcer not visible at surface
- Describe the condition of the wound/wound bed:
    Color: Color of tissue is an indication of tissue viability and oxygenation
    Odor: Odor may arise from infection present in the wound; it may also arise from necrotic tissue; some local wound care products may create/intensify odors and should be distinguished from wound/exudate odors
    Presence of necrotic tissue: Necrotic tissue is tissue that is dead and eventually must be removed before healing can take place. Necrotic tissue exhibits a wide range of appearance: thin, white, shiny, brown, tough, leathery, black, hard.
    Visibility of bone, muscle, or joints: In stage IV pressure, these structures may be apparent at the base of the ulcer. Note: Wounds may demonstrate multiple stages/ characteristics in a single wound (i.e., healthy tissue with granulation may be present along with necrotic tissue).
- Describe exudate/wound drainage:
    Presence of exudate: Exudate is a normal part of wound physiology and must be differentiated from pus, which is an indication of infection. Exudate may contain serum, blood, and white blood cells and may appear clear, cloudy, or blood-tinged.
    Amount of exudate: Amount may vary from a few cubic centimeters, which are easily managed with dressings, to copious amounts not easily managed. Drainage is considered "excess" when dressing changes are needed more often that q6hr.
- Assess the condition of surrounding tissue. *Surrounding tissue may be healthy or may have various degrees of impairment. Healthy tissue is necessary for use of local wound care products requiring adhesion to the skin. Presence of healthy tissue demarcates the boundaries of the pressure ulcer.*

THERAPEUTIC INTERVENTIONS

- Assure that all preventative measures necessary are in place (see also High risk for impaired skin integrity, p. 59), including appropriate pressure reduction or pressure relief surface, attention to nutritional needs, management of incontinence.
- ▲ Provide local wound care as follows:
    Stage I: The goal is to prevent further damage and shearing away of the epidermis.
        Apply a flexible hydrocolloid dressing (e.g., Duoderm, Sween-Appeal) or a vapor-permeable membrane dressing (e.g., Op-Site, Tegaderm) *to prevent friction and shear*
                                    or
        Apply vitamin-enriched emollient to skin every shift *to moisturize skin*
                                    or
        Apply topical vasodilator (e.g., Proderm, Granulex) *to increase circulation to skin*
    Stage II: The goal is to prevent further damage, protect from infection, and promote granulation and reepithelialization.
        Apply hydrocolloid dressing or vapor-permeable membrane dressing *to keep wound exudate at the site of the wound to promote moist wound healing.*

NURSING DIAGNOSES	EXPECTED OUTCOMES AND NURSING INTERVENTIONS / *RATIONALE* (■ = INDEPENDENT; ▲ = COLLABORATIVE)

THERAPEUTIC INTERVENTIONS—cont'd

Stage III: Accomplish débridement if necessary *to remove necrotic tissue* by using one of the following methods:

Consult plastic surgeon *to perform sharp débridement (surgical removal of eschar).*

or

Apply enzymatic débriding agent (e.g., Travase, Elase, Santyl) according to prescription. *These agents work by selectively digesting the collagen portion of the necrotic tissue; care should be taken to prevent damage to surrounding healthy tissue.*

or

Apply hydrocolloid **if no infection is present,** *to loosen eschar by autolysis.*

or

Apply wet-to-dry saline solution dressing *to loosen eschar.*

or

Apply dressings (Silvadene, Sulfamylon) *to loosen eschar and combat potential infection.*

or

Pack crater with absorption product (e.g., Bard Absorption).

or

Fill crater with gel (e.g., Carrington Gel) *to aid in débridement and maintenance of a moist wound bed.*

If a Stage III pressure ulcer is clean (as after débridement), carry out measures to promote moist wound healing:

Continue wet-to-dry dressings.

or

Pack with hydrocolloid granules, covered with hydrocolloid wafer.

or

Dress wound with calcium algienate, *which assists in healing through calcium-sodium ion exchange at the wound bed.*

Stage IV: The goal is to clean the ulcer bed and prepare it for skin and/or muscle flap closure. Stage IV ulcers have no base of epithelium and therefore cannot close without surgical intervention.

Apply any of the clean stage III recommended treatments, with the following modifications:

Granules should not be used, *because it may be impossible to retrieve all the granules placed in the wound as a result of tracting*

Dressings should use roller gauze (e.g., Kerlix) *to facilitate complete and easy removal of all dressing material*

High Risk for Infection

RISK FACTORS

Open pressure ulcer
Poor nutritional status
Proximity of sacral wounds to perineum

EXPECTED OUTCOMES

Patient remains free of local or systemic infection, as evidenced by absence of copious, foul-smelling wound exudate; normal body temperature.

ONGOING ASSESSMENT

■ Assess pressure ulcers for drainage, color of tissue, and odor. *All wounds produce exudate; the presence of exudate that is clear to straw-colored is normal. Purulent green or yellow drainage in large amounts typically indicates an infection, as does foul-smelling drainage. Infected tissue usually has a gray-yellow appearance without evidence of pink granulation tissue.*

▲ Monitor wound cultures, if available. *All pressure ulcers are colonized (i.e., will culture out bacteria, because skin normally has flora that will be found in an open skin lesion. All pressure ulcers are not, however, infected. Infection is present when there is copious foul-smelling drainage, and the patient has other symptoms of infection (fever, increased pain).*

· Assess patient for unexplained sepsis. *Pressure ulcers are frequently overlooked as the causative source of systemic infection (sepsis). When septic work up is done, the pressure ulcer must be considered a possible cause.*

▲ Assess nutritional status. *Patients who are seriously nutritionally depleted (e.g., serum albumin < 2.5 mg/dl) are at risk for developing infection produced by a pressure sore. Additionally, patients with pressure sores lose tremendous amounts of protein in wound exudate and may require 4000 cal/day or more in order to remain anabolic.*

· Assess for urinary and/or fecal incontinence. *Sacral wounds, because of their proximity to the perineum, are at highest risk for infection caused by urine and/or fecal contamination. It is sometimes difficult to isolate the wound from the perineal area.*

· Monitor temperature. *Fever is an indication of infection.*

Continued.

Integumentary Care Plans

NURSING DIAGNOSES	EXPECTED OUTCOMES AND NURSING INTERVENTIONS / *RATIONALE* (■ = INDEPENDENT; ▲ = COLLABORATIVE)

THERAPEUTIC INTERVENTIONS

▲ Provide local wound care as prescribed (see the section Impaired skin integrity).

■ Provide rigorous perineal hygiene after each episode of incontinence *to minimize pathogens in the area of sacral pressure ulcers.*

▲ Consult the dietician for assistance with a high-calorie, high-protein diet. *These patients, because of overall condition, frequently require enteral or parenteral nutrition in order to meet nutritional needs.*

▲ Provide aggressive nutritional therapy.

▲ Administer antibiotics as prescribed.

▲ Provide hydrotherapy as prescribed *to achieve wound cleansing and to promote circulation.*

High Risk for Impaired Home Maintenance Management

RISK FACTORS

Need for long-term pressure ulcer management

Lack of previous similar experience

Possible need for special equipment

EXPECTED OUTCOMES

Patient/family verbalize understanding of the following aspects of home care: pressure relief, wound care, nutrition, incontinence management

ONGOING ASSESSMENT

■ Assess patient's/significant other's understanding of long-term nature of wound healing of pressure ulcers. *Pressure ulcers may take weeks to months to heal, even under ideal circumstances. Wounds heal from the base of the ulcer up, and from the edges of the ulcer toward the center.*

■ Assess patient's/family's knowledge of and ability to provide local wound care. *Patients are no longer kept hospitalized until pressure ulcers have healed. This process and the need for local wound care may continue for weeks to months.*

■ Assess for availability of pressure reduction or pressure relief surface. *Patients may take thick, dense foam mattresses home from the hospital to place on their own bed. Rental provision of low-air loss (e.g., Flexicare, Kinair) beds and air-fluidized therapy (e.g., Clinitron, Skytron, FluidAir) beds may be arranged but often pose financial difficulty because few payor sources will cover the cost of these beds in the home.*

■ Assess understanding of and ability to provide high-calorie, high-protein diet throughout the course of wound healing. *Patients may require enteral feeding (via G-tube, nasogastric feeding tubes, or the oral route), which will require knowledge of preparation, use of special equipment (e.g., feeding pumps, administration sets).*

■ Assess patient's/family's understanding of the relationship between incontinence and further skin breakdown/complications of healing. *Managing incontinence may be the most difficult aspect of home management and is frequently the reason decisions for nursing home placement are made.*

■ Assess patient's/family's understanding of the prevention of further pressure ulcer development. *Patients who are incapable of independent movement will need frequent repositioning in order to reduce risk for breakdown in those areas that are intact.*

THERAPEUTIC INTERVENTIONS

▲ Involve social worker early in course of hospitalization *to plan for the details of discharge or to help patient/family determine whether discharge to the home is feasible or placement in an extended care facility is more realistic. Because many patients with pressure ulcers are elderly, it is often an elderly spouse who is available to provide care; as a result of the intensive nursing care needs of these patients, discharge to home is often unrealistic.*

■ Teach patient/family importance of pressure reduction/relief:
  Use of specialty surface. *If provision of specialty beds is a problem because of reimbursement issues, a waterbed may be a reasonable alternative.*
  Use of pressure reduction/relief surface where patient sits.
  Turning schedule that does not compromise other body areas.

▲ Include dietitian in teaching patient/family how to plan high-calorie, high-protein meals, or how to supplement regular meals with dietary supplements.

NURSING DIAGNOSES	EXPECTED OUTCOMES AND NURSING INTERVENTIONS / *RATIONALE* (■ = INDEPENDENT; ▲ = COLLABORATIVE)

THERAPEUTIC INTERVENTIONS—cont'd

- Teach patient/family how to manage incontinence:
  - Use of external catheters.
  - Use of underpads/linen protectors. *Reusable products made of cloth with a waterproof lining are better for the patient's skin and are more economical but require laundering.*
  - Use of moisture barrier ointments *to protect intact skin from excoriation.*
  - Care of indwelling catheters if no other option is feasible.
- Teach patient/family local wound care and provide opportunity for return demonstration.
- Teach patient/family to report the following signs indicating wound infection: purulent drainage, odor, fever, malaise.
- Consider/discuss with patient/family the need for in-home nursing care or homemaker services *to provide all or part of the patient's care.*
- Consider/discuss with patient/family the possible need for respite care. *Long-term responsibility for patient care in the home is very taxing; those providing the care may need help to understand that their own needs for relaxation are essential to the maintenance of health and should not be viewed as "shirking responsibility."*

See also:
Nutrition, Less Than Body Requirements, p. 44.
Enteral Tube Feeding, p. 303.
Body Image, p. 7.
High Risk for Individual/Family Coping, p. 17, 18.
Care-Giver Role Strain, p. 13.

By: Audrey Klopp, RN, PhD, ET
Mary McCarthy, RN, MSN, CS

Scleroderma

(PROGRESSIVE SYSTEMIC SCLEROSIS [PSS])

A chronic, inflammatory disease characterized by fibrous and degenerative changes in the skin, digital arteries, and internal organs, such as the esophagus, intestinal tract, lungs, kidneys, and heart. It can be a systemic disease or limited to a skin disease. The cause is unknown.

NURSING DIAGNOSES	EXPECTED OUTCOMES AND NURSING INTERVENTIONS / *RATIONALE* (■ = INDEPENDENT; ▲ = COLLABORATIVE)

Altered Skin Integrity

RELATED FACTORS
Inflammation
Vasoconstriction
Calcium deposition
Fibrosis

DEFINING CHARACTERISTICS
Change in skin texture, redness, swelling, tenderness, skin breakdown.
Lack of skin elasticity in affected areas, ulceration, drainage, pain.

EXPECTED OUTCOMES

The patient maintains optimal skin integrity within limits of disease, as evidenced by intact skin.

ONGOING ASSESSMENT

- Assess skin, noting color, moisture, texture, temperature; note redness, swelling, or tenderness. *In limited scleroderma skin changes occur primarily in the fingers. In contrast, in diffuse scleroderma skin changes can involve the hands and extend throughout the body.*
- Assess skin for any breaks in integrity. Note presence of ulcers, size, any drainage, and amount of necrotic tissue.
- Solicit patient's description of pain. *Usually expressed as itching or burning secondary to inflammation.*
- Assess interference with life-style. *Patients may develop contractures from their tight skin.*
- Assess interference with ADLs/lifestyle.

Continued.

NURSING DIAGNOSES	EXPECTED OUTCOMES AND NURSING INTERVENTIONS / *RATIONALE* (■ = INDEPENDENT; ▲ = COLLABORATIVE)

THERAPEUTIC INTERVENTIONS

- Provide prophylactic pressure-relieving devices (e.g., special mattresses, elbow pads).
- Maintain functional body alignment.
- Clean, dry, and moisturize intact skin with warm (not hot) water, especially over bony prominences; use unscented lotion (e.g., Eucerin or unscented Lubriderm). *Scented lotions contain alcohol, which dries skin.*
- Encourage adequate nutrition and hydration. *Hydration keeps the skin moist "from within."*
- Use nonaffected skin areas for injections and infusion of IV solution. *Affected skin is difficult to penetrate; once penetrated, it allows further skin damage.*
- Assist with ADLs as needed.
- Instruct patient to avoid direct contact with harsh chemicals (e.g., household cleaners, detergents), and to wear cotton-lined latex gloves when using them.

Altered Peripheral Tissue Perfusion

RELATED FACTORS

Raynaud's phenomenon: vasospasm, structural changes

DEFINING CHARACTERISTICS

Pain, numbness, cold sensations

Triphasic color changes: white, blue, red

EXPECTED OUTCOMES

The patient maintains optimal tissue perfusion, as evidenced by normal color to fingers and toes.

ONGOING ASSESSMENT

- Assess hands and feet for color, temperature, and skin integrity.
- Solicit patient's description of pain, numbness, and cold sensations.
- Assess interference with ADLs and life-style.

THERAPEUTIC INTERVENTIONS

- Remove vasoconstricting factors when possible.
- Keep extremities warm (socks, blankets, gloves, mittens).
- ▲ Administer vasodilating medications (calcium channel blockers) as prescribed. *Many patients benefit from treatment with these medications as seasons change and weather gets colder.*
- Instruct patient to avoid undue cold exposure:
  Wear oven mitts for refrigerator or freezer.
  Wear multiple layers of clothing (hat/cap, ear muffs, nose protector, mittens/gloves, socks) in cold environment.
  Wear items made of wool, cotton, down, or thinsulate *(provide most protection from cold exposure).*
- Instruct patient to avoid caffeine and nicotine *(cause vasoconstriction).*
- Instruct patient in stress management *(stress can precipitate vasospasm):*
- ▲ Refer to specialized program as needed.

Joint Pain

RELATED FACTORS

Inflammation early in disease

DEFINING CHARACTERISTICS

Pain
Guarding on motion of affected joints
Facial mask of pain
Moaning or other pain-associated sounds

EXPECTED OUTCOMES

The patient verbalizes a reduction in pain.
The patient appears comfortable.

ONGOING ASSESSMENT

- Assess for signs of joint inflammation (redness, warmth, swelling, decreased motion).
- Solicit patient's description of pain.
- Determine past pain-relief measures.
- Assess interference with life-style. *Pain is a chronic problem. If not adequately treated, it may significantly affect one's life-style.*

THERAPEUTIC INTERVENTIONS

- ▲ Administer antiinflammatory medication as prescribed; suggest first dose of day as early in morning as possible, with small snack. *Antiinflammatory drugs should not be given on empty stomach (can be very irritating to stomach lining and lead to ulcer disease).*
- ▲ Use nonnarcotic analgesic as necessary. *Narcotic analgesia appears to work better on mechanical than inflammatory types of pain and can be habit-forming.*
- Encourage anatomically correct position of joint. Do not use knee gatch or pillows to prop knees. Use a small flat pillow under head.
- Encourage use of ambulation aid(s) when pain related to weight bearing.

NURSING DIAGNOSES	EXPECTED OUTCOMES AND NURSING INTERVENTIONS / *RATIONALE* (■ = INDEPENDENT; ▲ = COLLABORATIVE)

THERAPEUTIC INTERVENTIONS—cont'd

- Encourage use of alternate methods of pain control such as relaxation, guided imagery, or distraction.
- Apply bed cradle *to keep pressure of bed covers off inflamed lower extremities.*
- ▲ Consult occupational therapist for proper splinting of affected joints. *Splints provide rest to the inflamed joint.*
- See also Pain, p. 49.

Joint Stiffness

RELATED FACTORS

Inflammation with early disease; contractures with advancing disease

DEFINING CHARACTERISTICS

Verbalized complaint of joint stiffness

EXPECTED OUTCOMES

Patient verbalizes a reduction in stiffness.
Patient demonstrates ability to perform required ADL.

ONGOING ASSESSMENT

- Solicit patient's description of stiffness:
Location: generalized or localized
Timing: morning, night, all day
Length of stiffness: Ask patient, "How long do you take to loosen up after you get out of bed?"Record in hours or fraction of hour
Relationship to activities; aggravating/alleviating factors.

THERAPEUTIC INTERVENTIONS

- Encourage patient to take 15-min warm shower/bath on rising. *Reduces stiffness, relieves pain. Water should be tepid. Excessive heat may promote skin breakdown.*
- Encourage patient to perform ROM exercises after shower/bath, two repetitions for each joint.
- Allow sufficient time for all activities.
- Avoid scheduling tests or treatments when stiffness is present.
- ▲ Administer antiinflammatory medication as prescribed; suggest first dose of day as early in morning as possible, with small snack. *The sooner patient takes medication, the sooner stiffness will abate. Many patients prefer to take medications as early as 6 or 7 A.M. Ask about normal home medication schedule; try to continue it. Antiinflammatory drugs should not be given on empty stomach.*
- Remind patient to avoid prolonged inactivity (*aggravates stiffness*).

High Risk for Altered Gastrointestinal Tract Function

RISK FACTORS

Inflammation
Stricture
Hypomotility
Atrophy

EXPECTED OUTCOMES

The patient verbalizes tolerance of food.
The patient maintains weight.
The patient has normal bowel pattern and consistency.

ONGOING ASSESSMENT

- Solicit patient's description of discomfort: pain, burning, regurgitation, constipation, diarrhea, or loss of appetite. *May occur as upper gastrointestinal (UGI) problem such as esophagitis or esophageal stricture. May also occur as lower gastrointestinal (LGI) problem. Patients with limited scleroderma experience decreased motility, which leads to constipation. Subsequent overgrowth of bacteria finally causes diarrhea.*
- Document patient's actual weight at admission (do not estimate). Reassess every week. *Important because patients lose weight secondary to malabsorption.*

THERAPEUTIC INTERVENTIONS

- Prevent reflux by elevating HOB at least 30 degrees, applying shock blocks to HOB, using pillows behind back for support.
- ▲ Administer medication (e.g., Zantac, Tagament, Pepcid, Prilosec) *to block gastric acid production and relieve burning/pain.*
- ▲ Administer antibiotics as prescribed. *Small doses used to treat symptoms of malabsorption; also help manage constipation/diarrhea.*
- Instruct patient to eat small frequent meals; avoid eating 2 hr before lying down; eat slowly, avoid spicy foods, fruit juices, alcohol, bedtime snacks, coffee, or other foods that produce symptoms of esophagitis.
- See also Nutrition, altered: less than body requirements, p. 44, Constipation, p. 16; Diarrhea, p. 19.

Continued.

NURSING DIAGNOSES	EXPECTED OUTCOMES AND NURSING INTERVENTIONS / *RATIONALE* (■ = INDEPENDENT; ▲ = COLLABORATIVE)

High Risk for Altered Dental Hygiene

RISK FACTORS

Microstomia
Sjögren's syndrome (dryness of mouth)

EXPECTED OUTCOMES

The patient maintains dental hygiene, as evidenced by decreased number of dental caries and good oral hydration.

ONGOING ASSESSMENT

- Assess patient's ability to open mouth wide. *Tight skin interferes with opening mouth.*
- Assess for obvious dental abnormalities: loss of teeth/gum disease/bleeding.
- Assess all mucous membranes/lips for moisture.
- Assess for salivary pools: have patient open mouth as wide as possible; with mouth open, patient puts tip of tongue to roof of mouth; look under tongue for signs of moisture. *Saliva protects teeth from caries and is necessary for digestion.*

THERAPEUTIC INTERVENTIONS

- Encourage frequent hydration.
- Provide lip moisturizer (e.g., petroleum jelly).
- Instruct patient to brush teeth after every meal. *Water pick may be beneficial.*
- Instruct patient to avoid high-sugar beverages and foods. Suggest sugar-free candy or beverages to moisten mouth *(may stimulate further salivary function). Saliva protects teeth from dental caries.*
- Instruct patient to inspect oral cavity daily. *Though it is difficult, patient must understand importance of this.*
- Instruct patient in ROM mouth exercises to increase oral opening.
- Suggest frequent visits to dentist familiar with scleroderma.
- ▲ Initiate dental consultation as appropriate.

High Risk for Hypertension

RISK FACTORS

Constriction of renal vessels
Scleroderma renal crisis
Usually found in patients with diffuse, rapidly progressive skin thickening

ONGOING ASSESSMENT

- Monitor for elevated BP. *Hypertension commonly accompanies scleroderma renal crisis. The renal crisis may progress into renal failure and require dialysis.*
- Initially assess blood pressure in both arms while patient is lying and sitting.
- Solicit presence/description of ankle/pedal edema, severe headaches, and fatigue. *These are signs of scleroderma renal failure.*
- Monitor and record I & O at least every shift.
- Weigh daily and record.
- ▲ Monitor blood chemistry. *Elevated blood urea nitrogen (BUN), creatinine levels are signs of altered renal function.*
- Monitor urine chemistry. *Proteinuria is a sign of altered renal function.*

THERAPEUTIC INTERVENTIONS

- ▲ Administer antihypertension medication as prescribed. Monitor blood pressure 30 min after administration of each dose. *Angiotensin-converting enzyme inhibitors (e.g., Captopril/Vasotec) are rapid-acting agents used to treat both renal failure and hypertension.*
- Provide uninterrupted rest periods throughout day (30 min 3-4 times/day) *to reduce blood pressure.*
- Instruct patient in accurate blood pressure measurement:
  Purchase a sphygmomanometer for home use to give valid, reliable measurement.
  Demonstrate correct use of patient's own BP monitoring equipment. Obtain return demonstrations until patient demonstrates correct technique and verbalizes confidence with skill level.
  Patient should monitor accuracy of own equipment q 6mo (can be done by comparing reading from home equipment with reading from standardized, calibrated in-hospital equipment).
- Instruct patient about the symptoms of scleroderma renal crisis:
- See also Hypertension, p. 122; Renal failure, acute, p. 436.

Fatigue

RELATED FACTORS

Increased disease activity
Anemia of chronic disease

EXPECTED OUTCOMES

The patient expresses increased energy level.
The patient appears rested.

ONGOING ASSESSMENT

- Solicit patient's description of fatigue: timing (afternoon or all day), relationship to activities, aggravating and alleviating factors.
- Determine night sleep pattern. *Pain may interfere with achieving restful sleep.*
- Determine whether fatigue is related to psychologic factors (stress, depression).

NURSING DIAGNOSES	EXPECTED OUTCOMES AND NURSING INTERVENTIONS / *RATIONALE* (■ = INDEPENDENT; ▲ = COLLABORATIVE)

DEFINING CHARACTERISTICS

Lack of energy, exhaustion, listlessness
Excessive sleeping
Decreased attention span
Facial expressions: yawning, sadness
Decreased functional capacity

THERAPEUTIC INTERVENTIONS

- Provide uninterrupted rest periods throughout day (30 min 3-4 times/day). *Patients often have limited energy supply.*
- Reinforce principles of energy conservation:
  Pacing activities (alternating activity with rest). *Patient often uses more energy than others to complete same tasks.*
  Adequate periods of rest (throughout day and at night)
  Organization of activities and environment
  Proper use of assistive/adaptive devices

If fatigue related to interrupted sleep:

- Encourage warm shower/bath immediately before bedtime. *Warm water relaxes muscles, facilitates total body relaxation; excessive heat may promote skin breakdown.*
- Encourage gentle ROM exercises (after shower/bath) *to maximize benefits of warm bath/shower.*
- Encourage patient to sleep in anatomically correct position. Do not prop up affected joints. Change positions frequently during night.
- Avoid stimulating foods (caffeine), activities before bedtime.
- Encourage use of progressive muscle relaxation techniques.
- ▲ Administer nighttime analgesic/long-acting antiinflammatory drug as prescribed.

Knowledge Deficit

RELATED FACTORS

New disease/procedures
Unfamiliarity with treatment regime
Lack of interest

DEFINING CHARACTERISTICS

Multiple questions
Lack of questions
Verbalized misconceptions
Verbalized lack of knowledge
Inaccurate follow-through of instructions

EXPECTED OUTCOMES

Patient verbalizes increased awareness of disease and treatment.

ONGOING ASSESSMENT

- Assess knowledge of scleroderma and its treatment.
- Assess degree to which discomfort interferes with learning.

THERAPEUTIC INTERVENTIONS

- Schedule educational sessions when patient is most comfortable. *Pain distracts patient and may lead to inability to absorb new information.*
- Introduce/reinforce disease process information: unknown cause, chronicity of scleroderma, processes of inflammation and fibrosis, skin and other organ involvement, remissions and exacerbations, control versus cure.
- Introduce/reinforce information on drug therapy. *Patient may be taking a regimen of drugs and needs to understand the different methods of administration and potential side effects to watch for.*
- Introduce/reinforce self-management techniques: ROM exercises, muscle strengthening exercises, pain management, joint protection, pacing activities, adequate rest, splinting, use of assistive devices, skin care, dental hygiene.
- Introduce/reinforce nutritionally sound diet.
- Stress importance of long-term follow-up. *Patient is living with long-term illness and requires ongoing treatment and emotional support.*
- Discuss unproven remedies; encourage to verify/discuss new treatments before use. *Patients may be vulnerable to fads/ads claiming curative effects of special vitamins/health foods.*

See also:
Anticipatory Grieving, p. 28.
Self-Care Deficit, p. 53.
Altered Sexual Patterns, p. 58.
Sleep Pattern Disturbance, p. 61.
Altered Nutrition: Less than Body Requirements, p. 44.
Impaired Gas Exchange, p. 27.
Decreased Cardiac Output, p. 12.
Ineffective Coping, p. 18.

By: Linda Ehrlich, RN, MSN
    Sue A. Connaughton, RN, MSN, Psy D Candidate

Psychosocial Care Plans

Anorexia nervosa

Syndrome characterized by an intense fear of fatness, severe weight loss, and disturbed body image occurring in otherwise normal, healthy individuals.

NURSING DIAGNOSES	EXPECTED OUTCOMES AND NURSING INTERVENTIONS / *RATIONALE* (■ = INDEPENDENT; ▲ = COLLABORATIVE)

Altered Nutrition: Less than Body Requirements

RELATED FACTORS

Inability to allow for adequate nutritional intake caused by fear of fatness

Excessive, irrational fear of fatness

Distorted body image

No other illness that would explain weight loss/prevent weight gain

DEFINING CHARACTERISTICS

Body weight 20% or more below ideal for height and frame

Self-restricted food intake despite hunger

Aversion to eating

EXPECTED OUTCOMES

Patient does not lose further weight.

Patient begins to gain weight.

Patient expresses some understanding of her abnormal eating pattern.

ONGOING ASSESSMENT

- Document patient's actual weight and height on admission. Weigh daily in a casual manner. *Reduces emphasis on weight.*
- Obtain accurate weight history, including reason for weight loss.
- Perform in-depth nutritional assessment:
  Diet history (reconstruction of typical 24-hr intake)
  Development of patient's beliefs and fears about food. *Focus on food may be a maladaptive means to deal with stress.*
  Level of nutritional knowledge
  Behaviors used to reduce energy intake (dieting), to increase energy output (exercising), and generally to lose weight (vomiting, purging, and laxative abuse)
- ▲ Assess electrolyte balance. *Provides data on the severity of malnutrition.*
- Monitor daily intake.

THERAPEUTIC INTERVENTIONS

- Closely supervise high-protein, high-calorie refeeding of approximately 1800 calories/day *to correct acute starvation phase.* Gradually increase daily caloric intake *to ensure steady weight gain until goal achieved.*
- Closely supervise bathroom use after meals if required *to decrease opportunity to vomit/dispose of food. Maintain consistency with this supervision.*
- Present and remove food without persuasion *to help separate emotional issues (e.g., approval) from eating behavior.*
- Set limits on excessive physical activity but allow daily activity *(over-restriction may induce severe/overwhelming anxiety).*
- Provide accurate nutritional information *to correct false ideas about food and weight gain.*
- Give assurances patient will not become overweight.
- Acknowledge patient's anger and feelings of loss of control caused by established eating program. *Patient may feel she is being punished. Therefore, staff need to clarify they are merely providing external controls that have not been internalized.*
- Provide supplemental feedings/nutrition as indicated.

Body Image Disturbance

RELATED FACTORS

Difficulty coping with maturation process

Failure to achieve unreasonable expectations of self

Alexithymia (channeling uncomfortable feelings into behaviors such as self-starvation)

DEFINING CHARACTERISTICS

Distorted perception of one's weight/body shape

Negative feelings about body

Self-loathing

Intense fear of gaining/not losing weight

EXPECTED OUTCOMES

Patient expresses a positive aspect of body/self.

Patient identifies a positive means to cope with current problems.

ONGOING ASSESSMENT

- Assess patient's perception of body image.
- Elicit patient's assessment of strengths and weaknesses.
- Assess patient's ability to identify feeling states.

THERAPEUTIC INTERVENTIONS

- Encourage patient to reexamine negative self-perceptions.
- Encourage identification, expression, and tolerance of unpleasant feeling states. *Anorectic patients have a need for control that they cannot express in other aspects of their life.*
- Help patient develop realistic, acceptable perception of body image and relationship with food. *Patients also need to understand the physical consequences of anorexia.*
- ▲ Refer for psychiatric counseling. *Eating disorders require specialized intervention.*
- ▲ Refer to support group. *Groups that come together for mutual support and guidance can be helpful.*

Continued.

Anorexia nervosa—cont'd

NURSING DIAGNOSES	EXPECTED OUTCOMES AND NURSING INTERVENTIONS / *RATIONALE* (■ = INDEPENDENT; ▲ = COLLABORATIVE)

Altered Family Process
 	
RELATED FACTORS
Developmental crisis of separation and family restructuring
 	
DEFINING CHARACTERISTICS
Family members unable to relate to each other for mutual growth and maturation as evidenced by patient's self-starvation and weight loss
	EXPECTED OUTCOMES
	Family members develop improved methods of communication.
	Family members express understanding of mutual problems.
	Family members identify resources for problem solving.
	
	ONGOING ASSESSMENT
	■ Assess type of interactional patterns used by family:
	    Enmeshment, *lack of generational boundaries between family members;*
	    Overprotectiveness, *demonstrated by exaggerated concern for welfare of others in family*
	    Rigidity, *emphasis on maintaining status quo*
	    Lack of conflict resolution via triangulation coalition *(parents collude with child to prevent conflict expression/resolution; e.g., child becomes symptomatic to deflect parental conflict)*
	    Involvement of the anorectic child in unresolved parental conflict
	
	THERAPEUTIC INTERVENTIONS
	■ Explore family's reasons for recurring problems *to deemphasize family's notion of patient as a problem.*
	■ Explore with family members effects of each individual's behavior on others.
	■ Identify interaction patterns among family members *to demonstrate how patterns engender dependence on environment for cues about regulation rather than fostering self-regulation.*
	■ Acknowledge and offer feedback to family's expressed feelings *to encourage direct expression and ownership of feelings.*
	■ Encourage participation in therapeutic group interaction, especially family therapy.

See also:
Ineffective Individual Coping,
p. 18.
Knowledge Deficit, p. 41.
Enteral Tube Feedings,
p. 303.
Total Parenteral Nutrition,
p. 324.
Altered Thought Processes,
p. 65.

By: Nancy Staples, RN, BSN

Bulimia

Bulimia is a syndrome characterized by ego-alien episodes of binge eating involving rapid consumption of large quantities of food within a discrete period. Feelings of guilt and pain follow from the lost sense of control, which trigger purging/dieting attempts to restore sense of control and weight mastery. The term normal weight bulimia (NWB) refers to those individuals whose weight has always been in the normal range or above; the term bulimia nervosa (BN) refers to the subgroup who have experienced a previous episode of, but who no longer meet the criteria for, anorexia nervosa.

NURSING DIAGNOSES	EXPECTED OUTCOMES AND NURSING INTERVENTIONS / *RATIONALE* (■ = INDEPENDENT; ▲ = COLLABORATIVE)

Altered Nutrition: More than Body Requirements

RELATED FACTORS

Intake exceeds metabolic needs

DEFINING CHARACTERISTICS

Dysfunctional eating pattern
Episodic binge eating
Eating in response to internal cues other than hunger
Weight gain

EXPECTED OUTCOMES

Patient does not gain additional weight.
Patient adopts/initiates adequate dietary habits.

ONGOING ASSESSMENT

- Obtain accurate history of weight fluctuations
- Assess height and weight; determine ideal body weight.
- Obtain accurate diet history, including daily intake, number and methods of dieting. *Patients frequently have experienced unsuccessful attempts at severely restrictive dieting followed by episodic, secretive consumption of large to enormous amounts of food (usually sweets or carbohydrates) within discrete period.*
- Determine type and frequency of binge-purge behavior, and associated feeling states. *Method of purging behavior (vomiting, laxatives, diuretics) may result in weight fluctuations, often greater than 10 lb.*
- Weigh patient twice weekly in same manner at same time; record. *More frequent weighing reinforces patient's preoccupation with body size.*

THERAPEUTIC INTERVENTIONS

- Establish reasonable weight range with patient.
- Devise diet plan that specifies number of calories (but not less than 1600/day) and includes all food groups. Plan should include three meals plus a light evening snack *as adequate intake alleviates effects of starvation (e.g., sleeplessness or waking during the night), preoccupation with thoughts of food, and tendency to binge behavior.*
- Give accurate information about nutrition, metabolic functioning, set-point theory, and role of deprivation in triggering binges, *to correct faulty ideas. Assure patient that all metabolic deficiencies can be corrected through proper nutrition.*
- Provide contact during, after meals *to encourage normal eating habits while interfering with potential impulse to vomit.*
- Encourage reasonable physical activity *to regulate weight and promote sense of well-being and control.*
- Be aware of potential for purging behavior, particularly weight shifts; if suspected, address issue directly. Use observation and supervision as necessary *to help patient interrupt cycle of purging behavior.*

Ineffective Individual Coping

RELATED FACTORS

Deficit in introspective awareness (i.e., difficulty identifying, articulating, and modulating internal states, e.g., hunger, satiety, and their effects)

EXPECTED OUTCOMES

Patient identifies own maladaptive coping behaviors.
Patient describes/initiates alternative coping strategies.

ONGOING ASSESSMENT

- Assess ability to differentiate and label mood states. *Binge/purge behavior is generalized to alleviate uncomfortable mood states (dysphoria).*
- Obtain detailed history of type, duration, and intensity of impulsive behaviors. *Multiple impulse disorders (e.g., alcohol/drug abuse, sexual promiscuity, stealing, and self-harm) may be present in response to psychosocial stressors (e.g., depression, stress, and anxiety)*

Continued.

Bulimia—cont'd

NURSING DIAGNOSES	EXPECTED OUTCOMES AND NURSING INTERVENTIONS / *RATIONALE* (■ = INDEPENDENT; ▲ = COLLABORATIVE)

DEFINING CHARACTERISTICS

Verbalizes inability to cope
Inability to problem solve
Alteration in societal participation
Potentially destructive behavior toward self
Inappropriate use of defense mechanisms

THERAPEUTIC INTERVENTIONS

- Instruct patient to keep a food journal; include before-, during-, and after-binge/purge activities. *Self-monitoring activities can begin association of mood states with binge-purge behavior.*
- Provide information on dieting, set-point theory, and role of deprivation in triggering binges *to help patient see how struggles with food are culturally and biologically influenced rather than are purely personal failures in "will-power."*
- Help patient develop list of alternatives to impulsive behavior (e.g., talking to someone, going for a walk). *By introducing technique of delay, impulse will lessen in strength; use of alternative strategies facilitates sense of mastery.*
- Encourage and accept patient's verbal expression of feelings. Maintain nonjudgmental attitude so as not to reinforce excessive feelings of guilt, shame, and helplessness.
- Review examples of cognitive distortion exhibited: magical thinking; dichotomous/all-or-nothing thinking; control fallacy; viewing self as externally controlled; magnification; overgeneralization.
- ▲ Refer for psychological counseling/intervention as indicated. *Eating disorders require specialized intervention.*
- Refer to support group. *Groups that come together for mutual support are beneficial.*

Body Image Disturbance

RELATED FACTORS

Feelings of inadequacy, worthlessness, criticalness
Shame and guilt caused by discrepancy between actual/ideal self

DEFINING CHARACTERISTICS

Body size dissatisfaction
Self-loathing
Negative feelings about body
Distorted perception of one's weight/body shape

EXPECTED OUTCOMES

Patient expresses a positive aspect about self/body.
Patient verbalizes/identifies a positive means to cope with current problems.

ONGOING ASSESSMENT

- Assess perception of body image as compared to ideal.
- Assess degree of impairment of life adjustments (i.e., work, interpersonal relationships) as result of symptomatic behavior. *It is not uncommon for patient's distorted sense of self to pervade all aspects of her life.*

THERAPEUTIC INTERVENTIONS

- Explore and encourage patient to introduce into life self-enhancing activities (e.g., exercising) *to disrupt isolation and withdrawal and increase self-esteem.*
- Encourage to use family/friends as source of support *to decrease social isolation and reduce fear of rejection from others.*
- Encourage to develop and use problem-solving skills *as a means of confronting perfectionistic self-expectations.*
- Focus on healthy aspects of personality. Give examples of how patient magnifies weight-related issues while minimizing or discrediting other personal assets.
- Listen to patient's concerns about self without minimizing them. *Maintaining positive regard can allow patient to experience self and others more acceptingly.*
- Encourage patient to join appropriate support group as adjunct to other treatment interventions, *to reinforce sense of community and provide additional structure.*

High Risk for Fluid Volume Deficit

RISK FACTORS

Fluid shifts caused by excess reliance on vomiting, laxatives, diuretics, severely restrictive dieting

EXPECTED OUTCOMES

Patient maintains optimal fluid volume, as evidenced by normal BP, normal heart rate, absence of arrhythmias, good skin turgor, electrolytes within normal limits.

ONGOING ASSESSMENT

- Monitor I & O.
- Assess for signs of dehydration.
- Monitor vital signs (*patient may be prone to hypotension and tachycardia*).
- ▲ Review lab results for electrolyte imbalance. *Hypokalemia is a common manifestation.*
- Observe for signs of unexplained diarrhea or persistent hypokalemia (*usually indicates continued vomiting/use of diuretics/laxatives*).
- Observe/monitor for dysrhythmias, *which may result from electrolyte imbalance.*

THERAPEUTIC INTERVENTIONS

- Provide adequate fluid *to remedy imbalances of fluid and electrolytes;* limit amounts of diet sodas consumed (*generally high in sodium*).
- Provide nutritional sources rich in needed electrolytes (e.g., Gator-ade).

By: Nancy Staples, RN, BSN

Depression

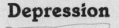

An affective disorder characterized by feelings of unworthiness, profound sadness, guilt, apathy, and hopelessness. A loss of interest and pleasure in usual activities is evident. Behavioral characteristics may include slowing of physical activity or agitation and alterations in sleeping, eating, and libido. Depression differs from sadness in that it is a disease rather than a feeling. Depressive features are seen in postpartum depression, premenstrual syndrome, alcohol and/or drug withdrawal, and involutional melancholia. Depression may also be reactive and situational, associated with grief and loss of health, job, and/or significant other. Depression features can be a component of mood disorders, including bipolar (manic-depressive) illness. Suicidal ideation and/or gestures, as well as psychotic thought processes, may be present.

NURSING DIAGNOSES

EXPECTED OUTCOMES AND NURSING INTERVENTIONS / *RATIONALE*
(■ = INDEPENDENT; ▲ = COLLABORATIVE)

Self-Esteem Disturbance

RELATED FACTORS

Ineffective or limited coping skills
Difficulties with relationship
Illness/disability
Significant losses
Decreased level of independence
Inadequate support systems
Cognitive/perceptual distortions
Lack of information about depression and treatment

DEFINING CHARACTERISTICS

Negative verbalizations about self
Neglect of appearance/personal needs
Excessive focus on failings/inadequacies
Poor eye contact
Feelings of helplessness
Ruminations

EXPECTED OUTCOMES

Patient uses positive self-statements to interrupt negative automatic thinking.
Patient begins to participate in treatment plan.

ONGOING ASSESSMENT

- Assess for presence of ruminations, negative thoughts, and feelings of inadequacy. *Depressed patients describe feelings of hopelessness and powerlessness so pervasive that they interfere with their ability to manage personal relationships and work-related responsibilities.*
- Assess understanding of depression and available treatment.

THERAPEUTIC INTERVENTIONS

- Assist patient in reviewing negative perceptions of self. *Provides basis for exploring the degree to which these perceptions are real.*
- Identify patient's positive personality features *to provide supportive feedback and validation of self-worth.*
- Encourage patient to be directly involved in treatment planning. *This will reduce sense of powerlessness.*
- Assist to identify self-defeating behaviors and to strategize ways to reinforce internal strengths. *Internalization of positive feedback will promote self-worth.*
- Instruct patient/significant other about causes of depression and specific treatment interventions: antidepressant medication, counseling, electroconvulsive therapy (ECT), hospitalization for increased protection. *A patient may feel guilty about being depressed and may not understand that it is treatable, and that symptoms can be managed (both behaviorly and pharmacologically).*

Social Isolation

RELATED FACTORS

Withdrawn and regressive behavior
Impaired communication
Low self-esteem
Disrupted personal relationships
Sexual dysfunction
Fear of rejection
Fear of failure

EXPECTED OUTCOMES

Patient develops a plan to be more involved with others.
Patient becomes actively involved with others, at least on a beginning level.

ONGOING ASSESSMENT

- Assess affect.
- Assess eye contact. *A depressed patient may maintain minimal eye contact as a result of fear of rejection.*
- Assess spontaneity and verbal frequency. *A depressed patient is seldom interactive.*
- Assess involvement with others.

Continued.

NURSING DIAGNOSES	EXPECTED OUTCOMES AND NURSING INTERVENTIONS / *RATIONALE* (■ = INDEPENDENT; ▲ = COLLABORATIVE)

DEFINING CHARACTERISTICS

Verbalizations limited in spontaneity and quantity
Depressed, dull affect
Rumination and preoccupation with negative thoughts
Feelings of unworthiness
Loss of interest in sexual activity

THERAPEUTIC INTERVENTIONS

- Encourage relationship with patient by spending time with him/her, providing supportive contact. *Patient's self-worth is enhanced by consistent, supportive staff presence.*
- Encourage participation in group activities as tolerated. Allow patient to leave group situations when contact with others is too anxiety-provoking. *Patient needs to feel some degree of control over environment.*
- Provide positive reinforcement when patient participates in group activities and interacts with others. *This reinforcement supports patient's efforts, and helps augment feelings of self-worth.*
- Acknowledge patient's involvement in daily activities. *This reinforces positive efforts.*

High Risk for Violence: Self-Directed

RISK FACTORS

Low self-esteem
Depressed mood
Hopelessness
Repeated failures in life activities
Reality distortion
Alcohol/drug abuse

EXPECTED OUTCOMES

Patient verbalizes suicidal ideation.
Patient participates in written contract/treatment plan to reduce risk of suicide.
Patient avoids impulsive behavior that could harm self.

ONGOING ASSESSMENT

- Interview patient to evaluate potential for self-directed violence. *Most people who are suicidal are ambivalent about wanting to end their life. The patient may see suicide as the only relief from emotional pain.* Ask:
  Have you felt like hurting yourself? *Suicidal ideation is the process of thinking about killing oneself.*
  Did you ever attempt suicide? *Suicidal gestures are attempts to harm oneself that are not considered lethal. Suicidal attempts are potentially lethal actions.*
  Do you currently feel like killing yourself? *This needs to be asked directly so the patient is assured of staff's comfort in hearing the response.*
  Do you have a plan to hurt yourself?
  What is your plan? What means do you have to carry out your plan? *Development of a plan and ability to carry it out greatly increases the risk of patient harming self.*
- Assess for the presence of risk factors that may increase potential for suicide attempts: *It is a myth that suicide occurs without forewarning. It is also a myth that there is a typical type of person who commits suicide. The potential for suicide exists in all people.*
  History of suicidal attempts. *Suicide may be seen as a ready option.*
  Mood/activity level that changes suddenly. *May signify that patient reached a decision to end life.*
  Giving away of personal possessions. *May represent finalization of affairs.*
  Male patient. *Males have higher incidence of successful suicide attempts.*
  Divorced, widowed, or separated individual
  Early stage of treatment with antidepressant medication during which patient's mood/energy elevates. *The significant increase in energy level predisposes the patient to act on previously felt impulses.*

THERAPEUTIC INTERVENTIONS

- Provide safe environment. *Suicide precautions are interventions taken to create a safe environment for the patient.* Protect patient from acting on self-destructive impulses. *Includes removing all potentially harmful objects: electrical appliances, sharp instruments, belts/ties, glass items. Maintaining patient safety is priority.*
- Provide close patient supervision by maintaining awareness of patient's whereabouts at all times. *The degree of supervision is based on the degree of risk the patient presents.*
- Develop verbal/written contract stating that he/she will not act on impulses to harm self. Review and develop new contracts as needed. *Patient needs to verbalize suicidal ideations with trusted staff. Written/verbal agreement also establishes permission to discuss subject, and to make a commitment not to act on impulses.*
- Encourage verbalization of feelings within appropriate limits. *Depressed patient needs opportunity to discuss thoughts/intentions to harm self. Verbalization of these feelings may lessen their intensity. Patient also needs to see that staff can tolerate discussion of suicidal ideations.*
- Spend time with patient *to provide sense of security, reinforce self-worth.*

| NURSING DIAGNOSES | EXPECTED OUTCOMES AND NURSING INTERVENTIONS / *RATIONALE*
(■ = INDEPENDENT; ▲ = COLLABORATIVE) |

By: Ursula Brozek, RN, MSN

Rape trauma syndrome

(SEXUAL ASSAULT)

Rape trauma syndrome is a response to the extreme stress and profound fear of death that almost all survivors (male or female) experience during the sexual assault. It refers to the acute or immediate phase of disorganization and the long-term process of reorganization that occur as a result of attempted or forcible sexual assault. Although every survivor of sexual assault has unique emotional needs and responses, all experience rape trauma syndrome. Current literature now refers to victims of sexual assault as "survivors" and is gradually replacing the term rape with sexual assault since sexual assault encompasses a broader range of abuse/violence. These phrases are used throughout this care plan.

| NURSING DIAGNOSES | EXPECTED OUTCOMES AND NURSING INTERVENTIONS / *RATIONALE*
(■ = INDEPENDENT; ▲ = COLLABORATIVE) |

Ineffective Coping (Survivor)

RELATED FACTOR
Sexual assault trauma

DEFINING CHARACTERISTICS
Acute:
Increased anxiety
Hostility, aggression
Guilt
Withdrawal
No verbalization of occurrence
  of assault/denial
Abrupt changes in relation-
  ships
Emotional outbursts
Sense of humiliation
Long-term:
Repetitive nightmares/reliving
  of assault
Phobias: fear of being indoors,
  outdoors, of crowds, of being
  alone, of men, of spouse, of
  lovers.

EXPECTED OUTCOMES
Patient demonstrates positive coping behaviors.
Patient verbalizes understanding of symptoms usually encountered on long-term basis.
Patient identifies a support person/system.

ONGOING ASSESSMENT
- Assess for signs of ineffective coping (see Defining Characteristics). *Defining characteristics are actually normal coping mechanisms that occur after sexual assault. However, if they persist and interfere with recovery, they become ineffective.*
- Identify previous coping mechanisms.

THERAPEUTIC INTERVENTIONS
- Provide calm, supportive environment. *Predominant emotion experienced by survivor is overwhelming fear/terror of death. Help to ease fear by assuring survivor of safety.*
▲ If available, contact sexual assault victim advocate. *Role of sexual assault victim advocate is to provide nonjudgmental support, immediate crisis intervention to sexual assault survivor.*
- Encourage survivor to express feelings about the experience. *The survivor will experience a profound loss of control over his/her body. Using the word survivor emphasizes that the survivor did what was necessary to survive the assault, and that this is most important.*
- Validate survivor's feelings; assist in channeling them appropriately.
- Allow survivor time to cope. Help survivor identify coping skills used successfully in past.
- Help survivor contact family/significant others (best support system).

Continued.

Rape trauma syndrome—cont'd

NURSING DIAGNOSES	EXPECTED OUTCOMES AND NURSING INTERVENTIONS / *RATIONALE* (■ = INDEPENDENT; ▲ = COLLABORATIVE)

DEFINING CHARACTERISTICS— cont'd

Reactivated life problems (i.e., physical/psychiatric illnesses)
Reliance on alcohol/drugs
Sleep pattern disturbances
Eating pattern disturbances
GI irritability
Sexual dysfunctioning
Depression/loss of self-esteem

THERAPEUTIC INTERVENTIONS— cont'd

- Help survivor regain sense of control over self/life. *At each stage of interaction, explain what you would like to do, why; ask permission. Asking for permission helps survivor feel in control.*
- Explain to survivor that in future mood swings, feelings of anger, fear, or sadness may be experienced; these are normal reactions.
- Provide anticipatory guidance regarding potential long-term sequelae of rape trauma syndrome (see Defining Characteristics). *Many of these long-term symptoms are experienced for months and years after the assault. They may also be triggered by situational crises later in life. Many long-term symptoms reflect the survivor's struggle to reorganize his or her life.*
- Facilitate survivor's decision-making process; use active listening techniques.
- ▲ Assure that the survivor does not go home alone when discharged. If no significant other is available, call Department of Human Services to escort patient.
- ▲ Provide community referrals for physical, emotional care.

High Risk for Ineffective Coping: Family/Significant Other

RISK FACTORS

Misunderstanding of events surrounding assault
Preoccupation with incident

EXPECTED OUTCOMES

Family/significant others express understanding of assault incidence and role of survivor.
Family/significant other identify ways to provide support to survivor.
Family/significant others use counseling resources as needed.

ONGOING ASSESSMENT

- Assess family/significant other for signs of ineffective coping: blaming of survivor for incident, expressions of guilt, inability to talk about incident, withdrawal, aggression, hostility, anger, embarrassment/humiliation.
- Assess current knowledge of situation.
- Observe family's current actions, and their effect on survivor. *How they respond will strongly impact survivor's coping ability.*
- Identify previous coping mechanisms. *They may not be effective for this situation/crisis.*

THERAPEUTIC INTERVENTIONS

- Encourage family to verbalize concerns, feelings. Identify importance of support, understanding to recovery. *Verbalized negative feelings (i.e., blaming survivor for assault) must be addressed. Survivor should not be made to feel responsible for assault; nothing justifies sexual assault.*
- Validate family's feelings; help them to channel them appropriately. Acknowledge the stress that they are experiencing.
- ▲ Provide support, counseling referrals. *Significant others may also exhibit emotional problems secondary to sexual assault and require counseling.*
- Discuss with family/significant others ways to support survivor: encouraging survivor to verbalize feelings; helping survivor resume usual life activities; avoiding overprotectiveness; being nonjudgmental; holding, touching survivor so as not to reinforce feelings of being unclean; helping mobilize survivor's anger; directing it at assailant. *Studies indicate that the type of emotional support the sexual assault survivor receives initially has direct bearing on recovery and long-term reorganization.*

High Risk for Associated Physical Injury

RISK FACTORS

Sexual assault trauma

EXPECTED OUTCOMES

Patient verbalizes relief or reduction in discomfort.
Patient has reduced complications from injury as a result of early assessment and intervention.

ONGOING ASSESSMENT

- Assess degree of injury sustained during the assault: bruises/swelling, lacerations/abrasions/scratches, muscle tension/general soreness, vaginal/oral/rectal irritation.
- Prepare woman for need for physical and pelvic exam. *Lab tests are needed to collect evidence, to verify presence of sperm in vagina, and to rule out sexually transmitted disease (STD) or pregnancy. Urine pregnancy test should be done on all female sexual assault survivors in childbearing years to identify preexisting pregnancy (alters type of medication prescribed).*
- Assess for need for medication *to relieve associated pain, nausea, vomiting, muscle tension.*

| NURSING DIAGNOSES | EXPECTED OUTCOMES AND NURSING INTERVENTIONS / *RATIONALE*
(■ = INDEPENDENT; ▲ = COLLABORATIVE) |

THERAPEUTIC INTERVENTIONS

- Obtain patient's written consent for examination and treatment. *This is necessary because the results of the examination will be considered evidence.*
- Collect, prepare evidence required by law. Refer to Sexual Assault Procedure in hospital policy.
- ▲ Medicate as prescribed for pain, nausea/vomiting, muscle tension, prevention of STDs, pregnancy.
- Perform wound care as needed.
- ▲ Give tetanus toxoid as prescribed.
- Provide follow-up care *to assess for and prevent complications (i.e., gonorrhea culture, Chlamydia culture, VDRL, pregnancy test in 4-6 wk, and HIV counseling).*

Self-esteem/Body Image Disturbance

RELATED FACTOR

Sexual assault trauma

DEFINING CHARACTERISTICS

Self-negating verbalization
Expressions of shame/guilt/
  embarrassment
Helplessness
Negative feelings about body
Preoccupation with assault
Withdrawal
Difficulty in relating to males

EXPECTED OUTCOMES

Patient verbalizes positive expressions of self-worth.
Patient verbalizes positive aspect about body.
Patient expresses understanding that she/he was not responsible for assault, but was a victim.

ONGOING ASSESSMENT

- Assess patient's current self-image.
- Assess reactions, feelings about sexual assault.

THERAPEUTIC INTERVENTIONS

- Show interest, respect, warmth, and nonjudgmental attitude. Avoid accusing, negative questions. *Much shame about sexual assault arises from mistaken belief that sexual assault is primarily sexual; thus survivor must in some way have provoked/enticed assailant. Sexual assault is crime of violence—not passion.*
- Listen attentively to convey belief in what survivor is saying.
- Acknowledge survivor's feelings. *Many survivors are filled with guilt, self-reproach. Remind survivor that she/he is in no way responsible for assault. Encourage survivor to direct negative feelings toward assailant, away from self.*
- Be aware of your own feelings and attitudes and effect on survivor. *The survivor feels very vulnerable and will sense the caretaker's own ambivalence, judgemental tone, or fear.*
- Provide anticipatory guidance to survivor/family.
- Determine, address survivor's special concerns/immediate needs (i.e., concerns about physical injury, pregnancy, STDs, AIDS).
- Encourage female staff member to stay with female survivor if possible, as advocate.
- Explain that patient's emotional, physical responses are normal; they may continue weeks after sexual assault trauma. *Sexual assault is ultimate invasion of privacy; much time (and usually counseling) needed before survivor feels safe, secure, in control.*

See also:
Anxiety, p. 5.
Knowledge Deficit, p. 41.
Powerlessness, p. 52.
Altered Sexuality Patterns,
  p. 58.

By: Evelyn Lyons, RN, BSN
  Anita D. Morris, RN
  Ursula Brozek, RN, MS

Substance abuse

(ALCOHOL AND DRUG ABUSE/DEPENDENCY AND
WITHDRAWAL)

Abuse is the inappropriate use of a potentially addictive substance. Prescription, over-the-counter, street drugs and alcohol may be abused. When the abuser becomes physically or emotionally dependent on the sensations that the drug causes, he or she is addicted. Commonly abused addictive substances include alcohol, narcotics, depressants, stimulants, hallucinogens, and cannobinols.

NURSING DIAGNOSES	EXPECTED OUTCOMES AND NURSING INTERVENTIONS / *RATIONALE* (■ = INDEPENDENT; ▲ = COLLABORATIVE)

Knowledge Deficit

RELATED FACTORS

Denial of problem
No experience with substance
abuse

DEFINING CHARACTERISTICS

Many questions
No questions
Incorrect information/
misconceptions

EXPECTED OUTCOME:

Patient verbalizes understanding of substance abuse and its treatment.

ONGOING ASSESSMENT

- Assess readiness to learn *(is necessary for taking in information.)* However, do not confuse readiness to learn with preparedness to change addictive behavior. They are not the same.
- Ascertain which significant others would benefit from attending information sessions. Provide information to friends/family when appropriate. *All are affected by the addicted member's behavior and can benefit from support and information.*
- Assess knowledge of physical and emotional dependency on alcohol, prescription, nonprescription, or street drugs.
- Assess knowledge of alcohol/drug abuse on the body, ability to think/process information, life-style (work, interpersonal relationships, self-concept, ability to maintain home).

THERAPEUTIC INTERVENTIONS

- Provide information about substance abuse in nonthreatening, matter-of-fact way. *Misconceptions/myths about substance abuse abound. Many abusers have beliefs that are much more accepting of their behaviors.*
- State information simply. *The aim is to present information. Refrain from trying to convince of facts, frighten into sobriety. This may only distance the person seeking help.*
- Expect patient to alternate between acceptance and rejection of information. *The patient is least likely to be able to absorb information while experiencing withdrawal/emotional longing for abused substance.*
- Communicate that with correct information and support the patient can choose detoxification and make decisions that will let him/her enjoy a healthier life.

Impaired Individual Coping

RELATED FACTORS

Coping behaviors never/
inadequately learned
No supportive others available
Social outlets all revolve
around drugs/alcohol

DEFINING CHARACTERISTICS

Frequent suicide attempts
Frequent overdoses
Binge drinking
Drug binging
Frequent psychiatric/medical
hospitalizations
Negative/counterproductive
behaviors: hostility; aggression; inadequate behavior;
physically abusive, lying,
antisocial/criminal behavior
Patient observed to verbalize
inability to cope, meet role
expectations

EXPECTED OUTCOMES

Patient demonstrates positive efforts at coping, one day at a time.
Patient begins to recognize own maladaptive behaviors.
Patient participates in a support group.
Patient refrains from drug/alcohol use.

ONGOING ASSESSMENT

- Assess for Defining Characteristics.
- Assess how long patient has had coping problems.
- Assess whether patient has any effective coping mechanisms.
- Assess character strengths, deficits *to establish framework for helping patient to develop coping mechanisms.*
- Determine to what degree lack of coping behaviors results from alcohol/drug abuse/dependency.
- Ask patient to identify behaviors that have most negative effects. Work to develop successful coping mechanisms for these behaviors first. *Patient will have greatest investment in meeting own priorities. Success may mobilize the patient to make other changes.*

THERAPEUTIC INTERVENTIONS

- Confront patient with unacceptable behaviors. Enlist friends/family members in providing feedback. *Provides immediate information. Patient may pause, reflect on impact on people in environment; also sets limits on behaviors others will tolerate.*
- Affirm insight whenever patient displays insight into own behavior. *Positive reinforcement may encourage patient to display more of same behavior.*

NURSING DIAGNOSES	EXPECTED OUTCOMES AND NURSING INTERVENTIONS / *RATIONALE* (■ = INDEPENDENT; ▲ = COLLABORATIVE)

THERAPEUTIC INTERVENTIONS—cont'd

- Gently confront patient with reality when he/she attributes problem to others/circumstances beyond control. *Allowing rationalizations to be unchallenged sanctions behavior.*
- Involve patient in support groups for recovering alcoholics/abusers.
- Do not overwhelm patient with global expectations. Expect short-term behavior changes. Do not make task impossible. *It is realistic to expect patient to refrain from alcohol/drugs one day at a time. Substance abuse is a disorder that can be marked by relapses.*
- Help patient develop substitute (positive) behaviors in lieu of negative ones.
- Help patient learn to identify feelings, express thoughts. *Articulating thoughts, feelings sometimes helps to diffuse them.*
- Reward positive behaviors. *This may help to sustain them.*
- Spend time with patient. Remain nonjudgmental. Avoid behaviors that reinforce an already low self-esteem.

High Risk for Self-directed/Other-directed Violence

RISK FACTORS

Withdrawal
Hopelessness
Depression
Hostility to others
History of injuring self/others
Psychosis/hallucinations that direct patient to hurt self/others

EXPECTED OUTCOMES

Patient verbalizes any suicidal/homicidal ideation.
Patient avoids impulsive behaviors that could harm self.

ONGOING ASSESSMENT

- Determine degree of suicidal/homicidal risk. *The degree of risk will determine degree of supervision/referral to psychiatric services.*
- Assess whether patient has the means or a plan to carry out act. *Development of a plan and ability to carry it out greatly increase the risk of the patient's harming self/others.*

THERAPEUTIC INTERVENTIONS

- Remove dangerous objects from environment. Ensure that the environment is safe for patients who may be impulse-ridden.
- Approach patient nonthreateningly; take time to introduce self, describe procedures. Accept patient's right to refuse procedures.
- Tell patient when you are going to touch him/her. *Paranoid/delusional patients may fear physical contact; may perceive it as personal threat.*
- ▲ Use medications to modify out-of-control behavior; treat delusional thinking; stabilize/reassure depressive features.
- See also Thought processes, altered, p. 65; Depression, p. 527.

Altered Health Maintenance

RELATED FACTORS

Alcohol/drug abuse/dependency
Economic/fiscal mismanagement
Presence of adverse personal habits
Withdrawal from physiologic dependence
Evidence of impaired perception
Lack of knowledge
Unavailability of services
Poor housing conditions
Inability to communicate needs adequately
Denial of need to change current habits

EXPECTED OUTCOMES

Patient begins to participate in healthy practices (i.e., improved nutrition, proper hygiene, adequate sleep).
Patient identifies available resources.
Patient uses available resources.

ONGOING ASSESSMENT

- Assess history of substance abuse.
- Assess last drug use; determine substance taken, amount, routes of administration. Assess amount of last alcohol ingestion, length of alcohol abuse.
- Assess history of adverse personal habits: smoking, poor diet, morbid obesity, poor hygiene, lack of exercise.
- Assess whether economic problems present barrier to maintaining health.
- Assess patient's hearing; orientation to time, place, and person to determine perceptual abilities.
- Assess past health history. *Substance abuse is closely related to specific medical complications.*
- Assess to what degree, environmental, social, interfamilial disruptions/changes correlate with poor health behaviors.
- Assess patient's knowledge of health maintenance behaviors.
- Determine patient's motives for failing to report symptoms reflecting health status changes.
- Discuss noncompliance with instructions/programs *to determine rationale for failure. Programs need to be constructed to support success.*
- Assess relationship with family/supportive others.

Continued.

NURSING DIAGNOSES	EXPECTED OUTCOMES AND NURSING INTERVENTIONS / *RATIONALE* (■ = INDEPENDENT; ▲ = COLLABORATIVE)

THERAPEUTIC INTERVENTIONS

- Provide rationales for importance of specific behaviors:

  Cessation of alcohol and drug abuse. *In addition to physical addiction, physical consequences of substance abuse mitigate against continued use.*

  Regular exercise/rest *to promote weight loss, increase agility and stamina*

  Proper hygiene *to decrease infection risk, promote maintenance and integrity of skin, teeth*

  Regular physical and dental checkups *to identify, treat problems early*

  Reporting of unusual symptoms to health professional *to initiate early treatment:* proper nutrition; regular inoculations; balanced low-cholesterol diet *to prevent vascular disease;* smoking cessation (*smoking directly linked to cancer, heart disease*)

- Follow-up clinic visits with telephone/home visits *to develop ongoing relationships with patient, vocalize support for patient.*
- Provide means of contacting health care providers available for questions/problem solution.
- Compliment patient on positive accomplishments to reinforce. Involve family/friends in health planning conferences.
- ▲ Ensure that other agencies (i.e., Department of Children and Family Services, social services, Visiting Nurses' Association, Meals on Wheels) follow through with plans.
- Refer to support group, Alcoholics Anonymous (AA), Narcotics Anonymous.
- See also Health maintenance, altered, p. 31; Cirrhosis, p. 295.

Noncompliance

RELATED FACTORS

Denial of substance abuse/ dependency

Ability to rationalize substance use

Lack of knowledge

Verbalized belief that treatment program does not meet personal needs

Lack of resources (financial, social, personal)

Physical limitations

Mental disability

Lack of satisfaction with outcomes

DEFINING CHARACTERISTICS

Behavior indicative of failure to adhere

Objective tests (lab tests inconsistent with compliance)

Missed appointments

Relapses

Evidence of exacerbation of symptoms

EXPECTED OUTCOMES

Patient adheres to therapeutic plan on a "one day at a time" program.

Patient demonstrates evidence of compliance by negative blood/urine culture results.

ONGOING ASSESSMENT

- Assess to what degree patient uses denial, rationalization to sustain habit.
- Assess secondary gains and reinforcement of maintaining present life-style (identify with fast/glamorous crowd, etc.).
- ▲ Perform blood/urine screens regularly *to test compliance.*
- Help patient identify most effective motivating factors.

THERAPEUTIC INTERVENTIONS

- Confront with laboratory findings that reflect ongoing drug use. *Rationalization and denial may obstruct a patient's ability to be honest with care providers. Truth and support form the basis of the therapeutic relationship.*
- Consider inpatient treatment during withdrawal. *Physical symptoms may require close surveillance during the withdrawal phase. Emotional support will need to be almost constant during this sensitive period.*
- Enlist friends'/family members' aid in achieving compliance. Be certain that they are not accepting of the addictive behaviors but supportive of *positive* behaviors.
- Follow up visits with telephone calls *to provide ongoing support.*
- Provide phone numbers of crisis intervention lines.
- Involve patient in Alcoholics/Narcotics Anonymous groups *to provide support. Such groups may assist the patient in gaining greater understanding of the benefits of treatment.*
- Encourage patient to take medications prescribed *to help minimize withdrawal symptoms.*
- Encourage patient to seek out new friendships/diversions *to reduce occasions for returning to abusive/addictive behaviors.*

NURSING DIAGNOSES	EXPECTED OUTCOMES AND NURSING INTERVENTIONS / *RATIONALE* (■ = INDEPENDENT; ▲ = COLLABORATIVE)

See also:
Altered Nutrition: Less Than
  Body Requirements, p. 44.
Powerlessness, p. 52.
Altered Family Processes,
  p. 23.
Impaired Home Maintenance
  Management, p. 34.
Caregiver Role Strain, p. 13.
Self-Esteem Disturbance,
  p. 55.

By: Deidra Gradishar, RNC, BS

Index

U

Ulcerative colitis; *see* Inflammatory bowel disease
Ulcers; *see* Gastrointestinal bleeding
Unresponsiveness; *see* Consciousness, altered level of
Urethritis; *see* Urinary tract infection
Urinary diversion, 475-479
Urinary elimination, altered pattterns of (incontinence), 71-74
Urinary retention, 74-75
Urinary tract infection/pyelonephritis, 480-481
Urokinase; *see* Thrombolytic therapy in myocardial infarction
Urolithiasis; *see* Renal calculi

V

VAD; *see* Ventricular assist device
Valve replacement; *see* Coronary bypass/valve surgery

Vascular access for hemodialysis, 456-458
Vascular surgery; *see* Carotid endarterectomy
Vasoocclusive crisis; *see* Sickle cell pain crisis
Ventricular assist device (VAD), 177-181
Ventriculitis; *see* Intracranial infection
Vulvectomy, 431-434

W

Wedge pressures; *see* Swan-Ganz catheterization
Weight loss; *see* Nutrition, altered: less than body requirements